Health Promotion in Nursing

Third Edition

Janice A. Maville, EdD, MSN, RN

Professor
Department of Nursing
The University of Texas-Pan American
Edinburg, Texas

Carolina G. Huerta, EdD, MSN, RN

Professor and Department Chair
Department of Nursing
The University of Texas-Pan American
Edinburg, Texas

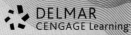

DELMAR
CENGAGE Learning

Australia • Brazil • Japan • Korea • Mexico • Singapore • Spain • United Kingdom • United States

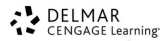

Health Promotion in Nursing, Third Edition
Janice A. Maville and Carolina G. Huerta

Vice President, Careers & Computing:
Dave Garza

Executive Editor: Stephen Helba

Associate Acquisitions Editor: Delia K. Uherec

Managing Editor: Marah Bellegarde

Editorial Assistant: Jennifer Wheaton

Vice President, Marketing: Jennifer Ann Baker

Marketing Director: Wendy E. Mapstone

Executive Marketing Manager: Michele McTighe

Associate Marketing Manager: Scott A. Chrysler

Senior Director, Education Production:
Wendy A. Troeger

Production Manager: Andrew Crouth

Senior Content Project Manager:
Kara A. DiCaterino

Senior Art Director: Jack Pendleton

For product information and technology assistance, contact us at
Cengage Learning Customer & Sales Support, 1-800-354-9706

For permission to use material from this text or product,
submit all requests online at **www.cengage.com/permissions**
Further permissions questions can be e-mailed to
permissionrequest@cengage.com

Library of Congress Control Number: 2011942793

ISBN-13: 978-1-111-64046-0

ISBN-10: 1-111-64046-7

Delmar
5 Maxwell Drive
Clifton Park, NY 12065-2919
USA

Cengage Learning is a leading provider of customized learning solutions with office locations around the globe, including Singapore, the United Kingdom, Australia, Mexico, Brazil, and Japan. Locate your local office at:
international.cengage.com/region

Cengage Learning products are represented in Canada by
Nelson Education, Ltd.

To learn more about Delmar, visit **www.cengage.com/delmar**

Purchase any of our products at your local college store or at our preferred online store **www.cengagebrain.com**

Notice to the Reader

Publisher does not warrant or guarantee any of the products described herein or perform any independent analysis in connection with any of the product information contained herein. Publisher does not assume, and expressly disclaims, any obligation to obtain and include information other than that provided to it by the manufacturer. The reader is expressly warned to consider and adopt all safety precautions that might be indicated by the activities described herein and to avoid all potential hazards. By following the instructions contained herein, the reader willingly assumes all risks in connection with such instructions. The publisher makes no representations or warranties of any kind, including but not limited to, the warranties of fitness for particular purpose or merchantability, nor are any such representations implied with respect to the material set forth herein, and the publisher takes no responsibility with respect to such material. The publisher shall not be liable for any special, consequential, or exemplary damages resulting, in whole or part, from the readers' use of, or reliance upon, this material.

Printed in the United States of America
1 2 3 4 5 6 7 16 15 14 13 12

CONTENTS

CHAPTER 3: THEORETICAL FOUNDATIONS OF HEALTH PROMOTION / 38

CHAPTER 4: THE ROLE OF THE NURSE IN HEALTH PROMOTION 53

SECTION II

Factors Influencing Health Promotion / 73

CHAPTER 5: COMMUNICATION / 74

CHAPTER 8: THE MIND-BODY-SPIRIT CONNECTION / 141

SECTION III

Promoting Health throughout the Life Cycle / 161

CHAPTER 9: PROMOTING MOTHER, INFANT, AND TODDLER HEALTH / 162

CHAPTER 10: THE CHILD / 202

CHAPTER 11: THE ADOLESCENT AND YOUNG ADULT / 223

CHAPTER 12: THE MIDDLE-AGED ADULT / 252

CHAPTER 13: THE OLDER ADULT / 272

CHAPTER 14: HEALTH PROMOTION THROUGH END-OF-LIFE / 297

SECTION IV

Health-Promotion Strategies and Interventions / 317

CHAPTER 15: EMBRACING PROPER NUTRITION / 318

CHAPTER 16: ENGAGING IN PHYSICAL FITNESS / 344

CHAPTER 17: CONTROLLING WEIGHT / 365

CHAPTER 18: AVOIDING TOBACCO, ALCOHOL, AND SUBSTANCE ABUSE / 388

CHAPTER 19: ENHANCING HOLISTIC CARE / 407

SECTION V

Health-Promotion Concerns / 435

CHAPTER 20: CONCERNS OF THE HEALTH PROFESSIONAL / 436

CHAPTER 21: ECONOMIC AND QUALITY CONCERNS / 455

CHAPTER 22: ETHICAL, LEGAL, AND POLITICAL CONCERNS / 466

PREFACE

Fundamental to any nursing education program are knowledge, concepts, skills, and practices necessary to address patient or client needs at the individual, family, group, and community levels. Nurses today must focus their practice on extending life while increasing the quality of life. The delivery of health care continues to shift from the hospital to the community and from disease treatment to prevention of disease and promotion of health. These trends, in addition to issues surrounding health care cost, quality, and access to care for people all over the world, implore an emphasis on health promotion that has become increasingly important if not urgent.

Nurses are a vital component to the success of any health-promotion endeavor to inspire, motivate, and educate patients or clients to achieve the highest level of health or wellness. Nurses are at the forefront to inspire others to envision the health or wellness they desire. They must then be able to motivate individuals, families, groups, or the community to take action to promote their health. Nurses must use current evidence-based knowledge to provide accurate information, interpret information, and educate at every opportunity to promote health. The intent of *Health Promotion in Nursing*, 3rd edition, is to inspire students to become involved in promoting health in self and others, to develop skills that motivate patients/clients, and to educate students using the most current information to develop a solid knowledge base in health promotion.

Health Promotion in Nursing, 3rd edition, has retained a nursing perspective and examination of biological, psychological, social, political, environmental, sexual, spiritual, and technological domains for a holistic approach to health and wellness. Philosophically, the approach taken for this book has been that health promotion encompasses the lifespan, including preconception to death, and is inherent within illness. Missing from previous editions was end-of-life care. For this reason, a new chapter, "Health Promotion through End of Life," has been added. Also new to this edition are two new features. In recognition that nations all over the world are striving for healthy populations, a *Global Highlight* feature in each chapter draws attention to activities, programs, or research in other parts of the world to emphasize that promoting health is a global endeavor.

Nursing practice is based on evidence-based research that is linked to an underlying theoretical basis. Therefore, another new feature, *Theory Link*, has been added to each chapter to connect the chapter content with a related theory.

This book is designed to prepare the beginning nurse with the basic principles of health promotion found in most health-promotion or wellness courses offered at the associate and baccalaureate levels. With more knowledge and information on health promotion, these nurses will be able to successfully confront and manage the challenges of health promotion. Realistic case studies in applicable chapters encourage readers to apply and synthesize the knowledge gleaned from the chapters. In today's world, a nurse must have an appreciation of the diverse nature of individuals, groups, and differing health practices. Accordingly, *Health Promotion in Nursing*, 3rd edition, places special emphasis on cultural variations inherent in health care. Nurses will also be more effective with others when there is a commitment to incorporate the principles of health promotion into their own lifestyles. Several resources as well as opportunities for self-examination and self-reflection are therefore included.

ORGANIZATION

Health Promotion in Nursing, 3rd edition, is composed of five sections broken down into 22 chapters.

SECTION I: CONCEPTUAL FOUNDATIONS AND THEORETICAL APPROACHES

Chapter 1 Health Promotion: Past, Present, and Future

This chapter provides the reader with an introduction to the concept of health promotion and factors influencing its emergence in the United States. Various definitions are examined along with social, economic, environmental, and political forces leading to the dramatic impact of health promotion on contemporary society. The concepts of health promotion and illness prevention are differentiated. *Healthy People 2020* initiatives and leading health indicators are strongly emphasized. The impact of terrorism is introduced.

Chapter 2 Nursing Concepts and Health Promotion

This chapter introduces concepts essential in defining the metaparadigm of nursing practice. Theoretical frameworks as underpinnings of the profession of nursing are included. Nursing educational levels and their relationship to health promotion are discussed. Assumptions basic to the integration of health promotion in nursing practice are emphasized.

Chapter 3 Theoretical Foundations of Health Promotion

This chapter discusses theoretical foundations and planning strategies related to health promotion. Major definitions of health are presented. Numerous theoretical models related to health promotion are detailed, including the Theory of Planned Behavior, Protection Motivation Theory, Health Belief Model, Transtheoretical Model of Behavioral Change, Consumer Information Processing Model, Diffusion of Innovations Model, PRECEDE-PROCEED Model, and the Pender Health-Promotion Model. The importance of self-responsibility in health promotion is examined in relation to theoretical concepts of human behavior. Guidelines to develop a health-promotion plan are introduced.

Chapter 4 The Role of the Nurse in Health Promotion

This chapter describes the important role of the nurse in health promotion for the individual, family, and community. Domains fundamental to nursing practice in health promotion are described. A collaborative, multidisciplinary approach for client empowerment is discussed. The application of the nursing process in health promotion is specifically addressed. Several classification systems used to support clinical decision making are included. Emphasis is placed on the holistic perspective of nursing practice in health promotion. Nursing diagnoses for health promotion are described and illustrated.

SECTION II: FACTORS INFLUENCING HEALTH PROMOTION

Chapter 5 Communication

This chapter explores the basic concepts of communication and provides an overview of the various models of communication. Topics include types of communication, specific communication techniques, barriers to communication, and the development of a therapeutic relationship to promote health. The influence of technology on communication is addressed. Coverage of the principles and strategies of teaching and learning is included.

Chapter 6 Cultural Considerations

This chapter focuses on the importance of cultural sensitivity in the promotion of health among various cultural groups. Cultural concepts are explained. Cultural competence, cultural awareness, and cultural sensitivity are differentiated. Specific ways of culturally advocating for clients are identified. Instruction on how to do a cultural assessment on self and others is included. Numerous opportunities for critical thinking and self-analysis are presented.

Chapter 7 Environmental Factors

This chapter examines the impact of environmental changes on health, how to prepare for them, and how to respond to them when they do occur. A discussion of global issues related to the environment is included. Natural disasters, air, water, noise, and waste result in a change in the health of individuals and communities. In addition, readers are given the opportunity to assess their home and work environments. Terror-related disasters and disaster planning are now specifically addressed.

Chapter 8 The Mind-Body-Spirit Connection

Psychoneuroimmunology has emerged as a field of science providing increasing evidence of the interrelatedness of psychological, neurological, hormonal, and immunological functions and their connections to health and well-being. This chapter provides an analysis of this concept and describes not only the what but the why of these interrelationships. The controversial nature of psychoneuroimmunology is presented. The link between spirituality/religion and health-related physiological processes is addressed. An emphasis is placed on the effect of stress on the neurological, endocrine, and immune systems.

SECTION III: PROMOTING HEALTH THROUGHOUT THE LIFE CYCLE

Chapter 9 Promoting Mother, Infant, and Toddler Health

Health promotion is an important aspect in the care of expectant mothers, infants, and toddlers. This chapter offers a wealth of information that addresses health promotion needs of women, beginning with preconception through pregnancy and postpartum. Special content is devoted to domestic violence and postpartum baby blues. By detecting health problems early in infants and toddlers, health status can be improved and future problems prevented. Screenings, immunizations, and health-promotion risk assessments for infants and toddlers provide a comprehensive look at these age groups.

Chapter 10 The Child

In addition to numerous health screenings for children, regular physical exams and the importance of health education in schools and community centers are emphasized. The importance of immunization against various diseases is presented. Programs for young children and school-age children that focus only on the negative outcomes of unhealthy behavior, but also programs that teach values, build self-esteem, and promote healthy lifestyles are addressed. Emphasis is placed on the growing health threat of obesity in childhood and detection of risk factors.

Chapter 11 The Adolescent and Young Adult

Adolescents and young adults are becoming increasingly interested in health promotion. This chapter focuses on specific topics such as pregnancy, teen pregnancy, smoking cessation, and drug rehabilitation. Information on the role of the nurse in promoting health in the adolescent and the young adult is presented. A health risk assessment tool has been added.

Chapter 12 The Middle-Aged Adult

The middle-aged adult is particularly receptive to the development of health promotion lifestyles. Topics such as general wellness, exercise, identification of personal risk factors, and education on chronic illness are addressed. The role of the nurse in promoting health in the middle-aged adult is presented.

Chapter 13 The Older Adult

Health promotion is an important part of the role of the nurse caring for the older adult. Studies indicate that the elderly are health-conscious and eager to adopt practices to improve their health. Activities that enable the older adult with chronic illness or disability or both to reach an optimum level of function are given. Physical fitness, nutrition, safety, and stress management are included. A new discussion has been added on health promotion in various settings, such as assisted living, home care, rehab facilities, long-term care, and nursing homes.

Chapter 14 Health Promotion through End-of-Life

End of life is part of the stages, experiences, and state of health that accompany one throughout life's journey. The primary focus of this chapter is to enlighten the reader in matters concerning health promotion and the end of life. An overview on various health promotion and end-of-life issues are discussed. Content related to loss, palliative care, hospice, pain management, spirituality, communication, decision making, and other concepts are included to focus the reader on promoting health and wellness at the end of life.

SECTION IV: HEALTH-PROMOTION STRATEGIES AND INTERVENTIONS

Chapter 15 Embracing Proper Nutrition

This chapter presents the concepts of nutrition and the role nutrition plays in maintaining health. The important role of nutrients such as fats, carbohydrates, proteins, and vitamins and minerals is discussed. General guidelines to meet daily nutrient needs are presented, along with charts and tables to depict nutrient needs and food sources. MyPlate, which has replaced the United States Department of Agriculture Food Guide Pyramid, is described. Issues and health-promotion strategies related to nutrition are discussed. The importance of cultural sensitivity in nutritional health is emphasized.

Chapter 16 Engaging in Physical Fitness

Physical fitness is an important aspect of health promotion. This chapter examines the relationship between physical fitness and health, benefits of exercise, types of exercise, and the nurse's role in promoting health through physical fitness. Practical problems related to exercise are discussed, along with practical tips for increasing activity and incorporating cultural sensitivity into care.

Chapter 17 Controlling Weight

The importance of weight control, theories of obesity, basic principles of weight control, and obstacles encountered in maintaining weight are presented. Recognition of dietary fads and their impact on weight control are newly included. Weight control strategies that incorporate cultural sensitivity and awareness are included, along with suggestions to overcome obstacles encountered and the role of the nurse in promoting weight control.

Chapter 18 Avoiding Tobacco, Alcohol, and Substance Abuse

This chapter presents an overview of the health risks associated with the use, abuse, and/or addiction to tobacco, alcohol, and other drugs. A discussion of drug effects and the basis of addiction is presented. Identification of risk and protective factors for individuals at risk for substance abuse has been added. The nurse's role in primary, secondary, and tertiary prevention strategies is addressed. A section discussing the nurse with a substance abuse problem is also included.

Chapter 19 Enhancing Holistic Care

Facilitating others in the promotion of their own well-being is essential for nurses involved in supporting the health of individuals, families, and aggregates. This chapter offers enhanced coverage of complementary and alternative medicine (CAM) and holistic techniques that nurses can incorporate when teaching clients self-care for health promotion. Included in this chapter are breathing and relaxation techniques, pressure and touch therapy, imagery and visualization, music therapy, aromatherapy, meditation, prayer, and other approaches. The effect of light, color, and sound on health is also addressed. Benefits, risks, and cautions for commonly used herbs and essential oils are detailed.

SECTION V: HEALTH-PROMOTION CONCERNS

Chapter 20 Concerns of the Health Professional

Nursing is a wonderful career choice. Benefits include caring for others and feeling as if you are making a difference in other people's lives. However, nurses and those who have chosen careers in the health professions often neglect their own health. This chapter addresses the effects of such neglect, including physical and psychological illness, burnout, and dropout from educational programs or from the profession. Health care reform and technology as sources of stress for nurses and other health care professionals are discussed. Practical strategies for enhancing health are provided for professionals and students.

Chapter 21 Economic and Quality Concerns

Advances in medical technology and increased life span have led to the escalation of health care costs. Policies made in the political arena dictate the financing of health care by the national and state governments. This chapter includes a focus on how health-promotion and health care costs relate to economic as well as quality issues. The importance of healthy lifestyle practices through health promotion as a means of controlling expenditures is discussed. The American Nurses Association Standards of Care are discussed in terms of safeguarding the quality of care delivered to clients.

Chapter 22 Ethical, Legal, and Political Concerns

Basic principles of ethics are identified. Students can examine ethical issues pertaining to health care costs, access to health care, and rationing of health care. The involvement by federal and state governments in health care delivery is presented. A discussion on HIPAA as a national framework for security standards and protection of client confidentiality is included.

OUTSTANDING FEATURES

Several key pedagogical features in *Health Promotion in Nursing*, 3rd edition, make the book user-friendly and draw readers' attention to some of the most critical points that will help them grow in their practice.

FEATURES

- **Nursing Alert:** Highlights serious or life-threatening signs or critical information that needs immediate attention.
- **Research Note:** Emphasizes relevant research on a particular issue. This helps readers understand the importance of grounding their practice in evidence-based research.
- **Spotlight On:** Introduces ethical controversies and clinical situations readers are likely to encounter, stimulating critical thinking.
- **Ask Yourself:** Encourages readers to examine their own views on a variety of issues so they may better understand the varying opinions they may soon encounter. These boxes encourage reflection on issues in a personal context and raise awareness.
- **Student Activities:** Stimulating activities for readers to do individually or in groups to enhance content presented in each chapter. Learning Activities, and multiple choice questions are included in every chapter for review of information and for self-assessment.

NEW TO THIS EDITION

Two new features have been added to each chapter.

- **Global Highlight:** Broadens the concepts, practices, and various issues of health promotion to include a world view. These boxes encourage readers to widen their global perspectives.
- **Theory Link:** Demonstrates to the reader how issues related to chapter content can be connected to a related theory. These boxes help to bridge the gap between theory and health promotion.

All chapters have been revised to reflect the most recent references, tables, charts, and graphs. Highlights of new content or information are presented for the following chapters:

Chapter 1 Health Promotion: Past, Present and Future
Healthy People 2020 and Table of Topic areas
Canada Health Act
UN Summit Millennium Development Goals
Introduction of Integrative Nurse Coach

Chapter 2 Nursing Concepts and Health Promotion
2010 ANA Scope and Standards of Practice
Doctor of Nursing Practice
Updated Health-Promotion Competencies for levels of nurse education preparation

Chapter 3 Theoretical Foundations of Health Promotion
Anticipatory guidance
Expansion on wellness concept

Chapter 4 The Role of the Nurse in Health Promotion
Nursing process expanded to include analysis of data for critical thinking
Current discussion on NANDA-I

Chapter 5 Communication
Discussion on communication as a vital key to meeting goals of *Healthy People 2020*

Chapter 6 Cultural Considerations
Greater emphasis on differentiation of ethnicity and race

Chapter 7 Environmental Factors
Biomonitoring is introduced
Revised table on everyday sounds and loudness
Effects of Haiti and Japan earthquakes and Gulf oil spill

Chapter 8 The Mind-Body-Spirit Connection
Addition of spirit to mind-body connection
Expanded section on stress and victims of natural disaster
New diagram of division of nervous system
New figure on endocrine system and function

Chapter 9 Promoting Mother, Infant, and Toddler Health
Expanded content on birth control

Chapter 10 The Child
Tumbling E chart for vision screening
New terms for obesity, underweight
Expanded section on nutrition
Emphasis on childhood obesity
Updated immunization schedules

Chapter 11 The Adolescent and Young Adult
Strategies to prevent obesity and eating disorders
Current data on substance use and abuse
Expanded section on violence in adolescence
Emphasis on teaching BSE for adolescents

Chapter 12 The Middle-Aged Adult
New section on promoting awareness of genetic/genomic issues
Revised table on risk assessment for middle-aged adults
Expanded information on adult immunizations

Chapter 13 The Older Adult
Expanded section on poverty and health care costs for elderly
New section on the elderly and disaster preparedness

Chapter 14 Health Promotion through End-of-Life
New chapter
The impact of health promotion and wellness in patients at the end of life
Focus on managing stress encountered by patients who are dying and loved ones who are experiencing grief due to loss

Chapter 15 Embracing Proper Nutrition

Greater emphasis on obesity epidemic

New section on dietary reference intakes

New USDA My Plate to replace Food Pyramid

Updated *Dietary Guidelines for Americans 2010*

Revised table of vitamins, mineral supplements, and health-promotion implications

Chapter 16 Engaging in Physical Fitness

Surgeon General's Vision for a Healthy and Fit Nation 2010

Social determinants of health

Healthy People 2020

Updated IOM *Dietary Reference Intakes for Electrolytes and Water*

Sparks & Taylor updated nursing diagnosis reference

Chapter 17 Controlling Weight

New statistics on obesity in Unites States and Canada

New graphic on complications of obesity in children

Content related to economics and weight management

New content on surgical options as a treatment option for obesity

New tips to confront the obesity epidemic

Chapter 18 Avoiding Tobacco, Alcohol, and Substance Abuse

Healthy People 2020

Chapter 19 Enhancing Holistic Care

Revised categories of practice and examples of associated modalities

Added new content on cognitive restructuring

Chapter 20 Concerns of the Health Professional

Updated information on professional nursing supply and demand

Content on electronic health records, Health Care Reform Affordable Care Act, and the Institute of Medicine & Robert Wood Johnson Foundation Report: *The Future of Nursing*

Chapter 21 Economic and Quality Concerns

Affordable Care Act

Additional information on factors driving health care costs

Updated information on health care spending

Expanded information on nurses' role in managed care

Chapter 22 Ethical, Legal, and Political Issues

Expanded discussion on new regulations with the Affordable Care Act

Case Studies (added to Chapters 8–20)

Provide students with the opportunity for critical thinking by featuring a real-life situation that focuses on health-promotion issues according to domains

STUDENT ANCILLARY

Premium Website Printed Access Card to Accompany Health Promotion in Nursing, 3rd edition, 978-1-111-64049-1

Premium Website Instant Access Code to Accompany Health Promotion in Nursing, 3rd edition, 978-1-111-64048-4

Access card free with every new book! The Website offers support to the reader by including:

- Answers to chapter questions enabling reading to check their comprehension of chapter concept.
- Glossary allows quick lookup of terms and can be used as a study tool!
- Chapter objectives allows reader to check their knowledge of the most important chapter concepts.

INSTRUCTOR COMPANION WEBSITE

This instructor companion Website is accessible via Cengage.com through an instructor account. It contains:

- Answers to the Case Studies, Learning Activities, and Multiple Choice questions from the book.
- Over 625 PowerPoint slides.
- A computerized testbank with 650 questions.
- Transition Guide to assist in updating your course to reflect *Health Promotion in Nursing,* 3rd edition.

CONTRIBUTORS

Beatriz G. Bautista, DNP, APRN, FNP-BC, CCD
Assistant Professor
Department of Nursing
The University of Texas-Pan American
Edinburg, Texas
Chapter 10

Patricia Bowden, MSN, RN
Clinical Instructor
College of Nursing and Health Sciences
The University of Texas at Tyler
Tyler, Texas
Chapter 9

Joyce Engel, PhD, M Ed
Associate Professor
Applied Health Sciences
Department of Nursing
Brock University
Ontario, Canada
Chapter 11

Alma Flores-Vela, PhD, MSN, RN
Clinical Instructor
Department of Nursing
The University of Texas-Pan American
Edinburg, Texas
Chapter 13

Diane Frazor, EdD, MSN, RN
Dean, School of Nursing
Wayland Baptist University
San Antonio, Texas
Chapter 21

Carolina G. Huerta, EdD, MSN, RN
Professor and Department Chair
Department of Nursing
The University of Texas-Pan American
Edinburg, Texas
Chapters 2, 3, 4, 15, 16, 17, 20, and 22

Janice A. Maville, EdD, MSN, RN
Professor
Department of Nursing
The University of Texas-Pan American
Edinburg, Texas
Chapters 1, 3, 5, 7, 8, 15, and 19

Jeanette McNeill, DrPH, RN
Professor
Ila Faye Miller School of Nursing and Health Professions
University of the Incarnate Word
San Antonio, Texas
Chapter 12

Beatriz Nieto, PhD, RN
Associate Professor
Department of Nursing
The University of Texas-Pan American
Edinburg, Texas
Chapter 14

Debra Otto, DM, RNP
Associate Professor
Department of Nursing
The University of Texas-Pan American
Edinburg, Texas
Chapters 18 and 21

M. Sandra (Sandy) Sánchez, PhD, RN
Professor and Coordinator
Bachelor of Science in Nursing Program
Department of Nursing
The University of Texas-Pan American
Edinburg, Texas
Chapter 6

Karyn Taplay, MSN, RNC
Lecturer
Applied Health Sciences
Department of Nursing
Brock University
Ontario, Canada
Chapter 13

REVIEWERS

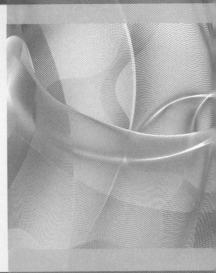

The authors would like to thank the reviewers of the third edition for their valuable feedback.

Max Alan Bishop, RN, MSN, BS Ed
ITT-Tech school of Health Sciences/Nursing
Phoenix, Arizona

Karen Bourgeois, DNS (c), FNP-BC, RN
College of Mount Saint Vincent
Riverdale, New York

Charity Dawson, BSN, RN
Henderson State University
Arkadelphia, Arkansas

Beverley Jones, MScN, MPA
St. Clair College
Windsor, Ontario, Canada

Anne Meyer, MS, FNP-BC
Instructor
Department of Nursing
Fitchburg State University
Fitchburg, Massachusetts

Marlena S. Primeau, MSN, CRNP, BSHECS
DV/SANE CERT
Clinical Assistant Professor
U.A. Huntsville College of Nursing
Huntsville, Alabama

Celeste Yanni, PhD, RN-CHPN
Quinnipiac University
Hamden, Connecticut

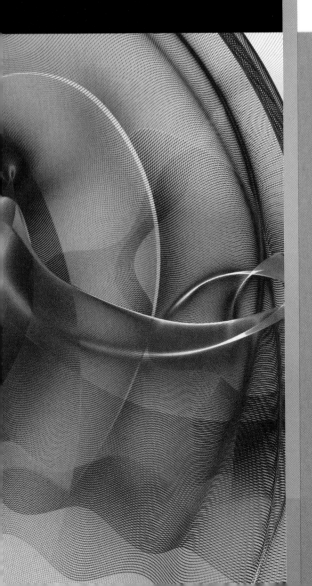

Section I

Conceptual Foundations and Theoretical Approaches

CHAPTER 1
Health Promotion: Past, Present, and Future

JANICE A. MAVILLE, EdD, MSN, RN

KEY TERMS

Code of Hammurabi	*Healthy People 2010*	Social Security Act
diagnostic-related groups (DRGs)	*Healthy People 2020*	terrorism
epidemiology	*LaLonde Report*	yang
health education	Medicaid program	yin
health promotion	Medicare program	
Healthy People 2000	*Nursing: A Social Policy Statement*	

OBJECTIVES

Upon completion of this chapter, the reader should be able to:

- Differentiate between health education and health promotion.
- Discuss three major movements contributing to the social mandate for health promotion in the nineteenth century.
- Relate scientific, social, economic, environmental, and political forces of the twentieth century contributing to the evolution of health promotion in the United States.
- Describe national, international, and world efforts for health promotion.
- Describe changes in contemporary nursing practice and policy resulting from health care reform.
- Examine the future of nursing in health promotion.

INTRODUCTION

Since the beginning of the 1990s, the explosion of interest and participation in health-promotion and wellness activities has resulted in a transformation in health care. Scientific findings, enthusiastic support from health care providers, and strong initiatives for disease prevention and health promotion at local, state, national, and global levels have fueled this evolution. Global and national mandates for promoting health have catapulted health-promotion activities to a high level of importance in the health care community and have caught the attention of many policy makers all over the world. Some health care programs focus exclusively on health promotion, and there is much hope for health-promotion legislation. In the new millennium, collaborative and cooperative efforts for health promotion among individuals, families, communities, health professionals, and government agencies will have dramatic effects on the health of the United States and the world.

Nurses have a rich history of practice and advocacy for health promotion. A knowledge of the heritage of health promotion is important in order to understand its powerful relationship to nursing. This chapter defines health promotion and differentiates this concept from health education. The history of health-promotion practices and sociopolitical developments is explored and related to a vision and a mission for nurses in the emerging collaborative practice paradigm of the future.

DEFINING HEALTH PROMOTION

Nations unite for it, programs are built on it, health professionals prescribe for it, and individuals either practice it or not. Yet a universally accepted definition of health promotion does not exist. In fact, health promotion is often confused with or used synonymously with health education. The confusion is the result of a change in the way of thinking about—or paradigm shift in—the concept of health (Chapter 2), which has undergone dramatic changes through the decades.

Not having a precise definition for health promotion may not be necessarily bad, though, because its absence allows for fluidity, flexibility, and diversity. It is important, however, to review pertinent definitions, to highlight the definition guiding this textbook, and to differentiate health promotion from health education. Other related concepts and theories will be explored in greater detail in Chapter 3.

HEALTH EDUCATION

Health education is a tool or mechanism for health-related learning resulting in increased knowledge, skill development, and change in behavior. Health education, then, is directed toward changing behavior aimed at achieving preset goals.

Health education can be expanded to include the society in which the individual functions. The knowledge that empowers individuals and promotes change for better health in the environment, economy, and society is essential for health promotion. In this sense, health education is not the same as, but is part of, the larger concept of health promotion.

HEALTH PROMOTION

In 1986, the World Health Organization sponsored the first International Conference on Health Promotion in which the Ottawa Charter was developed and adopted by 38 countries, with the object to "achieve Health for All by the Year 2000 and beyond" (Anonymous, 1986; Nutbeam, 1996). Health promotion, as presented in the Ottawa Charter, included enabling people to live healthy lifestyles by building healthy public policy, creating supportive environments, strengthening community action, developing personal skills, and reorienting health services. Furthering these objectives, the United States created *Healthy People 2000*, followed by *Healthy People 2010*, to provide a type of national road map to health for all Americans (U.S. Department of Health and Human Services, 2000; U.S. Public Health Service, 1990). Since 1986, health promotion has been described as a theme, an activity, a process, a principle, a strategy, a discipline, a philosophy, an art, and a science. It is no wonder that it has been difficult to arrive at a consensus for a definition.

Although a contextual analysis of the myriad of health-promotion definitions is beyond the scope of this chapter, four major themes provide for some unity: *empowerment*, *lifestyles*, *health enhancement*, and *well-being*. Embedded in these themes are issues of ethics, values, personal choice, responsibility, and potential. The definition guiding this textbook encompasses these themes and issues. Basically, **health promotion** is any endeavor directed at enhancing the quality of health and well-being of individuals, families, groups, communities, and/or nations through strategies involving supportive environments, coordination of resources, and respect for personal choice and values. Related concepts, including health education, health protection, and disease prevention, are part of the broader concept of health promotion. The definition that an individual or organization adopts depends on political, societal, and philosophical viewpoints.

The term "health promotion" was introduced in 1974 by Canadian Health Minister LaLonde (Macdonald & Bunton, 1992) and was not popular until the 1980s, when the World Health Organization began a campaign for global public health. Prior to that, efforts to improve health centered on education.

NURSING ALERT

Confusing Terms

Nurses and other health care providers have reached some agreement on the difference between the larger context of health promotion, with education as one of its components. Yet many administrators, policy makers, and health care providers still refer to "health *prevention*" activities when they actually mean "health *promotion*" activities. Certainly, no one wants to prevent health! Be alert for this misused and contradictory phrasing, and offer clarification when necessary.

ASK YOURSELF

Health Promotion and You

What does health promotion mean to you? How do politics, your personal philosophies, your culture, and your society affect your view of health promotion?

HEALTH PROMOTION: PAST

Today, society is composed of many cultures whose beliefs unite and sometimes conflict with modern professional health care practice. A contemporary example of the unity of belief and health care can be seen in the practice of drinking herbal teas. Previously thought to be part of folk or cultural lore, the benefits of many herbal teas have been confirmed, accepted, and recommended by professional health care providers. Health-promotion beliefs and practices from ancient cultures have evolved over time and influenced modern society.

BABYLONIA

Although evidence of medical records was discovered in Egypt around 3000 BCE (Ellis & Hartley, 2004), the earliest written reference to health is attributed to King Hammurabi of Babylonia (now Iraq), approximately 2000 BCE (2007). This written document was called the *Code of Hammurabi*, and it established standards and practices of living for Babylonians.

The regulations or laws in the *Code of Hammurabi* were based on promoting fairness and equality. A portion of this code regulated specific health practices and the conduct of physicians. With an eye-for-an-eye premise, some of the regulations seem drastic compared to present-day standards. For example, if a surgeon operated on a member of the wealthy upper class and saved the patient's life, the surgeon would be paid ten coins of silver for that service. If the same service was provided for a common person, the surgeon would be given five coins. If the patient was a slave, the surgeon would get two coins of silver. If the doctor made an error in performing the surgery and the patient died, then the surgeon's hand could be cut off (*Babylonia*, n.d.).

Although the promotion of health was not a primary focus of this document, the recorded laws support the understanding that health has always been broadly defined and that the community and individuals have shared responsibilities for it.

GREECE

The early Greeks are known for their practice of worshipping gods and goddesses who were believed to possess strength, beauty and/or power, all of whom were strong, beautiful, and powerful. Apollo was known as the god of health, and his son, Asclepius, was the god of healing. Hygeia, daughter of Asclepius, was the goddess of health, and another daughter, Panacea, was the restorer of health (Stanhope & Lancaster, 2004). In deifying these two goddesses, the Greeks signified their strong belief in keeping healthy. Striving to be more like the mythological gods they worshiped, the Greeks focused on health with an emphasis on personal health and hygiene, exercise, and healthy diets.

Hippocrates, born around 400 BCE, emphasized a natural cause for disease and initiated the scientific method for solving patient problems. He identified the importance of incorporating social, environmental, mental, and physical factors in treating the patient as a whole person (Guisepi, 2001). Hippocrates believed health to be dependent on equilibrium among the mind, body, and environment rather than on the whim of the gods. This belief, known as the holistic approach in health care practice today, continues to guide the practice of health care professionals and is a key element in understanding the concept of health promotion.

SPOTLIGHT ON

Ancient Use of Therapeutic Massage

The following was reported in a history of massage:

- Julius Caesar, ruler of Rome, underwent daily pinching of his body to ease chronic body aches.
- Prominent Greek physician Asclepiades advocated massage in place of medicines and discovered that massage could induce sleep.
- The Father of Medicine, Hippocrates, often prescribed massage for the treatment of joint dislocations. How do these ancient massage practices and philosophies compare to those used today?

ROME

Ancient Romans and Greeks lacked originality for health-promotion and disease-prevention practices. The medical practices of the Romans were obtained from their conquered regions, and physicians from these countries became slaves to the Roman Empire (Stanhope & Lancaster, 2004). Nonetheless, Roman accomplishments were directed mostly at public health with the establishment of regulations for sanitation, street cleaning, building construction, ventilation, and heating, among other areas (Clark, 2007).

From about 500 BCE to CE 500, the Romans' personal practices, which included exercise, massage, and therapeutic baths, were geared more to seeking luxury and personal indulgence than to the promotion of health. Elaborate bathhouses were built where the practices of therapeutic baths and massage were perfected.

Another similarity between the Greeks and Romans can be seen in their philosophies regarding health and illness. The Greek physician Hippocrates and the Roman physician Galen both viewed health as an interaction between a person and the environment. Galen is credited with formulating the beginnings of a definition of health that emphasized the ability of an individual to carry out the functions of daily life without hindrance or pain (Moore & Williamson, 1984).

CHINA

The Chinese were perhaps the greatest advocates of health promotion of all ancient cultures. They viewed a healthy life as one kept in harmony with the universe by maintaining a perfect balance between the dualistic forces of yin and yang (Eliopoulos, 2010). **Yin** was viewed as the female element, associated with negative energy, passiveness, destruction, the moon, darkness, and death. **Yang** was the male element, associated with positive energy, action, generativity, the sun, light, and the creativity of life. Maintaining this balance resulted in perfect health of the mind, body, and spirit. From the earliest records in 1400 BCE, the ancient Chinese philosophy of yin and yang has lasted throughout the centuries. It remains integral to the concepts of health and health promotion not only for the Chinese but for people in many other cultures in the modern world.

? ASK **YOURSELF**

Self-Assessment of Health/Illness Beliefs

What do you feel causes health or illness? Do you believe in a balance such as yin and yang? Have your beliefs changed from when you were younger? What has influenced your beliefs?

THE MIDDLE AGES, RENAISSANCE, AND EARLY AMERICA

Religious beliefs formed the basis for health concepts and practices in early civilizations and continue to have a great influence today. Over time, technology evolved within cultures and had a great impact on the development and practice of health promotion. Coinciding with evolving technology was the development of the field of study known as **epidemiology,** which examines the relationships among disease, the environment, the individual, and the community. Epidemiology has been defined in many ways, but it is essentially concerned with the time, place, and person components of disease, defect, disability, or death (Merrill & Timmreck, 2006). More specifically, epidemiology studies when disease occurs, how it is distributed in a population, the cause of the disease, the natural history or course of a disease, and factors influencing health promotion and protection. Table 1-1 shows the three major epochs of epidemiologic transition and how disease and life expectancy have changed over the last 700 years.

HEALTH PROMOTION IN THE MIDDLE AGES (CE 500–1500)

After the fall of Rome, during the period known as the Dark Ages, much of what was known about the health practices and medicine of ancient worlds was lost. Religious leaders and organizations claimed authority for the welfare of society, and suppression of medical science was not uncommon.

For nearly a thousand years (CE 500–1500), after the Dark Ages shifted into the Middle Ages, very little was accomplished to promote health or to treat illnesses. Not until the Crusades did a heightened sense of responsibility for health emerge when healthy warriors were needed to fight in religious wars (Clark, 2007). Although the emphasis on health by early Christians was on treating disease and illness, they did much to increase the public's awareness of health. The main accomplishment was the development of the quarantine in response to repeated epidemics of the bubonic plague during the latter part of the Middle Ages.

THE RENAISSANCE AND EARLY AMERICA (CE 1500–1800)

The European Renaissance (1500–1700) brought about the return to scientific thought with attempts to understand and control life. This changed the holistic view of health and illness, held by followers of Hippocrates, to a disintegrated view that the body was separate from the mind.

Interestingly, a renewed social consciousness emerged during this time; the responsibility of society for public health and welfare was at least recognized. Even so, most efforts related to health were directed to the improvement of medical technology. Other than that, in this relatively short span of time, little effort was made directly to the promotion of health.

During the European Renaissance, the colonies in America were being established. Compared to crowded European cities, the colonies were sparsely populated and remained isolated from one another for many years. Thus, early colonial health was good compared to that of the crowded Europeans, and the problems with communicable disease were minimal. In many respects, health promotion in colonial days was like that in ancient times: It was measured in terms of successful survival against the elements of nature.

The Industrial Revolution in the United States marked the transition of the country's economic foundation from

TABLE 1-1 Causes of Death, 1300–Present			
Epoch 1: 1300–1800	Age of pestilence	Endemic diseases, chronic undernutrition and malnutrition, periodic epidemics of infectious diseases (bubonic plague, smallpox, measles, malaria, typhus, typhoid, etc.), and famine	Life expectancy of 20 years
Epoch 2: 1800–1900	Age of declining pandemics	Declining epidemics, increase in endemic infectious diseases (tuberculosis, pneumonia, enteritis)	Life expectancy of 40–47.3 years
Epoch 3: 1900–Present	Age of degeneration and human-made diseases	Shift from infectious to chronic diseases (heart disease, cancer, stroke, injuries)	Life expectancy in 1900 of 47.3 years and in 2007 of 80.4 years for women and 75.4 years for men

Sources: Omran, A. R. (1971/2005). The epidemiologic transition: A theory of the epidemiology of population change. *The Milbank Quarterly, 83*(4), 731–757; McLeroy, K. R., & Crump, C. E. (1994). Health promotion and disease prevention: A historical perspective. *Generations, 18*(1), 9–17; Kramarow, E., Lentzner, H., Rooks, R., Weeks, J., & Saydah, S. (1999). *National Vital Statistics Reports (2010).* Deaths: Final data for 2007, 58(19), Hyattsville, MD: National Center for Health Statistics.

agriculture to industry. With this transition came the arrival of poor immigrants, shifting the population from rural to urban settings and resulting in inadequate living and working conditions. The general public health declined, and death from preventable diseases increased, especially among the children. In response to the health impact of low social and economic conditions, the social policy on health began to take form.

THE SOCIAL MANDATE FOR HEALTH PROMOTION

The social problems that flourished in the aftermath of the Industrial Revolution generated great interest in disease prevention, epidemiology, and community health. Three major movements in the late 1800s throughout Western Europe and America began to shape a social mandate for health promotion (Novak, 1988): (1) the developing consciousness of the people, (2) the changes occurring in medicine, and (3) the development of nursing as a profession. The social mandate for health promotion gained a strong foundation in these three major movements. Not only was social consciousness raised for the prevention of disease and the protection of health, but also the eyes of society were opened to the crucial role of nurses in what was the beginning of progressive health reform.

ASK YOURSELF

The Evolution of Health Technology

How has your own health been affected by discoveries made over 100 years ago? What recent discoveries have advanced health care even farther? Compare the state of health technology of underdeveloped countries to that of the United States and other developed countries. How do they differ? What accounts for the differences?

THE FIRST MOVEMENT

The first of the three major movements in the social mandate for promoting health was a greater sense of consciousness and reform from the wealthy of society. This segment of the population aimed to ease problems associated with poverty, substandard housing, child labor, poor prison conditions, and the undereducation of the general public.

A major contribution to this heightened consciousness in the United States can be attributed to the efforts of Lemuel Shattuck. A former teacher and book salesman, Shattuck worked for the passage of a law in Massachusetts establishing the statewide regulation of vital statistics (Novak, 1988). Shortly thereafter, in 1845, he published a census report of the city of Boston containing surprisingly high infant and maternity mortality rates. Recommendations were made in the report for organizing local and state boards of health, conducting surveys on sanitation, and educating nurses. Nearly ignored, the report's recommendations were not implemented for almost 20 years. Even so, the Shattuck Report is renowned as one of the first public health documents in the United States and earned Lemuel Shattuck the title of the Father of Public Health.

THE SECOND MOVEMENT

The attack on public health problems by the population prompted the second major movement for health promotion. The American Medical Association, founded in 1847, began responding to public pressure for disease prevention. As a result, medicine began shifting from an exclusive focus on the cure of disease to its prevention. Consequently, changes in the structure and function of the medical community began to take form.

Also of major importance during this time was new knowledge of the nature of infection and major discoveries that changed medical practice and education forever. For example:

- Louis Pasteur (1822–1895) discovered that heat killed bacteria.
- Joseph Lister (1827–1912) applied pasteurization and disinfection methodologies for surgical procedures.
- Robert Koch (1843–1910), a German physician, made the connection between specific organisms and specific infections.
- William Röentgen (1845–1923), also German, discovered x-rays.
- Ignaz Semmelweis (1818–1865), an Austrian obstetrician, was the first to identify handwashing as means to prevent infection.
- Pierre Curie (1859–1906) and his wife Marie Curie (1867–1934) discovered radium in 1898 (Kelly & Joel, 2002; Stanhope & Lancaster, 2004; Noakes, Borresen, Hew-Butler, Lambeart, & Jordaan, 2008).

ASK YOURSELF

The Wellness-Illness Continuum

Florence Nightingale believed that "the same laws of health" govern sickness and wellness. What does this statement mean to you? Do you feel it represents your belief about wellness and illness?

THE THIRD MOVEMENT

Although the practice of nursing has traditionally functioned in a framework of health promotion, the third movement, the evolution of nursing into a profession, can be largely attributed to the accomplishments of Florence Nightingale. During the Crimean War in Europe in the late 1850s, Florence Nightingale implemented her philosophy of nursing that included care for the well and the sick and numerous improvements in the health care of the military. She forged improvements in housing, sanitation, nutrition, physical fitness, and recreation for the military. As a result of her efforts, in only six months, the death rate in the military hospitals was reduced from 42% to 2.2% (Novak, 1988).

Nightingale's belief in health as a wellness-illness continuum is evident in her *Notes on Nursing,* originally published in 1859, in which she wrote that "the same laws of health or of nursing, for they are in reality the same, obtain among the well as among the sick" (Nightingale, 1859/1969, p. 10). She further wrote that the breaking of these laws "produces only a less violent consequence among the former than among the latter,—and this sometimes, not always" (Nightingale, 1859/1969, p. 10). She referred to disease as a "reparative process" of nature that resulted from lack of knowledge or attention (Nightingale, 1859/1969, p. 8). The education of clients and families, in her point of view, was a major responsibility of nurses and not limited to physicians only.

The works and deeds of Florence Nightingale spread to the United States in the early 1860s, greatly influencing nursing care during the Civil War years. They continue to affect nursing education and practice in the modern world.

SOCIOPOLITICAL INFLUENCES FOR HEALTH PROMOTION IN THE TWENTIETH CENTURY

Beginning in the twentieth century, scientific and sociopolitical events combined to become powerful determinants for reforming health care and stimulating political intervention into the twenty-first century. The epidemiology of disease shifted as hygienic and living conditions began to improve, antibiotics became routine for fighting infections, and scientific advancements were made in combating chronic illness. As a result, the morbidity from infectious diseases decreased, and the life expectancy of those with chronic illnesses increased.

The early 1900s saw enormous national and personal economic growth resulting from industrialization. In turn, great population shifts took place, with people leaving their rural lives for the promise of economic splendor in urban areas. This same hope for a better life attracted thousands of immigrants, especially from Europe.

The combined effects of rapid and uncontrolled industrialization, urbanization, and immigration resulted in congestion, poverty, malnutrition, and disease, setting the stage for renewed interest in promoting health. With this heavy health care burden, innovations in health care and mechanisms for government intervention were set into motion to reform how health care was provided in order to improve the health of all Americans.

HEALTH REFORM

An early contribution to reforming health care was a nurse-inspired innovation that resulted in the establishment of public health nursing and the endorsement of health promotion by insurance companies. In the early 1900s in New York City, Lillian Wald led the way for visiting nurses to incorporate health promotion in the form of education as they provided care at the Henry Street Settlement, treated children in public schools, visited sick workers in their homes, and treated the ill in rural areas. By enlisting the services of the nurses of the Henry Street Settlement, the Metropolitan Life Insurance Company was the first insurance company known to attempt to control costs by promoting the health of its policyholders (Novak, 1988).

The progressive movement of nursing and health reform toward health promotion in the United States was altered by the nation's involvement in World War I and again in World War II.

The medical model of disease treatment gained reemphasis during both wars with the finding that large percentages of military recruits were not fit for duty because of infectious diseases such as tuberculosis, typhoid fever, and gonorrhea. However, nurses during and after World War II made some progress toward health promotion when the role of the nurse was expanded to include caring for military families and veterans.

FEDERAL GOVERNMENT INVOLVEMENT IN HEALTH CARE

The concept that healthy mothers produced healthy children who become healthy adults spawned maternal and infant care programs throughout the 1920s and 1930s. Additionally, the increasing shift in illness from infectious to chronic diseases was also becoming apparent during this period. As a result, the involvement of the U.S. government in health issues increased with the enactment of legislation and the establishment of agencies designed for the improvement of the health of the nation's people. For example, Congress enacted the Sheppard-Towner Act of 1921 that funded maternal and child health services in 45 states (Novak, 1988). This legislation provided access to health care for entire families, resulting in increased health-education programs, the management of individual cases, and decreased infant mortality rates.

The hardships imposed by the stock market crash of 1929 prompted even more federal government intervention for the basic necessities of life for much of the population. As part of Franklin Delano Roosevelt's New Deal, help was made available through federal relief programs and government legislation. The most significant legislation was the **Social Security Act** of 1935. This legislation provided an immediate boost to the American family with public aid, social services, and aid to the elderly. The Social Security Act is significant not only because it provided immediate help for the American people but also because it marked the emergence of the federal government as a dominant force in health care delivery and finance.

Following World War II, the major advances in medical technology and disease control approached the miraculous. New drugs, diagnostic methods, and treatment regimes in the 1940s and 1950s heralded a new era in medical care, resulting in the saving of millions of lives and forever altering the practice of medicine and nursing. Penicillin and other antibiotics, limited to the military during the war, became available to the public; sulfanilamide was proven effective for fighting infections; antihistamines were discovered; cortisone was synthesized; anticoagulants were developed; psychotherapy advanced; polio vaccines were developed; the diagnosis and treatment of heart disease and heart failure were dramatically improved; and surgical techniques, including open heart surgery, were becoming more sophisticated (Kelly & Joel, 2005; Gourevitch, Caronna, & Kalkut, 2008). The boundaries for life itself were literally expanded. It is small wonder that the American public became enamored with medicine, doctors, and hospitals.

Not surprisingly, the wondrous advances in medicine and health care came with a heightened price tag. Hospitals began charging higher rates for services, and health insurance companies charged higher premiums for their policies. These costs were compounded by the fact that physicians' office visits were sparsely reimbursed, if at all, which led to increased admissions to hospitals and increased orders for diagnostic testing by physicians. Unfortunately, inherent in such a system is the potential for fraud with unnecessary admissions and diagnostic testing. Those who could afford insurance had access to care while the underinsured, poor, elderly, and chronically ill faced great difficulties.

MEDICAID AND MEDICARE

Coming to the rescue of those having difficulties with access to health care were Medicare and Medicaid, 1965 amendments to the Social Security Act, and their subsequent amendments. Not only did these amendments facilitate access to health care for the disadvantaged, but they also attested to the increasing magnitude of the federal government's involvement in financing health care costs. (Chapter 21 offers more detailed information on health care costs.)

The **Medicare program** was designed to provide hospital insurance and supplement medical insurance for people over age 65, people with disabilities who receive Social Security benefits, and clients in end-stage renal disease. The **Medicaid program** was designed to provide a share of payments made by state welfare to health care agencies caring for the poor, medically needy, aged, disabled, and their dependent children and families (Hoffman, Klees, & Curtis, 2006). Once the federal government began paying for services, health care costs soared. Enrollments and usage by participants spiraled upward, along with greed and fraud by providers. Additionally, the public began to consider health care as a basic right. Figure 1-1 depicts the spiraling health care expenditures in the United States between the years 1960 and 2009, showing these expenditures as an ever increasing share of U.S. gross domestic product (GDP), the government's primary measure of economic activity. Expenditures in the United States on health care were nearly $2.5 trillion in 2009, 23% more than in the previous four years. The expenditures in 2009 represent 17.6% of the gross domestic product; that level of spending translates into $8,086 per person (CMS, 2011). However, although the amount of expenditures has increased, the rate of spending per year has actually shown a decrease, the slowest annual rate of increase in health care dollars spent in the last 50 years (Martin, Lassman, Whittle, Catlin, & NHEA Team, 2011).

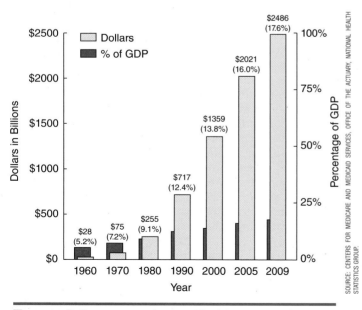

FIGURE 1-1 **Summary of national health care expenditures, population and share of the gross domestic product (GDP), 1960–2009.**

GOVERNMENT INITIATIVES FOR HEALTH PROMOTION IN THE TWENTIETH CENTURY

Beginning in the 1960s, as the United States was slowly awakening to the jolt of the economic crisis in health care, a movement toward the same concerns of the nineteenth century began to gain momentum. By the early 1970s, the public, who had become enraptured by the awesome advances in disease diagnosis and treatment, began to make the connections between health and lifestyles.

Facilitating these connections were major epidemiologic studies completed in the United States and Britain that provided valid evidence linking human behavior with chronic disease. Examples related to smoking and disease include the Framingham study, begun in Massachusetts in 1948, which linked cardiovascular disease to smoking, obesity, and hypertension (Gordis, 2009); the 1964 Doll and Hill study in Britain that associated smoking with disease (Chapman, 2005); and the 1964 U.S. Surgeon General's report *Smoking and Health,* which linked smoking with cancer (Parascandola, Weed, & Dasgupta, 2006).

In recognition of the effects of lifestyle and behavior on disease, the U.S. government established the Office of Disease Prevention and Health Promotion (ODPHP) in 1976 (Office of Disease Prevention and Health Promotion, 2011). Today, working within the framework of the U.S. Department of Health and Human Services (HHS), the ODPHP continues to be a vital federal health agency devoted to promoting the current and future status of the health of Americans.

CANADIAN INFLUENCE ON HEALTH PROMOTION

The United States, however, is not known to have taken the lead in the health-promotion movement. Canada has been recognized as having launched health promotion to the world and as having presented theoretical frameworks from which other countries have modeled their health-promotion programs. The government of Canada was the first to publicly acclaim health promotion as a major disease prevention strategy with the 1974 publication of *A New Perspective on the Health of Canadians,* known since as the *LaLonde Report.* In this classic document, Marc LaLonde, then the Canadian Minister of National Health and Welfare, introduced the idea that human biology, social and physical environments, lifestyle behaviors, and health care organizations share equal importance and should receive equal consideration as determinants in chronic illness and/or a healthy life (Graff & Goldberg, 2000). The report explicitly indicated that money spent on disease treatment could be saved if the disease could be prevented. The report gave rise to the concept of health care policy development and also to changing how health care professionals practice.

Another significant contribution from Canada was the Canada Health Act of 1984. This federal legislation identified five principals that health insurance plans in the nation's provinces and territories must respect in order to receive reimbursement: (1) public accountability by administration, (2) accessibility to insured services without paying fees, (3) comprehensiveness of care for necessary services, (4) universality to ensure care for all Canadians, and (5) portability for continued coverage for brief absences from a province (Canadian Nurses Association, 2000).

INTERNATIONAL GOALS FOR HEALTH

By shifting the emphasis of health care away from the medical model of treatment to a more holistic one of prevention, the *LaLonde Report* linked the individual with society and the world. This insight stimulated a cascade of major global and national social initiatives. The first major action was taken in 1977 by the World Health Organization (WHO) at the World Health Assembly at Alma-Ata in the Soviet Union. Along with the United Nations International Children's Education Fund, WHO issued the Alma-Ata Declaration, which committed member countries to the goal of "an acceptable level of health for all the people of the world by the year 2000" (WHO, 1978).

At the time of the Declaration, the health-for-all goal seemed achievable with strategies aimed at decreasing health disparities, increasing health technology, and providing primary health care for all. Health was envisioned as a human right. Three decades later, however, the achievement of the goal remains elusive. The efforts of the WHO are compounded by existing, new, and emergent infectious diseases.

The United Nations (UN) has also continued the quest for international health. The 2010 UN Summit on the Millennium Development Goals identified eight goals to be achieved by 2015 (UNDP, 2010). The goals are interlinked, with progress on one affecting all others:

1. Eradicate extreme poverty and hunger.
2. Achieve universal primary education.
3. Promote gender equality and empower women.
4. Reduce child mortality.
5. Improve maternal health.
6. Combat HIV/AIDS, malaria, and other diseases.
7. Ensure environmental sustainability.
8. Develop a global partnership for development.

? ASK **YOURSELF**

Government Involvement in Health Promotion

Do you think that the federal government should set goals in promoting health? How do you feel that such a level of government involvement affects the rights of individual citizens?

The United States and National Goals for Health

Subsequently, the United States Public Health Service published *Healthy People: Surgeon General's Report on Health Promotion and Disease Prevention* (U.S. Public Health Service, 1979). This classic document outlined three major strategies for reaching national goals for health: (1) preventive services for individuals provided by health professionals, (2) individual protection measures to be taken by the government and industries, and (3) health promotion actions to be taken by individuals and communities. Five priority areas

for health promotion across the life span were identified: (1) smoking, (2) hypertension, (3) alcohol and drug misuse, (4) poor nutrition, and (5) lack of exercise. The report identified the obligation that nurses have, along with other health care professionals, in providing health-promotion and disease-prevention services.

One year later, in 1980, in concert with the Surgeon General's report, 226 specific measurable objectives were identified to decrease mortality rates and disability from disease by the years 1990 and 2000 (U.S. Public Health Service, 1980). These objectives were developed even further with the publication of *Healthy People 2000: National Health Promotion and Disease Prevention Objectives, 1990* (U.S. Public Health Service, 1990). This document was developed by the U.S. Surgeon General, in conjunction with health care constituents across the nation, and it delineates 22 priority areas with 300 specific measurable objectives for health promotion, health protection, and surveillance and data systems for the United States to be achieved by the year 2000.

In the late 1990s, *Healthy People 2010* (U.S. Department of Health and Human Services, 2000) was similarly developed and organized into 28 specific focus areas and 467 related objectives with two major overarching goals: (1) to increase the quality and years of healthy life and (2) to eliminate health disparities for individuals who do not have access to quality health care. Although data on the achievement of the 2010 goals is currently being collected, preliminary results show that, for the major goals, only one of the two has been met. Life expectancy has increased by 1.2% when measured from birth and by 5.1% when measured at age 65, but the goal to eliminate health disparities was not met (Koh, 2010). Reports from various health agencies and organizations on the achievement of focus area goals are not promising and show that many objectives were not met. Analysis from the Center for Disease Control shows that only 18% of the nearly 1000 objectives have been achieved thus far and that, in fact, there were setbacks in 23% of the goals including increases in obesity, small and fragile infants, cesarean section births, tooth decay, and hypertension, just to name a few (Whittaker, 2010).

Healthy People 2020 has been developed to increase the achievement of goals and to reach more of the general public as well as health care providers and organizations. To facilitate those efforts, *Healthy People 2020* revised the categories of *Healthy People 2010* and added 10 new focus areas, 600 objectives, and 1300 measurements (U.S. Department of Health and Human Services, 2010). Table 1-2 lists the topic areas and identifies the 10 new areas added for 2020.

Healthy People 2020 expanded the two overarching goals from 2010 to four:

1. Attain high-quality, longer lives free of preventable disease, disability, injury, and premature death.
2. Achieve health equity, eliminate disparities, and improve the health of all groups.
3. Create social and physical environments that promote good health for all.
4. Promote quality of life, healthy development, and healthy behaviors across all life stages.

As depicted in Figure 1-2 *Healthy People 2020* has recognized that many factors influence the health of individuals and communities, including five major categories as determinants of health: policy making, social factors, health services, individual behavior, and biology and genetics.

TABLE 1-2 *Healthy People 2020 Topic Areas*

1. Access to Health Services
2. Adolescent Health*
3. Arthritis, Osteoporosis, and Chronic Back Conditions
4. Blood Disorders and Blood Safety*
5. Cancer
6. Chronic Kidney Disease
7. Dementias, including Alzheimer's Disease*
8. Diabetes
9. Disability and Health
10. Early and Middle Childhood*
11. Educational and Community-Based Programs
12. Environmental Health
13. Family Planning
14. Food Safety
15. Genomics*
16. Global Health*
17. Health Communication and Health Information Technology
18. Healthcare-Associated Infections*
19. Health-Related Quality of Life and Well-Being *
20. Hearing and Other Sensory or Communication Disorders
21. Heart Disease and Stroke
22. HIV
23. Immunization and Infectious Diseases
24. Injury and Violence Prevention
25. Lesbian, Gay, Bisexual, and Transgender Health*
26. Maternal, Infant, and Child Health
27. Medical Product Safety
28. Mental Health and Mental Disorders
29. Nutrition and Weight Status
30. Occupational Safety and Health
31. Older Adults*
32. Oral Health
33. Physical Activity
34. Preparedness*
35. Public Health Infrastructure
36. Respiratory Diseases
37. Sexually Transmitted Diseases
38. Sleep Health*
39. Social Determinants of Health*
40. Substance Abuse
41. Tobacco Use
42. Vision

*Denotes newly added areas for 2020.

Source: Healthy People 2010, *U.S. Department of Health and Human Services*. Retrieved from http://www.healthypeople.go/2020/topicsobjectives2020/default.aspx

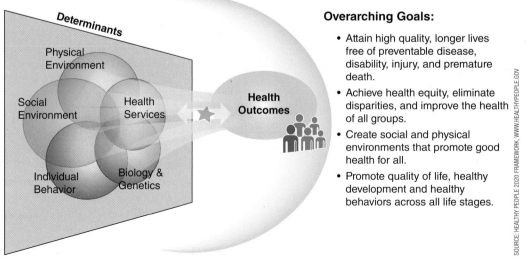

Healthy People 2020
A society in which all people live long, healthy lives

Determinants
- Physical Environment
- Social Environment
- Health Services
- Individual Behavior
- Biology & Genetics

Health Outcomes

Overarching Goals:

- Attain high quality, longer lives free of preventable disease, disability, injury, and premature death.
- Achieve health equity, eliminate disparities, and improve the health of all groups.
- Create social and physical environments that promote good health for all.
- Promote quality of life, healthy development and healthy behaviors across all life stages.

SOURCE: HEALTHY PEOPLE 2020 FRAMEWORK, WWW.HEALTHYPEOPLE.GOV

FIGURE 1-2 Healthy People 2020 Health Determinants and Goals.

GLOBAL HIGHLIGHTS IN HEALTH PROMOTION

Health Promotion and Politics in Australia

With concern for the health of Australians and the burden of health care on the country's health system, the Australian Health Promotion Association is calling for all politicians and political parties contesting the 2010 federal election to commit to progressing four initiatives that would (1) establish the National Preventative Health Agency, (2) implement a *Health in All Policies* approach across all sectors of government, (3) appoint a Minister of Preventative Health to direct the *Health in All Policies* agenda, and (4) increase investment in health-promotion and -prevention expenditures from 2.2% to 10% by the year 2015. New approaches are needed to address the entrenched causes of poor health and to reverse the trend of rising chronic conditions. Australia can become an international leader in health promotion and preventive health. A healthy society is a successful one. Health should be recognized as being central to achieving positive social, economic, and environmental outcomes for Australia as a whole.

The Australian Health Promotion Association—which represents individuals and organizations across Australia involved in the practice, research, and study of health promotion—has called for:

- Expediting the establishment of the National Preventative Health Agency.
- Implementing a *Health in All Policies* approach across all sectors of government.
- Appointing a Minister of Preventative Health with a brief to work across government to drive the *Health in All Policies* agenda.
- Increasing investment in health promotion and the prevention of ill health from the current level of around 2.2% of health expenditure to 10% by 2015.

Further detail in relation to these calls for action is provided in the Policy Reference: Australian Health Promotion Association. (2010). http://health-promotion.org.au/issues/276?task=view

HEALTH CARE COST CONTAINMENT

The mandate for cost containment, beginning in the 1980s, ushered in a new era of problems and challenges for both consumers and providers that continue today. **Diagnostic-related groups (DRGs)** were created in 1983 by physicians and contained 468 diagnoses to be used with the prospective payment system for Medicare to pay hospital services. As a result, those gaining admission into hospitals are often sicker due to delays in meeting criteria and are discharged earlier—and often more ill—than when they arrived. Whether inspired by technology or deemed medically necessary, the ordering of expensive procedures and diagnostic tests prevails in spite of containment efforts. Gaining access to health care has become confusing and unattainable for some individuals and groups. Reductions in hospital staff and early discharges have left many wondering about the quality of care provided. Cost, access, and quality have become the core issues affecting health care in America today.

CHANGES IN NURSING PRACTICE

A backlash from the effects of cost containment has actually resulted in many new and innovative actions with positive implications. Cost containment forced providers into increased competition, which, to some extent, has served to increase the quality of care. Also, more opportunities to provide for unmet health needs gave rise to an entirely new segment of health care: home health agencies and rehabilitation centers. Of major importance is the development of increased empowerment and professional entrepreneurship within the profession of nursing. With teaching and advocacy always at the heart of nursing practice, the empowerment has served to rejuvenate and legitimize the incorporation of health promotion in nursing practice. In essence, cost containment and efforts directed at health care reform redesigned how nurses practice. Community nurse-managed centers, models of nursing case management, and advanced practice models of nursing have replaced traditional modes of care (Stanhope & Lancaster, 2012). For example, home health care agencies, many of which nurses own and operate, seemed to literally spring forth overnight and practically on every corner in the 1990s. All these events, in combination with the changing paradigm for health care and nursing practice, have propelled the role of the nurse into one of high importance and extreme necessity in promoting the health of the American people.

As noted, the nursing profession has long advocated health promotion as integral to the practice of nursing. Client education and advocacy by nurses, unacceptable to many with a paternalistic and/or medical model orientation, was often accomplished in clandestine ways. Fortunately, the social initiatives set forth in 1980 for achieving national health goals by 1990 and 2000 called for the inclusion of health promotion, part of which consists of client education and advocacy, in the practices of all health professionals. Such inclusion not only legitimized this facet of care for nurses but also helped to extend nursing practice into new realms.

One exciting new area, for example, is the emergence of the integrative nurse coach. Nurses have a long history of advocating for and guiding patients on various health issues. In the newly identified role as nurse coach, however, nurses use their skills and knowledge within a wellness model of promoting health. The aim is to assist clients in coordinating, navigating, and finding balance in the complexities of health care and health care reform (Luck, 2010). With consideration of economics, nutrition, environment, social and cultural diversity, spirituality, and opportunities for integrative health care choices, skilled nurse coaches can have dramatic effect on the health of individuals and society because they are skilled in the use of evidence-based practice that embraces holistic and integrative modalities in a collaborative relationship with individuals, families, and groups for improved health outcomes.

CHANGES IN NURSING POLICY

By the end of the 1970s, the profession of nursing had undergone dramatic changes, including diversified educational preparation, the proliferation of specialty practice roles, practice control, and the restructuring of the professional organization. Such diversity resulted in confusion among nurses and the public regarding the nature and scope of nursing. In response to this confusion and in an effort to unify the profession, the American Nurses Association (ANA), in 1980, prepared the classic publication entitled *Nursing: A Social Policy Statement* (American Nurses Association, 1980). This document, prepared by leaders in the profession, was the first of its kind to describe nursing and the profession's responsibility to society. The definition of health provided in this document contained biological, developmental, environmental, and behavioral components. In 1995 the ANA published a revised policy statement titled *Nursing's Social Policy Statement* (American Nurses Association, 1995). The newer policy statement expands the definition of health and reflects an even greater commitment to the well-being of individuals in health and in illness.

These documents are significant in that they embody health promotion and disease prevention as unifying concepts for the profession. The ANA's social policy statements are closely aligned with the ethical guidelines set forth in the ANA's *Code for Nurses* and the International Council of Nurses' (ICN) *Code for Nurses*. Revised in 2005, the ANA's *Code for Nurses* reiterates the ethical commitment to health promotion that is inherent in the obligation of the nurse to the individual needs of the client and in the collaboration with other health professions and citizens. Through collaboration, nurses can work to promote efforts in communities and the nation to meet the health needs of the public.

The creators of the ICN's *Code for Nurses* used foresight in explicitly identifying the ethical commitment of nurses to the promotion of health. The ICN's *Code for Nurses* identifies the four major responsibilities of the nurse: (1) promoting health, (2) preventing illness, (3) restoring health, and (4) alleviating suffering. (See Chapters 2 and 22 for related information.) These responsibilities are further delineated in the nurse's responsibility to four entities: people, practice, coworkers, and the profession (International Council of Nurses, 2006.)

? ASK **YOURSELF**

Nursing's Commitment to Health Promotion

Imagine that you are a nurse interviewing for a new job. You learn that care in the agency focuses on disease treatment rather than on health promotion. How would you respond or react? What guides your response or reaction?

RESEARCH NOTE

A Delphi Study for Consensus on Health Promotion and Health Education

STUDY PROBLEM/PURPOSE

The author identified a lack of expert-based consensus that affects the ability and effectiveness of nurses in health promotion and educational activities. To examine constructs of health promotion and health education from international experts in order to arrive at a consensus.

METHODS

A two-round Delphi technique was used to first obtain concepts of health promotion and health education and perceptions of how these are operational in nursing education, practice, and policy setting. Participants were nurse experts in health promotion and health education from various nations, including Australia, Canada, China, Ireland, Korea, New Zealand, some Scandinavian provinces, South Africa, Taiwan, the United Kingdom, and the United States. The 134 statements received from the first round were sent as a second round to obtain consensus or agreement on a Likert scale ranging from 1 (strongly disagree) to 5 (strongly agree).

FINDINGS

Forty-nine of 62 experts completed both rounds of this study. Consensus was reached on 65 of the 134 original statements from round one. The ten highest-scoring statements for consensus were related to health promotion, not with health education. Nonconsensus was found with regard to the role of nurses working with other disciplines and agencies in health promotion and health education. Consensus was found on the expanding role of the nurse in health promotion education, driven by informed and empowered clientele. Agreement was apparent regarding nurse shortages in the workforce as a barrier to health-related reform. Contradictory statements existed that implied a lack of understanding of the difference between health promotion and prevention.

IMPLICATIONS

Although experts tend to agree on constructs of health promotion and health education, there is a lesser degree of consensus on implementation in practical and policy settings. It was suggested that, although experts may be knowledgeable on these issues, they may not be conveying their knowledge to others. The author noted that using a Delphi method does not result in indisputable facts and that experts in various parts of the world are influenced by such organizations as the World

Health Organization. Nonetheless, the study highlights the need for constructing a solid base for change in order to expand health promotion in nursing practice, theory, education, and policy.

Source: Whitehead, D. (2008). An international Delphi study examining health promotion and health education in nursing practice, education and policy. *Journal of Clinical Nursing*, 891–900. DOI: 10.1111/j.1365-2702.2007.02079.x.

HEALTH PROMOTION: WHERE IS IT GOING?

After decades of disease-oriented care, health promotion, as a descendant of the World Health Organization's goal of health for all, is now recognized as a powerful health care strategy for the enhancement of the quality of life. *Healthy People 2000* set the stage for the future of health promotion in the United States. But promoting health for all is not without its problems. Health promotion can be seen as an idealistic concept and, when viewed realistically, raises many issues reflecting the diversity of populations involved. Cost, access, and quality of health care for all people are emerging major issues as the government struggles with health care reform.

Because of the importance being placed on promoting health, and because the nurse is ever present in all phases and stages of health care, health promotion has been identified as the emerging frontier in nursing. As a profession, nursing has been greatly involved in the many changes, challenges, and opportunities for health promotion. Where is health promotion going? Will nurses be prepared to meet new challenges? How can we manage the changes? These are just a few of the questions that nurses who are looking to the future might ask.

FORCES SHAPING THE FUTURE OF HEALTH PROMOTION

Today, it is clear that forces shaping changes in health care will directly affect health-promotion needs and practices of the future. These forces include the changing dynamics of the demographics and behaviors of the people of the world and the impact of alterations in our physical world from climate changes, earthquakes, floods, oil spills, and other natural and human-caused disasters. For example, people are becoming better informed and are living longer, chronic health problems are increasing, the numbers of disadvantaged young and old are increasing, cultural diversity and varying lifestyles are increasing among the population, and the need for disaster preparedness and protection from violence is greater than ever.

Futurists have envisioned both encouraging and discouraging prospects for health in the twenty-first century. Industrialized countries have seen increased quality of health, not because of medical care but because of economic, social, and environmental improvements. This improvement can be attributed to the adoption of healthier lifestyles. However, environmental effects, such as global atmospheric changes, the depletion of natural resources, and pollution, have been identified as major health threats to the people of the world in the future.

Sociopolitical unrest, manifested in terrorism, has presented even greater threats to health and well-being. **Terrorism**

can be defined in many ways. Basically, it is the unlawful use of force and violence against persons or property to intimidate or coerce a government, the civilian population, or any segment thereof, in furtherance of political or social objectives (Griset & Mahon, 2003, p. 117). On Tuesday, September 11, 2001 (9/11), the world changed forever when a series of coordinated attacks were inflicted on the United States. Nineteen hijackers affiliated with al-Qaeda, an Islamic terrorist group led by Osama bin Laden, simultaneously took control of four U.S. domestic commercial airliners. The hijackers crashed two planes into the World Trade Center in Manhattan, New York City. A third hijacked plane crashed into the U.S. Department of Defense in the Pentagon, located in Arlington, Virginia. A fourth plane crashed into a rural field in Somerset County, Pennsylvania, following apparent passenger resistance. The official count records nearly 3000 deaths in the attacks, including the 19 hijackers (September 11, 2001 attacks, n.d.).

The 9/11 attacks are among the most significant events to have occurred thus far in the twenty-first century, affecting millions of people in a multitude of ways: physically, politically, psychologically, spiritually, and economically. The attacks, and the subsequent U.S.-led wars in the Middle East, have made U.S. homeland security concerns vastly more prominent than they were in the previous decade. (The effects of 9/11 in terms of health and health promotion are further addressed in Chapter 7.)

A FRAMEWORK FOR THINKING ABOUT THE FUTURE

Those who study health care offer frameworks that can be useful for envisioning the health promotion of the future and for planning its destiny. Using trends, scenarios, and vision is a proactive, rather than a reactive, approach to the future of health. Nearly three decades ago, Canadian futurist Norman Henchey (Henchey & Burgess, 1987) suggested thinking about the future in four distinct ways:

1. Possible future—What *may* happen, including so-called wild cards and everything possibly imaginable no matter how unlikely.
2. Plausible future—What *could* happen, integrating possible future events with what is currently known, creating a range of alternatives.
3. Probable future—What *will likely* happen, one of the plausible futures based on the current situation and the appraisal of likely trends.
4. Preferable future—What we *want* to have happen based on shared visions, empowering us to design the best future using our creative abilities.

? ASK YOURSELF

Consider the Future of Nursing

Using Norman Henchey's four ways of thinking about the future, what do you think about the future of nursing in health promotion in terms of what is possible, plausible, probable, and preferable?

Operating from a forward-looking viewpoint, organizations can use this proactive approach in planning for the future. From a narrow perspective, interventions through social control imply forced change that is focused on statistical analysis of the population, the identification of weaknesses, a health outcome, disease organization, and ways to motivate people. From a broader perspective, a more comprehensive view of health and well-being emerges, with foci on social-behavioral factors, the identification of strengths, health outcomes that extend into the community, and ways to incorporate the motives of the people that are transferred to future generations.

FACILITATING YOUR ROLE IN HEALTH PROMOTION

The effect of nursing practice on promoting health for all people in the future can be profound. Whether you are working in a rural or urban setting, hospital, clinic, home health agency, workplace, school, or community agency, you can influence the health of each and every one of your clients.

Challenges facing nurses and health-promotion practice today are numerous and varied. Among those challenges are keeping current with new knowledge, technology, and information systems; understanding the changing demographics of society and the world; engaging in partnerships and collaborative relationships with individuals, families, and groups; becoming involved in health-promotion policy development and implementation; participating in evidence-based practice; developing a worldview perspective; and embracing a proactive philosophy for professional practice.

The following measures can help nurses meet such challenges:

- *Expand the frontiers of your own knowledge.* By being knowledgeable about new research and technologies, you build a solid foundation to guide you in helping your clients. Keeping current with legislation affecting health care and your practice is also powerful knowledge.
- *Make collaboration with other providers a basic part of your practice.* Nurses have historically maintained a do-it-all attitude for client care. Most nurses have been educated to give total client care. Yet the overlap of care already exists with physicians, nutritionists, physical therapists, and others. Working in a complementary manner with other providers can strengthen the health plan for your clients. Remember, too, that empowering the client is important to the effectiveness of the collaborative network.
- *Place the emphasis of your care on outcomes, cost, and quality.* Because health care will continue to be cost-driven, you need to exercise a cost-conscious model of care while maintaining a focus on quality in achieving goals.
- *Enhance your sensitivities to biological factors, lifestyle choices, environmental factors, cultural diversities, and educational readiness of your clientele.* Rather than diagnosing and treating disease, health promotion is tailored to the individual.
- *Adopt a wellness focus to guide your practice.* Under the umbrella of wellness, health-promotion activities, including health maintenance and disease prevention, must be granted the same esteem and professionalism as nursing activities involved in caring for clients with disease diagnoses.

SUMMARY

This chapter has presented an overview of the historical, social, economic, and political developments that have forged the foundation for health promotion and provided direction for the future. Clearly, health promotion is a dynamic process in constant change. The health-promoting practices and policies of the past have gone through major alterations to adjust to the reality of the world today and to anticipate the future.

Nursing practice has also undergone major changes but has continually maintained a commitment to promoting health. Today, the nursing profession, with its varied roles and scope of practice, plays a vital part in the promotion of health that extends from individuals to families, groups, communities, and the world.

KEY CONCEPTS

1. Health promotion is a relatively recent term with various meanings among individuals and societies reflecting values, beliefs, politics, and philosophies. Health education is a major component of health promotion.
2. The history of health promotion is a tapestry woven from ancient cultures, practices based on beliefs and values of the population, changing health behaviors, the effects of technological and scientific advances, and powerful sociopolitical forces.
3. The heightened consciousness of society, the change of medical focus from disease treatment to illness prevention, and the development of nursing as a profession

were the major movements behind health promotion in the nineteenth century.
4. The contributions of science and the effects of economic, environmental, and sociopolitical forces in the twentieth century profoundly affected health promotion in the United States. World War II was a major catalyst in technology advancement, immunization development, and disease treatment that changed medical practice forever. The United States prospered with industrial technology, resulting in national and individual economic gains, shifts from rural to urban populations, alterations in disease epidemiology, and changes in lifestyles. The Social

Security Act provided the foundation for the socialization of health care, which was extended by Medicare and Medicaid. Government spending for health care brought relief to many people, as well as cost inflation and fraud. Cost, access, and quality have become major issues, prompting support for health promotion.

5. Canada was an early leader of nations for health promotion with the publication of the *LaLonde Report.* WHO enlisted the support of member nations in reaching the goals popularly known as "health for all by the year 2000." The United States has set new national goals for health, as described in *Healthy People 2010.*

6. The nursing profession, transformed by the social mandate for health promotion, continues to change in practice and policy to meet the dynamic needs of society. Consumer involvement, expanded roles for nurses, changing practice settings, and collaborative health care

management highlight the importance of health promotion in professional practices. The *Code for Nurses, Nursing's Social Policy Statement,* and *Standards for Clinical Nursing Practice* emphasize the commitment of the nursing profession to health promotion.

7. The health of nations is shaped by many influences, including economic, social, political, environmental, natural and human-caused disasters, and behavioral factors. Terrorism continues to be a major threat to the well-being of people of the world.

8. The future of health promotion and nursing practice will be affected by the manner in which nurses articulate their unique contributions. A personal commitment to increasing knowledge, collaboration, the individualization of health care, and the focus on wellness will expand to become a wide perspective of health promotion.

CHAPTER REVIEW

Learning Activities

1. Identify five examples of efforts to promote the health of people in your community.

2. Explain how nurses and other health professionals could be involved in these efforts.

3. Examine the new role of nurse coach and the effect you see on the health of clients in your area.

Multiple Choice

1. The Ottawa Charter was developed for which one of the following purposes?
   a. To achieve health for all by the year 2000 and beyond
   b. To expand health education for healthier lifestyles
   c. To guide Canada's health-promotion initiatives
   d. To solidify the United States and Canada in coordinated health care services

2. Dualism in health care, rooted in the past and currently existing, refers to the:
   a. combination of values, attitudes, and beliefs with modern health care practices.
   b. conflicts that exist between two different cultures regarding health care.
   c. differences between society's needs and programs developed by health care administrators.
   d. recognition that individuals are often multicultural.

3. A long-term study known for linking cardiovascular disease with smoking, obesity, and hypertension is:
   a. the Doll and Hill study.
   b. the Framingham study.
   c. *Healthy People 2000.*
   d. *Nursing: A Social Policy Statement.*

4. The influence of politics and government on health care in developed countries (United States, Canada, Britain, etc.) is:
   a. absent for the most part.
   b. extensive.
   c. focused on chronic disease.
   d. limited to financing issues.

5. The foundation for Medicare and Medicaid in the United States is attributed to which of the following?
   a. *Healthy People*
   b. *LaLonde Report*
   c. *Nursing: A Social Policy Statement*
   d. *Social Security Act*

6. Which of the following accurately describes diagnostic-related groups (DRGs)? They were:
   a. meant to provide for cost savings to clients.
   b. created by physicians to increase Medicare payments.
   c. designed by hospitals to increase the quality of care.
   d. developed by nurses to facilitate care.

7. Which of the following would you most likely be involved in as a nurse coach for an overweight female client with diabetes?
   a. Discussing her choices, options, preferences, and personal goals for optimum nutrition
   b. Joining an exercise group with her to accurately assess her commitment to weight management
   c. Making an appointment for the her to consult with a diabetes nutritionist
   d. Providing her with pamphlets on diet management and exercise routines

8. Your client wants to quit smoking. An appropriate component of teaching that represents a broad perspective of health promotion would include education on the:
   a. effect of secondhand smoke on family members.
   b. hazardous chemicals in cigarettes.
   c. policies related to smoking in the workplace.
   d. statistics on deaths from smoking.

ORGANIZATIONS AND WEBSITES

The Centre for Health Promotion: An internationally recognized organization that is committed to excellence in education, evaluation, and research through multidisciplinary collaboration to activate, develop, and evaluate innovative health promotion approaches in Canada and abroad: **http://www.utoronto.ca/chp/**

Healthy People 2020: Science-based, 10-year national objectives for promoting health and preventing disease for the United States: **http://www.healthypeople.gov/hp2020**

Office of Disease Prevention and Health Promotion: Works to strengthen disease prevention and health promotion priorities through a collaborative framework of Health and Human Services agencies: **http://odphp.osophs.dhhs.gov**

United Nations Development Programme: Explains the role of the UN Developmental Programme and provides detailed information on the eight Millennial Developmental Goals for 2015: **http://www.undp.org/mdg**

United States Army Center for Health Promotion & Preventive Medicine: Provides worldwide technical support for implementing preventive medicine, public health, and health-promotion/wellness services in all aspects of America's Army and the world community with a vision to be a world-class Center for Health Promotion and Preventive Medicine: **http://www.apgea.army**

U.S. Department of Health and Human Services: The U.S. government's principal agency for protecting the health of all Americans and providing essential human services through more than 300 programs covering a wide spectrum of activities: **http://www.hhs.gov**

REFERENCES

American Nurses Association. (1980). *Nursing: A social policy statement* (Publ. No. NP-63). Kansas City, MO: American Nurses Association.

American Nurses Association. (1995). *Nursing's Social Policy Statement* (Publ. No. NP-107). Washington, DC: American Nurses Publishing.

Anonymous. (1986). Ottawa charter for health promotion. *Canadian Journal of Public Health,* 77(6), 425–430.

Babylonia, a history of ancient Babylon. (n.d.). Retrieved from http://history-world.org/babylonia.htm

Bright, M. A. (2002). *Holistic health and healing.* Philadelphia, PA: F. A. Davis.

Canadian Nurses Association (2000, June). *Fact sheet: The Canadian health act.* Retrieved from http://cna-nurses.ca

Centers for Medicare and Medicaid Services (CMS), National Health Expenditure Data. (2011, November 4). *National health expenditure data historical.* Retrieved from https://www.cms.gov/NationalHealthExpendData/02_NationalHealthAccountsHistorical.asp#TopOfPage

Chapman, S. (2005). The most important and influential papers in tobacco control: Results of an online poll. *Tobacco Control, 14.* Retrieved from http://tobacco.health.usyd.edu.au

Clark, M. J. (2007). *Community health nursing: Caring for populations* (4th ed.). Upper Saddle River, NJ: Prentice Hall.

Cockerham, W. C. (1978). *Medical sociology.* Englewood Cliffs, NJ: Prentice-Hall.

Eliopoulos, C. (2010). *Invitation to holistic health: A guide to living a balanced life* (2nd ed.).Sudbury, MA: Jones & Bartlett.

Ellis, J. R., & Hartley, C. L. (2007). *Nursing in today's world* (8th ed.). Philadelphia, PA: Lippincott Williams & Wilkins.

Gordis, L. (2009). *Epidemiology* (4th ed.). Philadelphia: W. B. Saunders.

Gourevitch, M. N., Caronna, C. A., & Kalcut, G. E. (2008). Acute care. In A. R. Kovner & J. R. Knickman (eds.). *Health care delivery in the United States.* New York, NY: Springer, pp. 191–218.

Graff, P., & Goldberg, S. (2000). *The health field concept then and now: Snapshots of Canada.* Ottawa, ON: Canadian Policy Research Network.

Griset, P. L., & Mahon, S. (2003). *Terrorism in perspective.* Thousand Oaks, CA: Sage Publications.

Guisepi, R. A. (2001). *A history of ancient Greece.* Retrieved from history-world.org/ancient_greece.htm

Henchey, N., & Burgess, D. (1987). *Between past and future: Quebec education in transition.* Calgary: Detselig.

Hoffman, E. D., Klees, B. S., & Curtis, C. A. (2006, November). *Brief summaries of Medicare and Medicaid.* Retrieved from http://www.mindfully.org/Health/2005/Medicare-Medicaid-Summaries1nov05.htm

International Council of Nurses. (2006). *The ICN Code of Ethics for Nurses.* Geneva: ICN.

Kelly, L. Y., & Joel, L. A. (2005). *The nursing experience: Trends, challenges, and transitions* (5th ed.). New York, NY: McGraw-Hill.

Koh, H. K. (2010). A 2020 vision for healthy people. *New England Journal of Medicine.* Retrieved from http://www.nejm.org/doi/full/10.1056/NEJMp1001601

Kramarow, E., Lentzner, H., Rooks, R., Weeks, J., & Saydah, S. (1999). *Health and aging chart-book* (Library of Congress Catalog No. 76-641496, p. 30). Washington, DC: U.S. Government Printing Office.

Luck, S. (2010). Nurse coaches and changing the health of our nation. *Alternative Therapies, 16*(5), 78–80.

MacDonald, G., & Bunton, R. (1992). Health promotion: Discipline or disciplines? In G. MacDonald & R. Bunton (eds.). *Health promotion: Disciplines and diversity.* New York, NY: Routledge.

Martin, A., Lassman, D., Whittle, L., Catlin, A., & the NHEA Team. (2011). Recession contributes to slowest annual rate of increase in health spending in five decades. *Health Affairs, 30.* DOI: 10.1377.

McLeroy, K. R., & Crump, C. E. (1994). Health promotion and disease prevention: A historical perspective. *Generations, 18*(1), 9–17.

Merrill, R. M., & Timmreck, T. C., (2006). *Introduction to epidemiology,* 4th ed. Sudbury, MA: Jones & Bartlett.

Moore, P. V., & Williamson, C. C. (1984). Health promotion: Evolution of a concept. *Nursing Clinics of North America, 19*(2), 195–207.

National Vital Statistics Reports (2010). *Deaths: Final data for 2007, 58*(19). Hyattsville, MD: National Center for Health Statistics

Nightingale, F. (1859/1969). *Notes on nursing: What it is and what it is not.* New York, NY: Dover Publications.

Noakes, T. D., Borresen, J., Hew-Butler, T., Lambert, M. I., & Jordaan, E. (2008). Semmelweis and the aetiology of puerperal sepsis 160 years on: An historical review. *Epidemiology & Infection, 136*(1), 1–9.

Novak, J. C. (1988). The social mandate and historical basis for nursing's role in health promotion. *Journal of Professional Nursing, 4*(2), 80–87.

Nutbeam, D. (1996). Health promotion glossary. In *Health promotion: An anthology*. Washington, DC: Pan American Health Organization.

Office of Disease Prevention and Health Promotion, (2011). *Welcome*. Retrieved from http://odphp.osophs.dhhs.gov/

Omran, A. R. (1971/2005). The epidemiologic transition: A theory of the epidemiology of population change. *The Milbank Quarterly, 83*(4),731–757.

Parascandola, M., Weed, D. L., & Dasgupta, A. (2006, January 10). Two Surgeon General's reports on smoking and cancer: A historical investigation of the practice of causal inference. *Emerging Themes in Epidemiology, 3*(1). Retrieved from http://www.ete-online.com/content/3/1/1

September 11, 2001 attacks. (n.d.). Retrieved from en.wikipedia.org/wiki/September_11,_2001_attacks

Stanhope, M., & Lancaster, J. (2012). *Public health nursing: Population-centered health care in the community* (8th ed.). Philadelphia, PA: Mosby/Elsevier.

United Nations Department of Public Information. (2005, September). *2005 World summit outcome*. Retrieved from http://www.un.org/summit2005/presskit/fact_sheet.pdf

United Nations Developmental Programme (UNDP). (2010). *What will it take to achieve the millennium developmental goals?* New York, NY: UNDP.

U.S. Department of Health and Human Services. (2000). *Healthy people 2010*. Washington, DC: U.S. Government Printing Office.

U.S. Department of Health and Human Services. (2010) *Healthy people 2020*. Retrieved from http://www.healthypeople.gov/2020/about/objectiveDevelopment.aspx

U.S. Public Health Service. (1979). *Healthy people: Surgeon General's report on health promotion and disease prevention* (DHHS Publication no. 79-55071). Washington, DC: U.S. Government Printing Office.

U.S. Public Health Service. (1980). *Promoting health/preventing disease: Objectives for the nation*. Washington, DC: U.S. Government Printing Office. HE 20.2:D63/4.

U.S. Public Health Service. (1990). *Healthy people 2000: National health promotion and disease prevention objectives, 1990*. Washington, DC: U.S. Government Printing Office.

Whitehead, D. (2008). An international Delphi study examining health promotion and health education in nursing practice, education and policy. *Journal of Clinical Nursing, 17*(7), 891–900. DOI: 10.1111/j.1365-2702.2007.02079.x.

Whittaker, C. (2010). Journey to healthy people: A more realistic look at getting Americans healthy. *US Family Health Plan, 13*(2), 2.

World Health Organization (WHO). (1978). Declaration of Alma-Ata. International Conference on Primary Health Care, Alma-Ata, USSR, 6–12 September, 1978. Retrieved from http://www.who.int/hpr/NPH/docs/declaration_almaata.pdf

BIBLIOGRAPHY

Allender, J. A., & Spradley, B. W. (2005). *Community health nursing: Promoting and protecting the public's health*. Philadelphia, PA: Lippincott Williams & Wilkins.

Delaney, F. G. (1994). Nursing and health promotion: Conceptual concerns. *Journal of Advanced Nursing, 20*, 828–835.

Kalisch, P. A., & Kalisch, B. J. (2004). *American nursing: A history*. Philadelphia, PA: Lippincott Williams & Wilkins.

Kovner, A. R., & Knickman, J. R. (eds.). (2008). *Jonas and Kovner's health care delivery in the United States* (9th ed.). New York, NY: Springer.

Palmer, I. (1977). Nightingale: Reformer, reactionary, researcher. *Nursing Research, 22*, 101–110.

Spellbring, A. M. (1991). Nursing's role in health promotion: An overview. *Nursing Clinics of North America, 26*(4), 805–815.

Terris, M. (1996). Concepts of health promotion: Dualities in public health theory. In *Health promotion: An anthology*. Washington, DC: Pan American Health Organization.

CHAPTER 2
Nursing Concepts and Health Promotion

CAROLINA G. HUERTA, EdD, MSN, RN

KEY TERMS

adaptation

career ladder

concept

conceptual framework

cultural congruent care

general systems theory

holistic

homeostasis

metaparadigm

needs theory

paradigm

theory

transcultural nursing theory

OBJECTIVES

Upon completion of this chapter, the reader should be able to:

- Identify concepts essential in defining professional nursing practice.
- Describe how the concept of health promotion provides a framework for professional nursing practice.
- Explain how a metaparadigm is useful in defining a profession.
- Describe the four concepts central to nursing's metaparadigm.
- Describe nursing educational levels and their relationship to health promotion.
- List assumptions basic to integrating health promotion into nursing practice.
- Identify selected nursing theoretical frameworks.
- List various definitions of nursing.

INTRODUCTION

The concept of health promotion is not a new one to the nursing profession. Health promotion has evolved over the centuries and traces its roots to ancient times (see Chapter 1). In fact, Florence Nightingale's (1860) writings focused on health practices and health promotion in the context of the environmental impact on health. Nursing practice has long considered the concept of health promotion as integral to the prevention of disease, maintenance of health, identification of optimum health, and restoration of well-being.

A health-promotion focus provides nursing and health care professionals with a heightened consciousness in assuming responsibility for the personal health and welfare of those in their care, as well as the health and welfare of others in society at large. Unfortunately, lifestyle or behavioral changes needed to achieve a state of health are not easy tasks.

Implementing health-promotion strategies is extremely difficult if individuals lack motivation to do those things that will result in good health. In fact, many people, nurses included, are guilty of making lifestyle choices that seem to sabotage opportunities for achieving optimal health and living a long, prosperous life. Change, especially in relation to improving health, is difficult to achieve. Individuals need a lot of support and encouragement from knowledgeable health care professionals if they are to make lifestyle changes that will result in optimal health.

The previous chapter introduced the concept of health promotion and provided a historical perspective on its evolution and impact on contemporary society. This chapter focuses on nursing's metaparadigm, professional nursing today, and its relationship to health promotion. Nursing theories, health promotion as a conceptual framework, and the four concepts that define nursing's metaparadigm are described. Professional nursing practice's influence on personal as well as community health care behavior changes will be emphasized.

PROFESSIONAL NURSING PRACTICE AND HEALTH PROMOTION

The concept of health promotion is found in much of the current nursing literature. The interest in health promotion has risen because the idea of increasing levels of well-being, life expectancy, and health potential fits well with nursing as a caring discipline. Health-promotion strategies also decrease health care costs and morbidity. Because the concept of health promotion is integral to everything that nurses do, it provides a useful framework in defining and describing nursing. The nursing profession has always included health promotion in one form or another in its attempt to define itself and to identify the various nursing responsibilities.

The American Nurses Association's (ANA) *Code of Ethics for Nurses* (ANA, 2010a), for example, which was originally adopted in 1950, clearly indicates the profession's responsibility to the public in promoting efforts to meet health needs (Box 2-1). This document highlights nursing's responsibility for protecting, promoting, and restoring the health of the community it serves.

The ANA's *Scope & Standards of Practice* (ANA, 2010c), which addresses the profession's concern with the quality of nursing service and accountability, also highlights health promotion in nursing. These standards describe nurses' concern for ensuring that their actions provide for patient participation in health promotion, health protection, and optimization of health and that they assist patients in maximizing their potential. In fact, standard five in this document specifically

---

BOX 2-1
AMERICAN NURSES ASSOCIATION CODE OF ETHICS FOR NURSES

1. The nurse, in all professional relationships, practices with compassion and respect for the inherent dignity, worth, and uniqueness of every individual, unrestricted by considerations of social or economic status, personal attributes, or the nature of the health problem.
2. The nurse's primary commitment is to the patient, whether an individual, family, group, or community.
3. The nurse promotes, advocates for, and strives to protect the health, safety, and rights of the patient.
4. The nurse is responsible and accountable for individual nursing practice and determines the appropriate delegation of tasks consistent with the nurse's obligation to provide optimum patient care.
5. The nurse owes the same duties to self as to others, including the responsibility to preserve integrity and safety, to maintain competence, and to continue personal and professional growth.
6. The nurse participates in establishing, maintaining, and improving health care environments and conditions of employment conducive to the provision of quality health care and consistent with the values of the profession through individual and collective action.
7. The nurse participates in the advancement of the profession through contributions to practice, education, administration, and knowledge development.
8. The nurse collaborates with other health professionals and the public in promoting community, national, and international efforts to meet health needs.
9. The profession of nursing, as represented by associations and their members, is responsible for articulating nursing values, for maintaining the integrity of the profession and its practice, and for shaping social policy.

TABLE 2-1 ANA Professional Nursing Practice Standards/Statements and Their Relationship to Health-Promotion Concepts

STANDARDS/ STATEMENTS	PURPOSE OF DOCUMENT	RELATIONSHIP TO HEALTH PROMOTION
Scope & Standards of Practice (2010)	Outlines the expectations of the professional role of the registered nurse. Focuses on professional competence and the nurses' responsibility to maintain professional competence. Describes a means for determining the quality of nursing services received by patient. The standards reflect the values and priorities of the nursing profession.	Concerned with the health status of the patient, not just illness. Specifies that health status determines the nursing care needs and subsequent actions; highlights nursing's actions that promote, maintain, and restore well-being and health and that optimize health.
Code of Ethics for Nurses (2010)	Establishes a code of ethics that provides guidance for professional nursing conduct and responsibilities across all roles, levels, and settings.	Makes explicit nursing's values, duties, and commitments in relation to protecting, promoting, and restoring health in the care of individuals, families, groups, and communities. Delineates nursing's responsibility to assist patients in maximizing their own potential and requires them to participate in promoting their own health.
Nursing: A Social Policy Statement (2010)	Provides a framework for understanding professional nursing's responsibility in being uniquely accountable to society and its obligations for those receiving care. Expresses the social contract between society and the profession of nursing.	Focuses on nature of nursing and recognizes nursing practice as being restorative, supportive, and promotive. Conceptualizes the framework of nursing practice and emphasizes protection, promotion, and optimization of health. Nursing actions include promotion practices that mobilize health patterns of the body. Recognizes nurses' role of advocacy in the care of individuals, families, communities, and populations.

© Cengage Learning 2013

identifies a nursing plan of action that includes strategies to address health teaching and health promotion. According to the standards document, the registered nurse is to focus on health teaching that addresses health-promotion areas such as healthy lifestyles, risk-reducing behaviors, and preventive self-care.

The scope and standards document includes a description of the art of nursing that views patients holistically in all their dimensions. The goal of nursing is to promote and maintain health and to prevent or resolve disease, illness, or disability. The registered nurse thus uses strategies that are restorative, supportive, and promotive (ANA, 2010, p. 23). ANA's *Nursing's Social Policy Statement: The Essence of the Profession* (2010b) describes the social context in which nursing takes place. This document describes nursing as being concerned with the needs of individuals, families, communities, and populations. The nurse must address issues related to the promotion of health and wellness, to the promotion of safety and quality care, to the patient's physical, emotional, and spiritual comfort, and to pain and issues related to social policies and their effects on health.

The ANA documents are intended to reflect the scope of nursing practice and its theoretical or conceptual basis. Evidently, one of nursing's most highly prioritized responsibilities is to promote healthy behaviors among the constituents it serves. Table 2-1 identifies ANA documents important to

professional nursing and to their relationship to the concept of health promotion as a nursing goal. These documents are important to professional nurses in practice in that they identify nursing's role in the promotion of health.

NURSING AND HEALTH PROMOTION IN A GLOBAL COMMUNITY

Although there may be a tendency to be ethnocentric when it comes to the application of health-promotion concepts in the nursing arena, the concept of health promotion and the use of a health-promotion framework are not specific to nursing in the United States. In fact, as explained in the previous chapter, Canada has also had a rich legacy in utilizing health-promotion concepts in the provision of health care. Canada has long been a leader in introducing health-promotion concepts and integrating these concepts into nursing practice.

For example, the Public Health Agency of Canada (2010) has a website on health promotion covering such varied topics as community action programs for children, school health policies, healthy living topics, mental health, violence, and obesity, to name a few. This agency promotes strategies that focus on improving health among its citizens. A recent example on how

Canada is promoting health-promotion concepts in nursing practice is a current study that focuses on mental health during pregnancy. All mothers in a province are being screened by nurses for depression during pregnancy and the postpartum period. It is believed that, if mental health problems are caught early, strategies to promote mental health can be used and a multitude of adverse outcomes can be avoided, such as substance abuse and premature delivery (Canadian Nurses Association, 2011).

Other countries have made a major effort to integrate health-promotion concepts into health care, specifically nursing. International health promotion in nursing Web links offer multiple examples of current efforts taking place to integrate health promotion into nursing practice. These links demonstrate strategies to introduce health-promotion concepts in countries as varied as Ireland, England, Japan, Mexico, Switzerland, Slovenia, and Australia, to name a few. A commonality of international-health promotion strategies is the emphasis on the quality of life, prevention of injury and diseases, protection, and education to reduce the need for medical treatment or rehabilitation. Obviously, the integration of health-promotion concepts and strategies into health care delivery is of critical importance to nursing worldwide. For that reason, this text contains many references to global health promotion in nursing activities.

NURSING'S METAPARADIGM

Health promotion is an integral part of nursing practice and is essential in defining nursing as a profession. When viewing the nursing discipline on a broad basis, health promotion is always included in nursing's definition. It is part of what nurses do in nursing practice and is reflected in what is called the paradigm or metaparadigm of nursing. A **paradigm** is an example that serves as a pattern or model for something (Taber, 2009). A nursing paradigm provides a clear or typical example of nursing as a discipline. When used in the context of nursing theories, a paradigm is considered a group of related theories that share similar concepts and structural features or that provide a broad philosophical approach to nursing (Walker & Avant, 2011). Paradigms have been used in recent years by theorists to illustrate how concepts and theories fit into the actual practice of a discipline.

A **metaparadigm,** on the other hand, is typically used by an individual discipline to provide a global perspective of the field. It is viewed as transcending all paradigms (Walker & Avant, 2011). The prefix *meta* refers to a highly organized form at a later stage of development. A metaparadigm describes a later or more highly organized form of a paradigm. Nursing uses a metaparadigm as a unifying force to describe those common concepts specific to nursing. In fact, nursing theorists usually identify concepts that are congruent with their view of nursing and refer to these in their totality as nursing's metaparadigm. A metaparadigm is preferred to a paradigm because it is thought to represent a more organized framework than a paradigm. Nursing's metaparadigm helps to critically unify and evaluate the concepts that are characteristic of nursing. The metaparadigm of nursing summarizes the meaning of nursing and identifies the categories of knowledge relevant to nursing practice (Fawcett & Garity, 2009).

A description of nursing must include those concepts and theories that collectively or individually describe the profession. Definitions of nursing invariably include conceptual or theoretical frameworks that serve the purpose of explaining what nursing is and what actions are specific to nursing. For example, the concept of health promotion can be useful in defining or describing the nursing profession in relation to those nursing actions that assist patients, their families, or both to prevent illness, maintain health, and promote optimum well-being. A nursing metaparadigm that uses health promotion will then make certain that this concept is integrated throughout the description of the four concepts commonly used to organize nursing's metaparadigm. The four concepts that are found in theorists' descriptions of nursing's metaparadigm are *person, health, environment,* and *nursing* (Fawcett, 2005; Fawcett & Garity, 2009). These concepts are used in this chapter to define nursing and its relation to health promotion.

Prior to describing the profession in terms of nursing's metaparadigm, it is necessary to clarify the terms *concept, theory,* and *framework*. A **concept** is a generalized notion or idea that is useful in describing facts or occurrences. Person, environment, and health, for example, are major concepts used in defining nursing. Concepts provide a broad view or perspective of the nursing profession. **Theory,** on the other hand, is narrower and provides specificity in its description. Theory uses relational statements to present a systematic view of a phenomenon. It uses facts, definitions, and propositions to specify relationships among variables. Theories are useful for describing, explaining, predicting and controlling phenomena (Walker & Avant, 2011). Theory's primary purpose is to generate new knowledge and to make scientific findings meaningful and generalizable. Theory takes into account observable or empirical facts in the environment, relates these facts to each other, and makes sense out of them. The generation of theory, or theory building, is important to the discipline of nursing, which, for the most part, describes itself as an art and a science. As a science, nursing is expected to generate new knowledge and to expand existing knowledge by building theory. The linking of concepts and propositions through theory building makes the accumulated body of knowledge easily accessible and organized.

Nursing theory's primary purpose is to help us understand and further develop nursing practice. Theory provides a perspective that can be defined and described in various ways according to a person's individual experiences (Parker & Smith, 2010). As you might guess, theories of nursing are created by nurses. In most cases, these nurses do not set out to create theory or to become nurse theorists. Theories evolve out of nursing theorists' attempts to describe nursing and nursing practice, to identify choices and assumptions about the nature of nursing and nursing knowledge, and to describe what nurses do in the real world (Hickman, 2011a). Although they may not be aware of it, nurses use theory in their nursing practice daily. Theory undoubtedly provides value and support to the actions taken in nursing practice.

A framework is a structure that provides support in organizing and shaping something. It is much like the frame of a house that lends support to its roof, walls, and existing structures. A **conceptual framework,** also referred to as a conceptual model, is less formal in organizing phenomena than a theory. A conceptual framework or model describes and/or illustrates the concepts that are interrelated and central to the understanding of a phenomenon (Polit & Beck, 2012). This framework provides a way to shape nursing and nursing practice into a meaningful configuration. Frameworks used to define nursing may include theoretical frameworks that specify a certain theory or theorist or conceptual frameworks that identify the interrelated concepts important to nursing. A conceptual framework is less formal and less well developed than a theoretical framework. Because frameworks useful to describing nursing are not always based on a particular nursing theory, the terms *theoretical framework, conceptual framework,* and *conceptual model* are used interchangeably in this chapter.

DEFINING NURSING

Fawcett (2005) has attempted to conceptualize the essence of nursing in her description of nursing's metaparadigm. She has defined nursing in terms of the concepts that are central to nursing practice. Fawcett's metaparadigm provides organization in describing nursing as a practice discipline that has evolved from theory and nursing research. She uses the concept of person as the recipient of care (whether an individual, a family, or a group). She also includes the concepts of environment as encompassing both animate and inanimate objects, health to include the wellness and illness of the patient, and nursing actions to mean the actions taken by nurses in caring for a patient. Fawcett's metaparadigm is frequently used to define and delineate the scope of nursing. It has also been used to define the meaning of nursing research within the context of the meaning of nursing (Fawcett & Garity, 2009).

Nursing: A Social Policy Statement (ANA, 2010) illustrates how definitions of nursing include the promotion of well-being in the recipient of care. Nursing is defined as the actions that protect, promote, and optimize the health of individuals, families, communities, and populations. The document presents definitions that are congruent with nursing's metaparadigm and that also include human experiences, responses to health and illness, a knowledge base, and provisions for nurse-patient relationships that foster health and healing. The scope of nursing practice is continually evolving and is identified as one that includes practices that promote, attain, maintain, and restore health. The definition and scope of nursing in this ANA document demonstrate the connection of the four concepts described by Fawcett's metaparadigm on nursing. Nursing's definition and scope include the concept of person in relation to human responses, the concept of health and nursing's role in relation to its promotion, the environment as reflected by a person's experiences and responses to health problems, and the nursing actions that involve restoration, support, and the promotion of health.

PERSON, ENVIRONMENT, HEALTH, AND NURSING

Nursing's metaparadigm provides the substance and character of nursing as a profession. It is the strength on which nursing practice is built. Nursing's focus is on those actions and processes that are directed toward human beings and that take into consideration the environment in which human beings live and nurses practice (Fawcett & Garity, 2009). Figure 2-1 depicts nursing's metaparadigm and illustrates how the four concepts—person (human being), environment, health, and nursing—interact dynamically in practice.

PERSON

A thorough description of the concept of person is essential to providing direction for nursing as a practice discipline. The person as the recipient of care is perceived to possess attributes that must be considered in the performance of nursing actions. These attributes are useful in the professional nurse's assessment, planning, implementation, and evaluation activities.

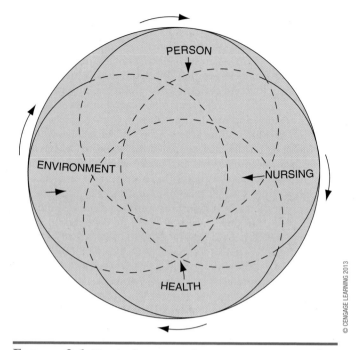

FIGURE 2-1 **Nursing's metaparadigm: interaction among the four concepts.**

Nursing models using a health-promotion approach describe recipients of care as human beings—holistic, biological, spiritual, psychological, and social beings made up of more than a sum of their parts. Person-centered nurses care for individuals in their totality as opposed to only the diseased areas. Because patients are also seen as capable of thinking critically, they are given the opportunity to have input into their own care. The patient is seen as interacting with the environment, having energy, and being dynamic and is perceived as constantly changing and adapting. Patients are cultural beings whose uniqueness sets them apart from all others, even though they may possess a shared culture. In the performance of nursing care, the nurse considers persons in a **holistic** manner, in their totality, and places great importance on their life experiences. People's experiences are a part of their very essence of being, and thus a knowledge of their past, present, and possible future experiences must be considered when planning their care and health-promotion activities. Knowing patients holistically and recognizing that they are the primary participants in the nursing process is essential to the provision of quality nursing care and is the central focus of nursing practice (Huerta & Sánchez, 2009).

Individual uniqueness, in terms of total functioning, must also be considered when planning and performing patient care. As recipients of nursing care, patients are entitled to full disclosure and to active participation in the development of their health promotion or nursing care plans. A person is perceived as having many needs and as being capable of achieving and maintaining optimum health. For example, Maslow (1970, 1999), a social psychologist, describes persons as social beings having many common needs that motivate their behavior. The meeting of these needs is important to the maintenance of health throughout the life span.

MASLOW'S HIERARCHY OF NEEDS

Maslow identifies what he calls the *hierarchy of needs* that encompass the physiological, safety and security, love and belonging, self-esteem, and self-actualization needs of all people.

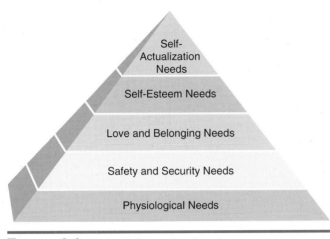

FIGURE 2-2 Maslow's hierarchy of needs.

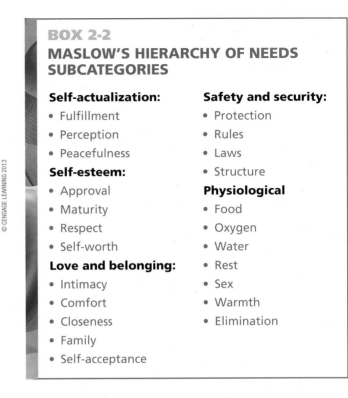

These needs are ranked in relation to their importance. Figure 2-2 illustrates a pyramid depicting the hierarchy of needs.

Imagine that the pyramid has a staircase consisting of five flights to the top. If the intent is to get to the top, then a person must climb each step. Maslow's hierarchy of needs can be described in the same manner in that needs at one level must be met before a person can reach the next level. These physiologic needs form the base of the staircase: basic life-sustaining needs such as food, water, air, rest, sleep, and activity. If basic needs are met, the individual is ready to climb the next flight. The needs at the next level are safety and security. The satisfaction of these needs allows the person to meet the love and belonging needs found on the third level and the self-esteem needs found on the fourth level of the staircase.

Ascending this fourth flight of stairs does not ensure that the person will make it to the top. Maslow describes this top of the pyramid as the highest level and as representative of a person's self-actualization needs. Many barriers prevent most people from reaching this fifth level, but, according to Maslow, people continuously strive to achieve this level. The fifth level is represented as the top level because it is elusive and difficult to achieve. Box 2-2 depicts the specific needs that might surface within each category of needs.

Many factors can influence a patient's pursuit of optimum health. It is nursing's responsibility to identify some of these factors and to assist patients in determining the steps that can be taken to achieve the optimum health state. The self-prioritization of needs by patients, for instance, occurs all of the time and may impact their health-related outcomes. For example, a mother may choose to provide the only available water to her child so that the child's thirst may be satisfied. In doing this, she has chosen to satisfy her need for love and belonging instead of meeting her own physiological need for water. Fortunately, people have the ability to communicate, think independently, and prioritize because these characteristics are essential to meeting needs and promoting health. Knowledge of a human needs framework is useful in nursing practice because this framework provides a method for prioritizing patient care activities, as well as a means for understanding the nurse's personal behavior and that of the patient.

Nursing attests to the importance of the concept of person by caring for, educating, directing, and assisting people in their attempt to achieve optimum health. The concept of person in nursing's metaparadigm focuses on individuals' ability to direct their own health and determine the most favorable actions to acquire it.

BOX 2-2
MASLOW'S HIERARCHY OF NEEDS SUBCATEGORIES

Self-actualization:
- Fulfillment
- Perception
- Peacefulness

Self-esteem:
- Approval
- Maturity
- Respect
- Self-worth

Love and belonging:
- Intimacy
- Comfort
- Closeness
- Family
- Self-acceptance

Safety and security:
- Protection
- Rules
- Laws
- Structure

Physiological
- Food
- Oxygen
- Water
- Rest
- Sex
- Warmth
- Elimination

ENVIRONMENT

The environment is a major influence on a person's overall functioning and health-promotion activities. As a result, it is critical for nurses to understand how the internal as well as external environments impact a patient's everyday life. Nurse theorists throughout the history of modern nursing have identified the environment as an important concept in determining what nursing is and what nurses do. In fact, Florence Nightingale, who is recognized as the founder of contemporary nursing, described her whole philosophy of nursing in terms of environmental factors that influence health and disease. In her *Notes on Nursing* (1860/1969), which Nightingale wrote in 1859, she delineates symptoms of disease as environment related and expounds on environmental factors that cause or prevent disease. Pure water, fresh air, light, cleanliness, and efficient drainage are described as environmental factors essential to disease prevention.

The environment consists of both internal and external environments that continuously interface with each other. People's internal environments include their ideas, biological makeup, emotions, and the psychosocial elements that influence them. Included in this psychosocial entity are a person's spiritual, cultural, and social needs and experiences. A person's internal biological environment includes bodily mechanisms that control such functions as heart rate, temperature, and blood pressure.

On the other hand, the internal psychosocial environment may consist of emotional responses, such as to crisis or stress. Responses to crisis or stress are reflected internally in the biological functioning of the human body. For instance, a person living in a stressful environment may worry excessively. This worry state may result in reactions by the internal environment that might lead to hypersecretion of hydrochloric acid by the stomach, resulting in stomach ulcers or other symptoms. The internal response to this stress may also result in an increase in blood pressure and heart rate. Obviously, many factors can upset a person's internal environment.

The external environment consists of more than the physical surroundings. It consists of all events and influences that occur externally and that impact a person's health status and functional abilities. Responses to our external environment are contextually based and reflect our own individual interpretation of the environment. Reactions to the external environment may or may not lead to health-promoting changes. Persons, for example, who live in a highly polluted area of a metropolitan city may decide to move to a less polluted area in order to improve their health. Other people, because of their living conditions, believe that they can do little to effect healthy changes. These people, however, can be self-directed and do as much as possible to change their external environment. For example, people living in filthy and drug- or cockroach infested housing projects or tenements are impacted by these conditions. They may not have the choice to move elsewhere or change very much about their living conditions, but they can implement changes that impact their health, such as cleaning their homes. People can be catalysts in changing the external environment and thus promote changes in themselves and others.

Recognition of the interdependence and continuous interaction between the internal and external environments is important. This interdependence and subsequent interaction can lead to either health promotion or illness. People's choices impact them and their environment. These choices are reflected internally (e.g., poor eating habits) or externally (e.g., overexposure to the environment or our relationships with our family, peers, friends, and society). Figure 2-3 demonstrates how our external environment can affect our well-being.

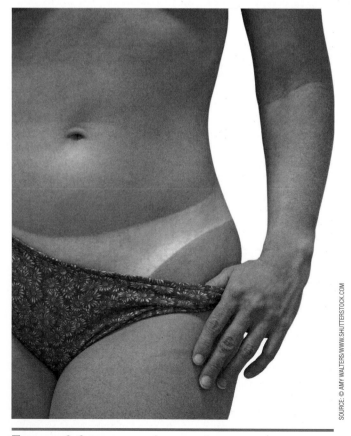

SOURCE: © AMY WALTERS/WWW.SHUTTERSTOCK.COM

FIGURE 2-3 **Excessive exposure to the sun can be harmful to our health.**

HEALTH

Although the concept of health is essential to defining nursing's metaparadigm, there is no current consensus on what actually constitutes good health. In fact, there is probably more agreement on what constitutes poor health. Within the last three decades, the view of health has changed dramatically. In the late 1950s and the 1960s, for example, the health care field was influenced by Dunn's (1959) definition of health. This definition indicated that the concepts of health and illness were two diametrically opposed views; that is, a person who had experienced any symptoms of disease, whether in an acute or a remission state, could not be considered healthy. Since that time, the definition of health has evolved to include the view that health and illness exist on a continuum ranging from health and wellness on one end to illness and death on the other. Accordingly, then, health and illness exist in degrees. Most contemporary nursing leaders agree with this view.

The concept of health is central to nursing because all the actions and responsibilities integral to nursing involve aspects of health. Health is a central concept because nurses and patients interact when there is a health need. Today's nurse is taught to view health as an always changing, never static state that is determined by internal or external influences. These influences can be self-directed, as in the case of a young woman who decides to smoke although she is aware of the risks. Other influences are external, such as in the case of the youth who decides to drink or do drugs because of peer pressure. In any case, these internal and external influences can result in health or illness depending on the value the individual places on health.

DEFINITIONS OF HEALTH

There are several approaches to describing the health status of an individual. One approach is to describe health in terms of the role of the person in society. This approach views persons as being healthy if they are able to meet their role obligations; that is, a person who can still work or assume the role of a parent is considered healthy. Other approaches to defining health include determining health status by finding out whether a person is free from disease or can adapt to changes in the internal or external environment. In a positive view of health, the focus of health is on whether an individual has strengths, resiliencies, resources, and potential. This view of health emphasizes human capabilities, not pathology (Pender, Murdaugh, & Parsons, 2011). Nursing, too, usually describes health in relation to a person's functioning in society. A person who is functioning at the best level possible is considered healthy.

Family functioning is also an important consideration when defining health. Family health is seen as the abilities and resources available to a family to accomplish its developmental tasks. If the family is able to perform effectively as a unit, then the family is healthy. Other definitions of health focus on the community. Community health is dependent on individual health as well as on the social, physical, and political arenas that are present to support a healthy life (Pender, Murdaugh, & Parsons, 2011).

Health is not only a state of physical functioning but also a concept that encompasses the total functioning of a person; that is, health refers to the ability of persons to function effectively physically, socially, psychologically, and spiritually. In this context, effective physical functioning refers to the ability of the body structures to change and adapt, resulting in a positive health status. Effective social functioning relates to the ability of a person to interact in a meaningful fashion and to form relationships with others, recognizing that people are all different and come from diverse backgrounds.

Likewise, an individual who is in a positive state of psychological health has the ability to problem-solve, manage stress and crisis, and respond in an appropriate emotional manner to situations. A positive health status also includes the spiritual domain of a person. The belief in a higher power, whether it is God or some other power source, is essential to maintaining overall health. Spirituality also includes other aspects of a person's total health, such as ethical standards, moral character, and values. This total positive functioning of a person within these domains constitutes a healthy state, leads to a fulfilling life, and results in **homeostasis,** or a state of equilibrium within the body.

NURSING

The last concept found in nursing's metaparadigm is probably the most important. Although it is difficult, if not impossible, to use a concept to describe itself, nurse theorists usually describe nursing in terms of what the nurse does for the patient (Fawcett, 2005). Nursing is the reason nurses come together with patients and interact with them. Although it is important to consider the concepts of person, environment, and health, the interaction among these three concepts becomes the focus of nursing care.

Nurses work with culturally diverse people in a variety of settings and assist in meeting the health care needs of individual patients, groups, society, and the world community. As such, nursing practice extends into all areas of the health care delivery system. Nursing provides a service that assists people in increasing their knowledge, preventing illness, maintaining or regaining an optimum state of health, or coping with death and the dying process. Obviously, nurses have multiple responsibilities and assume the roles of care provider, teacher, counselor, helper, and health-promotion resource in addition to the roles commonly associated with the profession. See Chapter 4 for the roles that nurses commonly assume when engaged in health promotion.

NURSING AS A PROFESSION

The characteristics of the discipline of nursing fit well with criteria commonly found in a profession. Nursing is considered to be a profession in that it is based on a body of knowledge, abides by its own ethical code, has established professional standards, and requires that nurses assume accountability for their actions. In addition, professional nursing is taught in institutions of higher learning, usually a university or college, whose curriculum includes education in the research process and the science of inquiry. Nursing is a profession that is considered to be scientifically based and self-governed; that is, nursing requires a theoretical knowledge base in addition to the nursing practice skills (Wilkinson & Treas, 2011). Nursing also has its own professional associations, which espouse the principles of the profession and safeguard nursing's interest. The most recognized of these associations is the American Nurses Association. Other broad nursing associations include the National League for Nursing and the American Association of Colleges of Nursing, the primary voice for baccalaureate and graduate education.

NURSING EDUCATIONAL LEVELS AND HEALTH PROMOTION

The knowledge and competencies of registered nurses directly relate to educational preparation. Nurses function to meet the demands placed on them by society and the nursing profession according to their educational background. Education has a significant impact on the competencies and knowledge base of nurse clinicians (American Association of Colleges of Nursing, 2010a). Employers are urged to take note of and capitalize on the education and experiences provided by the various educational programs that lead to the registered nurse designation. Nurses should be employed according to their educational capacities.

There are several routes to becoming a registered nurse. These educational pathways are diploma, associate degree in nursing, and baccalaureate degree programs. Graduates of all RN programs sit for the same National Council Licensure Exam-RN (NCLEX-RN). Baccalaureate nursing programs, however, encompass all of the materials covered in both associate and diploma programs and provide more in-depth information about the sciences, nursing research, community health nursing, and nursing management (American Association of Colleges of Nursing, 2010a). Education for these RN pathways can take place in a variety of settings.

The registered nurse with a diploma or associate degree can be further educated through a **career ladder,** or a degree completion program. A career ladder approach focuses on transitioning from one educational level to the next. Registered nurses choosing a career ladder approach can expect to improve their nursing care and general nursing practice. A career ladder approach leads to a better educated nursing workforce. Clinical competencies and improved patient outcomes can be expected with additional nursing preparation.

All registered nurse preparation programs include a foundation of basic sciences and focus on critical thinking, problem-solving skills, leadership skills, and health promotion. The amount of preparation on each concept depends on the type of program undertaken. The acquisition of knowledge on health-promotion concepts, skills, and behaviors can be differentiated according to the competencies of the program graduates.

Graduate nursing education programs also differ in terms of the expected competencies related to health promotion. Graduate nursing education programs include master of science in nursing (MSN) and doctoral nursing preparation programs with a specific focus area. MSN programs may be clinical practice oriented or may be more theoretical or research directed. Nursing doctoral programs may be practice based or research based. The doctor of philosophy (PhD) in nursing programs are more research oriented and prepare students to pursue intellectual inquiry (American Association of Colleges of Nursing, 2011). Nursing doctoral programs that are practice based, called the doctorate in nursing practice (DNP), emphasize the impact of nursing practice and interventions that influence health care outcomes. The DNP is equipped to implement the science developed by research-focused doctorates in nursing (American Association of Colleges of Nursing, 2010b).

As noted, nurses can choose from several pathways to receiving a doctorate. Doctoral programs are varied and may include a PhD in nursing (PhD), a doctor of nursing science degree (DNS, DSN, or DNSc), a nursing doctorate degree (ND), and the doctorate in nursing practice (DNP) degree. In 2004, AACN members endorsed a position statement that is expected to move the current levels for master's prepared advanced practice nurses to the DNP by 2015. Table 2-2 demonstrates how health-promotion competencies differ according to educational preparation.

INTEGRATING HEALTH-PROMOTION CONCEPTS INTO NURSING PRACTICE

Any definition of nursing includes activities that are specific to nursing. These definitions focus on what nurses do for patients, their families, and significant others, and they usually include such activities as caring for patients, assisting those that cannot do so for themselves, and teaching patients how to care for themselves. All these activities involve the concept of health promotion and lead to the formulation of several assumptions essential to integrating health promotion into nursing practice. These assumptions help blend health promotion with the concepts found in the metaparadigm on nursing and are an eclectic view of some of the assumptions described by several nursing theorists, including Imogene King, Dorothea Orem, Martha Rogers, and Sister Callista Roy (see Box 2-3).

ASSUMPTIONS

The first assumption listed in Box 2-3 is critical to professional nurses engaging in health-promoting activities. Nurses who are effective in implementing health-promotion strategies realize that people are self-directing and make important decisions daily that have long-lasting consequences. These decisions can make the difference in terms of achieving optimum health. The fact that people can direct their own life means that, for the most part, they can promote or destroy their health. The ability to think abstractly and critically is found only in humans and is essential to making appropriate decisions. Choices affecting health can range from simple to very complex.

For example, a patient's health-promotion decision can be as simple as deciding to exercise for 30 minutes a day. On the other hand, a patient's decision to undergo coronary bypass surgery instead of conservative treatment with cardiotonic

---

BOX 2-3

ASSUMPTIONS ESSENTIAL TO INTEGRATING HEALTH PROMOTION INTO NURSING PRACTICE

1. People have the capacity for self-direction, abstraction, and critical thinking.
2. The environment can affect a person's ability to live a long and prosperous life.
3. People are capable of learning and adapting and can be made aware of the things that promote well-being.
4. As open systems, people are capable of change.
5. People are biological, psychological, social, and cultural beings who form families and/or networks.
6. Communication, both verbal and nonverbal, is essential to the achievement of health throughout the life span.

---

drugs is infinitely more complex. The nurse's knowledge of the consequences associated with any of the patient's choices is essential. A nurse who recognizes professional responsibilities in promoting health must provide patients with accurate information that may influence their decisions and ultimately their lives.

Professional nurses engaged in health-promotion activities should also recognize the influences of the environment on patient outcomes. As stated in the second assumption in Box 2-3, the effects of the environment can have longstanding consequences on a person's health; that is, if the environment is not a healthy one that is conducive to promoting quality of life, health promotion may no longer be possible unless certain changes occur in the environment. A positive environment increases quality of life and adds to inner and outer stability and wellness. A household environment, for example, where there is constant bickering or strife or one that has mentally ill members can be very stressful. Long-term stress can have deleterious effects on the body and mind (Selye, 1974; Townsend, 2006). The nurse who recognizes the impact of environmental factors on patients understands the importance of treating people in a **holistic** manner, that is, in their unique totality.

The assumption that everyone is capable of learning and adapting (assumption 3) is critical to promoting health in our society. However, although human beings are quite capable of learning, several factors can limit learning. For example, if people are not motivated to learn the things that will lead to healthy and productive lives, their capacity to learn is irrelevant. People decide what they need to know and are willing to do or not do regardless of any disabilities (Craven & Hirnle, 2009). Additionally, the ability to adapt internally or externally can be either effective or ineffective. A reason for stressing people's capacity to learn and adapt in this assumption is that a major nursing focus is to improve the health behaviors of patients and to assist them in adjusting to changes in their lives. Nurses impact health behaviors of patients through their roles as caregivers and patient educators.

Everyone is capable of changing his or her behavior (assumption 4), whether in a positive or negative direction.

TABLE 2-2 Nursing Educational Preparation and Health-Promotion Competencies

PROGRAM PREPARATION	TYPICAL YEARS OF STUDY	EDUCATIONAL SETTING	SELECT HEALTH PROMOTION COMPETENCIES
Associate Degree	2	Community college	Provide safe, compassionate, comprehensive nursing care to patients and families through an array of health care services.
			Implement a plan of care for patients and/or families, taking into consideration disease prevention, wellness, and promotion of healthy lifestyles.
			Develop, implement, and evaluate teaching plans for individuals, families, or both concerning health promotion and maintenance and the restoration of health.
			Refer patients/families to resources that facilitate the continuity of care: health promotion, maintenance, and restoration.
Diploma	3	Hospital (Diploma programs are hospital-based and single-purpose schools of nursing.)	In addition to the preceding health-promotion competencies.
			Diploma nursing schools' missions and philosophies vary from those of an associate degree program, but both are expected to achieve same competencies.
Baccalaureate degree	4	Senior college or university	In addition to the preceding health-promotion competencies.
			Provide safe, compassionate, comprehensive nursing care to individuals, families, populations, and communities.
			In-depth knowledge of health-promotion concepts.
			Implement comprehensive teaching plans to meet the health-promotion learning needs of patients, families, populations, and communities.
			Perform comprehensive assessments relative to factors impacting health status and needs.
			Possess a holistic understanding of health care and approaches to health care, including health promotion.
Master of science in nursing	2–3 years following BSN	Senior college or university	In addition to the preceding health-promotion competencies.
			Use epidemiological, social, and environmental data in assessing the health status of populations (individuals, families, groups, and communities).
			Develop and monitor holistic plans of care addressing the health-promotion and disease-prevention needs of populations (individuals, families, groups, communities). Incorporate theories and research in developing strategies to promote and preserve health.
			Empower populations (individuals, families, groups, communities) in attaining and maintaining functional wellness.
Nursing doctorate	3–6 years following MSN	University	In addition to the preceding health-promotion competencies.
			Influence regulatory, legislative, and public policy to promote health and preserve healthy communities.
			Incorporate theories and research in developing strategies to promote and preserve health.
			Empower populations (individuals, families, groups, communities) in attaining and maintaining functional wellness.

Sources: American Association of Colleges of Nursing. (2010a). *The impact of education on nursing practice*; American Association of Colleges of Nursing. (1995). *A model for differentiated nursing practice*; The Texas Board of Nursing. (2010). *Differentiated essential competencies (DECs) of graduates of Texas nursing programs evidenced by knowledge, clinical judgments, and behaviors.*

SPOTLIGHT **ON**

Holistic Health Care

People are complex beings made up of physical, social, cultural, and psychological properties and should be viewed in a holistic manner. This concept of holism provides a view of people in their complex entirety. A holistic approach to health care recognizes the interactions that occur among body, mind, emotions, and spirit. Nurses should always strive to provide holistic nursing care.

? ASK **YOURSELF**

Using Communication Skills in a Global Society

How would you communicate with a patient who was from a different country, whose culture is different from yours, and who spoke a language different from your own? Would you know what your patient needs? Would you be able to interpret the patient's needs if you did not speak the same language or share the same culture? What other forms of communication could you use? What can you do to prepare for taking care of the patient with different cultural and communication needs in an ever more global society?

Belief in this assumption is vital for nurses and their patients to effectively carry out health-promotion activities. People never remain static but are always interacting and communicating with their environment. The ultimate goal is the achievement of homeostasis or stability while continually adjusting and changing. Nurses promote positive changes in patients through patient teaching, patient advocacy, caregiving, and consulting and collaborating with other members of the healthcare team.

Assumption 5 recognizes that people have sociocultural characteristics and cannot be cared for in isolation. The word "patient" does not necessarily refer only to the person receiving the care but may include the person, the family, significant others, a social group, or a community. For instance, dietary teaching for a diabetic patient might be ineffective if the patient is the only one to receive instruction. To increase the effectiveness of instruction and future compliance with the diet, the lesson on diabetic diet planning logically may include the patient, spouse, family, significant other, or anyone else who cares and cooks for the patient.

Communication ability is essential to promoting a healthy lifestyle (assumption 6). One of the unique characteristics of people is their ability to communicate both with words and with actions and expressions. This ability allows them to communicate their needs to others and proves to be useful in satisfying needs. Appropriate communication skills can assist people in achieving optimum well-being. This ability to communicate also provides a means to interact socially, an essential component of a full and productive life.

We rely primarily on our verbal communication skills as well as those of our patients to obtain an adequate interpretation of a situation. For a competent nurse, the ability to determine what a patient has said or not said or to interpret other forms of nonverbal communication enhances caring skills and assists in achieving the desired outcomes for patient care. The astute observation of the patient's verbal and nonverbal behaviors is essential to providing quality nursing care. Likewise, remember that the nurse's own verbal and nonverbal behaviors can communicate many things to the patient as well. The quality of the nurse–patient relationship is related to the quality of communication between the nurse and the patient (Craven & Hirnle, 2009). Chapter 5 further discusses the impact of communication skills on educating others about health promotion.

RESEARCH

NOTE

Study Problem/Purpose: Optimism and Healthy Behaviors in First-Time Mothers

STUDY PROBLEM/PURPOSE

To see whether first-time mothers' optimism helps them participate in health-promoting behaviors. First-time mothers are thought to experience much stress that might impact their previous healthy behaviors. This study examined whether a relationship exists between perceived stress and health-promoting behaviors. The study also included the concept of optimism to see whether optimistic first-time mothers had less stress and better health-promoting behaviors than those that were not optimistic.

METHODS

This study used an ex post facto cross-sectional design. The sample consisted of 174 primiparous mothers who had given birth within the previous 12 months. The sample was given an online questionnaire, the Health Promotion Lifestyle Profile II scale, and the revised Life Orientation Test.

FINDINGS

Stress was found to relate to fewer health-promoting behaviors among the mothers in the sample. Stress and health-promoting behaviors were found to be mediated by the optimism displayed by the moms.

IMPLICATIONS

Decreased stress levels and optimism may be the keys to increasing health-promoting behaviors in first-time mothers. Awareness of new mothers' stress levels by health care professionals may prompt them to find stress-relieving activities and educational strategies helpful to first-time mothers.

Gil, R. M., & Loh, J. (2010). The role of optimism in health-promoting behaviors in new primiparous mothers. *Nursing Research, 59*(5), 348–355.

THEORETICAL FOUNDATIONS

Theoretical or conceptual frameworks that encompass some of the assumptions discussed in the preceding section and that define nursing and its metaparadigm are useful in delineating health-promotion activities. These theoretical/conceptual frameworks not only guide the nursing profession by addressing the four central concepts found in nursing's metaparadigm, but also serve as the bases for hypotheses testing that adds to nursing's body of knowledge. These frameworks, then, can serve as a springboard for nursing research through theory building and their application in problem solving. Several theoretical frameworks and conceptual models are commonly used in defining nursing. Although the following theoretical frameworks are found in most of the literature describing nursing, they are not totally inclusive. Among the most common conceptual models/frameworks is Pender's Model of Health Promotion (Pender, 2011; Pender, Murdaugh, & Parsons, 2011). This model is covered briefly here and will be covered in more detail in Chapter 3. Other theoretical frameworks used and described in this chapter are systems theory, adaptation theory, needs theory, human becoming and human care theory, and transcultural theory.

PENDER'S MODEL OF HEALTH PROMOTION

A text on health promotion in nursing would not be complete without the inclusion of Pender and her Health Promotion Model (HPM). In developing her model, Pender defined health promotion as "behavior motivated by the desire to increase well-being and actualize human health potential" (Pender, Murdaugh, & Parson, 2006, p. 7). Pender's HPM proposes a framework that nursing can use to determine which factors influence health-promoting behaviors.

A key concept in the HPM is that of motivation. Motivation is thought to propel individuals to engage in health-enhancing behaviors. The concepts of self-efficacy and expectancy are also included in the HPM and are borrowed from social-cognitive theory. Self-efficacy refers to the feelings that we get when we believe that we can do something or engage in a certain type of behavior. The expectancy concept involves feelings that what we are doing is of value to us. Obviously feeling that we can do something that is of personal value to us is an important consideration when developing a health-promotion plan. Social-cognitive theory also emphasizes self-direction, self-regulation, and perceived self-efficacy—all concepts related to engaging in health-promoting behaviors and that are essential to the HPM (Pender, 2011). The HPM is helpful to nurses who are developing strategies that will enhance health-promotion behaviors among their patients. Chapter 3 will offer a more detailed explanation of Pender's Health Promotion Model.

SYSTEMS THEORY

General systems theory was described by Von Bertalanffy in 1968 and has been helpful to nursing theorists in describing the relationship among people, health, and their environment. This theory focuses on the exchange of energy between the individual and the environment and has as its central concept that a person is whole and greater than a sum of the parts. The person interacts with the environment continuously in a reciprocal and open manner; that is, people influence and change their environment, and the environment influences and changes people. Health-promotion activities thus result from patient self-direction. The environment has an impact on the health-promotion activities and direction that an individual chooses to take. An overweight person, for example, can choose to diet and stock only healthy foods in the refrigerator and pantry or choose to ignore obesity and keep fattening foods available for snacking. Regardless of the choice, the person's environment includes choices of healthy or unhealthy foods that influence the individual's health. Systems theory proposes that change is self-directed, that the environment influences the course of this direction, and that change occurs continuously. Change creates energy fields, and these energy fields include the patient and his or her internal and external environments. The energy fields created by change are always evolving and never remain static (Fawcett, 2005). A patient's choices of what foods to eat, such as in the obesity example, create these energy fields that eventually result in changes in health status.

Systems theory identifies systems and subsystems, proposing that these can interact and exchange energy with the environment. For example, Dorothy Johnson's Behavioral Systems Model (1980) conceptualizes a nursing patient as a behavioral system. The system is seen as being orderly, repetitive, and organized with interrelated and interdependent biological and behavioral subsystems. The recipient of care (the patient) is seen as a collection of behavioral subsystems that interact with other subsystems to form the behavioral system (Holaday, (2010). In systems theory, the individual, patient, group, society, and community are considered to be systems. Other theorists have also incorporated aspects of this theory in their frameworks describing nursing.

ADAPTATION THEORY

Adaptation theory has also been used by several nurse theorists to describe and define nursing. The major concepts in this theory are change, adaptation, and coping. **Adaptation,** in this context, is the process of changing behavior in response to external or internal stimuli or surroundings. That is, the patient is seen as an adaptive system, capable of controlling individual responses. The environment, whether it is internal or external, stimulates the individual to respond or change accordingly. The environment consists of all of the conditions, influences, and events that affect people (Roy & Zhan, 2010). Everyone has unique and constantly changing adaptation levels. Not all of the adaptive responses, however, are considered appropriate or effective. Health and illness are responses to the adaptation process. Sister Callista Roy's *Adaptation Model* is based on adaptation theory and focuses on how this process affects nursing and health (Gallagher-Galbreath, 2011).

Adaptation theory is useful in describing why people behave in certain ways and in explaining why people choose or do not choose to participate in their own health promotion. The example of the overweight person is useful in demonstrating how this person might adapt and also illustrates the relationship between adaptation theory and health promotion. If an overweight male cannot climb a flight of stairs without experiencing difficulty catching his breath, he may respond or adapt by taking the elevator instead of the stairs next time. In much the same way, this person's internal environment makes several attempts to adapt. The increased effort required to climb stairs forces the lungs to increase their respiratory efforts and thus provide needed oxygenation for the entire body. This obvious adaptive response results in the overweight person's huffing and puffing and experiencing facial flushing while climbing the stairs.

NEEDS THEORY

Needs theory may be used interchangeably with goals theory or self-deficit theory. This theory describes all people as having common needs that must be met and that are essential for maintaining optimum health. People's needs may sometimes be confused with what they want, but needs and wants are two separate concepts. A need is usually defined as a requirement that has not been met. A want is something desirable but not essential. **Needs theory** describes people as whole, with many complex needs that motivate behavior. Everyone meets his or her needs in a unique way and may defer satisfying needs if they are not viewed as a priority at that time. Health-promotion activities and needs are person centered unless they cannot or will not be met by the person.

Needs theory may be used to explain health-promotion activities because such behaviors are driven by need. For example, a student may stay up all night to cram for an exam on the following day. This student may respond to the need for sleep by going home to bed after the exam. Or maybe not. Health behaviors are also influenced by individual values. If another important exam is coming up the next day, the student may choose to forego sleep in favor of staying awake and studying. Dorothea Orem's Self-Care Deficit Theory (2001) is based on needs theory.

HUMAN BECOMING THEORY AND HUMAN CARE THEORY

Human becoming and human care theories, developed in the late 1980s, have common philosophical roots. Both theories are useful in describing the nature of nursing and are rooted in humanistic and existential philosophy. These theories may also be useful in describing nursing's metaparadigm.

Rosemarie Parse's theory is based on human becoming and existence. Her book *Illuminations: The Human Becoming Theory in Practice and Research* (1995) was developed from her theory entitled *Man-Living-Health* (1981). This theory, in turn, evolved from some of Martha Rogers's principles and concepts, stated in her *Science of Unitary Human Beings Theory* (Hickman, 2011b). Parse's theory revolves around the concept of person and a person's interactions within the environment. Parse sees people as having choices in providing meaning to situations and as bearing responsibility for decisions. Parse maintains that people choose values, have their own way of living, and grow more diverse and complex in time (Fawcett, 2005).

Many caring conceptual frameworks are based on Jean Watson's original work. Watson is best known for her theory on caring, in which she sees the nursing role as a collective caring-healing role (1979). She is one of the first theorists to support the concept that people have souls and a spiritual dimension to their being. The essence of her theory of human

> **SPOTLIGHT ON**
>
> **Culture and Society**
>
> In certain cultures, the role of the woman is to be subservient to her spouse. Speaking up to her spouse and expressing a contrary opinion is considered disrespectful, and she might be held in contempt by other members of that culture and society. Consequently, women of that cultural sect are expected to abide by the cultural mores if they want to be accepted by their society.

caring, also referred to as Watson's Theory of Transpersonal Caring (1996), is authentic caring that preserves dignity and the wholeness of humanity. The major conceptual elements of the theory are transpersonal caring, ten carative factors, and caring in general (Kelly & Johnson, 2011).

In some respects, both the human becoming and caring theories are central to the discipline of nursing. Concepts in these theories can be easily incorporated into nursing practice. These theories provide a framework for working with human beings, taking into consideration the each person's uniqueness.

TRANSCULTURAL THEORY

According to George (2011), Madeleine Leininger was the first nurse theorist to use the term *transcultural nursing* (p. 490). Since then, **transcultural nursing theory** has become popular and reflects nursing's and society's beliefs regarding the importance of culture and its effects on the total functioning of an individual. The major concepts in this theory are human care, the influence of culture, the worldview of individuals, cultural congruence, commonality of needs, and diversity.

Transcultural theory focuses on the individual and describes how culture influences and provides meaning to everything that a person does, thinks, feels, or hears. A person is perceived to be a complex biological, psychological, social, spiritual, and caring being with meaningful patterns that vary among cultures. A person's culture provides meaning to health and illness, and the nurse must appreciate it when assisting patients with their health-promotion activities and behaviors. If the person's culture is not considered in planning care, noncompliance with treatment occur and results in a further delay in recovery.

According to this theory, health and illness cannot be defined because these concepts have no universally accepted definitions. Transcultural theory, however, proposes that health and illness are determined by the views of individual cultures. Human behavior is influenced by the cultural context within which it occurs. The nurse's responsibility is to bring cultural congruence and **cultural congruent care** to patients by utilizing the patient's cultural lifeways and norms. Cultural congruent care is care that is provided to fit with an individual's, group's, or institution's values, beliefs, and lifeways. Cultural congruent care is necessary to provide meaningful and satisfying health care services to those in need of them (Leininger, 2001). Transcultural theory maintains that nurses are responsible for linking the patient's culture with the health care delivery system. The nursing arena is so complex that the role of the nurse in providing holistic, culturally competent care is difficult at times. Many health care needs are culturally based and not adequately addressed in health care. Patients from diverse cultures seek nursing care, and nurses must adjust their delivery of care to include culturally congruent nursing care (Huerta & Sánchez, 2009). Transcultural nursing theory can be used in planning this patient care and in promoting, restoring, and maintaining health. Competent nurses use a transcultural theory framework in all aspects of their professional role.

ORGANIZING NURSING THEORY

One of the goals of nursing theory is to describe nursing's metaparadigm in terms of the concepts essential to professional nursing practice. These same concepts are useful in organizing the theoretical frameworks previously described and may be useful in the development of a personal definition or philosophy of nursing.

NURSING'S METAPARADIGM AND NURSING THEORY

The various nursing theorists have used the concepts of person, environment, health, and nursing in their development of nursing theory. Virginia Henderson (1966), for example, in her development of a definition for nursing, viewed the human being as a biological, psychological, spiritual, and social being. She refers to people as having basic needs that can be categorized into 14 components of nursing functions. In much the same way, King (1971), in her Theory of Goal Attainment, describes the person as a social, sentient, rational, reacting, perceiving, time-oriented, cognitive human being. Pender (1996), the leading nurse proponent of a health-promotion model, states that people are capable of determining their own health status and that they create conditions to express their uniqueness. Other theorists view the concept of person as just described but include cultural characteristics as well as transcultural variances of human beings (Leininger, 1978). All of the major nursing theorists organize their theories by addressing nursing's metaparadigm concept of person.

Likewise, nursing theory addresses the concept of environment. King (1971), for example, sees people and their environment as being in continuous interaction. She identifies the environment as consisting of both a person's internal and external environments. Likewise, Sister Callista Roy (1974a, 1974b), in her adaptation model, describes the interactions between people and their environment. She, too, sees the environment as consisting of all that surrounds or influences a person. According to Callista Roy, the environment can be described as including both the internal and external environments. Martha Rogers, too, focused on the role of the environment and included this concept in her Science of Unitary Human Beings Theory (Rogers, 1970). Rogers identified people and their environment as energy fields interacting as whole entities and having their own identities. People and their environmental fields are integral to one another.

The concept of health is also described by nursing theorists. King (1971) describes health as a dynamic state occurring in all life cycles. Roy (1974a, 1974b, 1999) also describes health and illness as part of life's processes. She believes that if people adapt to their surroundings, then health is achieved.

SPOTLIGHT **ON**

Providing Cultural Congruent Care

A Mexican-American mother brings her irritable baby to the clinic. In talking to the nurse, the mother states that her baby has been sick since she took him to a birthday party where he was admired by all of the guests but no one touched him. She fears that he has been given *mal de ojo*, or evil eye. The mother has attempted to cure him through prayer and rubbing his body with an egg. The nurse assesses the child and takes into consideration what the mother has told her and the mother's cultural beliefs. A nurse who accepts the patient's own approach to health care is accepting of the patient and family's cultural worldview and is providing cultural congruent care.

Only when adaptation does not occur does a person become ill. Nursing theorists have also described health as being defined according to society's perception. For instance, in some societies, obesity is an acceptable norm. Leininger (1978, 2001) recognizes society's influence on health and notes that health is primarily culturally defined. She describes health as being influenced by the value that the culture places on a person's abilities to perform certain tasks. Pender, Murdaugh, and Parsons (2011), on the other hand, focus on the concept of health in relation to health promotion. They state that being free of symptoms of disease does not necessarily mean that a person is healthy. Pender (2011) states that a definition of health must be a holistic one. This definition necessitates that social aspects be considered to gain a real understanding of health. The definition also acknowledges that a healthy status provides a sense of empowerment. She believes that a person engaging in health-promoting behavior can achieve health and ultimately can be quite powerful in achieving life's goals. Chapter 3 will discuss Pender's and other nurse theorists' models of health and health promotion in more detail.

The concept of nursing, of course, is of major importance in developing and organizing nursing theory. A generally held belief is that nursing is an art and a science. The art of nursing requires the skills that are used in administering care to patients. The science of nursing relates to the ability of the discipline to apply knowledge of scientific principles when caring for patients and to generate new knowledge through research. Orem's (2001) description of nursing seems to capture the essence of this concept. She defines nursing as a service that helps human beings who are unable to help themselves. Nursing is based on actions deliberately selected and performed by nurses to help individuals or groups to maintain or change their conditions (Renpenning & Taylor, 2003). King (1971), on the other hand, sees nursing as a process of action, reaction, interaction, and transaction used to meet basic needs of individuals. The major nursing theorists describe nursing concerns, goals, and functions. Table 2-3 describes selected nurse theorist's views of nursing's metaparadigm and the relationship of health promotion to each.

TABLE 2-3 Nursing's Metaparadigm and Health Promotion: Selected Nurse Theorists' Views

NURSE THEORIST	CONCEPT OF PERSON	CONCEPT OF ENVIRONMENT	CONCEPT OF HEALTH	DEFINITIONS OF NURSING	RELATIONSHIP TO HEALTH PROMOTION
Florence Nightingale's (1860) environmental theory of nursing	Consists of physical, intellectual, spiritual, and social attributes. Concept of person defined only in terms of the individual's relationship with her or his environment.	Environment is major cause of disease.	Emphasizes impact of environmental factors on health. Symptoms of disease are due to the lack of fresh air, light, cleanliness, pure water, and efficient drainage.	The goal of nursing is to "put the patient in the best condition for nature to act upon him" (p. 75). "Nursing ought to assist the reparative process" (p. 6).	Health promotion is primarily environment and nurse centered. Disease occurs because of nature. "Real knowledge of the laws of health alone can check this" (p. 73). Health promotion focuses on eliminating environmental factors that cause disease.
Virginia Henderson's (1966, 1991) Needs Theory	Biological, psychological, spiritual, social being. The individual is a whole person with various fundamental needs. The person has 14 basic needs.	No major emphasis placed on the environment; however, she states that friends and family impact health status.	Health is present if a person is not deprived of what he values or needs and is then able to maintain independence.	"The unique function of the nurse is to assist the individual sick or well, in the performance of those activities contributing to health or its recovery (or to peaceful death) that he would perform unaided if he had the necessary strength, will, or knowledge. And to do this in such as way as to help him gain independence as rapidly as possible" (1991, p. 21).	Health promotion is person centered. Individuals are responsible for own health promotion. If individual is unable to perform the duties that promote health, a nurse assists the patient by providing what is lacking, carrying out the prescribed treatment, and reducing discomfort if death is imminent.
Martha Roger's, (1970, 1990) Science of Unitary Human Beings Theory	Open systems, composed of more than the sum of their parts and characterized by their energy systems, and capacity for abstraction, imagery, language, and thought.	People and their environment are central to one another and are defined as energy fields. Environmental fields are whole, irreducible, indivisible, and characterized by wave patterns that change continuously.	Health is a value term and consists of those behaviors valued by individuals or cultures. Health and sickness are part of life processes.	Nursing science is the study of unitary, irreducible, indivisible human and environmental fields (1990).	In order to promote health, people must be considered in their totality, which must include the environment. Health promotion focuses on people and their environment. Health-promotion activities are patient-centered.

NURSE THEORIST	CONCEPT OF PERSON	CONCEPT OF ENVIRONMENT	CONCEPT OF HEALTH	DEFINITIONS OF NURSING	RELATIONSHIP TO HEALTH PROMOTION
Imogene King's (1971) Theory of Goal Attainment	Responsive, perceptive, goal-directed, time-oriented, cognitive, social being. Utilizes mind, body, and energy in reacting to past and present experiences and events. A person functions in social systems through interpersonal relationships in terms of individual perceptions that influence his or her life and health.	Continual exchange between people and their environment. Environment consists of both internal and external environments. All of society must be involved in achieving health.	Health is a dynamic state that occurs as a result of continuous adaptation to stress. Health is an ever-changing state of being; it cannot be completely achieved because it is not a static state.	"Nursing is a process of action, reaction, interaction, and transaction whereby nurses assist individuals of any age and socio-economic group to meet their basic needs in performing the activities of daily living and to cope with health and illness at some particular point in the life cycle" (p. 25).	The importance of health promotion to a person is dependent on his or her perceptions of its value. Health promotion consists of the utilization of resources to achieve maximum potential.
Dorothea Orem's (2001) Self-Care Theory	Persons who provide their own self-care or care for others have specialized capabilities for action. All human beings have requisites for self-care, some of which are common to all human beings.	The total environment consists of psychosocial and physical environments.	Self-care requirements that are not met constitute a health deviation. Health describes the state of wholeness or integrity of human beings. Temporary indispositions do not mean a person is not healthy.	"Nursing has as its special concern the individual's need for self-care action and the provision and management of it on a continuous basis in order to sustain life and health, and recover from disease or injury, and cope with their effects."	Person-centered health promotion consists of self-care activities that sustain life and regulate disease. Health-promotion activities consist of knowledge-seeking actions, assistance if necessary, control of external factors, resource-using actions, and self-control.
Rosemarie Parse's (1995) Theory of Human Becoming	Humans are open, unitary; they freely choose meaning in situations and bear responsibility. Humans are central to human becoming theory. They coexist while forming rhythmical patterns with the universe.	People and the universe are continuously interacting, constituting patterns of relating. Human beings and the universe are inseparable, complementary, and evolving together. The universe is made up of everything in a person's lived experience.	Health is people's lived experience. It can be defined as a way of living, a personal commitment. It is a continuously changing process mutually cocreated through the human-universe experience.	Nursing is a basic science whose practice is a performing of art. Nursing involves innovation and creativity. Nursing's responsibility to society is to guide individuals in choosing possibilities in changing the health process.	Health promotion must consider the total lived experiences of an individual. Health promotion does not involve prescriptive approaches; rather, the patient is the authority figure in the relationship and the prime decision maker in areas involving personal health.

(continued)

TABLE 2-3 Nursing's Metaparadigm and Health Promotion: Selected Nurse Theorists' Views (*continued*)

NURSE THEORIST	CONCEPT OF PERSON	CONCEPT OF ENVIRONMENT	CONCEPT OF HEALTH	DEFINITIONS OF NURSING	RELATIONSHIP TO HEALTH PROMOTION
Jean Watson's (1979, 1996) Theory of Transpersonal Caring	A human is a valued person greater than and different from the sum of his or her parts. A person can use the mind to attain higher levels of consciousness. People need each other in a caring way.	The environment is considered in the context of the human-environment field, perceived within a specific context, such as social or physical, or within the greater context of interacting within a phenomenological field.	Health refers to unity and harmony within the mind, body, and soul; health is the degree of congruence between the perceived self and the self as experienced. Disease results from incongruences.	Nursing is carried out through human care and caring. Caring is the moral ideal of nursing, with the goal of helping another to gain self-knowledge, control, and healing.	The goal of health promotion is human care. Health promotion is directed toward care of the physical body within the context of the unity of mind, body, spirit, and nature.
Pender's (1996, 2011) Health Promotion Model	Person is a complex biopsychosocial being. A person seeks to actively regulate behavior thus delivering personal benefit; takes active role in choosing lifestyle changes to promote health.	A person interacts with the environment, progressively transforming the environment and being transformed over time.	Health empowers: Includes biopsychosocial spiritual, environmental, cultural dimensions.	The goal of nursing is to assist the recipient of care in choosing behaviors that improve well-being.	Health promotion is not illness or disease specific. It seeks to expand positive potential for health.

SUMMARY

Health promotion is an essential concept within contemporary society not only in the United States but worldwide. This concept is continuously highlighted by the various health professions and is a driving force in the establishment of initiatives useful to the achievement of optimum health. The importance of this concept to nursing is evident by the number of documents that cite the promotion of health as a nursing goal. These documents clearly identify nursing's responsibility in promoting efforts to meet the community's health needs.

Health promotion as a conceptual framework is useful in defining nursing practice and is reflected in nursing's metaparadigm. This metaparadigm uses concepts and theories that collectively or individually describe the profession, and it organizes nursing's metaparadigm around four central concepts: person, health, environment, and nursing. A nursing metaparadigm integrating health-promotion concepts describes the profession in relation to activities that assist individuals and families, prevent illness, maintain health, and promote optimum well-being.

Several assumptions are critical to integrating health-promotion concepts into nursing practice. These assumptions are primarily related to characteristics inherent in human beings. To successfully incorporate health promotion into practice, nurses must assume that a person is self-directing, is capable of learning, is capable of change, possesses a complex makeup, and is able to communicate individual needs. Also, the environment can have a dramatic effect on a person's optimum health and life span.

Theoretical frameworks are useful in defining nursing and its metaparadigm and in delineating health-promotion activities. These frameworks form the bases for hypotheses testing and for formal nursing research, and they add to nursing's body of knowledge through research findings. Among the most common frameworks used are systems theory, adaptation theory, needs theory, human becoming and human care theory, and transcultural theory.

The concept of health is central to nursing because all actions integral to nursing involve aspects of health. Nursing is the reason we come together with the patient. The interaction of the concepts of person, environment, and health becomes the focus of our nursing care. Nursing provides a service that assists people in increasing their awareness, preventing illness, maintaining or regaining health, or coping with death and the dying process.

KEY CONCEPTS

1. The concept of health promotion is essential to the prevention of disease, the maintenance of health, and defining optimum health.
2. Health promotion provides an organizing framework useful in defining nursing
3. Health promotion is not a concept exclusive to the United States; other countries consider the importance of health promotion in providing health care to patients.
4. Metaparadigms provide a global perspective of nursing and help to critically evaluate concepts characteristic of the nursing discipline.
5. Nursing theories utilize the four concepts described in nursing's metaparadigm: person, health, environment, and nursing.
6. People are holistic, biological, psychological, social, and spiritual beings with common needs.
7. The environment consists of internal and external influences that can affect personal functioning.

8. There is no consensus on what constitutes health; health may be viewed as a continuum or as the opposite of illness.
9. Knowledge of health-promotion concepts, skills, and behavior can be differentiated according to graduate competencies.
10. Systems theory focuses on exchanges of energy between systems and subsystems and/or between people and their environment. Adaptation theory focuses on change and effective adaptive responses. Needs theory can explain patient and nurse behaviors. Human becoming and human care theories focus on humanistic and existential philosophies. Transcultural theory focuses on the cultural meaning of health and illness.
11. The characteristics of the nursing discipline fit well with criteria commonly describing a profession.
12. Nursing theorists organize nursing theory by addressing nursing's metaparadigm concepts.

CHAPTER REVIEW

Learning Activities

1. Describe your nursing philosophy in writing. List at least 10 statements that reflect this philosophy.
2. Categorize the statements in part 1 in relation to the four concepts found in nursing's metaparadigm. (Some statements may fit more than one category.)

   Person   Health   Environment   Nursing

3. Describe why you selected the preceding categories for your belief statements. Be specific in your rationale by stating why the statement fits.

Multiple Choice

1. ANA's Standards of Nursing Practice:
   a. describe a means of determining the quality of nursing services received.
   b. establish a code of ethics that guides practice.
   c. set competency levels for clinical only.
   d. provide a framework for understanding nursing's relationship to society.
2. Of the following, which nurse is the most likely to incorporate theories and research in developing strategies to promote and preserve health?
   a. A nurse with an associate degree in nursing
   b. A nurse with a bachelor of science in nursing degree
   c. A nurse with a doctorate in nursing
   d. A nurse with a master of science in nursing degree

3. General systems theory focuses on:
   a. goals and self-deficits identified by patient.
   b. changing behaviors through an adaptation process.
   c. complex needs that motivate behavior.
   d. the exchange of energy between an individual and the environment.

4. Transcultural nursing theory was originally described by which of the following nursing theorists?
   a. Sister Callista Roy
   b. Dorothea Orem
   c. Madeleine Leininger
   d. Martha Rogers

5. The concept of health promotion is:
   a. a relatively new concept dating to the 1990s.
   b. rarely found in the nursing literature.
   c. specific to the medical profession.
   d. used internationally by health care professionals.

6. ANA's Scope and Standards of Practice are:
   a. expectations outlined for the professional nursing role.
   b. used by all health care professionals.
   c. focused primarily on patient illness rather than on patient wellness.
   d. summary statements describing nursing's ethics code.

7. The nursing's metaparadigm:
   a. describes the standards for clinical nursing practice.
   b. demonstrates how nursing theories and concepts are interrelated.
   c. is less well organized than a nursing paradigm.
   d. provides a global perspective of nursing as a discipline.

8. The concept of health is:
   a. essential in defining nursing's metaparadigm.
   b. easily defined as to what health is.
   c. not as important as the concept of nursing.
   d. totally separate from the concept of illness.

ORGANIZATIONS AND WEBSITES

American Association of Colleges of Nursing (AACN): The national voice for America's baccalaureate and higher-degree nursing education programs; addresses education, research, advocacy, and data collection and provides a search site map for publications relevant to professional nursing: **http://www.aacn.nche.edu**

American Nurses Association (ANA): The only full-service professional organization representing the nation's 3.1 million registered nurses through its constituent member nurses association and its organizational affiliates, the ANA provides information on ANA services, programs, and publications, and includes a search site map for items, articles, and issues of interest to professional nursing: **http://www.nursingworld.org**

Canadian Nurses Association (CNA): The national professional voice of registered nurses in Canada. A federation of 11 provincial and territorial nursing associations and colleges representing 139,893 registered nurses, CNA advances the practice and profession of nursing to improve health outcomes and to strengthen Canada's publicly funded, not-for-profit health system: **http://www.cna-nurses.ca**

International Union for Health Promotion and Education (IUHPE): A world-wide independent and professional association of individuals and organizations committed to improving the health and well-being of people through education, community action, and development of healthy public policy: **http://www.IUHPE.org**

National Council of State Boards of Nursing: For not-for-profit organizations whose members include the boards of nurse examiners for 50 states, the District of Columbia, and the five U.S. territories: **http://www.ncsbn.org**

REFERENCES

American Association of Colleges of Nursing. (1995). *A model for differentiated nursing practice.* Retrieved from http://www.aacn.nche.edu/Publications/DIFFMOD.PDF

American Association of Colleges of Nursing. (2010a). The impact of education on nursing practice. *AACN Media Fact Sheets.* Retrieved from http://www.aacn.nche.edu

American Association of Colleges of Nursing. (2010b). The Doctor of Nursing Practice. *AACN Media Fact Sheets.*

American Association of Colleges of Nursing. (2011). The research-focused doctoral program in nursing: Pathways to excellence. *Report from the AACN Task Force on the Research-Focused Doctorate in Nursing.*

American Nurses Association (ANA). (2010a). *Guide to the code of ethics for nurses.: Interpretation and application.* Silver Spring, MD: Nursesbooks.org. Publisher.

American Nurses Association. (2010b). *Nursing's social policy statement: The essence of the profession.* Silver Spring, MD: Nursesbooks.org.

American Nurses Association. (2010c). *Scope & standards of practice: Nursing* (2nd ed.). Silver Spring, MD: Nursesbooks.org.

Canadian Nurses Association (2011). Perspectives: Making mental health a priority. *Canadian Nurse, 107*(1), 9.

Craven, R. F., & Hirnle, C. J. (2009). *Fundamentals of nursing: Human health and function* (6th ed.). Philadelphia, PA: Walters Kluwer Health//Lippincott Williams & Wilkins.

Dunn, H. (1959). High level wellness for man and society. *American Journal of Public Health, 49,* 786–792.

Fawcett, J. (2005). *Contemporary nursing knowledge: Analysis and evaluation of nursing models and theories.* Philadelphia, PA: F. A. Davis.

Fawcett, J., & Garity, I. (2009). *Evaluating research for evidence-based nursing practice.* Philadelphia, PA: F. A. Davis.

Gallagher-Galbreath, J. (2011) Roy adaptation model: Sister Callista Roy. In J. B George (ed.), *Nursing theories: The base for professional nursing practice,* 6th ed. Upper Saddle River, NJ: Pearson Education, pp. 291–337.

George, J. B. (2011). Theory of culture care diversity and universality: Madeleine M. Leininger. In J. B George (ed.), *Nursing theories: The base for professional nursing practice.* Upper Saddle River, NJ: Pearson Education, pp. 404–434.

Gil, R. M., & Loh, J. (2010). The role of optimism in health-promoting behaviors in new primiparous mothers. *Nursing Research, 59*(5), 348–355.

Henderson, V. (1966). *The nature of nursing: A definition and its implications for practice, research, and education.* New York, NY: Macmillan.

Henderson, V. (1991). *The nature of nursing: Reflections after 25 years.* (Publ. No. 15-2346). New York, NY: National League for Nursing.

Hickman, J. S. (2011a). An introduction to nursing theory. In J. B. George (ed.), *Nursing theories: The base for nursing practice* (6th ed.). Upper Saddle River, NJ: Pearson Education, pp. 1–22.

Hickman, J. S. (2011b). Human becoming school of thought: Rosemarie Rizzo Parse. In J. B. George (ed.), *Nursing theories: The base for nursing practice*, 6th ed. Upper Saddle River, NJ: Pearson Education, pp. 479–509.

Holaday, B. (2010). Dorothy Johnson's behavioral system model and its applications. In M. E. Parker & M. C. Smith (eds.), *Nursing theories & nursing practice* (3rd ed.). Philadelphia, PA: F. A. Davis Company, pp. 104–112.

Huerta, C., & Sánchez, S. (2009). Influence of culture on knowing persons. In R. C. Locsin & M. J. Purnell (eds.), *A contemporary nursing process: The (un)bearable weight of knowing nursing.* New York, NY: Springer, pp. 481–503.

Johnson, D. (1980). The behavioral system model for nursing. In J. P. Riehl & C. Roy (eds.). *Conceptual models for nursing practice* (2nd ed.). New York, NY: Appleton Century Crofts), pp. 207–216.

Kelly, J. H., & Johnson, B. (2011). Theory of transpersonal caring: Jean Watson. In J. B. George (ed.). *Nursing theories: The base for nursing practice*, 6th ed. Upper Saddle River, NJ: Pearson Education, pp. 454–478.

King, I. (1971). *Toward a theory of nursing: General concepts of human behavior.* New York, NY: Wiley.

Leininger, M. M. (1978). *Transcultural nursing: Concepts, theories, and practice.* New York, NY: Wiley.

Leininger, M. (2001). *Culture care diversity and universality: A theory of nursing.* Boston, MA: Jones & Bartlett.

Maslow, A. (1970). *Motivation and personality.* New York, NY: Harper & Row.

Maslow, A. (1999). *Toward a psychology of being.* New York, NY: Wiley.

Nightingale, F. (1860/1969). *Notes on nursing: What it is and what it is not.* London: Gerald Duckworth.

Orem, D. E. (1980). *Nursing: Concepts of practice* (2nd ed.). New York, NY: McGraw-Hill.

Orem, D. (2001). *Nursing: Concepts of practice.* St. Louis, MO: Mosby.

Parker, M., & Smith, M. C. (2010). Nursing theory and the discipline of nursing. In M. E. Parker & M. C. Smith (eds.), *Nursing theories & nursing practice* (3rd ed.). Philadelphia, PA: F. A. Davis Company, pp. 3–19.

Parse, R. (1981). *Man-living-health: A theory of nursing.* New York, NY: Wiley.

Parse, R. (1995). *Illuminations: The human becoming theory in practice and research.* New York, NY: National League for Nursing Press.

Pender, N. J. (1996). *Health promotion in nursing practice* (3rd ed.). Norwalk, CT: Appleton & Lange.

Pender, N. (2011). Health Promotion Model. In J. B. George (ed.), *Nursing theories: The base for nursing practice*, 6th ed. Upper Saddle River, NJ: Pearson Education, pp. 544–576.

Pender, N., Murdaugh, C. L., & Parsons, M. A. (2011). *Health promotion in nursing practice* (6th ed.). Upper Saddle River, NJ: Pearson Education.

Pender, N., Murdaugh, C.L., & Parsons, M.A. (2006). *Health promotion in nursing practice* (5th ed.). Upper Saddle River, N.J: Prentice-Hall.

Polit, D. F, & Beck, C. T. (2012). *Nursing research: Generating and assessing evidence for nursing practice.* Philadelphia, PA: Wolters Kluwer/Lippincott Williams, & Wilkins.

Public Health Agency of Canada. (2010). http://www.phac-aspc.gc.ca/index-eng.php.

Renpenning, K. M., & Taylor, S. G. (2003). *Self-care theory in nursing: Selected papers of Dorothea Orem.* New York, NY: Springer.

Rogers, M. (1970). *The theoretical basis of nursing.* Philadelphia, PA: F. A. Davis.

Rogers, M. (1990). Nursing: Science of unitary, irreducible, human beings: Update 1990. In E. A. M. Barrett (ed.), *Visions of Rogers' science-based nursing.* New York, NY: National League for Nursing, pp. 5–11.

Roy, C. (1974a). *Introduction to nursing: An adaptation model.* Upper Saddle River, NJ: Prentice Hall.

Roy, C. (1974b). The Roy adaptation model. In J. P. Riehl & S. C. Roy (eds.), *Conceptual models for nursing practice.* New York, NY: Appleton & Lange, pp. 135–144.

Roy, C. (1999). *The Roy adaptation model.* Stamford, CT: Appleton & Lange.

Roy, C., & Zhan, L.(2010). Sister Callista Roy's adaptation model. In M. Parker & M. Smith (eds.), *Nursing theories* (3rd ed.). Philadelphia, PA: F. A. Davis, pp. 167–181.

Selye, H. (1974). *Stress without distress.* Philadelphia, PA: Lippincott.

Taber. (2009). *Taber's cyclopedic medical dictionary* (21st ed.). Philadelphia, PA: F. A. Davis.

The Texas Board of Nursing. (2010). *Differentiated essential competencies (DECs) of graduates of Texas nursing programs evidenced by knowledge, clinical judgment, and behaviors.* Author. Retrieved from http://www.bne.tx.us

Townsend, M. (2006). *Psychiatric mental health nursing: Concepts of care in evidence-based practice.* Philadelphia, PA: F. A. Davis Company.

Von Bertalanffy, L. (1968). *General systems theory: Foundations, development, and application.* New York, NY: Braziller.

Walker, L. O., & Avant, K. C. (2011). *Strategies for theory construction in nursing.* Boston, MA: Pearson.

Watson, J. (1979). *Nursing: The philosophy and science of caring.* Boston: Little, Brown.

Watson, J. (1996). Watson's theory of transpersonal caring. In P. Hinton Walker & B. Neuman (eds.). *Blueprint for use of nursing models.* New York, NY: NLN Press, pp. 141–184.

Wilkinson, J. M., & Treas, L. S. (2011). *Fundamentals of nursing: Theory, concepts, and applications.* Philadelphia, PA: F. A. Davis.

BIBLIOGRAPHY

Alligood, M. R. (Ed.). (2010). *Nursing theory: Utilization and application.* St. Louis, MO: Mosby.

Alligood, M. R., & Tomey-Mariner, A. (Eds.). (2010). *Nursing theorists and their works.* Maryland Heights, MO: Mosby/Elsevier.

Andrews, H. A., & Roy, C. (1986). *Essentials of the Roy adaptation model.* Norwalk, CT: Appleton-Century Crofts.

Chesnay, M. (Ed.). (2008). *Caring for the vulnerable: Perspectives in nursing theory, practice, and research.* Sudbury, MA: Jones & Bartlett.

Chin, P., & Kramer, M. K. (2008). *Integrated knowledge development in nursing* (7th ed.). St. Louis, MO: Mosby Elsevier.

Hood, L. J. (2010). *Leddy and Pepper's conceptual bases of professional nursing* (7th ed.). Philadelphia, PA: Wolters Kluwer Health/Lippincott Williams & Wilkins.

King, I. (2007). *Middle range theory development using King's conceptual system.* New York, NY: Springer Publishing.

Leininger, M., & McFarland, M. R. (2002). *Transcultural nursing: Concepts, theories, research, and practice* (3rd ed.). New York, NY: McGraw-Hill.

Leininger, M. M., & McFarland, M. (2006). *Culture care diversity & universality: A worldwide nursing theory* (2nd ed.). Sudbury, MA: Jones & Bartlett.

Roy, C., & Andrews, H. A. (1999). *The Roy adaptation model: The definitive statement.* Norwalk, CT: Appleton & Lange.

Tannahill, A. (2009). Health promotion: The Tannahill model revisited. *Public Health, 123,* 396–399.

CHAPTER 3
Theoretical Foundations of Health Promotion

Janice A. Maville, EdD, MSN, RN
Carolina G. Huerta, EdD, MSN, RN

KEY TERMS

anticipatory guidance
Consumer Information Processing Model (CIP)
Diffusion of Innovations Model
disease prevention
health

Health Belief Model
health-promotion plan
health protection
high-level wellness
models
Pender Health Promotion Model

PRECEDE-PROCEED Model
Protection Motivation Theory
self-efficacy
Theory of Planned Behavior
Transtheoretical Model (TTM)

OBJECTIVES

Upon completion of this chapter, the reader should be able to:

- Explore the meaning of health.
- Examine definitions of health promotion.
- Differentiate health promotion from wellness, disease prevention, and health protection.
- Compare and contrast theories and models of human behavior, human behavior and health, and human behavior and health promotion.
- Relate theoretical concepts of human behavior to the promotion of health.
- Discuss the application of theories and models for health-promoting behavioral outcomes.
- Describe strategies for the development of a health-promotion plan.

INTRODUCTION

Society today is plagued with many health-related issues that impact our quality of life: the alarming statistics on obesity in children and adults, the post-traumatic stress experienced by our returning war veterans, the natural disasters like those in Haiti in 2010 and Japan in 2011 and their sequelae, and the sustainability of our environment, just to name a few. As a result, the promotion of health assumes ever increasing importance today. Health promotion is continuously highlighted by nurses and other health care professionals through the establishment of initiatives that are vital to the achievement of optimum health and wellness. Before these health-promotion initiatives can be applied to nursing practice, however, we need to examine the how health promotion has been defined and differentiated from other health-related concepts, as well as how theories and models have been developed to explain this concept. In doing so, a firm foundation may be established on which practice can be implemented. This is the nature of a profession. This is the nature of nursing.

Health promotion and the issues instrumental in its development were discussed in Chapter 1. Chapter 2 introduced the metaparadigm of nursing and emphasized assumptions basic to the integration of health promotion in nursing care. This chapter focuses and expands on the many definitions of health and differentiates health promotion from wellness and disease prevention. Chapter 2 introduced nursing theories and their relationship to health promotion in general. This chapter explains various theories and models as they relate to health promotion. The guidelines essential to developing a health promotion plan are introduced.

CLARIFYING TERMS

Defining health and describing what constitutes a healthy status is complex because there are many varying perspectives. As discussed in Chapter 2, there is no consensus on what constitutes health. There is agreement, though, that **health** encompasses the total functioning of an individual. To attain a state of health, individuals must effectively function in a number of areas: physical, psychological, social, cultural, environmental, and spiritual. Viewed in this manner, health reflects the holistic nature of individuals. Although the health status of an individual can be described in several ways, there is usually no one definition for the terms *health* and *health promotion*. In fact, several terms related to health and health promotion that are used frequently in nursing and health care and throughout this text need clarification. For example, health promotion is different from wellness. Likewise, health promotion and disease prevention are not necessarily the same. *Health protection* and *health promotion* are also terms that do not necessarily mean the same thing, yet may be used to describe the same phenomenon. The following section attempts to clarify some of the terms related to health promotion.

WELLNESS

The concept of wellness has existed for over five decades, yet this term is still a difficult one to define. This concept was heavily influenced by Dunn (1959), who recognized that health and illness were often described as being direct opposites of each other, when in fact they could be viewed on a continuum that includes high-level wellness. Dunn's theory of high-level wellness has served as a focal point for the discussion of health

---

SPOTLIGHT **ON**

A Small Word with Big Implications

The word *health* has only six letters, but there are as many definitions as people asked to define it. This complexity is increased by considering the meaning of health as it relates not only to individuals but to families, communities, and nations. For example, to a student, being healthy may mean being able to go to school and meet school-related obligations. To other individuals, being healthy may mean being free from any type of disease.

---

promotion and is frequently described to differentiate it from the concept of health.

If health refers to effective personal functioning, then wellness refers to this effective functioning and more. Wellness is multidimensional, and its definition usually includes the characteristics of wellness. The various dimensions in its definition may include social, occupational, spiritual, physical, intellectual, emotional, environmental, financial, mental, and medical wellness (Definitions of Wellness, 2011). Wellness includes individual functioning at the highest potential and can be viewed as the actualization of the human potential (Pender, Murdaugh, & Parsons, 2011). *Wellness* is an expanded term that is not as restricting as *health*. Accordingly, **high-level wellness** describes the dynamic state of wellness that occurs at the individual, environmental, cultural, and social levels. Key to this state are the capability and potential of the individual.

Dunn (1973) perceived high-level wellness as a step above health. This concept of high-level wellness is congruent with systems theory in that individuals are seen as open systems interacting continuously with their environment (refer to Chapter 2 for a discussion on systems theory). This interaction involves energy. People are made up of various forms of dynamic energy, including expendable energy that is used to carry out daily activities of living. According to Dunn, high-level wellness involves progress toward a higher level of functioning, the challenge to live at our full potential, and the integration of the whole being, including body mind and spirit, into the functioning process There is no one optimal level of wellness; however, all people are capable of moving toward a personal level of wellness. A wellness approach requires a holistic view of people and may include many degrees of wellness.

DISEASE PREVENTION AND HEALTH PROTECTION

Like the term *wellness*, the terms *disease prevention* and *health protection* are frequently used when discussing health and health promotion. Although the concept of wellness has a positive connotation with a focus on the individual's expanded potential for health, **disease prevention** has a negative connotation because it focuses on the reduction and severity of disease. Disease prevention thus looks at actions that modify the environment, behaviors, or bodily defenses in eliminating, slowing, or changing a disease process. **Health protection**, which is frequently used interchangeably with disease prevention, also reflects a disease-related focus that is consistent with the medical model supported by the discipline of medicine.

ASK **YOURSELF**

Health and Wellness—Two Different Concepts?

A friend of yours is 40 pounds overweight and rarely reports any ailments. She states that she considers herself quite healthy, although she knows she is overweight. You are aware that her weight limits her participation in several activities and believe that she would be healthy if she lost the extra weight. What do you think the word *health* means to your friend? How do you define health for yourself? Do you see a state of wellness as different from health? Is it possible to be healthy without being well?

Because both disease prevention and health protection activities are aimed at the prevention of disease or disorder, their focus is on particular groups or individuals at risk for the development of a disease or disorder rather than on all people, whether as individuals or as a family, society, or community. As such, these terms do not imply a positive representation of health that moves forward; they are concerned with maintaining the status quo of certain individuals or groups by reducing their risks for disease.

Describing health and health promotion by using such terms as *disease prevention* and *health protection* implies that others are expert at knowing what is best for an individual. These experts use strategies such as health education to persuade individuals to assume responsibility for their own health. In turn, knowledge may be gained, skills may be learned, and behaviors may be changed to avoid disease, but health may not be enhanced in the same way as when using a health-promotion approach.

Human behavior incorporated into lifestyle is responsible for the health status of most individuals. The World Health Organization (WHO) reviewed 24 lifestyle-related health risks and concluded that poor childhood nutrition, unsafe sex, alcohol abuse, bad sanitation and hygiene, and high blood pressure are responsible for approximately 25% of the 60 million deaths that occur around the world each year (2009). Other statistics reported by the Centers for Disease Control and Prevention (2011) show that in 2007 nearly 70 percent of deaths in the United States resulted from seven leading causes: heart disease (25.4%), cancer (23.2%), stroke (5.6%), chronic lower respiratory disease (5.3%), accidents (5.1%), Alzheimer's (5.1%), and diabetes (3.0%). Six of the seven diseases listed are directly related to lifestyle behaviors and choices.

HEALTH PROMOTION

Although *wellness, disease prevention*, and *health protection* are terms used individually in defining health, they are all also used

---

GLOBAL HIGHLIGHTS IN HEALTH PROMOTION

Unhealthy Lifestyles and Lifespan

A British study found that millions of Britons have such an unhealthy lifestyle that the effect on their bodies is the same as adding 12 years to their actual ages, causing them to age prematurely. The study included 5000 British adults and found that four unhealthy habits (smoking, poor diet, lack of exercise, and drinking too much alcohol) increased the risk of dying early by as much as the equivalent of 12 years. The study found that a third of those who admitted having these four habits died during the 20-year duration of the study compared to those who did not have those habits.

Source: Kvaavik, E., Batty, G. D., Ursin, G., Huxley, R., & Gale, C. R. (2010). Influence of individual and combined health behaviors on total and cause-specific mortality in men and women. *Archives of Internal Medicine, 170*(8), 711–718.

---

in defining health promotion and the activities that promote health. These terms are thus in concert with the concept of health promotion as defined in Chapter 1 because the definition includes any activity useful in enhancing the quality of health and well-being of individuals, families, groups, communities, and nations. Certainly the activities necessary to achieve high-level wellness enhance the quality of health. These activities can also include endeavors directed toward disease prevention and health protection. Thus, the concepts of wellness, disease prevention, and health protection are subsumed in the definition of health promotion.

The major themes of empowerment, lifestyle change, health enhancement, and well-being, as described in Chapter 1, are central to defining health promotion. Health promotion differs from wellness, disease prevention, and health protection in that it seeks to empower people to change through personal choices regarding their lifestyles and health enhancement and well-being activities. The major difference is in the underlying motivation for the behavior. Whereas terms such as *disease prevention* and *health protection* imply behavior that avoids disease or maintains the status quo, health promotion is motivated by the desire to increase wellness and actualize human health potential (Pender, Murdaugh, & Parsons, 2011). Health promotion thus includes any activity that helps people adopt or maintain lifestyles that support a state of optimal health or a balance of physical, emotional, social, spiritual, and intellectual health. Nurses can facilitate health promotion by using **anticipatory guidance** that involves the preparation of patients or clients for an anticipated developmental and/or situational crisis (Bulecheck, Butcher, & Dochterman, 2008).

THEORETICAL FOUNDATIONS

Individuals have their own thoughts and perceptions. People use their impressions of what is going on within and around them to form ideas or concepts about a phenomenon or area of interest such as health. These concepts can become connected or related to form a theory that helps to explain a phenomenon or area of interest. (See Chapter 2 for further clarification on theory and theoretical frameworks.) **Models** are visual representations of the concepts that work together to become a theory.

Researchers who have studied human behavior have developed and tested theories that help to explain why people behave in a certain manner. Researchers who have analyzed human behavior and health have developed theories that seek to explain factors and interactions among factors influencing the health of individuals or a group of individuals. Building on these factors, researchers interested in health promotion have developed theories and models to explain human behavior for the enhancement of health. Predominant theories and models relative to each of these areas are presented in the following sections.

THEORIES OF HUMAN BEHAVIOR AND HEALTH

Promoting health has been part of national and international agendas over the past 30 years. Governments can make laws designed to protect individuals from harm, such as seat belt and helmet laws. But, at a more fundamental level, the individual determines personal health status and what they can do to improve it. Planning strategies for health promotion depends on having an understanding of human behavior.

Many theories and models have been developed by researchers interested in studying factors related to health behaviors in particular. Selected for discussion are the Theory of Planned Behavior, Health Belief Model, and the Protection Motivation Theory, as well as the Transtheoretical Model of Behavior Change. Because of their emphasis on risks and threats of disease, these theories and models are strongly aligned with health protection rather than with health promotion.

THEORY OF PLANNED BEHAVIOR

The Theory of Planned Behavior was developed by social psychologist Icek Ajzen (Ajzen, 2002). Prior to this theory, others had explained how attitudes and intentions influenced behavior. Building on this, the **Theory of Planned Behavior** took into account that the control of behavior is not always voluntary and that a type of behavior control continuum exists with lack of control at one end and total control at the other. If people have the resources, support, or skills needed for a certain behavior, they are at the control end of the continuum.

Perception of control of behavior was also an important element of this theory. In later theories and models, this concept is expressed as **self-efficacy**, or self-conviction or the belief that one can be successful in achieving the desired behavior. For example, Figure 3-1 shows how the Theory of Planned Behavior might be applied in a real-life situation. If a person

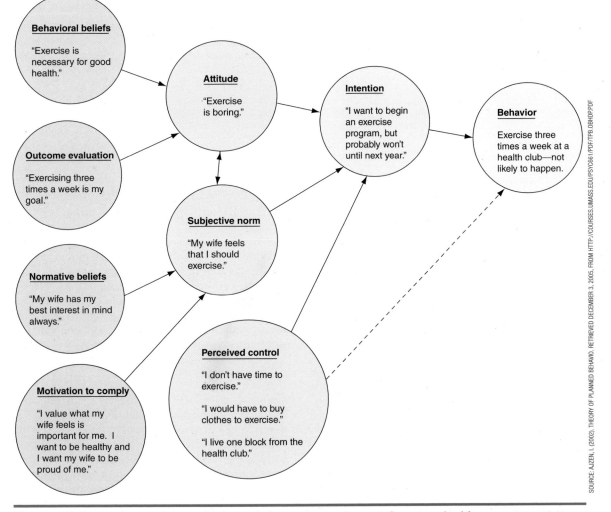

FIGURE 3-1 The Theory of Planned Behavior helps to examine factors influencing a health-promoting activity such as exercise.

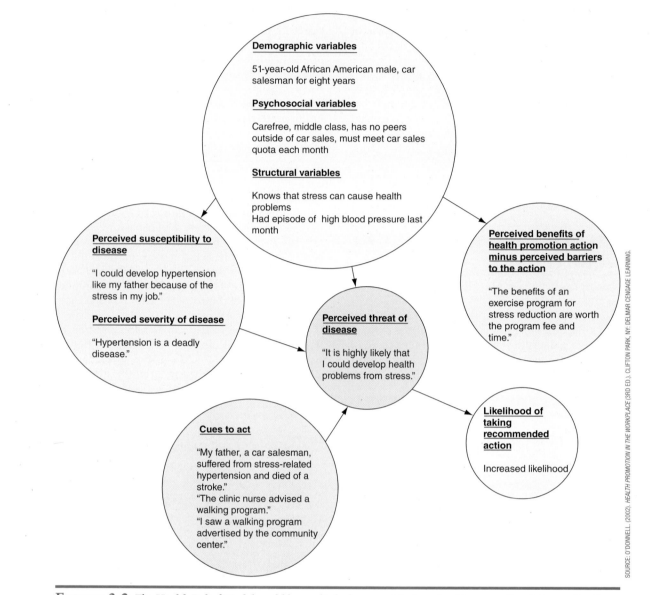

FIGURE 3-2 The Health Belief Model could be applied when considering a health-promotion intervention for a disease risk factor such as stress.

knows that exercise as the outcome expectation (behavior) is necessary to promote health (subjective norm), the attitude toward exercise and the individual's self-efficacy (perceived control) influence the intention to carry out this behavior.

HEALTH BELIEF MODEL

The **Health Belief Model** is a well-known model that became significant because of its emphasis on predicting individual preventive health behavior. It was developed by four social psychologists—Hochbaum, Kegeles, Leventhal, and Rosenstock—for the U.S. Public Health Service in order to offer an explanation for nonparticipation by people in disease prevention programs (O'Donnell, 2002). Consequently, this theory is based on an individual's ideas about and appraisal of perceived benefits compared to the perceived barriers and costs of taking a health action. The Health Belief Model suggests that a person's susceptibility to a health threat and its seriousness influence the decision to engage in a preventive health behavior.

The model helps to identify the strengths as well as the weaknesses of the individual that could affect the success of a plan of action for disease prevention. The model assumes that individuals value health. The original model, developed in the 1950s, was later revised to include nonhealth reasons, such as finances, knowledge about disease, or personality, that could modify perceptions about susceptibility to disease. Although intended as a disease-prevention model, the Health Belief Model could be applied when considering stress as a disease risk factor, as shown in Figure 3-2.

PROTECTION MOTIVATION THEORY

The **Protection Motivation Theory**, developed in the mid-1970s, is a fear-driven model. It proposed that a perceived threat to health activates thought processes regarding the severity of the threatened event, the probability of its occurrence, and coping mechanisms (Rogers, 1975). The motivation to protect results from the perception of the threat and the conviction or belief that one can be successful in achieving the desired behavior known as **self efficacy**. The Protection Motivation Theory is oriented more toward disease prevention than health promotion. The theory contains components of the Health Belief Model (vulnerability, severity, and response efficacy) and the social learning theory (self-efficacy).

The major areas where the Protection Motivation Theory has been applied are alcohol use, healthy lifestyle enhancement, the promotion of diagnostic health behaviors, and disease prevention. The original theory and model have been revised many times. A schematic representation of this model for smoking cessation is shown in Figure 3-3.

TRANSTHEORETICAL MODEL OF BEHAVIOR CHANGE

The **Transtheoretical Model (TTM)** was the result of smoking cessation research in adults by Prochaska and DiClemente (2005). These researchers concluded that changes in health behaviors progress through five distinct stages containing the elements of thought, action, and time (Table 3-1). Adjunct to this model are nine processes of change that affect the individual across all stages of change. These processes of change are categorized as experiential (what the individual is experiencing in relation to self, the environment, and others) and behavioral (the processes that enhance success for change). These two categories include the following factors (Fahrenwald & Walker, 2003):

1. Experiential:
   a. Consciousness raising.
   b. Dramatic relief.
   c. Environmental reevaluation.
   d. Social liberation.
2. Behavioral:
   a. Counterconditioning.
   b. Helping relationships.
   c. Reinforcement management.
   d. Self-liberation.
   e. Stimulus control.

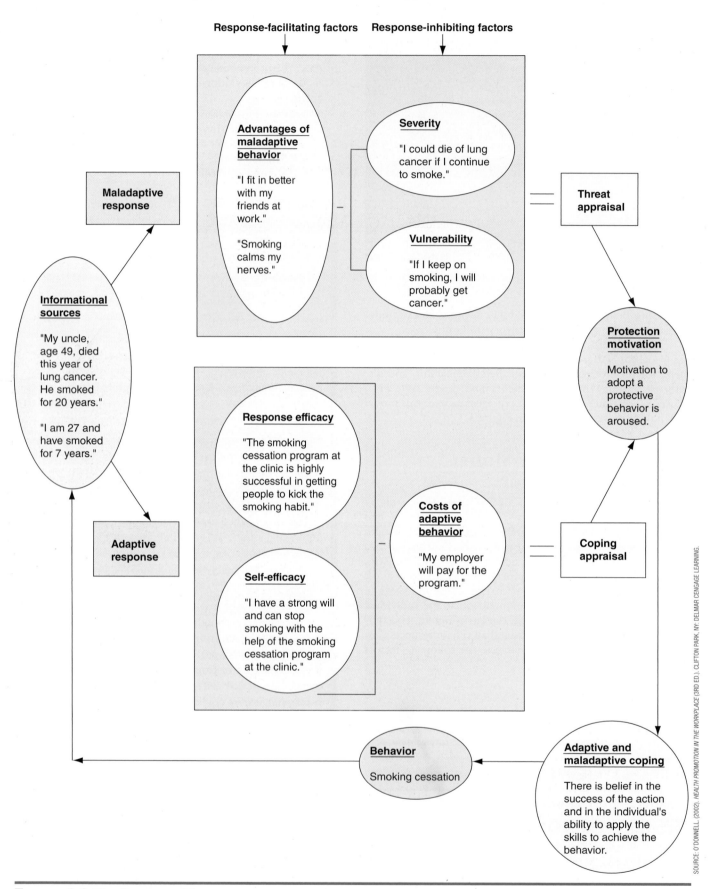

FIGURE 3-3   This illustration of the Protection Motivation Theory shows how elements related to threat of disease and coping could affect a health-promotion activity such as smoking cessation.

SOURCE: O'DONNELL. (2002). *HEALTH PROMOTION IN THE WORKPLACE* (3RD ED.). CLIFTON PARK, NY: DELMAR CENGAGE LEARNING.

TABLE 3-1 Summary of Stages of the Transtheoretical Model of Behavior Change

STAGE	THOUGHT	ACTION	TIME
Stage 1: Precontemplation	No thought to making a change	No action planned	Not within the next six months
Stage 2: Contemplation	Thoughts of making a change	Actions considered	Within the next six months
Stage 3: Preparation	Seriously thinking of making a change	Actions identified	Within the next month
Stage 4: Action	Involved in the change	Actively involved in the behavior change	Involved in the change for six months
Stage 5: Maintenance	Processing effects of change	Continuation of behavior change	Indefinite

Source: Adapted from Prochaska, J. O., & DiClemente, C. C. (2005). The transtheoretical approach. In J. C. Norcross & M. R. Goldfried (eds.), *Handbook of psychotherapy integration*. New York: Oxford University Press, pp. 147–171.

The Transtheoretical Model is valuable in helping to understand why individuals do or do not become involved in making a healthy behavior change, in evaluating their personal situations, and in tailoring efforts and strategies according to each individual's stage of change.

MODELS FOR GROUPS, ORGANIZATIONS, AND COMMUNITIES

Most theories and models for behavior change and health have focused largely on the individual. A few, however, offer structures to guide families, groups, communities, and even nations in making changes for healthier environments. Those selected for discussion are the Consumer Information Processing Model, the Diffusion of Innovations Model, and the PRECEDE-PROCEED Model.

CONSUMER INFORMATION PROCESSING MODEL

The **Consumer Information Processing Model (CIP)** (Bettman, 1979) incorporates concepts related to the use of information and the motivational effect of using this information in making choices. Although its initial intention was to explain consumer behavior, its applicability is appropriate in examining how choices are made that affect health. Essentially, this model recognizes that individuals (1) have limits on the amount of information they obtain, use, and recall; (2) actively search for information based on their motivation, attention, and perception; (3) create rules for more rapid decision making; (4) base future decisions on the outcome of choices made; and (5) desire information that is relevant and convenient.

Although this model may seem to be individual-specific, its application is most helpful to families and communities. A prime example is the information presented to consumers regarding food. Applying the concepts of the CIP model, the labels are for the most part concise and pertinent. Information needed to make a selection, such as "low salt" or "sodium-free," is relatively easy to locate and compare with other items. Health-promotion information, similarly, needs to be available, useful, and designed for convenient cognitive processing by the consumer.

? ASK YOURSELF

Consumer Information Processing and Point of Purchase

What purchases have you made lately that were related to promoting your health or that of your family? How did you use the components of this model in making your decision to make the purchase or not to purchase?

DIFFUSION OF INNOVATIONS MODEL

The **Diffusion of Innovations Model** addresses how new ideas, products, and social practices spread within a society or from one society to another (National Cancer Institute, 2005; Rogers, 2003). Decisions by organizations and communities to adopt new programs or practices (innovations) depend on how successful they were in other areas.

Diffusion is the communication process that is vital to the dissemination of information about the innovation, whether it is an idea or a product or a practice. The communication method is vital to the actual adoption. Involving community leaders, using mass media, and choosing interpersonal modes of communication enhance the likelihood of practice adoption.

The Diffusion of Innovations Model reflects the characteristics of innovations that can impact their adoption:

1. Relative advantage—The extent to which an innovation is seen as better than the idea or practice it is replacing.
2. Compatibility—The extent to which the innovation fits with existing values, habits, experience, and needs.
3. Complexity—The extent to which the innovation is understood.
4. Trialability—The extent to which the innovation can be tried or practiced before it is adopted.

5. Observability—The extent to which results of the innovation can be seen or observed (National Cancer Institute, 2005)

Time, communication systems, the social structure, and the innovation itself intertwine to create a complex model designed for long-range change on a broad-based level. The Diffusion of Innovations Model has been used successfully in communities the world over for smoking cessation campaigns. Most recently it has been found successful for use in a community inhalant abuse project (New England Inhalant Abuse Coalition, 2011), in a worksite sun protection program in the outdoor recreation industry (Buller, 2005), and as a framework for a diabetes management program (De Civita & Dasgupta, 2007).

PRECEDE-PROCEED Model

The **PRECEDE-PROCEED Model** evolved over the past 50 years from two separate frameworks created by Green, Kreuter, and colleagues (Green & Kreuter, 2005). These frameworks unite to form a model to guide the development of health-promotion programs for groups, communities, states, and nations. Over time, the intent of this model has shifted from health education program planning to health-promotion planning. The purpose is to focus on the outcomes of, rather than the inputs for, program planning. Simply put, the outcome of quality of life forms the beginning of the model, which then works backward to determine the components for success in the following order:

1. Assessment of health, behavior, lifestyle, and environment.
2. Analysis of factors that predispose, reinforce, and enable the project or program.
3. Implementation of educational or health-promoting program(s) with evaluation of influences by health policy organizations and regulations.

The PRECEDE portion of the model was developed between 1968 and 1974. The model's title is an acronym for its components: *p*redisposing, *r*einforcing, and *e*nabling *c*onstructs in *e*ducational/ecological *d*iagnosis and *e*valuation. The focus of PRECEDE is to use a multidimensional approach in diagnosing a problem in a target population in order for appropriate health education to be implemented as an intervention. Because this model is founded in the social/behavioral sciences, epidemiology, administration, and education, it recognizes that health and health behaviors have multiple causations that must be evaluated in order to assure appropriate intervention. Table 3-2 lists the five phases of the PRECEDE portion of the model.

The PROCEED portion of the model (*p*olicy, *r*egulatory, *o*rganizational *c*onstructs in *e*ducational and *e*nvironmental *d*evelopment) was added in the 1980s to encompass the wider environmental, policy, and organizational factors that Green and Kreuter had recognized during their involvement with national programs of community health promotion. The intent of the model shifted from an educational program planning approach to one that is centered on population health promotion. At its core is the belief that behavior change will occur when the people involved have become empowered with the understanding, motivation, skills, and active engagement in community affairs that improve their quality of life.

Note that, in Table 3-2, the administrative diagnosis is the final planning step to PRECEDE implementation. From there, PROCEED is activated to implement the plan or policy in phase six. Phases 7, 8, and 9 evaluate the process for factors that enhance or impede it, organize the resources and services as required by the plan or policy, assess achievement of objectives that are established for each phase, and evaluate the overall objective relating to quality of life. The addition of PROCEED extends the model beyond educational interventions to the political, managerial, and economic areas for action that are necessary to create social environments that are more conducive to healthy lifestyles.

According to Green and Kreuter (2005), the PRECEDE-PROCEED Model has been applied, tested, studied, extended, and verified in nearly a thousand published studies and in thousands more of unpublished projects in community, school, clinical, and workplace settings over the last 15 years. Its multidimensional, multilevel nature creates a complexity that is

Table 3-2 Phases of the PRECEDE-PROCEED Model

PRECEDE		PROCEED	
Phase 1	Social diagnosis: Evaluation of social problem(s)	Phase 6	Implementation: Operationalization of program
Phase 2	Epidemiological Diagnosis: Analysis of health problem(s)	Phase 7	Process evaluation: Evaluation of the process used to implement the program
Phase 3	Behavioral and environmental diagnosis: Identification of health practices linked to problem(s)	Phase 8	Impact evaluation: Assessment of the achievement of objectives
Phase 4	Education and organizational diagnosis: Identification of learning objectives	Phase 9	Outcome evaluation: Measurement of overall goal achievement and effect on quality of life
Phase 5	Administrative and policy Diagnosis: Analysis of policies, resources, and management components		

GLOBAL HIGHLIGHTS IN HEALTH PROMOTION

Using the PROCEED Model to Understand Mental Health–Promoting Behaviors in Japan

Researchers Mo and Mak (2008) in Hong Kong applied the PROCEED model to examine factors associated with behaviors that promoted mental health and to gain insight into how these behaviors affected mental well-being and quality of life among 941 Chinese adults. It was found that a sense of coherence (predisposing factor), social support (reinforcing factor), and daily hassles (enabling factor) were significantly related to mental health–promoting behaviors, which are associated with mental well-being and quality of life. Research such as this will be increasingly important in addressing mental health issues in countries around the world, especially in the aftermath of catastrophic events.

compounded by time and effort by those involved at every phase. Although it is specifically suitable for broad-based interventions with long-term goals, it has been successfully implemented in a variety of settings and target populations. Recent examples of implementation are health-promotion research on dietary versus intuitive eating behaviors in military spouses (Cole & Horacek, 2010), the development of a health-promoting hospital in Africa (Delobelle, Onya, Langa, Mashamba, & Depoorter, 2010), and mammography use among low-income minority women (Kratzke, Garzon, Lombard, & Karlowicz, 2010).

HEALTH-PROMOTION MODELS

Chapter 1 described how health promotion evolved from global concerns of the World Health Organization nearly 40 years ago and how efforts have grown at the local, national, and international levels. Several models of health promotion have been developed as a result of this concern. One such contribution is the Tannahill Model of Health Promotion, developed by Scottish scholar Andrew Tannahill in the early to mid-1980s. In the United States, the leading health-promotion model is the Health-Promotion Model developed and later revised by nurse researcher Nola Pender.

? ASK **YOURSELF**

Personal Health-Promotion Model

How do you believe your individual characteristics and experiences have affected your perceptions and feelings about your health-promoting behaviors? If you had to design your own personal health promotion model, what would it look like?

PENDER MODEL OF HEALTH PROMOTION

In spite of all the efforts to explain why people behave as they do, internal and external variables included, no one theory has been developed to integrate or link all the diverse circumstances into one health-promotion theory. Psychologist and nurse educator Dr. Nola Pender, however, has developed a model that integrates perspectives from the areas of behavioral science and nursing.

Since its inception in 1982, the Pender Health Promotion Model has been used exclusively in nursing practice and research. Due to its comprehensive, integrative, and holistic approach, it has been applied by various researchers, health care practitioners, and community leaders in countries around the world in multitudes of health-promotion activities. These activities have included the preparation of health-promotion plans for individual clients, for worksites, and for communities. Additionally, the Health-Promotion Model has been used and studied in scores of health-promotion research endeavors.

The **Pender Health Promotion Model** integrates concepts from the expectancy-value model of human motivation and social cognitive theory to form the theoretical basis (Pender, Murdaugh & Parsons, 2011). In other words, people work toward what they feel is of value to them and are influenced by unique internal and external factors. Self-efficacy is predominant in the model. What makes this model unique, however, is its holistic perspective, which is integral to professional nursing care.

The Health-Promotion Model variables are grouped into three major categories: (1) individual characteristics and experiences, (2) behavior-specific cognition and affect, and (3) behavior outcome. As such, the Health-Promotion Model shows how individual characteristics, including prior related behavior, personal factors, and biopsychological social factors, have a direct effect on the desired health-promoting behavior. These same characteristics have an indirect effect on behavior-specific cognitions and affect, or the perceptions and feelings a person has regarding benefits and barriers of the action, self-efficacy, and sensitivity to the desires and demands of others. All of this combined directly affects the individual's commitment to a plan of action and ultimately the performance of the health-promoting behavior. Figure 3-4 shows the application of this model for an individual whose behavioral outcome is weight loss.

DEVELOPING A HEALTH-PROMOTION PLAN

The theories of health promotion and human behavior described in the previous sections provide nursing with the tools necessary to develop a comprehensive health-promotion plan for clients, as individuals, families, communities, and groups. A **health-promotion plan** looks beyond the client to the family and the community because the client does not exist in isolation.

The health-promotion plan focuses on achieving wellness and, along with the client (identified as an individual, a family, or a community), determines the activities necessary to achieve optimum health. The plan examines the client's vulnerability to health imbalance, assesses client weaknesses and strengths, and determines the potential for illness. Unlike the nursing process plan, which includes existing or potential health problems, the

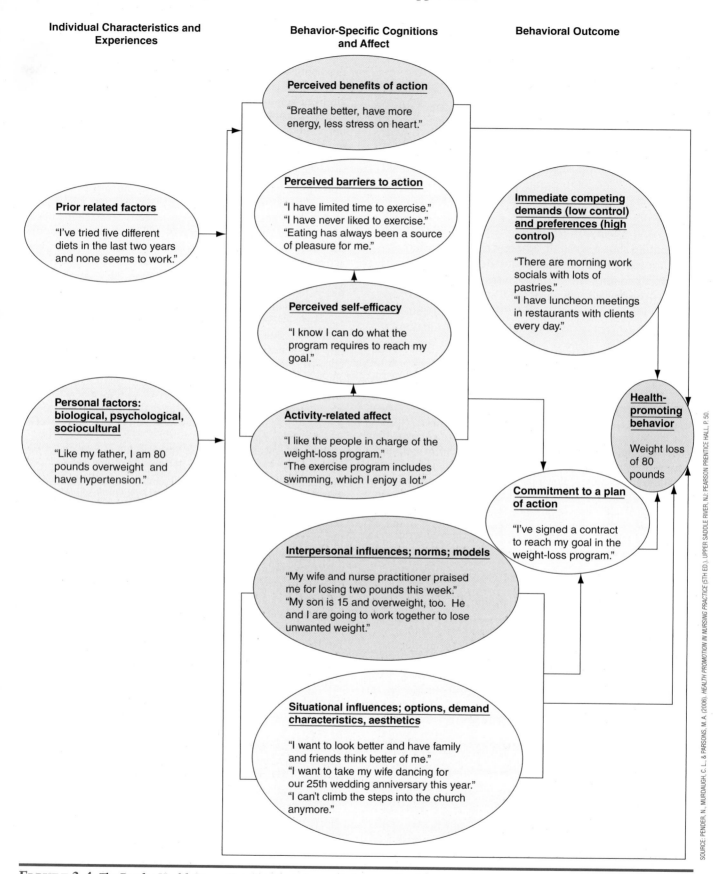

Individual Characteristics and Experiences

Behavior-Specific Cognitions and Affect

Behavioral Outcome

Perceived benefits of action

"Breathe better, have more energy, less stress on heart."

Prior related factors

"I've tried five different diets in the last two years and none seems to work."

Perceived barriers to action

"I have limited time to exercise."
"I have never liked to exercise."
"Eating has always been a source of pleasure for me."

Immediate competing demands (low control) and preferences (high control)

"There are morning work socials with lots of pastries."
"I have luncheon meetings in restaurants with clients every day."

Perceived self-efficacy

"I know I can do what the program requires to reach my goal."

Personal factors: biological, psychological, sociocultural

"Like my father, I am 80 pounds overweight and have hypertension."

Activity-related affect

"I like the people in charge of the weight-loss program."
"The exercise program includes swimming, which I enjoy a lot."

Health-promoting behavior

Weight loss of 80 pounds

Commitment to a plan of action

"I've signed a contract to reach my goal in the weight-loss program."

Interpersonal influences; norms; models

"My wife and nurse practitioner praised me for losing two pounds this week."
"My son is 15 and overweight, too. He and I are going to work together to lose unwanted weight."

Situational influences; options, demand characteristics, aesthetics

"I want to look better and have family and friends think better of me."
"I want to take my wife dancing for our 25th wedding anniversary this year."
"I can't climb the steps into the church anymore."

SOURCE: PENDER, N., MURDAUGH, C. L., & PARSONS, M. A. (2006). *HEALTH PROMOTION IN NURSING PRACTICE* (5TH ED.). UPPER SADDLE RIVER, NJ: PEARSON PRENTICE HALL, P. 50.

FIGURE 3-4 The Pender Health Promotion Model can be applied to many health-promotion activities, including weight loss.

health-promotion plan emphasizes the achievement of optimum health outcomes for clients.

Critical to the development of a health-promotion plan is the nurse's recognition that clients are the experts regarding their own health needs. They have the right to be a active participants in the determination of their health. Consequently, client participation in the planning process is essential if the goals of the plan are to be attained. Also important is that the nurse has an understanding of the motivation for human behavior and for changing health behaviors. The successful health-promotion plan identifies the interactions among all the factors that influence the health of the individual (Pender, Murdaugh, & Parsons, 2011). The development of a health-promotion plan involves the collection of assessment data; the recognition of resources, supports, and constraints or barriers to the achievement of goals; and the identification of outcome measures, planning/implementation, and evaluation. These phases of the Health-Promotion Model are reflected in the composition of a comprehensive health-promotion plan.

ASSESSMENT AND DATA COLLECTION

The collection of data to be used in making a client assessment is a critical phase in the development of a health-promotion plan. This phase involves looking at the client holistically. The client's health status is viewed not only in terms of physiological needs but also in terms of total biological, psychological, social, spiritual, cultural, intellectual, and environmental functioning. The assessment phase goes beyond the individual client to the family, community, and related influences. The family assessment is important in order to assess the client's ability to handle a health problem or an activity aimed at eliminating a risk factor such as smoking. The community assessment is essential because the community is where the client exists, and changes to the surrounding community may be necessary (Pender, Murdaugh, & Parsons, 2011).

RESOURCES, SUPPORTS, AND CONSTRAINTS OR BARRIERS/ OUTCOME MEASURES

The assessment phase identifies the resources and individual supporting systems available to the client. Barriers or constraints that may prevent the client from achieving health-promotion goals are also identified. The identification of resources, supports, and constraints is critical in that these may enhance or limit the client's ability to accomplish activities in the health-promotion plan. The incentives for client change are also identified. The client's health, health beliefs, and behaviors are also assessed because these provide the data for the identification of outcome measures needed for achieving optimal health (Pender, Murdaugh, & Parsons, 2011). These outcome measures, as determined by the client together with the nurse, must be measurable and realistic.

PLANNING AND IMPLEMENTATION

The health-promotion planning phase looks at possible problems and weaknesses of the client that increase health risks. The planning phase is based on the assessment data collected and on the outcome measures determined. Again, the plan capitalizes on the resources and supports previously identified in order to enhance the client's ability to change health behaviors. Active participation by the client in planning the care is important. Both the client and the nurse identify health priorities and objectives and determine a time frame that is reasonable for achieving the previously identified outcome measures. Nursing facilitates learning, provides support, assists in identifying possible plan options, and decreases barriers to the achievement of goals (Pender, Murdaugh, & Parsons, 2011).

EVALUATION

Determining whether the health-promotion plan achieves the needed behavior changes—whether in client lifestyle, health beliefs, or practices—calls for evaluation. The nurse and client review and evaluate the client's progress. They then determine whether the identified outcomes were achieved and whether they were achieved in a timely manner. If the goals or outcome measures were not achieved, the question of what needs to be included in the plan or eliminated must be asked. The last step in the evaluation phase is the determination of whether any plan revisions are needed. According to Pender, Murdaugh, & Parsons (2011), periodic revisions of the plan provide a systematic approach to moving a client toward a higher level of health. Once the plan for health promotion is developed, the implementation of the nursing process can begin. For information on how the health-promotion plan and nursing process can be used in planning client care, refer to Chapter 4. Table 3-3 provides an example of a health-promotion plan for the community. This format may also be used in health planning for individuals and families.

SUMMARY

The promotion of health is extremely important today. Nurses and other health care providers are involved in identifying needed changes in behavior, lifestyle, or both for the achievement of optimum health or wellness. Defining the terms used in describing health is important in identifying health-promotion outcomes, and the terms used in defining health must reflect the holistic nature of individuals. High-level wellness, for example, involves a dynamic state of wellness that occurs at the individual, environmental, cultural, and social levels. Key to high-level wellness is an understanding of the capacity and potential of the biological, psychological, sociological, cultural, and spiritual human being. The concepts of wellness, disease prevention, and health protection are subsumed in the definition of health promotion.

Theoretical frameworks provide structure and guidance for applying the abstract concepts of theory to a vast array of real circumstances for promoting health for individuals, groups, and communities. Several theories have been developed to explain, describe, or predict human behavior and how this behavior is related to health outcomes and the promotion of health. Each one of us is an individual with unique characteristics, personalities, qualities, intentions, and motivations.

TABLE 3-3 Sample Health-Promotion Plan for the Community

Health-promotion need: Need for community program to augment retirement life for older adults.

Assessment data: Community of 35,000 with 30% over age 65 (United States has average of 13% over age 65). There is one community center but no programs for older adults and no senior citizen centers.

Outcome measure(s): The community will establish a program to enhance retirement life for older adults.

PLAN OF ACTION: OBJECTIVES	IMPLEMENTATION	RESOURCES	SUPPORTS/ CONSTRAINTS	EVALUATION
1. Identify retirement issues of older adults in the community	Form a task force Develop a needs assessment survey Recruit volunteers to conduct survey	Churches, garden club, and barber shop Community newspaper, volunteered printing and copying	Several older adults among city leaders Lack of monetary resources	Task force of six members formed, including two city leaders 600 needs assessment surveys completed at seven churches, four supermarkets, and two hardware stores
2. Develop program to address retirement issues	Establish a community action committee Develop program Present program to City Council	Financial planner, community health nurse, recreation coordinator, and retirees willing to develop program	Community center has space and time for planning and conducting meetings and program No budget for program	Program developed addressing six major retirement issues Program presented to city council and approved with allocation of budget
3. Implement program	Develop schedules, market program, and implement program	Part-time program coordinator hired with city council funds to manage implementation	Community action committee to serve as advisory to coordinator	Use questionnaires to evaluate program effectiveness

There is no one exactly like us in the entire world. As a result, no one theory or model can be applied universally. Theories and models, however, are not only useful but necessary in providing a foundation for practice that is grounded in science. There are theories and models that attempt to explain:

1. Human behavior and health (Theory of Planned Behavior, Health Belief Model, Protection Motivation Theory, Transtheoretical Model).
2. Organization and community health promotion (Consumer Information Processing Model, Diffusion of Innovations Theory, PRECEDE-PROCEED Model).
3. Individual health promotion using the Pender Health Promotion Model.

The theories and models of health promotion provide nursing with the tools necessary to develop comprehensive health-promotion plans for clients, families, and communities. These health-promotion plans are developed jointly with clients because clients are considered the experts regarding their own health. The client's plan focuses on wellness and determines the factors that act in concert to influence health. Development of the health-promotion plan involves assessment, identification of outcomes, planning, and implementation and evaluation phases.

KEY CONCEPTS

1. Defining what constitutes health is complex. There is agreement that health encompasses the total functioning of an individual.
2. The concept of health refers to high-level personal functioning; the concept of wellness refers to high-level functioning and more.
3. High-level wellness challenges individuals to live to their full potential in all areas involving the whole being.
4. Health promotion is any activity useful in enhancing the quality of health and well-being of individuals, families, groups, and communities.

5. The terms *wellness*, *health protection*, and *disease prevention* are all subsumed under the concept of health promotion.

6. The theories and models focusing on human behavior originated in the field of behavioral psychology in an attempt to explain or predict why humans do what they do. Health care researchers added a disease-prevention/health-protection focus. The recent emphasis on the promotion of health has resulted in the generation of theoretical frameworks and models aimed at enhancing health and well-being. Biological, psychological, cultural, and social factors are predominant in these theories and models.

7. Personal responsibility and a sense of control in the client (individual or group) are key concepts for the promotion of health. Belief in the ability to do what is required for the desired health-promoting behavior (self-efficacy), along with the necessary skills, resources, and support, is a major component influencing the behavioral outcome.

8. Theories and models can be used in planning for the health-promoting behavioral outcomes of individuals, families, groups, communities, or nations. For nurses, using a systematic approach, or a combination of approaches from different theories or models, empowers the client through introspection, communication, and the coordination of resources directed toward commitment to the achievement of a health-promotion outcome.

9. Strategies for the development of a health-promotion plan include empowerment of the client through active involvement in development of the plan, collection of data for assessment, and recognition of resources useful in supporting the plan.

10. A positive nurse-client relationship is important in the promotion of client health.

11. The nurse facilitates client learning, provides support for clients undergoing behavioral and lifestyle modifications, and identifies options in the achievement of client health-promotion goals.

CHAPTER REVIEW

Learning Activities

1. Describe your personal definition of health. Remember at least three different situations or occasions when you felt extremely healthy. Include how you felt during those times in your personal definition of health.

2. Develop a health-promotion plan for Mr. and Mrs. M, a young couple in their early 20s with a 1-month-old daughter. This couple wants to know how to keep themselves and their baby healthy. There is a history of cancer on the wife's side. They do not seek regular screenings in relation to their health risks.

3. Think about a specific time when you tried to improve your health by focusing on a specific health-related outcome (e.g., quit smoking, losing weight). How did your feelings of self-efficacy help you achieve your health goal? Make a list of prior related factors that influenced your ability to achieve the health outcome goal. Identify personal and biopsychosocial factors that had a direct effect on achieving the desired health-promoting behavior.

Multiple Choice Questions

1. Which one of the following terms is defined as any activity useful in enhancing the quality of health and well-being of individuals, families, groups, and/or nations?
   a. Disease prevention
   b. Health protection
   c. Health promotion
   d. High-level wellness

2. Which one of the following models conceptualizes change in behavior through a five-stage progression that incorporates thought, action, and time?
   a. Consumer Information Processing Model
   b. Health-Promotion Model
   c. PRECEDE-PROCEED Model
   d. Transtheoretical Model

3. Which of the following statements most accurately represents a health-promotion plan as opposed to a nursing process plan?
   a. A health-promotion plan includes existing or potential health problems.
   b. A health-promotion plan emphasizes the achievement of optimal health outcomes.
   c. A health-promotion plan recognizes the health care provider as the expert regarding the client's health needs.
   d. A health-promotion plan focuses on process rather than on outcomes.

4. You are a member of a community group seeking to adopt a new program that creates a bicycle lane along a popular main street in town. Which of the following model are most appropriate for this project?
   a. Consumer Information Processing Model
   b. Diffusion of Innovations Model
   c. Health-Promotion Model
   d. PRECEDE-PROCEED Model

5. Using the Pender Model of Health Promotion, which of the following comments indicate a commitment to action in a client whose goal is to reduce personal stress?
   a. "I know I can learn to do relaxation meditation."
   b. "I want to feel more relaxed."
   c. "My husband and I are going on a vacation in two months."
   d. "My yoga class begins next Tuesday."

ORGANIZATIONS AND WEBSITES

National Cancer Institute: Theory at a Glance provides an overview of health-promotion theories and describes their importance in planning, implementing, and evaluating health-promotion programs: **http://www.cancer.gov/cancertopics/cancerlibrary/theory.pdf**

Ontario Health Promotion e-Bulletin: A weekly online newsletter for people interested in health promotion. It provides information on education opportunities, projects, issues, and resources: **http://www.ohpe.ca/node**

PRECEDE-PROCEED Model: Web page of the originator: **http://www.lgreen.net/precede.htm**

REFERENCES

Ajzen, I. (2002). *Theory of planned behavior.* Retrieved from www.people.umass.edu

Anderson, R. N., & Smith, B. L. (2005, March 7). Deaths: Leading causes for 2002. *National Vital Statistics Reports, 53*(17). National Center for Health Statistics. Retrieved from http://www.cdc.gov/nchs/data/nvsr/nvsr53/nvsr53_17.pdf

Bettman, J. R. (1979). *An information processing theory of consumer choice.* Reading, MA: Addison-Wesley.

Bulecheck, G., Butcher, H. & Dochterman, J. (eds.). (2008). *Nursing interventions classification (NIC),* 5th ed. St. Louis, MO: Mosby/Elsevier.

Buller, D. B. (2005). Randomized trial testing a worksite sun protection program in an outdoor recreation industry. *Health Education & Behavior, 32*(4), 514–535.

Bumsted, M. M., Smith, S. N., Cross, P. S., Cochran, T. M., Bromm, M. M., & Jensen, G. M. (2003). Using the PRECEDE-PROCEED model to improve health and wellness of American Indian elders. *Journal of Geriatric Physical Therapy, 26*(3), 41.

Centers for Disease Control and Prevention. (2011). Leading causes of death. *Faststats.* Retrieved from http://www.cdc.gov/nchs/fastats/lcod.htm

Cole, R. E., & Horacek, T. (2010, May–June). Effectiveness of the "My Body Knows When" intuitive-eating pilot program. *American Journal of Health Behavior, 34*(3), 286–297.

De Civita, M., & Dasgupta, K. (2007, June). Using diffusion of innovations theory to guide diabetes management program development: An illustrative example. *Journal of Public Health, 29*(3). Retrieved from http://jpubhealth.oxfordjournals.org/content/29/3/263.short

Definitions of Wellness. (2011). Retrieved from http://www.definitionofwellness.com/index.html.

Delobelle, P., Onya, H., Langa, C., Mashamba, J., & Marie Depoorter, A. (2010). Advances in health promotion in Africa: Promoting health through hospitals. *Global Health Promotion, 17*(2 Suppl). Retrieved from http://ped.sagepub.com/content/17/2_suppl/33.full.pdf+html

Dunn, H. L. (1959). High-level wellness for man and society. *American Journal of Public Health, 49,* 786–792.

Dunn, H. L. (1973). *High-level wellness.* Arlington, VA: Beatty.

Eshah, N., Bond, E., & Froelicher, E. S. (2010). The effects of a cardiovascular disease prevention program on knowledge and adoption of a heart healthy lifestyle in Jordanian working adults. *European Journal of Cardiovascular Nursing, 9*(4), 244–253.

Fahrenwald, N., & Walker, S. N. (2003). Application of the transtheoretical model of behavior change to the physical activity behavior of WIC mothers. *Public Health Nursing, 20*(4), 307–317.

Godin, G., & Kok, G. (1996). The theory of planned behavior: A review of its applications to health-related behaviors. *American Journal of Health Promotion, 11*(2), 87–95.

Green, L. W. (2005). *The Precede-Proceed Model of health program planning and evaluation.* Retrieved from http://lgreen.net

Green, L. W., & Kreuter, M. W. (2005). *Health program planning: An educational and ecological approach,* 4th ed. New York, NY: McGraw-Hill Higher Education.

Karsh, B. (2004). Beyond usability: Designing effective technology implementation systems to promote patient safety. *Quality & Safety in Health Care, 13*(5), 388–394.

Kratzke, C., Garzon, L., Lombard, J., & Karlowicz, K. (2010). Training community health workers: Factors that influence mammography use. *Journal of Community Health, 35*(6), 683–688.

Lafferty, C. K., & Mahoney, C. A. (2003). A framework for evaluating comprehensive community initiatives. *Health Promotion Practice, 4*(1), 31–44.

McGinnis, J. M., Williams-Russo, P., & Knickman, J. R. (2002). The case for more active policy attention to health promotion. *Health Affairs, 21,* 78–93.

Mo, P. K., & Mak, W. W. (2008). Application of the PRECEDE model to understanding mental health promoting behaviors in Hong Kong. *Health Education Behavior, 35*(4), 574–587.

National Cancer Institute. (2005). *Theory at a glance: A guide for health promotion practice.* Retrieved from http://www.cancer.gov/cancertopics/cancerlibrary/theory.pdf

New England Inhalant Abuse Coalition. (n.d.). *New England Inhalant Abuse Coalition: Our Approach.* Retrieved from http://www.inhalantprevention.org/coalition/background/intro.html

O'Donnell, M. P. (2002). *Health promotion in the workplace* (3rd ed.). Clifton Park, NY: Delmar Cengage Learning.

Pender, N., Murdaugh, C. L., & Parsons, M. A. (2011)). *Health promotion in nursing practice* (6th ed.). Upper Saddle River, NJ: Pearson Education.

Prochaska, J. O. & DiClemente, C. C. (2005). The transtheoretical approach. In J. C. Norcross & M. R. Goldfried (eds.), *Handbook of psychotherapy integration.* New York, NY: Oxford University Press, 147–171).

Prochaska, J. O., Redding, C. A., & Evers, K. E. (1997). The transtheoretical model and stages of change. In K. Glanz, F. M. Lewis, & B. K. Rimer (eds.), *Health behavior and health education: Theory, research, and practice.* San Francisco: Jossey-Bass, 60–82.

Rogers, E. M. (2003). *Diffusion of innovations* (5th ed.). New York, NY: Free Press.

Rogers, R. W. (1975). A protection motivation theory of fear appeals and attitude change. *Journal of Psychology, 91,* 93–114.

World Health Organization. (2009). *Global health risks: Mortality and burden of disease attributable to selected major risks.* Retrieved from http://www.who.int/healthinfo/global_burden_disease/GlobalHealthRisks_report_full.pdf

CHAPTER 4
The Role of the Nurse in Health Promotion

CAROLINA G. HUERTA, EdD, MSN, RN

KEY TERMS

advocate
community
coordinator of care
culture broker
domains

empowerment
expected outcomes
interventions
nursing diagnosis
nursing process

primary disease prevention
secondary prevention
spiritual health
taxonomy
tertiary prevention

OBJECTIVES

Upon completion of this chapter, the reader should be able to:

- Identify domains fundamental to nursing practice in health promotion.
- Describe how the technological domain impacts the domains fundamental to nursing practice in health promotion.
- Define holistic nursing practice in relation to health promotion.
- Describe the role of the professional nurse in health promotion for the individual, family, and community.
- Describe the steps of the nursing process in health promotion.
- Define specific nursing responsibilities for promoting health during each phase of the nursing process: assessment, analysis of data, diagnosis, planning, implementation, and evaluation.
- Utilize the nursing process in promoting health in individuals, families, and communities.
- Identify risk factors or potential problems influencing health.
- Identify current factors affecting nursing roles in health promotion.

INTRODUCTION

The role of the nurse in health promotion has expanded over time. Nursing's role in the care of patients has evolved from a physician-focused model of medical management to one that includes independent nursing function and practice, advocacy, and leadership with the goal of promoting individual, family, and community health. Today's nurse is practicing in exciting yet challenging times.

The focus on the discipline of nursing is intense and provides nursing with the opportunity to strengthen its voice and to practice to its full extent. This increased scrutiny on the discipline of nursing has led to important reports such as the Institute of Medicine of the National Academies' *Future of Nursing* (2010) that is helping nursing respond effectively to the rapidly changing health care system and the role of the nurse in providing and promoting quality care to all. Health promotion in nursing is a continual, active process necessary to achieve and maintain the condition of wellness. Health promotion is a multi- and transdisciplinary practice whose aim is to improve and maintain health and that has been an integral part of nursing practice throughout history. Health promotion must be delivered holistically and encompass care delivered by other health care professionals as well (Blue & Black, 2008).

Promoting health has been a fundamental goal of nursing and has been emphasized in the public arena as a key to optimum wellness. The desired outcome has obvious benefits for individuals and society as a whole. Not only does the concept of health promotion decrease medical costs and morbidity, but its focus on health maintenance also increases the quality of life and life expectancy. By limiting the number of people requiring hospitalization, treatment, and continued care, health promotion and maintenance provide a solution to the health care dilemma. Nursing's role in health promotion, although expanded, has changed little over time. Technological developments have impacted the delivery of nursing care, yet nursing's focus continues to be the alleviation of suffering and the enhancement of health and wellness.

Previous chapters have defined health promotion, identified nursing concepts related to health promotion, and addressed health-promotion models and theoretical foundations related to health promotion. This chapter focuses on domains fundamental to nursing practice and health promotion, concepts related to health and wellness, holism, nursing roles in health promotion, and the nursing process.

DOMAINS FUNDAMENTAL TO NURSING PRACTICE IN HEALTH PROMOTION

Many factors can influence whether an individual achieves a state of optimal health or wellness. These factors consist of internal and external influences that can be considered separately or combined. These internal and external factors can be classified in terms of domains and dimensions that provide the nurse with a holistic approach to nursing practice. These **domains**, or areas of concern affecting optimal health, are fundamental to health promotion and include biological or physiological, psychological, sociological, environmental, political, spiritual, intellectual, sexual, and technological factors. Figure 4-1 depicts domains and dimensions affecting optimal health. These

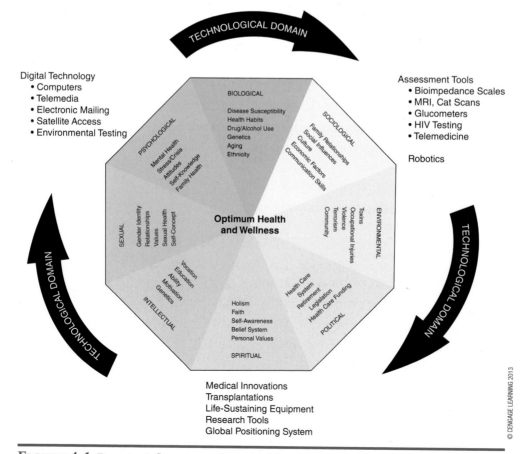

FIGURE 4-1 Domains influencing optimum health and wellness.

domains are described in this chapter and referred to throughout this textbook.

BIOLOGICAL DOMAIN

Physiological and genetic composition predisposes individuals to disease or wellness. Biological factors can influence our susceptibility to disease and serve as predictors of potential health problems. No disease is entirely ethnicity-specific, and some have more to do with genetics; however, many health problems are identified among specific ethnic groups. For instance, persons from African American and Native American populations are more likely to experience hypertension. A higher incidence of diabetes mellitus has been found among the African American, Native American, Mexican American, Filipino, and Jewish American populations. Stomach cancer is more prevalent among Japanese and Korean populations than in any other racial or ethnic group (Parker, Johnson-Davies, et al., 2008). Individuals' health, then, may be dependent on conditions that are beyond their control and that have more to do with genetics and the genomic interactions with the environment and other psychococial and cultural factors (Calzone, Cashion, Freetham, Jenkins, Prows, Williams, & Wung, 2010). Of course, individuals may respond to health-promoting lifestyle changes. It is becoming apparent among health care workers that lifestyle education may promote health among all people. For more on the influence of genetics on health, refer to Chapter 12.

PSYCHOLOGICAL DOMAIN

The psychological domain, or the mental health, of an individual plays a significant role in promoting wellness and preventing disease. Feelings of depression can make the difference between whether a person gets up and goes to school or work or stays in bed and calls in sick. A person's perceptions of health and well-being are reflected in behavior and attitude. The relationship between psychological factors and physical illness is recognized when individuals respond to stress. Persons who are compulsive, obsessively clean, and prompt are more likely to develop ulcerative colitis than persons who are not perfectionists. Self-knowledge and desire are necessary to initiate healthy behaviors (Craven & Hirnle, 2009). For example, persons with hypertension and high cholesterol who exercise regularly and follow prescribed dietary instructions likely recognize the potential health problems that could develop without changes in lifestyle. People who have negative perceptions about their body limitations resulting from illness, such as heart failure or cancer, may not be so able to comprehend instructions and may not benefit as much from health teaching.

People use their developmentally determined sense of self-esteem and identity to meet their basic needs. Obviously, individuals respond to crisis depending on their personal development and individual needs All health-promotion planning, then, should be based on the broad participation of patients and all those involved in their health-promotion activities (Bartholomew et al., 2011). Nurses are in a unique position to facilitate the processes of adapting and coping in their interactions with patients.

SOCIOLOGICAL DOMAIN

How a person relates to others in the family, community, or society influences individual responsiveness to health-promotion

---

SPOTLIGHT **ON**

Health Domains and Nursing's Metaparadigm

Consideration of all the domains that might affect a person's health is essential to providing nursing care and adds to our understanding of nursing's metaparadigm, as described in Chapter 2. For example, in caring for a 65-year-old Hispanic male who has little formal education and who is receiving home health services for congestive heart failure, the nurse must consider all of the domains that might be affected. The nurse notes that the patient's current physiological impairments relate to his previous physiological state (biological domain) that includes diabetes and cardiovascular disease. The limits imposed by his illness may affect his psychological functioning, especially if he has led a very active life. The sociological impact of his illness on his family and perhaps his cultural and spiritual needs are important in planning care. The effect of the technological domain on the other domains must also be considered. For example, if the patient has little awareness of how to access health-related information from computers, he must depend on health care professionals to provide the information and education needed to alleviate symptoms. All of the domains must be considered in providing an individualized health-promotion plan.

---

activities. Social mores often affect the health practices of an individual within a community. For instance, some African Americans or Mexican Americans may seek guidance from folk healers before seeking assistance from local health professionals. Trusting in the health care professional and valuing one's health are the foundation of health-promotion practices (Dayer-Berenson, 2011).

Accessibility to health care is an additional sociological factor influencing positive or negative outcomes of health promotion. Economic factors must also be considered. In low-income

---

? ASK **YOURSELF**

Mental Status and Health Promotion

Will the person who is hospitalized for cardiac problems and now suffering from depression be readily responsive to information on how to promote a healthy lifestyle? How does a person's psychological outlook affect nursing needs?

families, transportation or money may not be available to seek medical attention or to buy food or medication. The lack of information is also a barrier to health care for persons living in rural, underdeveloped communities.

As mentioned in Chapter 2, many nursing theorists consider sociological influences as integral parts of their theoretical frameworks. These theorists view people holistically and recognize that a person is a biological, psychological, social being. One theorist who focused extensively on the influence of sociological as well as cultural factors is Madeleine Leininger (1978), whose theory recognizes society's influence on health and its cultural definitions.

ENVIRONMENTAL DOMAIN

Primary environmental hazards are found in the home, workplace, and community. Obviously, safety is a chief concern in all these areas, but awareness of it is especially important in the home. Potential hazards are often overlooked until an accidental drowning, fall, or burn occurs. Most individuals think their home is poison proof or that firearms are stored properly. People seldom think of garbage, radon, lead, formaldehyde, carbon monoxide, and tobacco as home hazards. Yet statistics show that the home is often the most dangerous place of all. Far from unusual are accounts of child poisonings or accidental shootings in the news. For example, accidents were the fifth leading cause of mortality reported in our country in 2007 (Centers for Disease Control and Prevention, 2011).

Educational programs and community assessments by health care professionals on the hazards found in our own backyard could prevent thousands of accidents that occur yearly and take people's lives. For example, 14 children died when their school bus was sideswiped by another car and went over a ravine into a creek. Obviously, a protective fence around the creek or the use of seat belts could have saved some of these lives. Perhaps if the school district or the community health care workers had conducted an assessment of potential hazards along the bus routes, such a senseless tragedy could have been avoided.

At the workplace, in addition to the obvious hazards (such as sanitation and chemicals), other conditions pose threats: noise, temperature, infectious agents, physical agents (such as motor vehicles), radiation, and psychological stress. Environmental toxins and pollutants can affect our health status. The 2011 major earthquake in Japan and its concomitant threat of radiation exposure is one example of the importance of addressing the environmental domain (Roan, 2011). The community may provide public information describing environmental hazards and safety precautions. A nurse with a holistic approach is in a unique position to raise awareness of the importance of environmental factors in promoting health. For further description on how the environment relates to health promotion, refer to Chapter 7.

POLITICAL DOMAIN

Bureaucratic policies influence and are directly responsible for funding health care programs, and government policy directly affects community health goals. In the past three decades, policies influencing health care have changed drastically. The decentralization of health care has led to the duplication of services and excessive health care costs. Today, health care programs are often limited or eliminated. Limited funding is a major concern to the public as well as to health care professionals. Federal,

state, and local fund reductions may limit or totally eliminate specific health care programs.

Health care professionals provide the health-promotion activities needed in the community and require political support for them. Professional nurses may be involved in health promotion at the national and local government levels through lobbying and actively participating in national nursing organizations and in community or regional health task forces. Disease prevention is the primary focus of the health care system today. The government is focusing on health promotion and prevention to encourage a healthy society and to reduce health care costs. *Healthy People 2020* (U.S. Department of Health and Human Services, 2010) describes health problems and objectives for health promotion for the United States. This document has proven beneficial in providing a political impetus for the creation, expansion, and funding of health care legislation and programs in the United States.

SPIRITUAL DOMAIN

An individual's beliefs and value systems may affect decisions regarding health and life. Spiritual values and beliefs may be barriers to health care among certain population groups. For example, Jehovah's Witnesses do not believe in blood transfusions or the injection of blood products. Caring for patients of faiths different from ours may necessitate a personal spiritual assessment and perhaps the development of alternate approaches to nursing problems. All nurses should identify individual beliefs to ensure that any barriers to health are identified and preventive measures are implemented.

Spiritual health may be identified as a balance between self and others. Spiritual distress may occur when there is an imbalance. Individual faith and hope promote health and foster coping ability in times of stress. Nurses must consider the spiritual domain because unresolved spiritual distress may lead to hopelessness, anxiety, and depression (LeMone, Burke, & Bauldoff, 2011). The nurse should recognize a person's need for rituals and respect family roles.

? ASK **YOURSELF**

Spiritual Domain and Decision Making

As a pediatric nurse, could you work with a patient's family whose religious beliefs did not permit the administration of medications for their critically ill child? Would your own spiritual beliefs and biases affect your nursing care?

The health-promoting nurse recognizes that all people have diverse spiritual and family role needs. Professional nurses may care for patients whose beliefs are much different from their own; consequently, they should perform a spiritual self-assessment to reveal their biases as well as spiritual strengths. Only through an honest recognition of personal spiritual beliefs can nurses assist others in their health-promoting decision making.

RESEARCH NOTE

Improving Health Outcomes in Grandmothers Raising Grandchildren

STUDY PROBLEM/PURPOSE

To examine the effects of an intervention program aimed to improve the health of grandmothers who are raising their grandchildren in parent-absent homes.

METHODS

A convenience sample of 529 female caregivers, primarily African Americans, agreed to participate in the study. Inclusion criteria for the study included grandmothers or great-grandmothers raising one or more grandchildren 16 years of age or younger in parent-absent homes. A longitudinal pretest-posttest design was used. Data were collected prior to the intervention and again at 12 months when the intervention was complete. The intervention involved home visits by registered nurses and social workers. A survey was used to assess physical and mental health, using eight multi-item scales.

FINDINGS

A comparison of pre- and posttest mean scores on the survey indicated significantly improved mean scores for vitality, physical effects on role functioning, emotional effects on role functioning, and mental health. The findings suggest that grandmothers raising grandchildren may benefit from a home-based intervention designed to improve health.

IMPLICATIONS

The study provided support for the use of nurse-based interventions to address the health challenges experienced by grandmothers who are raising grandchildren.

Source: Kelley, S., Whitley, D. M., & Campos, P. E. (2010). Grandmothers raising grandchildren: Results of an intervention to improve health outcomes. *The Journal of Nursing Scholarship, 42*(4), 379–386.

INTELLECTUAL DOMAIN

In considering the domains influencing nursing practice and health promotion, it is important to recognize the influence of the intellectual domain. A person's intellect may determine his or her understanding of illness, needed lifestyle changes, and hospitalization.

People are born with certain intellectual abilities that are primarily defined genetically and subsequently cultivated by their environment. The intellectual domain is also influenced by psychological and biological factors. Individuals are born with some degree of intellectual ability, yet a person's desire or motivation to achieve or not achieve may determine the level to which the ability is developed. Environmental influences within the home, school, and community contribute to an individual's perception of success or failure. Although nurses do not perform IQ tests on their patients, they need to recognize the impact of the intellect on all health-promotion activities.

SEXUAL DOMAIN

The sexual domain is private and may or may not be openly discussed. Values based on upbringing and social influences, perhaps, may underlie sexual identity. Sexual expression, attitudes, and orientation may change or become more evident as one matures from adolescence to young adulthood; consequently, health risks associated with sexual activities increase (Belcher, 2008). The health professional demonstrates a nonjudgmental attitude toward a person's sexuality in order to promote trust and confidence. However, sexual identity and sexual history should be determined in order to recognize potential health problems not only for the individual but for others as well. For example, nurses working with a population at risk for human immunodeficiency virus (HIV) would be remiss if they did not include an assessment of a person's sexual practices that may, in turn, affect health practices and lifestyle behaviors.

TECHNOLOGICAL DOMAIN

Although considered a separate domain in this text, the technological domain affects all the others. As depicted in Figure 4-1, technology can affect biological, psychological, sociological, environmental, political, intellectual, spiritual, and sexual functioning. For example, technology affects the biological domain by influencing outcomes brought about by life-threatening situations. Technology is largely responsible for organ transplantation, a fairly common procedure that can lead to a longer and fuller life for those afflicted with a debilitating organ injury or failure. The psychological domain, too, is influenced by technology that allows viewing of the structures of the entire brain, thus assisting in the diagnosis of causes for defects in psychological functioning. In the sociological and intellectual domains, technology has made it possible for individuals to research symptoms and conditions on the

GLOBAL HIGHLIGHTS IN HEALTH PROMOTION
International Focus on Health Promotion

A health-promotion focus is not unique to United States health professionals. Nurses and health professionals in other countries are also expected to educate patients in health-promotion activities. The South Asian Institute of Health Promotion, for example, is affiliated with the India Research Institute specializing in public health and education. This is a nonprofit, nongovernmental organization that strives toward health promotion and the prevention of infectious and noncommunicable diseases through multidisciplinary cross-cutting research and awareness, and the generation and dissemination of pertinent health-promotion information.

Source: South Asian Institute of Health Promotion (SAIHP), India. Global Development Network. Retrieved from http://cloud2.gdnet.org/cms .php?id=organization_details&organization_id=2979

Internet, communicate with health care specialists, and socialize via email with their peers and family members who may not be with them during their illness.

Innovations such as computers, digital technology, tele-media, email, satellite access, various assessment tools, robotics, and other medical discoveries have influenced the achievement of health promotion and wellness. The popular use of electronic health records technology has revolutionized care because patient records are readily accessible to the health care team, and the planning of care is focused on safety and efficiency. Technological advances increase learning and the speed of processing information. Globalization and knowledge sharing are expanding through technology.

HOLISTIC PHILOSOPHY

The holistic philosophy views the total individual in all domains in an accepting, caring manner to promote optimum health and wellness. Health promotion from a holistic perspective involves the total person, biological and psychological, affected by numerous external and internal influences. An individual may have multiple nursing diagnoses that represent separate systems or domains, yet holistic practice continues to look at the person as a whole being.

HOLISTIC NURSING PRACTICE

As described in Chapter 2, the holistic approach to nursing refers to a view of people in their entirety or totality. Holistic nursing practice, then, involves caring for individuals in their entirety, including all the aforementioned domains. **Nursing process**, on the other hand, refers to a problem-solving method for developing an appropriate plan of care and wellness outcomes for patients. Nursing care is delivered through this process, and the given subject matter (individual, family, and community) is viewed in a systematic manner with the ultimate goal being individualized care (Craven & Hirnle, 2009). Holistic nursing centers on the individual and family and on an individual's rights and ability to cope. All domains are considered in order to provide holistic care.

The cultural, spiritual, psychosocial, intellectual, and biological domains contain differences that must be addressed

to selectively and purposefully meet individual needs. Each domain possesses a dichotomy in that health promotion can be helped or hindered, depending on the characteristic found or adhered to by the individual patient or aggregate. Because cultural influences may block positive actions toward healthy lifestyle changes, the nurse must be knowledgeable regarding cultural variables and individual beliefs. This knowledge is vital to formulate positive health action plans.

In a holistic approach, the nurse recognizes how spiritual beliefs may influence health-promoting actions by individuals and act accordingly. Understanding spiritual beliefs enables the nurse educator to collaboratively select appropriate approaches to promoting care with individuals. Although some spiritual beliefs may limit health-promotion choices (e.g., no exercise from sundown Friday to sunup Sunday for Seventh Day Adventists), other beliefs expand options.

A holistic approach also recognizes psychosocial influences. An astute nurse is well aware that an individual's psychosocial status may affect how health and wellness are viewed. For example, financial strain limits the frequency of physician visits for routine health evaluations for some individuals; however, persons with insurance or financial resources may visit health care settings more frequently than necessary. Some individuals may not visit health care settings because they do not understand the need even though the financial means are present. Differences may create interest in one area of health promotion and less in another.

Probably one of the most important domains to consider when the nurse cares for a patient holistically—yet one that might be ignored—is the psychological domain. This domain includes mental as well as intellectual variables that also affect individual perception of health and health-promoting activities. For example, special populations such as the mentally challenged may require that patient education by nurses be addressed according to the individual levels of understanding of the patient. This population may also require special learning activities and more frequent assessments.

Biological differences may predispose persons to a weak or strong constitution. Susceptibility to specific disease may be prevalent among some ethnic groups. The African American population is more likely to suffer from sickle cell anemia than are European Americans (De, 2008). A holistic nurse practitioner is aware of individual biological differences and incorporates these differences into the plan of care.

An effective nurse focuses on interest areas first to encourage compliance and trust. As a result, the patient is ready to accept additional information regarding the disease processes and potential health hazards. Looking at individuals holistically provides a nonbiased, personal approach to health and disease prevention.

ROLES OF THE NURSE IN HEALTH PROMOTION

The role of the nurse in health promotion is complex, enveloping several roles into one (see Box 4-1). The nurse involved in health promotion assumes the usual roles commonly identified with the nursing profession: change agent, advocate, educator, empowering agent, coordinator of care, leader or member of the profession, provider of care, research user, and role model. In a health-promotion approach, the nurse empowers patients to care for and maintain their own health. Nurses need to shift from simply fulfilling their traditional functional roles

---

HEALTH PROMOTION THEORY LINK

Virginia Henderson's (1991) definition of nursing and health-promotion domains takes into account the domains fundamental to nursing practice. She sees the nurse as assisting individuals who are sick or well in any activities that contribute to health, recovery, or a peaceful death (p. 21). Nurses help patients to achieve independence as rapidly as possible. Henderson sees the person (patient) as being a biological, psychological, spiritual, social being, and she identifies 14 basic needs that address the biological, psychological, sociological, environmental, and spiritual domains that affect optimal health.

BOX 4-1
ROLES OF THE NURSE IN HEALTH PROMOTION

1. Activist/proactive change agent
2. Advocate
3. Educator
4. Empowering agent
5. Communicator
6. Consultant
7. Coordinator of care
8. Leader/member of a profession
9. Provider of care/caregiver
10. Research user
11. Health-promotion models researcher
12. Role model

to assuming greater responsibility in a much wider arena of action focusing on healthy people, on healthy environments, and on the challenges that occur in trying to transform nursing (Kearney, 2008). Consequently, the roles of the nurse involved in health promotion include those of empowering agent, proactive change agent, consultant, and, for those nurses with doctoral degrees, researcher testing health-promotion models.

ACTIVIST/PROACTIVE CHANGE AGENT

Inherent in the role of the nurse in health promotion is functioning as an activist and proactive change agent. Nurses should view themselves as clinical practitioners as well as social activists who can bring about social change (Wilkinson & Treas, 2011), which is essential in transforming the future. Nurses can make a difference beyond the clinical level by challenging institutional and political barriers that impede the progress toward wellness and health-promotion goals. The nurse who embraces a health-promotion approach to nursing care recognizes that a person is capable of initiating change and is competent in knowing self-needs. In the role of proactive change agent, the nurse performs a thorough assessment of the patient, family, and community. Once strengths and weaknesses are identified, the proactive change agent nurse builds on those strengths, enhances existing resources, and fosters support systems that enhance the person's ability to change (Pender, 1996).

ADVOCATE

The nurse represents the patient and the patient's needs at all times. An **advocate** is one who takes the patient's side and provides complete information to allow him or her to make decisions concerning individual health care (Craven & Hirnle, 2009). When a person's condition warrants an immediate appointment, the nurse may act as a referral agent and assist in obtaining the care deserved. As such, the nurse is the patient's representative. The nurse is responsible for facilitating the patient's well-being and for maintaining the patient's best interest. As an advocate, the nurse implements evidence-based measures to reduce risks and to promote quality care and a safe environment for the patient, self, and others [The Texas Board of Nursing (TBON), 2010].

EDUCATOR

The nurse-educator role does not require a specific setting. Education may occur in formal or informal places, in the hospital, home, or community. The role of the nurse as educator is one of the most important. Education to remedy health-promotion deficits is essential for solving problems. Posthospital telephone contact, for example, may lead to clarification and information pertaining to medication or diet regimen. Questions asked in the physician's office or clinic also afford the nurse the opportunity to instruct and explain health-promoting activities. Formal education programs may be offered to the public regularly so that public awareness of potential and actual health risks is heightened.

EMPOWERING AGENT

In contrast to other approaches to health care that focus on fear or threats to motivate behavior changes, the health-promotion model considers personal values and people's feelings about their ability to achieve goals as the primary motivation for health behavior changes (Pender, Murdaugh, & Parsons, 2011). Individuals receiving health care are thus empowered through their ability to self-direct and self-regulate. Nurses who recognize their responsibilities in health promotion also assume the role of empowering agents. As an empowering agent, the nurse emphasizes the active role of the recipient of care by including the individual in every aspect of it. The nurse empowers the patient, the family, the community, and other groups that may relate to the patient's situation. This empowering process can be the impetus for improving the health of communities and the quality of life for individuals, families, and communities (Pender, Murdaugh, & Parsons, 2011).

COMMUNICATOR

The role of the nurse as a communicator is especially important and is closely linked to the role of the nurse as empowering agent. **Empowerment**, in relation to health promotion, is the process of helping others to help themselves. For the nurse, this involves persuasion, support, and encouragement, all of which are conveyed through various modes of communication. Empowerment can best be accomplished through education, which is communicated in many ways to a patient. The role of the nurse as a communicator also involves communication with all who are involved in the patient's care. This collaborative, multidisciplinary approach to patient empowerment requires that the nurse be skillful in communicating. In fact, health promotion and health education cannot be achieved without the power of the nurse as a communicator. See Chapter 5 for further information on concepts related to communication in teaching/learning.

CONSULTANT

In the management of patient care, the nurse may be frequently called on to act as a consultant if a patient is unable to solve a personal health problem. The role of the nurse can include being a formal or informal consultant. In the role of consultant, the nurse assesses the problem situation, collects information, identifies the actual problem, and, in conjunction with the patient, determines appropriate solutions.

COORDINATOR OF CARE

The nurse acts as a **coordinator of care** to assure the appropriate sequence of events in the patient's plan of care.

Leadership skills are required to coordinate the plan of care and to refer patients to appropriate sources when indicated. In the role of coordinator of care, the nurse also functions as a facilitator by directing care within the health care system to meet patient needs and to prevent the duplication of services. As the coordinator of care, the nurse is expected to communicate and collaborate with members of the interdisciplinary health care team to promote and maintain the optimal health status of patients and their families (TBON, 2010). The nurse is knowledgeable regarding nursing issues and trends, societal changes, and community resources. A working relationship between the nurse and the individual, family, and community may determine whether the health care goals are achieved.

LEADER/MEMBER OF THE PROFESSION

Nurses are responsible for their own actions, for being health care advocates, and for serving as leaders of the nursing profession. Nurses assume responsibility and accountability for quality nursing care provided to patients and their families (TBON, 2010). To ensure accountability, nurses must keep their education in the field of practice current and implement research findings in day-to-day nursing. Leaders maintain the standards of care and edify the professional practice of nursing. Nurses apply the historical development of the profession to current trends in order to direct the profession to meet societal changes. As a leader, the nurse promotes ethical and legal standards, innovative practices, and service to the public to maintain a positive image for nurses.

Registered nurses are skilled in using a systematic approach in providing or coordinating health promotion, maintenance, and restoration. Nursing management and nursing care supervision are two responsibilities of the nurse.

PROVIDER OF PATIENT-CENTERED CARE

As a caregiver for health restoration, the nurse is actively involved in the nursing process, a problem-solving method for developing an appropriate plan of care and wellness outcomes for a patient, while continually assessing the person's responses to nursing interventions. Direct patient care may be delivered in the home, hospital, or community setting. The nurse assesses all domains of the individual, family, or aggregate populations and develops a plan of care, recognizing that the patient is the center focus of all nursing actions. Through the inclusion of the patient in the planning process, the caregiver better understands the community composition and resources available that may be influencing the outcomes of care. The plan of care is implemented after the nurse and patient establish appropriate, realistic goals. Through direct care, the nurse can evaluate the patient and determine whether needs are being met. After analysis and evaluation, the plan of care may be restructured at any time to further promote patient comfort and well-being.

RESEARCH USER AND HEALTH-PROMOTION MODELS RESEARCHER

As a research user, the nurse can play a significant role in advancing a theoretical knowledge base for health promotion and in facilitating patient outcomes utilizing contemporary, current knowledge and practice. Statistical evidence of nursing theory supports nursing actions and expands nursing science.

The conscientious nurse continues to use research findings, increase personal knowledge, and thereby improve patient care. The graduate level-educated nurse, usually one prepared at the doctoral level, can assume the role of a researcher who empirically tests health-promotion models, thus increasing the predictive value of health promotion in health care.

ROLE MODEL

Nurses represent the standards and quality of care defined within the limits of education, experience, and state licensing bodies. The general public has the right to expect safe, conscientious practice from nurses. Professionally, optimal standards of practice must be maintained for the achievement of the desired health care outcomes. As role models, experienced nurses exemplify the highest ideals of nursing practice, and they command admiration, trust, and respect from all health care professionals and persons receiving care.

Although nurses rarely view themselves as role models for future nurses, they must be seen by others as just that. As students and later on as professionals, these individuals are expected to abide by the highest standards of care and to show, through their actions, that they are truly worthy of the professional title "registered nurse."

OVERVIEW OF THE NURSING PROCESS

The nursing process is a problem-solving method that involves gathering and interpreting data to formulate a plan of care. The nurse is significant in determining the needs of the patient and in representing the individual. The nurse and patient jointly must identify nursing needs before the health-promotion nursing process plan can be formulated.

Nursing theories may be used in clinical practice within the nursing process to further the development and understanding of nursing practice and to provide the theoretical knowledge base for practice (Smith & Parker, 2010). Nursing theorists describe the various steps of problem solving as the nursing process. Although the process has a number of steps, they can be broadly categorized as (1) the assessment of the patient, (2) the identification of a need or potential need (analysis and diagnosis), (3) the development and implementation of a health care plan, and (4) evaluation of all areas.

The nursing process is a continual, ongoing process used to determine whether a health problem or potential health problem exists. The steps of the nursing process supported by the majority of nursing theorists and subsumed by the preceding four steps are:

1. Assessment
2. Analysis
3. Nursing diagnosis
4. Outcome identification
5. Planning
6. Implementation
7. Evaluation (American Nurses Association, 2010)

Patient responses are continually monitored to determine the effectiveness of care. Using the data collected, the nurse and patient determine what action is needed to provide the correction or prevention of the patient's condition. The nursing process in health promotion utilizes the steps of assessing, analysis and diagnosing, planning, implementing, and evaluating. The primary foci in the nursing process when utilized for health promotion appear to be its emphasis on wellness without a primary physical or mental condition, the empowerment of the individual, the promotion of lifestyle changes, and health enforcement. Health promotion seeks to expand positive potential for health with emphasis on strength, resiliencies, capability, and resources rather than on existing pathology (Pender, Murdaugh, & Parsons, 2011). The nurse looks at potential illnesses or problems and then seeks to provide preventive measures. For the nurse to be instrumental in health promotion, nurses must consider potential risk factors within the individual, family, or community. Among teenage girls, for example, the nurse would consider potential risk factors such as smoking, sexually transmitted diseases (STDs), and pregnancy, along with their potential effects on the individual, family, community, and society. Use of the nursing process in health promotion is congruent with the Pender Health Promotion Model (Pender, 1996) in that it seeks to increase wellness and actualize human potential.

ASSESSMENT (ACQUIRING INFORMATION)

The first step is the assessment of an individual, family, or community. The term **community**, when used in a health-promotion context, refers to a collection of like-minded people who work with each other and who have common traits and interests such as language, certain rituals, and special customs (Wilkinson & Treas, 2011). Members of a community identify themselves as such. They participate in activities to improve their community through planned change (Pender, Murdaugh, & Parsons, 2011). Assessment includes data collection, asking questions to learn as much as possible about the person, the identification of resources, and the recognition of barriers to goal achievement. Past medical history is important in formulating a diagnosis and developing a plan of action. Environment, culture, family background, educational level, social standing, and gender may contribute to the individual's perception of health or illness (Pender, Murdaugh, & Parsons, 2011). Assessment involves observing, questioning, inferring, and clarifying information to determine the appropriate nursing action.

Observation begins when the nurse first sees the individual seeking care. Skin color, gait, poise, demeanor, facial expression, and speech are among the characteristics to be noted. Psychiatric or neurologic impairment may be suggested on this first encounter.

Interviewing the individual gives inside information into the person's personal habits, perceptions, current state of mind, medical history, and spirituality. The nurse should ask open-ended questions and give the person time to speak. The nurse needs to be an active listener. A trusting, friendly rapport encourages a relaxed atmosphere.

Questions (who, what, where, when, why) are helpful in assessing the patient. Who is the patient? Who else lives in the home? Who is the caretaker? What symptoms are present? What has the patient done to relieve the problem? Where does he work? Where was the patient when symptoms began? When did symptoms begin? When did the patient first seek treatment? Why is the patient here? Why has previous treatment not been successful? Numerous assessment forms can be used. Institutions may choose to develop forms specific to their patient population.

ANALYSIS OF ASSESSMENT DATA (USING CRITICAL THINKING)

Although most textbooks describing the nursing process include nursing diagnosis as the step following assessment, merely collecting data in the assessment phase is not enough. The data collected must be critically examined prior to arriving at a nursing diagnosis. The data collected must be analyzed, synthesized, sorted and grouped according to commonalities and clustered in order to make sense of what it all means. The analysis of data provides the support needed to arrive at the nursing diagnosis. For example, in arriving at a nursing diagnosis of *hopelessness related to a personal loss*, a nurse caring for a patient with this diagnosis might have clustered the patient's data to include the following: a decrease in patient's affect, a decreased appetite, no patient verbalization, and decreased sleep. Other data that provides support for the nursing diagnosis of hopelessness might be included as well (e.g., death of a child or a history of antidepressant medication use). Data such as the patient's occupation, her vital signs, and level of education, for example, may have little relevance to support the diagnosis and therefore may not be clustered with the other items.

The analysis of data requires critical thinking on the part of the nurse, which involves the use of reason and judgment and a flexible, nonjudgmental, inquisitive approach (Wilkinson & Treas, 2011). In the analysis phase, the nurse must distinguish data that is relevant from that which is irrelevant and unimportant (Le Mone, Burke, Bauldoff, 2011). The analysis phase, then, is critical to the correct identification of a nursing diagnosis and the subsequent plan of care.

NURSING DIAGNOSIS

The **nursing diagnosis** consists of the actual identification of a patient's need and is formulated as described in the previous section after "the nurse establishes a database that includes the simultaneous consideration of the dynamic interactions of physiologic, psychological, sociocultural, developmental, and spiritual variables" (Fawcett, 2005, p. 178). Based on nursing knowledge and the patient history, the professional nurse establishes one or more specific nursing diagnoses.

The nurse does not confuse the nursing diagnosis with the medical diagnosis. The nursing diagnosis is specifically developed from the nursing perspective and is separate from the physician treatment plan. The diagnosis leads to the plan of care that the nurse will implement. The nursing diagnosis identifies a patient's needs and forms the basis for adopting a plan for nursing action.

Organizations such as the North American Nursing Diagnosis Association International (NANDA-I) develop terminology to describe important clinical decisions made by nurses for individuals, families, and communities (NANDA, 2009). The nursing diagnosis may be an actual need identified or a potential need that could develop in the future. According to NANDA-I (2009), nursing diagnoses provide the basis for determining nursing interventions needed to achieve outcomes for which the nurse assumes responsibility. NANDA-I has developed one of the most recognized classification systems with a listing of approved diagnoses. These nursing diagnoses are crucial to the selection of interventions and outcomes. Because of this, NANDA-I provides a **taxonomy**, or common classification structure that links nursing diagnoses, interventions, and outcomes. *The NNN Taxonomy of Nursing Practice* has been created and refined within the last several years to link nursing diagnoses, interventions, and outcomes. It was developed through the NNN Alliance of NANDA International, the Nursing Interventions Classification (NIC), and the Nursing Outcomes Classification (NOC). Box 4-2 lists several classification systems, including NANDA-I, used to support clinical decision making and to organize and categorize nursing phenomena.

Not all institutions have adopted the NANDA-I–approved diagnoses, but many have. The three parts of the nursing diagnosis for actual problems are (1) diagnosis, (2) cause, and (3) sign/symptom. Previous work by the NANDA focuses primarily on describing illness problems. For example, the actual nursing diagnosis for the patient with a decubitus ulcer should state: "Impaired skin integrity (diagnosis) related to decreased circulation (cause) as evidenced by an open sore on sacral area (sign/symptom)." For potential problems, only the first two parts of the nursing diagnosis are necessary. The potential nursing diagnosis for a patient with a family history of breast cancer should state, "Ineffective health maintenance (diagnosis) related to knowledge deficit regarding self-breast examinations (cause)."

Nursing theorists view health promotion and health maintenance as two distinct concepts. Previously, NANDA-I (2007) focused on health maintenance as well as health promotion; however, the latest NANDA-I (2009) is more focused on health promotion and has developed nursing diagnoses that incorporate health maintenance.

These nursing diagnoses look at health promotion as well as the concept of self-management (self-health maintenance) and include ineffective self-health maintenance, impaired home maintenance, readiness for enhanced immunization status, and self-neglect. Of the steps in the nursing process, assessment is the key determining factor for establishing nursing diagnoses and determining outcomes that are focused on the provision of a safe and effective plan of care.

PLANNING

From the nursing diagnosis, a plan of care is formulated and implemented. Outcome identification, or goal setting, is an important part of the planning stage. Once a nursing diagnosis is established, the nurse determines what outcomes are important to resolving the patient's problems. **Expected outcomes** are measurable goals set by the nurse and the patient, and they are derived from the patient's nursing diagnosis (Sparks-Ralph & Taylor, 2011). Outcomes or goals are either short or long term. Short-term outcomes are those directed toward immediate problems. "Long-term goals take more time to achieve and usually involve prevention, patient teaching, and rehabilitation" (Sparks-Ralph & Taylor, 2011, p. xvi). The patient's setting may also dictate the type of outcome expected. A goal for a patient in the emergency room, for example, might differ from one for the same patient receiving home health care.

The nursing care plan represents the goal or outcome that the individual patient should reach. Realistic goals are stated specifically and within a designated time frame. For example, a correctly stated goal reads: "Patient will breathe deeply and cough to remove secretion during the postoperative hospitalization period" or "Patient will reduce the number of cigarettes smoked from two packs to one pack per day within two weeks' time." The goal should be stated in measurable terms for evaluation purposes.

The nursing care plan is developed with potential problems or needs in mind. Appropriate nursing interventions and expected outcomes are identified. A quality nursing care plan decreases the risks of poor or incorrect care, gives direction by determining patient outcomes, provides for continuity of care, and serves as a method of communication on the health care team (Sparks & Taylor, 2011).

IMPLEMENTATION

Interventions, which are based on the nursing diagnoses, are nursing actions that enable the person to achieve the desired goal. Interventions for health promotion and/or health protection are identified during the implementation phase. Interventions directed at health promotion are motivated by the desire to increase wellness, whereas health-protection interventions are motivated by a patient's desire to avoid illness (Wilkinson & Treas, 2011). Patient interventions are determined by primary, secondary, or tertiary prevention. In **primary disease prevention**, high-level wellness is the goal. Primary disease prevention includes activities and lifestyle factors that can be changed or maximized. Ensuring adequate nutrition, exercising, taking immunizations, and preventing stress are good examples of primary disease prevention. **Secondary prevention** focuses on screenings that identify

---

BOX 4-2

SELECT CLASSIFICATION SYSTEMS

North American Nursing Diagnosis Association (NANDA)

North American Nursing Diagnosis Association International (NANDA International)

Nursing Interventions Classification (NIC)

Clinical Care Classification (CCC)

Nursing Outcomes Classification (NOC)

Nursing Management Minimum Data Set (NMMDS)

Patient Care Data System (PCDS)

International Classification for Nursing Practice (ICNP®)

abnormalities within a population and includes all health screenings and assessments. **Tertiary prevention** seeks to address the situation once symptoms have occurred. It is directed toward minimizing disease or disability and optimizing health (Wilkinson & Treas, 2011). Educating individuals about primary prevention may involve addressing unhealthy behaviors and mutually determining a plan to achieve wellness or optimum health. Secondary prevention involves assessing individual awareness of the importance of health screenings, such as lab tests for the assessment of diabetes or cholesterol. Tertiary prevention focuses on helping the ill person get well or live within certain limitations. Individual variables affect the lines of defense among physiological, psychological, sociological, developmental, or spiritual domains.

Critical to using the nursing process in health promotion is consideration of the interactions among all the factors influencing the health of the individual, the family, the community, or society at large (Pender, Murdaugh, & Parsons, 2011). In health promotion, interventions may occur either less or more frequently. Immunizations may be given to adults and children once a month in a community clinic. Nutrition classes for heart-healthy living or diabetes education may be conducted weekly or monthly. Interventions for health promotion may occur in the clinical setting or in the community. Tables 4-1 and 4-2 describe nursing diagnoses and interventions over the life span.

EVALUATION

The plan of action and the results of implementation should be evaluated regularly to determine whether the desired goals have been achieved. Accurate record keeping is essential to establish reference logs. Evaluation occurs after action has been implemented. Did the action do what was intended? Does the action need to change? Is the patient worse? The evaluation process is ongoing.

Any change in the patient's condition warrants a look at the current implementation of care and its merit. Has the goal been achieved? What has been accomplished? In all settings for health promotion, the nursing care plan is used for evaluation. The care plan may change hourly, daily, weekly, or monthly, depending on the patient's progress toward goal achievement.

NURSING PROCESS AND HEALTH PROMOTION FOR THE INDIVIDUAL, FAMILIES, AND COMMUNITIES

The nursing process involves looking at all domains affecting individuals, families, and communities. Motivation to seek action is determined by a desire to protect health, avoid illness, or enhance one's level of health regardless of illness (Pender, Murdaugh, & Parsons, 2011). The culture and social environment of the community influence health promotion for individuals, families, and communities. The models of health promotion described in Chapter 3 focus on preventive measures, educational efforts, policy making, and personal empowerment. All of these measures and concepts should be included in the nursing process health-promotion plan.

INDIVIDUAL

The individual may be viewed separately from the family and community as a sole being with unique physiological

and psychological complexity. The individual's perception of health and health risks determines specific health-seeking behaviors. In assessing an individual, careful attention must be focused on the health history regarding previous diseases or disabilities, lifestyle patterns, and knowledge of health condition/status. The individual may live alone or be a member of a family unit.

FAMILY

The family may be considered a separate open population system composed of a varying number of individuals. Families may be defined as couples, nuclear, blended, or extended. Relationships within the family among one or more individuals form subsystems within the family as a whole. Interpersonal relationships affect the family dynamics and create an atmosphere of stress or tranquility. Crises occur at differing frequencies and intensities among families. Coping abilities are represented in families with strong organization, positive personal values, and purposeful lifestyles. Dysfunctional families may promote disorganization within the family unit and create disharmony among its members. The nursing process, applied to the family unit, assesses the family structure, relationships, risk factors, and health education.

COMMUNITY

A community is a population of people with common interests and common values. A community may be determined by geographical proximity or by a common functional focus of individuals interacting as social units and sharing common interests (Pender, Murdaugh, & Parsons, 2011, p. 68). Examples of a community are pregnant teenage girls, persons who smoke cigarettes, and persons with tuberculosis. The assessment of communities includes a careful history, demographic information, lifestyle, and knowledge of health risks. Program planning that is focused on community health promotion utilizes steps similar to those of the nursing process: (1) assessing and identifying a problem or need, (2) diagnosing the problem, (3) creating a strategic action plan, (4) implementing the plan to achieve the desired outcome, and (5) evaluating the plan of action (Engelke, 2008).

RISK FACTORS AND HEALTH PROMOTION

A risk factor can include any personal habits, behaviors, environmental conditions, or inborn or inherited traits that affect a health-related condition (Harkness & DeMarco, 2012).

Risk factors may or may not be controllable. For example, cigarette smoking, blood pressure, weight, exercise, cholesterol, and stress may be controllable, but factors such as age, heredity, and gender cannot be. Health risk appraisal tools assist the nurse in the assessment of potential health problems by identifying specific factors that increase the risk of impairments or disabilities (Hulton, 2008). An example of a health risk appraisal tool utilizing domains is shown in Figure 4-2.

Some risk factors to be considered in the area of health promotion are environment, work, socioeconomic level, education, gender, cultural influences, and spiritual beliefs. The role of the nurse as educator is essential to resolving patient problems and providing direction on how to decrease risk factors.

TABLE 4-1 Sample Health Promotion Nursing Diagnoses across the Lifespan

AGE LEVEL	NURSING DIAGNOSIS EXAMPLES	INTERVENTIONS
Infant (Birth–1)	Ineffective breast-feeding pattern related to mother's deficient knowledge	Assess the mother's knowledge regarding breast-feeding. Identify barriers that may impact successful breast-feeding. Demonstrate appropriate breast-feeding technique. Assess mother's level of anxiety. Educate on anxiety-reducing techniques. Provide written information regarding successful breast-feeding practices. Evaluate baby's sucking ability. Keep baby awake and alert during feedings.
Children (1–14)	Risk for injury related to delayed developmental skills	Identify motor, mental, sensory, or musculoskeletal deficits. Include parents in educational session describing risks in the child's environment. Orient child to home environment. Instruct child and family on how to avoid accidents. Caution parents regarding dangers of playground and home, including information on the use of electrical equipment, water from the bathtub, placing toxic chemicals out of child's reach. Promote early childhood development programs. Begin educating children on lifelong health-promotion habits and health protection.
Adolescent and young adult (15–24)	Risk for poisoning related to lack of knowledge on risks associated with substance abuse	Provide information to adolescent and parents on the harmful and potentially lethal effects of abusing drugs and alcohol. Discuss consequences of peer pressure. Provide appropriate written materials related to abuse of drugs. Help identify potential stressors, depression, and related family issues. Provide available community resources to prevent or treat substance abuse. Discuss differences between medications that are prescribed and those available without a prescription. Listen nonjudgmentally.
Adult (25–64)	Risk for ineffective health maintenance related to chronic disease, stress, cardiovascular disease, and smoking	Discuss need for health maintenance routine. Encourage regular exercise, fitness, and sound nutritional practices. Provide information on appropriate health screenings for age. Teach effective stress reduction and coping skills. Involve person in decision making by providing choices. Identify barriers to performing activities unassisted. Review dietary habits. Educate on risk factors associated with a sedentary lifestyle.
Older adult (65 and older)	Activity intolerance related to deconditioned status	Mutually establish realistic goals for activity levels. Identify assistive devices helpful in increasing activity (e.g., cane, walker, shopping cart on wheels, or trapeze). Encourage rest period in between exercise activity. Establish progressive goals to increase activity. Encourage person to take part in exercise and social activities. Monitor for signs of weakness or fatigue. Educate on home safety to prevent accidents and reduce risk of falls.

TABLE 4-2 Nursing Diagnoses for the Individual, Family, and Community

INDIVIDUAL

Diagnosis: Decreased Cardiac Output

Interventions:	• Educate patient re: diet, exercise, medical screenings. • Provide activity information re: type of exercise, time required for effective prevention.	• Counsel patient re: diet and cholesterol. • Monitor vital signs, blood cholesterol at regular intervals.
Evaluation:	• What lifestyle changes are observed? • Does patient exercise regularly? • Are nutritional goals met? Is weight desirable?	• Does patient seek regular physical exams and attend wellness/illness clinics?

Diagnosis: Ineffective Health Maintenance Related to Uncontrolled Diabetes

Interventions:	• Educate patient re: disease, medication, diet, exercise. • Provide information re: community resources.	• Advise patient re: necessity for regularly scheduled appointments with health personnel. • Counsel patient.
Evaluation:	• Does patient follow medication regimen? • Can patient correctly describe the diet, exercise, and health regimen to follow and parameters for blood glucose?	• Does patient seek resources for assistance?

FAMILY

Diagnosis: Ineffective Health Maintenance Related to Safety Hazards in the Home

Interventions:	• Determine ages of family members. • Stress health-promotion activities.	• Educate family re: risk factors (wet floors, toys, visual disturbances, fire hazards, motor vehicle safety, etc.).
Evaluation:	• Lifestyle changes? • Is family demonstrating health-seeking behaviors?	• Does family attend safety seminars in the community or call for assistance?

Diagnosis: Impaired Parenting Related to Loss of Spouse

Interventions:	• Counsel patient re: primary role of lost partner. • Determine roles within family.	• Refer to counseling center.
Evaluation:	• Do child and parent communicate daily? • Does child behave appropriately?	• Does parent discipline and seek assistance in caring for child?

COMMUNITY

Diagnosis: Ineffective Community Coping Related to Increased Levels of Teen Pregnancy

Interventions:	• Counsel community regarding issues related to teen pregnancy. • Determine knowledge base of community.	• Implement outreach program to raise community awareness of the need to deal with teen pregnancy as a community problem.
Evaluation:	• Is community teen population demonstrating health-seeking behaviors?	• Is community demonstrating understanding of prevention?

Diagnosis: Ineffective Health Maintenance Related to Deficient Knowledge Regarding Smoking Risk Factors

Interventions:	• Provide information re: risk factors related to smoking. • Educate community re: ways to reduce risk factors.	• Provide health screenings (chest x-rays). • Monitor individuals' and community's willingness to reduce smoking hazard.
Evaluation:	• Is community demonstrating health-seeking behaviors?	• Do community members seek regular physical exams and attend wellness/illness checks?

Health Risk Appraisal According to Domains

Please complete the following:

Client Profile

Name _____   Age _____
Gender _____   Ethnicity _____
Occupation _____   Marital Status _____
Height _____   Weight _____
HDL _____   LDL _____
Total cholesterol _____   B/P _____

Biological Domain

Usual source of health care _____
Present health problem _____
Current perception of health (poor, fair, good, excellent) _____
List home treatment/complementary therapies _____
Current medications _____
Immunization status   DPT _____ Influenza _____ MMR _____
                      Varicella _____ Hepatitis _____ Polio _____
                      Pneumonia _____ Others _____
Screening tests   HIV _____ TB _____ PSA _____
                  Mammogram _____ Cervical Pap Smear _____
                  Other _____
Date of last health exam _____
Date of last dental exam _____
Date of last vision exam _____
Exercise routine _____
Numer of times exercise per week _____
Intensity of exercise (mild, moderate, intense) _____
Diagnosed   Diabetes _____ Heart disease _____ Other _____
Smoker (Yes/No)   No. of cigarettes per day _____

page 1 of 3

Psychological Domain

Engage in therapy (Yes/No) _____ Meditation _____ Yoga _____
Sleep patterns _____
Description of activities of daily living _____
Patterns of coping (poor, good, excellent) _____
Coping activities _____

Social Domain

Annual income _____
Living arrangements _____
Alcohol use (Yes/No) _____
Drug/substance use (Yes/No) _____
Coffee drinker/Cola drinker (Yes/No) _____ Amount _____
Recreational activities _____
Frequency of travel _____
Meal patterns _____
Person who cooks (self, mother, spouse, other) _____

Environmental Domain

Allergies (Yes/No) _____ To what _____
Home environmental concerns _____
Neighborhood concerns _____
Work-related risks _____
Sun exposure (never, occasionally, often) _____
History of violence (domestic, self-inflicted, other) _____
Number of accidents/speeding tickets in last year _____

Political Domain

Use of seatbelts (Yes/No) _____
Use of child safety seats _____
Use of helmet when on ATV, motorcycle, etc. _____
Insurance (Yes/No) _____
Medicare/Medicaid (Yes/No) _____

page 2 of 3

Spiritual Domain

Religion _____
Religious restrictions (describe) _____
Religious beliefs/practices _____

Intellectual Domain

Educational background _____
Reading proficiency _____
Language(s) spoken _____
Preferred language _____

Sexual Domain

Monogamous (Yes/No) _____
Number of sexual partners in previous year _____
Last Pap smear _____
Last mammogram _____
Last testicular exam _____

Technological Domain

Use of assistive devices (wheelchair, walker, cane, prosthesis, etc.) _____
_____
Any hearing aids, glasses, LASIK surgery _____
Computer literate (Yes/No) _____
Email, Internet accessibility _____

page 3 of 3

FIGURE 4-2 Health risk appraisal according to domains.

ENVIRONMENT

The environment often predisposes a person to disease processes. Living conditions may promote illness. For instance, among the bacterial and viral infections, tuberculosis is more prevalent in crowded living conditions. Persons in areas of contaminated water are at an increased risk for intestinal infections if sanitation measures are neglected. The role of advocate requires that nurses be cognizant of the environmental risk factors that exist and speak up to alleviate them.

WORK

Work influences health and wellness. Many employers—such as hospitals, factories, and large institutions—today provide health screenings and health prevention programs for employees. Work safety is imperative for optimum health and wellness. The number of dependents living in the home and the head of the household play a large part in the status of the family and of the individuals within the household.

The nurse may take an active role in developing community programs for individuals and their families. Often the small business owner is not able to provide health education programs routinely. The nurse may collaborate with small business owners to provide the needed information to employees.

SOCIOECONOMIC LEVEL

The socioeconomic level of an individual influences the affordability of health care and health-promotion activities. Often, funds are limited and the resources are unavailable to access the care required for optimum health. Persons may delay seeking treatment or information due to a lack of money. Nutrition and living conditions may affect the health risk of the individual as well.

EDUCATION

Education may influence the level of understanding among the public. Laypersons often do not have the knowledge base to know what causes a disease, much less how to prevent its development. Public education announcements and offerings of health information provide a beginning knowledge level and promote further learning. Education must be simple, clear, and understandable. Intellectual differences may influence the type and length of educational offerings. Nurses should speak at the educational level of their patients, communicating the message in simple terms. The caregiver may also require explicit information regarding patient needs. This information should be given at the educational level of the caregiver.

Health-seeking behavior is critical to implementing health promotion. For instance, a person who does not believe immunizations are necessary will probably reject them. Health-seeking behavior is more readily enhanced through education. The level of education and ability to learn may influence the success or failure of health promotion. A nurse must first know the audience and recognize its needs. Information should be presented in simple terms, using appropriate pictures, vocabulary, and literature for the education level of the recipient. Often health promotion is not achieved because the general public does not know the requirements for good health.

Providing information through community, private, and corporate educational facilities generates public knowledge.

Media presentation is an excellent means of disseminating information. The types of media useful for health education are radio, television, and the Internet. Persons may be contacted via media at the rural, urban, district, regional, state, national, and international levels. To achieve the maximum outcome of health promotion and wellness in the world, individuals must be educated. Nurses are influential in their individual communities and should network with other health professionals to enhance the public knowledge of health and wellness.

GENDER

Individuals are susceptible to gender-specific health alterations. Males develop testicular cancer and females uterine/ovarian cancer due to genetic composition. Women have a higher incidence of breast cancer. Men develop cancer of the head and neck more often than women. Men experience high blood pressure more often than women until the age of 45 when high blood pressure becomes more prevalent in women. Women encounter the health care system more frequently than men because of issues centered on their social definition as women, such as reproduction and child rearing (Black & Hawks, 2009).

CULTURAL AND SPIRITUAL INFLUENCES

Knowledge of various cultural beliefs regarding health, religion, and wellness enables the nurse to prepare an appropriate teaching tool relevant to specific cultures and religions. Cultural and spiritual differences must be recognized to enhance learning and to allow for the development of appropriate health prevention measures for an individual. Christian Scientists rely on prayer to heal, while some cultures observe rituals to rid the body of "evil spirits" (see Chapter 6). Cultural "brokering" may be required. A **culture broker** is a go-between, one who advocates on behalf of an individual, family, or community. Cultural brokering is an effective approach to inform health care providers about the effects of culture on health and behavior (Miller, 2008). The culture broker mediates, or bridges, interactions between individuals and groups of varying cultural backgrounds. A culture broker promotes cultural understanding and reduces cultural conflicts (Harkness & DeMarco, 2012). Most patients respond to a nurse's suggestion if the nurse first listens carefully. The nurse must first understand cultural beliefs before stating the reasons for intervention. Listening sessions can present opportunities to educate the patient and to adapt the program accordingly. Nurses seeking to reach compromises with the patient build trust and ultimately community support for educational programs. Community support of educational programs may be difficult for some persons to follow if cultural differences abound.

CURRENT FACTORS AFFECTING NURSING ROLES IN HEALTH PROMOTION

Health promotion is the key phrase in the health care workplace today. Nurses are essential for promoting public health. Factors influencing health promotion today are (1) the health care system, (2) nursing roles, (3) increasing technology, (4) the economic environment, and (5) individual behavior.

HEALTH CARE SYSTEM

Nursing is at the forefront of the changing health care system today. The Institute of Medicine's *Future of Nursing* report (2010) has placed nurses front and center in transforming the health care system. This report indicates that nurses can provide seamless, affordable, quality care accessible to all and thus improve health care outcomes. The report was commissioned in an attempt to transform nursing roles and the nursing profession. Nurses are expected to play a pivotal role in the implementation of the 2010 Affordable Care Act, which represents the broadest health care overhaul since 1965 when Medicaid and Medicare programs were created. The health care system is changing rapidly due to the rising cost of medical care and treatment. Different approaches to health care concerns have resulted in managed care. Insurance parameters, hospital regulations, and physician diagnoses regulate individual health care. To reduce the costs of medical care, hospitals are encouraged to provide optimum care to expedite discharge from the unit as soon as possible. The hospital is reimbursed a set dollar amount for each patient admission. Extended stays in the hospital result in less monies for care.

NURSING ROLES

New nursing roles are developing as the profession expands with the changing health care environment. Until recently, nurses carried out physicians' orders and worked predominantly in hospitals at the patient's bedside. The role of the nurse today has expanded with specialization and increasing health information. Nurses may become certified in their areas of expertise, such as cardiology, medical-surgical, critical care, pediatrics, or neonatology. Increased knowledge enhances the nursing role. Some nurses today are educated to be nurse practitioners to work in underserved areas of the country. Nurse practitioners work in rural settings, hospitals, or clinics and provide services parallel to the physician specialist: family practice physician, pediatrician, cardiologist, or gynecologist. Nurse practitioners may be educated at the doctoral level (doctorate in nursing practice) and are expected to play a major role in transforming health care.

Nurses are available to assess additional patients for the physician, making health care easier for persons to access. The nurse works in collaboration with the physician and provides similar services. Nurse practitioners work in family planning clinics, neonatal units, and physicians' offices. In many areas, the nurse has prescriptive authority to dispense medications when indicated. Increased knowledge leads to increased responsibility and community esteem. Nurses are the leaders in health-promotion activities.

Leadership will be vital to the success of health promotion involving the appropriate integration with health care systems. The nurse collaborates with other disciplines to achieve the desired results for the patient . Networking will be a selected tool to design and distribute information throughout the country to determine whether outcome criteria have been established.

INCREASING TECHNOLOGY

Technological advances have greatly impacted the role of the nurse in health promotion. Technology has advanced so much that sometimes keeping up with the latest developments is difficult. For example, using digital technology, individuals now have a wealth of information literally at their fingertips. Some medical practices are offering results of physicals, electrocardiograms, and other diagnostic tests that can be loaded on a thumb or jump drive. Records can then be updated on visits to specialists and beamed to other health caregivers. Websites such as WebMD and HealthRecord.com let individuals manage their own and their family's health history. Data can be gathered and stored and then shared with physicians, nurses, and other members of the health care team (Wilkinson & Treas, 2011). Computer technology also helps consumers research their health concerns and email their providers questions related to their health care.

High-tech equipment is also available for specific diagnostic testing and treatment. Mammography, magnetic resonance imaging, and computerized axial tomography visualize specific tumors and their size and depth. Radiation and nuclear medicine are two modes of treatment for persons with diagnosed disease.

Equipment is available to monitor diseases such as diabetes and/or cholesterol levels. One example is the One-Touch Glucometer that reads the blood sugar level and that may be carried in a small, transportable case for home or hospital use. The test results are immediately displayed.

Health promotion may be achieved more rapidly through technology. Media channels and interactive computer networks are tools to reach a greater number of persons in areas where accessibility to health care is limited or where there is a lack of information. Schools, libraries, and many homes have televisions and computers that can be used for the transfer of information.

ECONOMIC ENVIRONMENT

Rising medical expenses, health maintenance organizations, and managed care reflect the increasing cost of maintaining health. Public awareness of the state of health care in this country is high today. The federal government is attempting to implement the national health plan. The aging population is increasing. There are dwindling funds to support the aged population when health needs are the greatest. See Chapter 21 for further information on health care cost and quality issues.

INDIVIDUAL BEHAVIOR

Individuals must assume responsibility for their own health. Genetic predisposition to specific diseases may influence health. Nurses educate individuals about health maintenance and disease when a genetic predisposition exists. For example, the African American population has a predisposition to develop sickle cell anemia, and hereditary factors predispose Hispanics to diabetes. Predisposition is beyond a person's control; however, knowing that a predisposition exists is imperative in preventing serious medical consequences. The perceived benefit of behavior is valued for promoting health (Pender, Murdaugh, & Parsons, 2011).

SUMMARY

Many factors can influence the achievement of optimal health or wellness. These factors can be classified according to domains that allow the nurse to view the patient holistically. The domains affecting optimal health are fundamental to health promotion and are biological or physiological, psychological, sociological, environmental, political, spiritual, intellectual, sexual, and technological.

Health maintenance and promotion may occur in a variety of settings such as the hospital, home, and community. Types of health-promoting activities include counseling, screening, and education. These activities may occur in any area of health promotion. In the hospital, the nurse addresses the patient family, or caregiver. Factors regarding precipitating symptoms, health history, and support system are obtained at this time. At home, the patient , family, and nurse may interact to determine nursing process plans to address problems with the individual or within the family unit. A primary goal of the nurse in the home, hospital, or community is to develop rapport and trust with the individual, family, or community.

An accepting, trusting relationship between the nurse and patient leads to compliance and respect for the health care profession, while empowering the individual. If nurses can give patients empowerment for the direction of health and wellness in their lives, it will be passed to the next generation. When the individual assumes personal responsibility for health, the value of health and well-being is also recognized.

Nurses are in the forefront today to encourage health values and responsibility. As a result, disease can be detected earlier with less treatment cost, and health and wellness can increase among general populations. Health services are becoming increasingly accessible in urban and rural areas. Health promotion may occur in any setting at any time when initiated by a qualified health care professional. Resources, public awareness, and public interest for improving quality of life create a positive health perspective for the twenty-first century. Nurses lead the parade in promoting the wellness of future generations.

KEY CONCEPTS

1. The domains fundamental to effective nursing practice are biological, psychological, sociological, environmental, political, spiritual, intellectual, and technological.

2. Health promotion is a continual, active process designed to achieve and maintain wellness.

3. Holistic nursing practice views health care in terms of the whole individual.

4. The role of the nurse is complex and includes activist/advocate, educator, coordinator of care, leader/member of the profession, provider of care, research user, role model, empowering agent, and change agent.

5. The nursing process is the accepted guide for developing appropriate nursing care and wellness outcomes for persons. The phases of the nursing process are (1) assessing data, (2) analyzing data and establishing a nursing diagnosis, (3) planning, (4) implementing, and (5) evaluating.

6. Health promotion is designed to prevent illness before it begins and to maintain current health status.

7. Promoting individual responsibility for health is significant for long-term health outcomes and compliance.

8. Nursing responsibilities for promoting health care should include understanding the (1) political and social changes in the government process, (2) risk factors for potential health problems and their respective preventive measures, and (3) health education resources.

9. Risk factors to be considered in developing a health-promotion plan are environment, work, socioeconomic level, education, gender, culture, and spiritual beliefs.

10. Current factors influencing health promotion are (1) the rapidly changing health care system, (2) the expanded role of the nurse, (3) technology, (4) the economic environment, and (5) individual behavior.

CHAPTER REVIEW

Learning Activities

1. Describe five situations that you have experienced that influenced your achievement of an optimal state of health.

2. Categorize your answer to question 1 in terms of the domains described in the chapter.

3. Take one of the following situations and utilize the nursing process in:

   Listing two factors to be assessed.

   Identifying one nursing diagnosis for each.

   Describing three actions to alleviate the nursing diagnosis.

   Evaluating each action and its efficacy in solving the nursing problem.

Situation A

Mr. Jones, a 55-year-old male, borderline diabetic, is 5 ft., 11 in. tall and weighs 200 lb. His physician reported elevated cholesterol levels and recommended a fitness and weight reduction program. Mr. Jones states he works at a "high-pressure" job and eats snacks a lot.

Situation B

Mrs. Smith, an 80-year-old female, lives alone since the death of her spouse two months ago. The family is not able to persuade Mrs. Smith to participate in her usual activities such as grocery shopping and needlework. Her daughter Sue also states Mrs. Smith skips meals, is anemic, and cries a lot.

4. Using the following case study, categorize the data according to the identified domain. Describe how each of these domains influences health promotion.

> Laura is a 35-year-old single mother of three who has recently been diagnosed with Type 2 diabetes. She is a college-educated finance broker for a large company, and she works 50 hours per week. She has few hobbies but does like to read and spend time outdoors with her children. She and her children live in a large apartment complex, and she knows very few of her neighbors. She has low self-esteem and does not like to go out, not even to church, because she has gained 30 lb. over the years. She is computer literate, and she does email old friends occasionally. She knows how to use the Internet to research her newly diagnosed condition.

Multiple Choice Questions

1. When discussing a health-promotion plan for an individual recently diagnosed with diabetes, the nurse explains to the family that the term *health promotion* means:
   a. achieving optimal health.
   b. being free of all disease processes.
   c. maintaining the health status quo.
   d. protecting health.

2. Of the following, which role of the nurse is *essential* when using a health-promotion approach to patient care?
   a. Coordinator of care
   b. Empowering agent
   c. Member of a profession
   d. Provider of care

3. Immunizations to prevent diphtheria, polio, and tetanus are considered which of the following?
   a. Initial intervention
   b. Primary prevention
   c. Secondary intervention
   d. Tertiary prevention

4. When initially treating a known problem, the nurse is working at which of the following levels of prevention?
   a. Intermediate prevention
   b. Primary prevention
   c. Secondary prevention
   d. Tertiary prevention

5. In the nursing process, critical analysis of data occurs in which of the following stages?
   a. Assessment
   b. Planning
   c. Implementation
   d. Evaluation

6. In arriving at a nursing diagnosis, the nurse:
   a. determines a taxonomy of data classifications.
   b. identifies resources and barriers to goal outcome achievement.
   c. synthesizes, sorts, and groups data according to commonalities.
   d. identifies specific patient outcomes and goals.

7. A culture broker:
   a. increases the incidence of cultural conflicts.
   b. mediates and bridges interactions between cultural groups.
   c. relies on prayer to resolve cultural conflicts.
   d. shares cultural beliefs with patients and their families.

8. In the role as advocate, the nurse:
   a. defers the medical team concerns to the patient.
   b. provides all the care needed by the patient.
   c. relays other nurses' concerns to the patient.
   d. represents the patient's needs to all health care workers at all times.

ORGANIZATIONS AND WEBSITES

Health and Wellness Resource Center and Alternative Health Module: An online go-to-medical-reference center that provides access to references in libraries everywhere: **http://galenet.galegroup.com**

ILSI Center for Health Promotion (CHP):
   2900m Chamblee-Tucker Road, Building 2
   Atlanta, GA 30341-4128
   Phone: (770) 455-9435 /Fax: (770) 455-1826
Nonprofit research and education organization dedicated to the promotion of health in individuals and populations on a global basis.

NANDA International:
   PO Box 157
   Kaukauna, WI 54130-0157
Develops terminology to describe the important judgments nurses make in providing nursing care.

Nursing Informatics and Technology Resources for Nurses and Families: Online site provided by the University of California–San Francisco that offers nursing references, nursing center, teaching, writing, and search engine resources: **http://pegasus.cc.ucf.edu**

Online Journal of Issues in Nursing: Provides access to online articles related to professional nursing: **http://www.ana.org**

Stanford Prevention Research Center:
   Stanford University School of Medicine
   Medical School Office Building
   251 Campus Drive, Mail Code 5411
   Stanford, CA 94305-5411
   Phone: (650) 723-6254 /
   Fax: (650) 725-6906
Disseminates information on disease prevention and control. Research conducted through the Center seeks methods to improve the overall level of community health by favorably modifying the social and personal factors known to influence chronic disease incidence: nutrition, physical activity, tobacco use, social and economic factors, and stress.

REFERENCES

American Nurses Association. (2010). *Nursing: Scope and standards of practice* (2nd ed.). Silver Springs, MD: Nursesbooks.org.

Bartholomew, L. K., Parcel, G. S., Kok, G., Gottlieb, N. H., & Fernandez, M. E. (2011). *Planning health promotion programs: An intervention mapping approach* (3rd ed.). San Francisco, CA: Jossey-Bass.

Belcher, A. S. (2008). Maternal and child populations. In L. L. Ivanov & C. L. Blue (eds.). *Public health nursing: Leadership, policy, & practice.* Clifton Park, NY: Delmar Cengage Learning, pp. 478–494.

Black, J. M., & Hawks, J. H. (2009). *Medical surgical nursing: Clinical management for positive outcomes* (8th ed.). St. Louis, MO: Saunders Elsevier.

Blue, C. L., & Black, D. R. (2008). Principles of health promotion. In L. L. Ivanov & C. L. Blue (eds.), *Public health nursing: Leadership, policy, & practice.* Clifton Park, NY: Delmar Cengage Learning.

Calzone, K. A., Cashion, A., Freetham, S., Jenkins, J., Prows, C. A., Williams, J. K., & Wung, S. F. (2010). Nurses transforming health care using genetics and genomics. *Nursing Outlook, 58,* 26–35.

Centers for Disease Control and Prevention. (2011). Leading causes of death. *Faststats.* Retrieved from http://www.cdc.gov/nchs/fastats/lcod.htm

Craven, R., & Hirnle, C. (2009). *Fundamentals of nursing: Human health and function* (6th ed.). Philadelphia, PA: Wolters Kluwer Health/Lippincott Williams & Wilkins.

Dayer-Berenson, L. (2011). *Cultural competencies for nurses: Impact on health and illness.* Boston, MA: Jones & Bartlett.

De, D. (2008). Acute nursing care and management of patients with sickle cell anemia. *British Journal Of Nursing, 17*(13), 818–823.

Engelke, M. K. (2008). Public health nursing research. In L. L. Ivanov & C. L. Blue (2008). (eds.). *Public health nursing: Leadership, policy, & practice.* Clifton Park, NY: Delmar Cengage Learning, pp. 390–404.

Fawcett, J. (2005). *Contemporary nursing knowledge: Analysis and evaluation of nursing models and theories.* Philadelphia, PA: F. A. Davis.

Harkness, G. A., & DeMarco, R. (2012). *Community and public health nursing: Evidence for practice.* Philadelphia, PA: Wolters Kluwer/Lippincott Williams & Wilkins.

Henderson, V. (1991). *The nature of nursing: Reflections after 25 years.* (Publ. No. 15-2346). New York, NY: National League for Nursing.

Hulton, L. J. (2008). Health risk appraisal. In L. L. Ivanov & C. L. Blue (2008). (eds.). *Public health nursing: Leadership, policy, & practice.* Clifton Park, NY: Delmar Cengage Learning, pp. 241–252.

Institute of Medicine of the National Academies. (2010). *The Future of nursing:Leading change, advancing health.* Washington, DC: The National Academies Press.

Kearney, R. (2008) . *Advancing your career: Concepts of professional nursing.* Philadelphia, PA: F. A. Davis.

Kelley, S., Whitley, D. M., & Campos, P. E. (2010). Grandmothers raising grandchildren: Results of an intervention to improve health outcomes. *The Journal of Nursing Scholarship, 42*(4), 379–386.

Leininger, M. M. (1978). *Transcultural nursing: Concepts, theories, and practice.* New York, NY: National League for Nursing.

LeMone, P., Burke, K., & Bauldoff, G. (2011). *Medical surgical nursing: Critical thinking in patient care* (5th ed.). Boston, MA: Pearson Education.

Miller, A. M. (2008). Immigrant and refugee populations. In L. L. Ivanov & C. L. Blue (eds.). *Public health nursing: Leadership, policy, & practice.* Clifton Park, NY: Delmar Cengage Cengage Learning, pp. 553–574.

North American Nursing Diagnosis Association International (NANDA). (2007). *NANDA nursing diagnoses: Definitions and classification 2007–2008.* Philadelphia, PA: North American Nursing Diagnosis Association.

North American Nursing Diagnosis Association International (NANDA). (2009). *NANDA international nursing diagnoses: Definitions and classifications 2009–2011.* Oxford: Wiley-Blackwell.

Parker, S. L., Johnson-Davies, K., Wingo, P. A., Ries, L. A., & Heath, C. W. (2008). Cancer statistics by race and ethnicity. *CA: A Cancer Journal for Clinicians, 48*(1), DOI:10.3322/canjclin.48.1.31.

Pender, N. J. (1996). *Health promotion in nursing practice* (3rd ed.). Norwalk, CT: Appleton & Lange.

Pender, N., Murdaugh, C. L., & Parsons, M. A. (2011). *Health promotion in nursing practice* (6th ed.). Upper Saddle River, NJ: Pearson Education.

Roan, S. (2011). Radiation exposure and the effects on human health. *Los Angeles Times.* Retrieved from http://articles.latimes.com

Smith, M. C., & Parker, M. E. (2010). Nursing theory and the discipline of nursing. In M. E. Parker, & M. C. Smith (eds.), *Nursing theories & nursing practice* (3rd ed.). Philadelphia, PA: F. A. Davis.

South Asian Institute of Health Promotion (2010). *India global development network.* Retrieved from http://cloud2.gdnet.org/cms.php?id=organization_details&organization_id=2979

Sparks-Ralph, S., & Taylor, C. (2011). *Sparks and Taylor's nursing diagnosis reference manual* (8th ed.). Philadelphia, PA: Wolters Kluwer/Lippincott Williams & Wilkins.

Texas Board of Nursing (TBON). (2010). *Differentiated essential competencies (DECs) of graduates of Texas nursing programs evidenced by knowledge, clinical judgments, and behaviors. Vocational (VN), Diploma/associate degree (diploma/ADN), Baccalaureate degree (BSN).* Austin, TX: TBON.

U.S. Department of Health and Human Services. (2010). *Healthy people 2020.* Washington, DC: U.S. Government Printing Office.

Wilkinson, J. M., & Treas, L. S. (2011). *Fundamentals of nursing* (2nd ed.). Philadelphia, PA: F. A. Davis.

BIBLIOGRAPHY

Anderson, E. (2011). *Community as partner: Theory and practice in nursing.* Philadelphia, PA: Wolters Kluwer/Lippincott Williams & Wilkins.

Cashion, A. (2009). The importance of genetics education for undergraduate and graduate nursing programs. *Journal of Nursing Education, 48*(10), 535–536.

De Sevo, M. R. (2010). Genetics and genomics resources for nurses. *Journal of Nursing Education, 49*(8), 470–471. 16(1), 12–17.

Goodman, C., Davies, S. L., Dinan, S. Tai, S. S., & Iliffe, S. (2011). Activity promotion for community-dwelling older people: A survey of the contribution of community care nurses. *British Journal of Community Nursing,16*(11), 120–117.

Ivanov, L. L., & Blue, C. L. (2008). *Public health nursing: Leadership, policy, and practice.* Clifton Park, NY: Delmar Cengage Learning.

Jitramontree, N., & Schoenfelder, D. P. (2010). Evidence-based practice guideline. Exercise promotion: Walking in elders. *Journal of Gerontological Nursing, 36*(11), 10–18.

Wallace, J. P., Taylor, J. A., Wallace, L. G., Cockrell, D. J. (2010). Student focused oral health promotion in residential aged care facilities. *International Journal of Health Promotion & Education. 48*(4), 111–114.

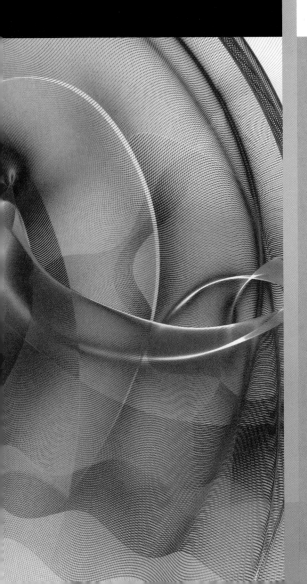

Section II

Factors Influencing Health Promotion

CHAPTER 5
Communication

JANICE A. MAVILLE, EdD, MSN, RN

KEY TERMS

active listening
agraphia
alogia
andragogy
ataxic aphasia
auditory amnesia
auditory aphasia
authenticity
body language
caring
communication
decoder

empathy
empowerment
encoder
expressive aphasia
feedback
global aphasia
kinesics
message
motor aphasia
nonverbal communication
nonverbal vocalizations
paralanguage

pedagogy
personal presentation
proxemics
sensory channel
therapeutic communication
touch
unconditional positive regard
verbal communication
visual aphasia
word blindness
word deafness

OBJECTIVES

Upon completion of this chapter, the reader should be able to:

- Define communication.
- Discuss the six elements of communication.
- Contrast the two types of communication.
- Relate human behavior to communication.
- Explain the importance of communication in therapeutic relationships as found in selected nursing theories.
- Describe four nurse characteristics that promote effective communication.
- Identify therapeutic techniques for effective communication.
- Discuss the role of the nurse in the use of communication for health promotion.

INTRODUCTION

A school nurse is teaching the dangers of steroid use to a group of exceptionally healthy athletes at the prime of their lives. A nurse in a hospital rehabilitation unit holds out her arms to a 4-year-old boy as he practices walking with crutches for the first time since his amputation. A hospice nurse strokes the hands of a man dying of AIDS. These are common scenes of nurses doing what all nurses must do well. They are teaching, they are encouraging, and they are caring as they seek to promote higher levels of health in their patients. But, they are all doing something even more basic. These nurses are communicating. And, in communicating, they are engaging in one of the cornerstones of health promotion, one of the basic activities on which all other health-promoting activities are built. Improving health communication is essential to promoting individual and population health.

COMMUNICATION, NURSING, AND HEALTH PROMOTION

Communication is the process of conveying ideas, thoughts, opinions, or facts from one person to another. In the work setting, nurses communicate most with patients, with their patients' families, and with others on the health care team. When considering nursing care and the human interactions involved, it is difficult to think of anything a nurse does that does not involve communication.

Effective communication is important at all times because breakdowns may cause ill feelings and have other negative consequences. Poor communication might even have a devastating effect on a patient's health. Not surprisingly, health promotion depends to a great extent on communication between nurse and patient.

To improve communication skills, nurses must at all times be aware of the messages they are sending. This is not an easy task. Some basic theories, models, and concepts have been created or adapted by nurses to improve communication. These theories, models, and concepts were generated by a number of individuals from disciplines inside and outside nursing. Nurses should be able to use these in a very practical way to promote the health of others.

NURSING **ALERT**

Strengthening Communication

To strengthen your own communication at the level of message formation, do not start to talk just to fill an uncomfortable silence. You may fill the void with just empty talk. Don't be vague or seem confused. Get your thoughts in order. Know what you want to say before you begin to speak. Patients need clear and confident communications—especially patients in acute situations.

One widely accepted model suggests that communication consists of six generally accepted elements:

1. **Message**—the content (idea, thought, opinion, or fact) one person wishes another person to receive. Unfortunately,

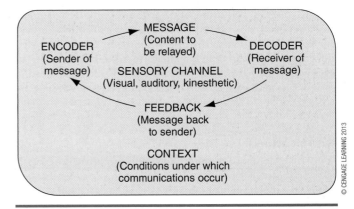

FIGURE 5-1 The elements of communication.

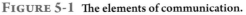

this content cannot be relayed directly from brain to brain. It must be put into a transmissible and receivable form.

2. **Encoder** (sender)—the person who initiates communication by placing a message in a form that is understandable to the intended recipient.

3. **Sensory channel**—the means by which a message is sent. There are three primary routes: the visual (sight), auditory (hearing), and kinesthetic (touch) channels. Sometimes all three channels are used together, such as when a nurse leans toward an accident victim, looks her in the eye while squeezing her hand, and says, "I can help you."

4. **Decoder** (receiver)—the intended recipient of the original message. This person must decode the encoded message to understand the sender's intended thought, opinion, or fact.

5. **Feedback**—the process whereby the overall communication is evaluated for effectiveness. This is the encoding and sending of a message from the receiver back to the original sender in order to let the sender know the message was received. Feedback says, in effect, "I read you loud and clear" or "I'm afraid I didn't quite get your message. Can you repeat it for me?" Without feedback, the sender can never really be certain the intended communication occurred.

6. **Context**—the conditions under which communication occurs.

Figure 5-1 is a graphic representation of the elements of communication. Awareness of these elements and how they work helps nurses and other health care professionals avoid misunderstandings and can strengthen the communication process. A closer look at the six elements provides a glimpse of how awareness may help a nurse in daily communication.

THE MESSAGE

Communication breaks down when the content (idea, thought, opinion, or fact) of a message is incomplete. The person who starts to talk without knowing (or before thinking through completely) what she or he wants to say often sends a garbled message. Consider, for example, the patient with Alzheimer's disease who clutches at a nurse's arm to convey a feeling of discomfort. This patient may be incapable of understanding the source of distress—disorientation, loneliness, or something else altogether. The message is vague because the patient's thoughts and ideas are confused.

Vague messages are extremely frustrating to the receiver. A nurse who is unable to understand the message is likely to be unable to help. Health care providers must understand that patients may be communicating without completely understanding their own thoughts. Understanding that communication is breaking down at the point of message formation helps nurses consider ways to help patients focus or relax in order to clarify their thoughts. When this is not possible, nurses must try to think for a patient. What has happened that affected the patient's ability to communicate clearly?

ENCODING

For a variety of reasons, communication can break down with encoding. Much depends on the skill of the encoder. For example, the nurse may intend to ask about a patient's stress management and asks, "How have you been?" Instead of responding about stress management, the patient may interpret the question as a social greeting and respond with, "Fine. How are you?" The message the nurse wished to send differed from the actual encoded message sent. In this case, the problem lies in faulty encoding.

Nurses need to understand when communication is breaking down at the point of encoding rather than at message formation. If a patient is unable to form a coherent thought, a nurse's approach to that patient is quite different from the approach to a patient who is, for example, speaking a foreign language. When the encoder is using an unfamiliar term (or entire coding system), nurses need to let the person know that she or he is using an indecipherable code. An alternative code has to be found.

As the encoder, a nurse must know that the receiver will understand the message. A common language, vocabulary, or code must be used. The patient should also be able to understand any abstractions used and be able to concentrate. For example, when communicating with patients, health care professionals will find it useful and to use lay terms in their speech and to avoid the use of medical terminology or jargon.

THE CHANNEL

Communication also breaks down if inappropriate sensory channels are used. For example, patients may try to tell you that they feel pain. They may have the ability to think clearly but lack the ability to speak (expressive aphasia), as, for example, when they are recovering from a stroke. Such patients may try to form the word for "pain," and it comes out as "plant" or "fly." Because they lack the ability to form words appropriately, they are incapable of vocally expressing that they have pain. Worse still, they cannot express where that pain is being experienced. For one lacking verbal encoding ability (the ability to form words), the auditory channel is obviously not the best option.

In such cases, a nurse should understand that communication is breaking down at the auditory channel. Other channels should be explored. Is body language reflective of additional communication? Can the patient write out the message? In worst case scenarios, patients might be able to nod or blink in response to "yes" or "no" questions. In other situations, a nurse might try the kinesthetic channel and touch a patient, feeling for areas of increased warmth where inflammation might be present.

Any communicator should consider all possible channels and the receiver's ability to use them. If the auditory channel is used to convey a message, the receiver's sense of hearing must be unimpaired. The nurse may have to move closer to the patient or augment auditory deficits by verifying that a patient's hearing aid is in place, is turned on, and contains a working battery.

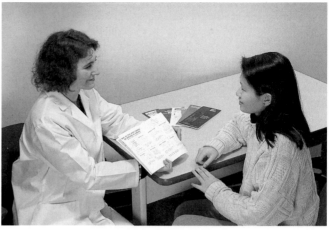

FIGURE 5-2 Using visual materials enhances the messages the nurse wants to convey and increases the client's understanding.

If the visual channel is used, the receiver must have the eyesight to see the message at the distance it is displayed. The lighting must also be adequate. An astute nurse ensures that needed eyeglasses or contact lenses are clean and in place.

If the kinesthetic channel is used, the receiver's reactions to touch should be assessed. This may be an ideal channel for certain messages, but, for some individuals, touch may be intrusive. Violating a patient's sensibilities may result in a complete rejection of intended communications. Nurses must always seek permission to touch a patient.

In summary, use more than one channel, as necessary, to communicate clearly. When teaching, for example, even clear verbal messages may be enhanced with charts, graphs, outlines, and other visual aids. The nurse in Figure 5-2, for example, is using the auditory channel and the visual channel. When teaching, the nurse might also use the kinesthetic channel when appropriate and desirable.

DECODING

Breakdowns in communication also occur if the receiver is unable to correctly decode the message. Often, the inability to comprehend a message is the result of a breakdown in an earlier step in the communication process (i.e., an inappropriately encoded message or an ill suited channel); however, breakdown may occur even if all else goes well in the communication process. The recipient may not pay attention—a very frequent occurrence in health care. The patient may be worried about a family problem, may be depressed or in pain, or may be otherwise distracted. Additionally, the decoder may be so anxious about the expected message that she or he jumps to unwarranted conclusions. Nurses need to note communication blocks and work to overcome them.

FEEDBACK

Communication also breaks down without appropriate feedback. Frequently, this stems from a desire to avoid embarrassment. Consider, for example, a patient who may nod in apparent understanding when the physician explains measures to lower cholesterol. As soon as the physician leaves the room, the patient turns to the nurse and asks, "What did the doctor mean by 'lower my lipid level'?"

? ASK **YOURSELF**

Enhancing Message Decoding

When receiving messages, do you ask for clarification whenever necessary? Do you pay close attention to the sender, or do you fail to hear what is being said because you are thinking about what you will say next? Always focus on what is being said, and really listen to the entire message before you start to formulate a response.

CONTEXT

Finally, communication may break down because of surrounding conditions. Context affects all other elements of communication. Think about what a blizzard would do to the communication between a couple stranded in a stalled car. They might be too distracted by the cold to think or speak clearly. Words sent over the auditory channel might be drowned out by the roar of the wind outside. Environmental context also applies in the health care arena. Role relationships and emotional factors frequently come into play in emotionally charged situations. For example, a parent may be so anxious about her child that she never even hears a nurse's attempts at communication.

Contextual variables affecting communication include:

1. The surrounding environment, including the geography, climate, weather, and ambient temperature.
2. The social, cultural, and ethnic expectations for individuals as they communicate.
3. The social, work, and educational positions and roles of the participants in the interaction.
4. The history and experiences of the participants.
5. The physical, mental, and emotional states of the participants.
6. The goals and expectations of the participants.
7. The effects of current events on the situation.
8. The time constraints imposed on the participants.

✳ NURSING **ALERT**

Validating That Messages Are Understood

As a nurse who suspects a block in communication at the point of feedback, you should be able to assess the patient's understanding by asking specific questions to verify understanding. Do not simply ask whether the patient understands. A good idea is to ask a question that cannot be answered with a simple yes or no. A good example of this type of question is, "Tell me how you can alter your diet to reduce your cholesterol level."

Each of these factors may have positive or negative effects on communication. Most allow for intervention by the alert nurse who is aware of ways to enhance communication by taking the context into consideration.

TYPES OF COMMUNICATION

Communication theorists generally accept that there are two types of communication: verbal and nonverbal. **Verbal communication** is the use of words to convey messages. Often, these words are written or spoken, but they may be formed in other ways, such as by the use of the keyboard, sign language, or Braille. **Nonverbal communication** is the conveyance of messages without the use of words. Nurses can be more effective communicators if they are consciously aware of both the nonverbal and the verbal communication occurring between themselves and others.

VERBAL COMMUNICATION

Verbal communication, it would seem, should be very clear because of the use of a common language made up of defined words. Unfortunately, like all communication, the verbal arena is subject to faulty message formation, encoding, channel selection, reception, decoding, and feedback.

Speakers vary in their ability to use language to convey precise content. Additionally, dictionaries differ in their definitions of words. Worse yet, many words have more than one meaning, and those meanings often change over time and geography. For example, in 1958, a teenager might have asked for a "pop" in Toledo, Ohio; a "soda" in Beacon, New York; or a "phosphate" in Boston, Massachusetts. All three references indicate a carbonated beverage in a generic sense. Similarly, a teenage girl in the 1950s would likely refer to her steady date as her "boyfriend," but her grandmother would refer to him as her granddaughter's "beau." Some words last beyond their time. Some become generalized, and some become more specific over time. In some respects, it is a wonder that verbal communication does not break down far more frequently than it does.

Interestingly, the ability to use verbal communication is so important that an inability to verbally communicate is considered a disease. Table 5-1 lists terms related to the inability to communicate via various channels.

Teaching is a very large part of nursing. In teaching, verbal communication can be vital (but not essential). Think of how difficult it likely was for the teacher of Helen Keller. First, she had to teach her student to communicate verbally by touch before she could really begin her much wider education. In teaching, sending verbal messages over more than one channel at the same time is often helpful. Educators, for example, make wide use of computers, movies, videos, television, slide-tape presentations, and lectures with the use of an overhead projector.

In addition to augmenting the spoken word with pictures, diagrams, music, and other nonverbal messages, audiovisual technologies are frequently used to present words in both speech and print. This reinforcement uses both visual and auditory channels for the same verbal content and is helpful in communication and in learning retention. For example, a video might feature a speaker who is introduced only by the title "Doctor" and a last name, which might be spelled "Wallick," "Walluch," "Walluck," "Wallach," or "Wallack." Presenting the

TABLE 5-1 Communication Channels, Deficits, and Descriptive Terms

CHANNEL	DEFICIT	DESCRIPTIVE TERM
Auditory, expressive	Ability to think without the ability to speak Types include: • A general inability to speak. • An inability to coordinate the muscles responsible for speech.	**Expressive aphasia** **Alogia** **Motor aphasia, ataxic aphasia**
Auditory, receptive	Ability to think and hear without the ability to understand the spoken word heard	**Auditory aphasia (auditory amnesia, word deafness)**
Visual, expressive	In a literate person, the inability to co-ordinate hand muscles sufficiently to produce handwriting	**Motor aphasia (agraphia)**
Visual, receptive	In a literate person, the inability to de-code the written word	**Visual aphasia (word blindness)**
Mixed auditory and visual, receptive	In a literate person with the ability to think, an inability to understand the spoken or the written word	**Aphemesthesia**
All channels	In a literate person, an inability to ex-press or receive verbal messages in any form	**Global aphasia**

© Cengage Learning 2013

speaker's name visually in a subtitle enables the viewer to later find books or articles written by the speaker.

When teaching one to one, the nurse should reinforce the spoken word with the written word whenever possible. A printed handout or booklet allows the patient to review key points in the message, and it allows the patient to take the message home upon discharge from the health care facility, if needed. A handwritten message can do the same.

SPOTLIGHT **ON**

Generational Differences in Expressing Feelings

Each generation is unique in how they approach verbal communication and in what they allow themselves to express. Baby boomers (born between 1946 and 1964) and younger persons have lived and are living in decades when freedom of expression is encouraged. They are apt to reveal their feelings and share them with others. Older persons, on the other hand, may find it difficult to share their true feelings, especially with someone they do not know well.

NURSING **ALERT**

Working with an Interpreter

Interpreting for people with hearing impairments is very physical. The task involves almost constant movement of the arms, hands, and fingers of the interpreter, resulting in the expenditure of a great deal of energy. Allowing for intervals of rest is important, especially when interpretation is needed for extended periods of time.

Special attention needs to be paid to patients with impaired receptive channels. The visually impaired have much less trouble with verbal communication than do the hearing impaired. Communication with a receiver who is hearing impaired is often time-consuming, as is feedback. To avoid confusion, the nurse sometimes has to communicate through a third person, or interpreter, whose hearing is intact and who has the ability to use sign language (sign). The interpreter listens to a hearing speaker, interprets the words into sign language for the patient with impaired hearing, and reverses the process for feedback to the sender. If no interpreter is available, the patient with impaired hearing is usually able to either read lips to some degree or read written language.

Patients who are hearing impaired and who use a sign language or system make up a very diverse population. Their diversity is reflected not only by their hearing impairment but also by individual differences in age, gender, race, ethnicity, national origin, religion, sexual orientation, and socioeconomic status, as well as the sign language/system that they use. In the United States, it is estimated that 100,000 to 1 million people use American Sign Language (ASL) as their primary language. Many of these people experience inequities in accessing health care and health information, thus affecting their ability to achieve optimal health for themselves, their families, and their communities (Barnett et al., 2011).

In some situations, the nurse may have to use a sign language interpreter to facilitate communication and better serve the health needs of patients who are hearing impaired. Those who sign use their hands to spell out letters of the alphabet or to indicate entire words. Signing letters one at a time is termed finger spelling and can be laborious. Even so, to learn to sign entire words, learning to fingerspell is a first step—much like learning the alphabet to read words. See Additional Resources at the end of this chapter for resources helpful in learning to fingerspell and sign.

Writing is also an option when lip reading and signing are not. It is slow but a good alternative. Paper and pencil should always be readily available for nurses to use with patients who are hearing impaired.

? ASK **YOURSELF**

Personal Presentation

Think about a female acquaintance you know fairly well. With this person in mind, think about your reaction if she shaved her head. What would this behavior communicate to you? For this individual, would this behavior have a specific meaning?

Is she the type who is merely looking for attention? Does she have a health problem, such as a skin condition, that requires shaving for treatment? Is she joining a religious cult? Is she protesting something? Did she lose a bet? Is she self-mutilating because of a mental illness? Does she have a role in a play or movie? Taking into consideration all that you know about her, you might make a correct guess. But your conclusion would be only a guess until confirmed.

NONVERBAL COMMUNICATION

It is well-known that over 90 percent of communication is nonverbal. No matter how hard we try, we cannot avoid communicating in a nonverbal manner. Our appearance, facial expressions, body language, and other behaviors all relay a message. How receivers interpret that message can vary. Theorists agree that most communication takes place without the use of words. A large number of variables may alter messages, so they must be interpreted with caution.

Nonverbal communication consists of body language and paralanguage. **Body language** is the use of nonverbal communication behaviors that include personal presentation, proxemics, kinesics, and touch. **Paralanguage** is the use of the nonverbal components of spoken language, which consist of nonverbal vocalizations that alter the meaning or quality of verbal messages.

PERSONAL PRESENTATION

Personal presentation is how individuals show themselves to the world. It includes dress, grooming, and the use of cosmetics, perfumes, and deodorants. Personal presentation creates an identity that an individual wishes to portray to the outside world. Details may vary depending on where individuals are going and whom they might see. For example, people may choose to present themselves differently when going to school than when going out for a formal dinner.

Those who fail to meet societal expectations or who alter their normal pattern of personal presentation are communicating something to others. Maybe a health care need is communicated. For example, someone who has not attended to personal appearance may indicate a lack of needed resources (time, money, or energy). This behavior may also be communicating a change in the level of health. Failure to attend to normal grooming frequently signals a lack of energy that may indicate a depression. Bear in mind, however, that changes in grooming may result from a number of factors, as may any change in behavior. The meaning of nonverbal behavior, including presentation of self, cannot be interpreted with certainty without verification by the message sender.

PROXEMICS

Proxemics is how we use the personal space around us, the distances we maintain from others. The scientific study of proxemics in humans began with Hall (1966), who theorized that people are surrounded, at all times, by a space considered to be an extension of themselves. This is "personal space." Most individuals allow only a select few—such as children or a spouse—to enter this space. They become very uncomfortable if others intrude into it. Most people tend to behave in ways designed to protect their space from accidental intrusion. The size of this personal space is culturally determined and varies considerably. In the United States, for example, most of us maintain personal distances of approximately 18 in. Of course, there are also individual variations.

Most activities and relationships are governed by concepts of space. People tend to place themselves at socially and culturally determined distances from each other according to their relationships and according to their activities at the time. These distances have been determined to be approximately as follows (see Figure 5-3):

1. Intimate distance (0 to 1.5 ft)—the distance allowing touch and very close communications, usually with only a select few persons.
2. Personal distance (1.5 to 4.0 ft)—the distance allowing personal communications with persons known fairly well.
3. Social distance (4 to 12 ft)—the distance allowing casual, social-level communications with acquaintances.
4. Public distance (12 to over 25 ft)—the distance allowing formal communication among one person and a larger number of persons, as might occur with public speaking in an auditorium.

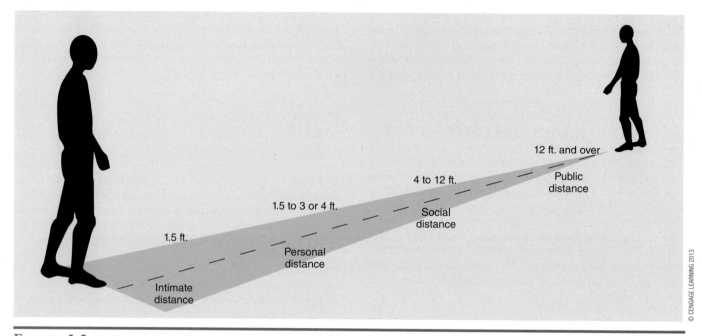

FIGURE 5-3 Distances in communication proxemics.

A person who fails to adhere to unwritten rules concerning appropriate distances for communication may be demonstrating a lack of socialization to cultural norms. Alternatively, a person who feels her or his personal space is being violated often feels threatened. The normal response is to back away and thus increase personal space. Most people can read this subtle body language and back away from someone's personal zone after an accidental intrusion. Failure to back away frequently causes extreme discomfort, especially if the person is, for example, confined to a hospital bed and cannot back away. Intrusions into personal space can result in unexpected behavior. In extreme cases, persons may even become violent as they seek to protect themselves.

Nurses need to be aware of space. They work closely with patients at intimate distances, meeting personal needs in a matter-of-fact manner. It is important to understand that individual patients have varying levels of tolerance for such closeness and intrusion into their space. Nurses must therefore be ever aware and respectful of the personal space needs of patients. This requires being alert to slight body movements. It requires explaining to a patient what will be done before making an intrusive action. It often requires asking permission.

ASK **YOURSELF**

Knowing Your Kinesics

To be constantly aware of your kinesics is difficult, but trying can be well worth the effort. Ask a trusted friend for feedback about your body positioning, facial expressions, and gestures. Are you coming across as bored, rude, overly anxious, aloof, or angry? Are your gestures annoying or distracting? How can you change your image for the better?

KINESICS

Kinesics is the conscious or unconscious movement of the body, including changes in body posture, facial expressions, and gestures. As with other types of body language, kinesics may be conscious or unconscious, voluntary or involuntary. Kinesics are therefore not easy to interpret with precision. Is a person with a ramrod spine sitting up so straight because she is alert and on the defensive, or has she merely spent a lifetime learning to maintain excellent posture?

People communicate a variety of emotions with their bodies, eye contact, and facial expressions. These communications are often culturally determined. For example, a young Asian woman who lowers her eyes when talking to an adult is showing respect. On the other hand, a young American woman who lowers her eyes when talking to an adult is often thought to be indicating dishonesty, guilt, or shame.

TOUCH

Touch is the manner in which people come into bodily contact with one another. It can be seen as a special way of moving your body or gesturing, or it may be seen as the most intimate distance in the study of proxemics. Touch is a very important part of human communication and indeed of human health and even human life. Touch can be comforting and pleasurable when it communicates caring, as seen in Figure 5-4, or it may cause physical and emotional pain. A firm handshake may communicate trust and the offer of friendship, whereas a limp handshake, on the other hand, may flag boredom or distaste.

PARALANGUAGE

Paralanguage is the use of sounds with and without words (verbal language). It is an intermediate area between nonverbal and verbal communication; it consists of **nonverbal vocalizations** (such as grunts, groans, sighs, and sobs) that alter the quality of verbal messages.

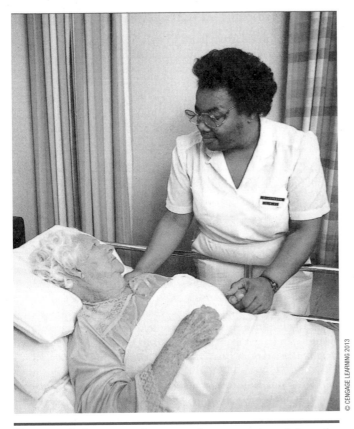

© CENGAGE LEARNING 2013

FIGURE 5-4 **A sense of caring can be communicated through touch.**

Vocalizations that accompany verbal messages (such as accent, intensity, intonation, nasality, pause, pitch, range, rate, rhythm, stress, and volume) are closely associated with, and often support and strengthen, the accompanying verbal message. It is best when the verbal message and other vocalizations agree. However, this is not always so, and the verbal message and its accompanying paralanguage message may disagree. Consider the person who rapidly snaps, "Oh, I just don't care. Do what you want to do!" Obviously she *does* care and cares enough to be angry about it.

COMMUNICATION AND THE THERAPEUTIC RELATIONSHIP

Nurses are expected to use communications with patients in a manner designed to promote health. The interactions with patients should be therapeutic relationships. The role of the nurse varies in interaction with the needs of individuals, groups, families, and communities. To facilitate the therapeutic relationship, the nursing role must adapt to the situation and change with the roles played—resource person, teacher, leader, counselor, and so on.

NURSE CHARACTERISTICS THAT PROMOTE COMMUNICATION

Certain characteristics of nurses tend to promote communication. An astute nurse cultivates these characteristics as personal attitudes to strengthen communication with patients.

UNCONDITIONAL POSITIVE REGARD

Unconditional positive regard is an attitude that Carl Rogers (1942), the renowned psychotherapist, believed to be necessary for any therapist to have if therapy was to have positive results. Nursing has adopted this value. Showing **unconditional positive regard** for your patients means accepting and respecting them as fellow human beings without imposing any conditions for that acceptance.

⊕ HEALTH PROMOTION THEORY LINK

King's Theory of Goal Achievement

Imogene King developed a conceptual framework for nursing in the 1960s that she further clarified throughout the 1970s and 1980s (Alligood & Marriner-Tomey, 2010). It initially consisted of four systems that are universal to nursing: social systems, perceptions, interpersonal relationships, and health. Communication was inherent within each of these systems and a major concept in the interpersonal systems.

In 1981, King expanded her framework to include goal attainment, which addressed how nurses interact with patients for health goal achievement (Alligood & Marriner-Tomey, 2010). She added the concepts of personal space, learning, and coping. If communication is important in health goal achievement, then the nurse must place emphasis on human characteristics and interaction for all ages, genders, ethnicities, and individual health characteristics.

Nurses display this characteristic in verbal and nonverbal ways. By saying "I'm so glad to see you today," the nurse accepts patients and encourages them to be themselves. Using touch, such as a pat on the hand or back, offers further encouragement.

Unconditional positive regard is a characteristic that promotes trust between the patient and nurse. When the nurse has this attitude, patients will feel more freedom to express themselves without anticipation of rejection.

EMPATHY

Empathy, or empathetic understanding, means identifying closely with a patient because you can imagine yourself in the patient's situation. Offering comments such as "I think I understand how you feel" or mirroring the patient's facial expressions are examples of verbal and nonverbal ways of displaying empathy. When there is empathy, there is harmony between the nurse and patient.

AUTHENTICITY AND GENUINENESS

Authenticity means being real or genuine, as opposed to hiding behind a mask of professionalism. Being authentic helps to further establish trust with the patient. Authenticity requires openness and sharing true feelings. For instance, if an obese teenager on a weight management program sets a goal of losing 10 lb in 10 days, it is honest to say "I think it would be better if we looked at a more realistic time frame" instead of "I just know you can do it!"

CARING

Caring is more than just the respect and valuing that occurs with unconditional positive regard. **Caring** is having a personal interest in the patient; it is *feeling* for the patient; it is an investment of the self. Caring is exhausting, however. It entails a substantial drain of emotional energy. Many nurses become disappointed or hurt when a patient's health care outcomes are not attained.

But there are rewards for caring. Nurses experience much relief or happiness as they see a patient progress a great deal. Caring involves a risk but it can be one of the most beneficial aspects of nursing.

Caring can be shown in many ways, both verbally and nonverbally. Just saying "I care about you" establishes a climate of acceptance and encouragement. Merely paying attention shows a sense of caring for a patient.

ACTIVE LISTENING

Active listening is the act of perceiving what is communicated verbally as well as nonverbally. Active listening is critical to true communication between the patient and nurse. Listening becomes active when it moves beyond merely hearing the spoken word and into an involvement with the patient, whereby feelings, meanings, or intentions behind spoken words are reflected by the nurse. In this sense, active listening helps the patient to clarify and further articulate inner thoughts. For example, a patient may say, "I can't follow this diet." A typical response could be "Don't worry; many people are successful with this diet." An active listening response could be "I understand that you feel you can't follow this diet. Could you tell me what makes you feel this way?" Active listening relays to the speaker that you understood not only what was said but also the underlying feelings.

Active listening has many advantages. First, it enhances the relationship between the nurse and the patient by creating a sense of mutual trust. Second, it minimizes the chances for misinterpretation. Third, it creates an atmosphere of acceptance that encourages patients to verbalize more than they might otherwise do.

In using active listening, nurses must be cognizant of the verbal and nonverbal messages being conveyed by patients in order to respond appropriately. Nurses must understand that their personal characteristics, their choice of communication techniques, and the manner and timing of their use of communication techniques can all affect communication (Estes, 2009).

✺ NURSING ALERT

Communicating Therapeutically

Never assume that, because you are using one type of therapeutic technique, you are communicating therapeutically. Nurse theorist Peplau (Parker, 2009) noted that nurses must be able to use a wide range of therapeutic techniques and, more important, be able to identify which technique they are using at a given time. Conscious awareness of interactions remains vital to therapeutic communication.

SPECIFIC TECHNIQUES THAT PROMOTE COMMUNICATION

Therapeutic communication requires the use of verbal and nonverbal techniques that are focused on patient needs. It also requires the avoidance of unhelpful or nontherapeutic techniques.

The ability to use these techniques may be developed only if practiced. Table 5-2 provides a list of therapeutic communication techniques, their definitions, and examples of how they can be used in various age groups. Table 5-3 identifies some of the non-verbal and verbal barriers to communication that can interfere with the therapeutic relationship between the patient and nurse.

TABLE 5-2 Therapeutic Communication Techniques

TECHNIQUE	DESCRIPTION/DEFINITION	EXAMPLE
Provide broad opening	The nurse invites the patient to select a topic.	Nurse with child: "What would you like to tell me about yourself?" Nurse with adolescent: "Tell me what's been on your mind." Nurse with adult: "I'm interested in hearing about issues of concern to you."
Provide silence	The nurse allows the verbal conversation to stop to provide a time for quiet contemplation of what has been discussed, for formulation of thoughts about how to proceed, or for tension reduction.	[Silence] Nurse: Observes patient's behavior for what is not being expressed verbally. Child: Looks down at floor. Adolescent: Eyes well with tears. Adult: Fidgets with hands, adjusts in chair, and eyes dart around the room.
Select focus	The nurse selects a topic for exploration from among several possible topics presented by the patient.	Nurse with child: "You said you hate all of your brothers. Tell me about Melvin first." Nurse with adolescent: "You've briefly mentioned three different suicide attempts. For now, I'd like to focus on just what was going on with you at the time of the first attempt." Nurse with adult: "Let's return to the last point you made and talk more about that."
Clarify	The nurse lets the patient know that what was said was unclear. If necessary, the nurse asks for clarification or provides input regarding how to make the message clearer.	Nurse with child: "You say you fell in a hole. Tell me what you mean by this." Nurse with adolescent: "I didn't understand what you meant then. Can you say that in different words?" Nurse with adult: "Let me repeat back to you what I think I heard you say."
Interpret	The nurse pulls facts together to come to a conclusion and then verifies that with the patient.	Nurse with child: "OK, your two friends pushed you into the slide, and that's how you got the scar on your head." Nurse with adolescent: "Your stomach pains seem to happen whenever you have to give a report in class." Nurse with adult: "Your food and sleep diary shows that you sleep better when you have a light snack around 9 p.m."
Restate	The nurse rephrases what the patient has said. The rephrased message lets the patient know the nurse is attentive and allows for further dialogue.	Child: "Ugh! That's yucky!" Nurse: "You don't like how the medicine tastes, right?" Adolescent: "I upchucked, and it grossed me out." Nurse: "You vomited and it upset you." Adult: "I'm up and down all night." Nurse: "You are having difficulty sleeping."
Validate	The nurse attempts to verify with the patient that a certain term means the same thing to both parties.	Nurse with child: "You want 'moo moo'? Does 'moo moo' mean milk?" Nurse with adolescent: "When you say your brother is crazy, does the word 'crazy' mean 'kind of wild'?" Nurse with adult: "Tell me if we both understand the term 'nap' the same way."

Source: Adapted from Estes, M. E. Z. (2006). *Health Assessment & Physical Examination* (3rd ed.). Clifton Park, NY: Delmar Cengage Learning.

TABLE 5-3 Barriers to Effective Communication

NONVERBAL BARRIERS OF PATIENT OR NURSE		VERBAL BARRIERS
PHYSICAL	PSYCHOLOGICAL	CONVEYED BY NURSE
Speech impairment	Personal perceptions	Giving orders, advice
Hearing impairment	Personal prejudices	Threatening patient
Vision impairment	Fear of person, environment, subject	Lecturing
Cognitive impairment	Lack of interest	Criticizing, blaming, shaming
Environmental distractions or disruptions		Overly praising
		Too much or too little information

© Cengage Learning 2013

USING COMMUNICATION FOR HEALTH PROMOTION

The organizing framework for achieving the goals for health promotion is the nursing process (discussed in Chapter 4). For health promotion, this involves collaboration with the patient to identify needs, determine desired outcomes, plan actions, implement the plan, and evaluate the actual outcomes. Obviously, effective communication is vital in this collaborative process between the nurse and the individual, family, group, or community.

COMMUNICATION AND *2020*

As discussed in Chapter 1, *Healthy People 2020* is a national health initiative for Americans with four major goals: (1) to attain high-quality, longer lives free of preventable disease, disability, injury, and premature death; (2) to achieve health equity, eliminate disparities, and improve the health of all groups; (3) to create social and physical environments that promote good health for all; and (4) to promote quality of life, healthy development, and healthy behaviors across all life stages (U.S. Department of Health and Human Services, 20011a).

Healthy People 2020 provides for a framework for the prevention of threats to the health of individuals, groups, communities, and the nation.

Programs to meet the goals of *Healthy People 2020* are directed at preventing disease and promoting health. Prevention involves nurses working with patients individually or in groups to prevent disease by providing counseling and education on health issues. It may also include expertise in performing and interpreting the results of screening tests, administering immunizations, and giving medications aimed at preventing disease. Promoting health becomes both challenging and rewarding when nurses endeavor to encourage and empower people to adopt or adhere to healthy lifestyles.

Communication is not only a necessity but also a vital key in meeting the goals of *Healthy People 2020*, whether the nurse is actively participating in a formal health program for many patients or caring for an individual patient in a clinic, an institution, or the patient's home.

In their various roles, nurses communicate with patients. Whether acting as a resource person (answering questions and interpreting technical information), teacher (developing novel learning experiences for patients), leader (encouraging the democratic process in patient groups), and/or counselor (facilitating the patients' self-directed actions and promoting experiences leading to health), using appropriate therapeutic communication is integral to achieving the goals of *Healthy People 2020*. It is important to remember that, within each of these roles nurses may communicate with patients or clients who are individuals, couples, families, small groups, or larger groups in communities or societies. Often the nursing goal is to change the behavior of these patients. Changes may include:

- Encouraging patients to behave in a manner more consistent with attaining higher levels of wellness.
- Or discouraging them from behaving in a manner that could cause them to become ill.

THE HEALTH-PROMOTION MODEL AND COMMUNICATION

Pender's Health Promotion Model and Revised Health-Promotion Model (Pender, Murdaugh, & Parsons, 2010), as described in Chapter 3, is often used by nurses to assist patients in altering their health-related behaviors. This model is helpful in facilitating a change in behavior and in making decisions about health. It proposes that individual characteristics (biological, psychological, and sociocultural) and experiences (past health behavior) have both a direct and an indirect effect on the likelihood of an individual's engaging in health-promoting behaviors. What the individual perceives about the health-promoting behavior (its benefits and barriers to action, perceived control of health, and perceived self-efficacy) and what influences exist (family, peers, societal norms and models, and personal and work environment) have a direct effect on the patient's commitment to a plan of action and the health-promoting behavior. Table 5-4 identifies some specific communication-related interventions by domain.

When using Pender's Health Promotion Model and Revised Health-Promotion Model, nurses use a variety of therapeutic techniques of communication to draw information from patients. They thus discover their patients' definition of health, the importance of health, the perception of the control of health, the ability to control personal health, and interpersonal as well as situational influences and support. A great deal of this information may be new even to the patient.

TABLE 5-4 Communication-Related Nursing Interventions Categorized by Domain

DOMAIN	INTERVENTIONS
Biological	Assess patients for intact sensory perception abilities (vision, hearing, touch). Make sure patients use hearing aids or eyeglasses if available. Assess patients for physical conditions that may cause communication difficulties or limitations, including loss of sensory perception, stroke, injuries, disease, or birth defects. Monitor energy levels and expenditure during communication. Allow for rest periods as needed. Arrange for an interpreter if needed. Modify visual materials as necessary.
Psychological	Assess each patient's readiness to communicate. Assess each patient's understanding of messages sent or information provided. Provide clarification as necessary.
Sociocultural	Recognize the customs, beliefs, and values of each individual patient. Modify communication to accommodate cultural beliefs and customs.
Spiritual/religious	Recognize that spiritual and religious beliefs have varying influences on the patient's perceptions of health and control of health.
Environmental	Ensure an environment conducive to good communication, including adequate lighting, comfortable temperature, and freedom from distracting noise.
Technological	Choose the appropriate technology for communicating: video, audiotape, computer-interactive, teleconference, email.

© Cengage Learning 2013

EMPOWERING THROUGH COMMUNICATION

Empowerment, in relation to health promotion, is the process of helping others help themselves. For the nurse, this requires much persuasion, support, and encouragement. But empowerment can best be accomplished through education. In fact, many perceive health promotion and health education as synonymous.

The rising cost of health care and the abundance of information on related issues, made available to individuals from a variety of sources, are two major forces driving the increased demand by patients for knowledge and skills about self-care and the prevention of disease (Bastable, 2007). The Internet has become a medium for both information and misinformation. Nurses can help to empower patients through introducing new information, clarifying misinformation, and validating patients' interpretations of information.

Achieving the goals of *Healthy People 2020* requires effective communication by all health professionals with all categories of clientele, whether they are children, adults, families, or groups in the community. Understanding what to teach, how learners learn, the learning environment, and the technological aspects of communication is important for nurses as they communicate for the purpose of education. For the teaching to be effective, it must be tailored to the learner.

WHAT TO TEACH

In some work settings, nurses teach content or programs integral to the health agency or facility. For example, a clinic nurse teaches about the clinic's immunizations and chemoprophylaxis (drug therapy). The specific content taught to each individual or group depends on the patients' needs for specific information. Patients want to know about the things that have relevance or personal meaning for them, such as information that helps them avoid trouble, solve their problems, or live a better life.

HOW LEARNERS LEARN

Adults learn differently than children. Malcolm Knowles, renowned adult learning theorist, in his classic text, *The Modern Practice of Adult Education: Andragogy Versus Pedagogy* (1970), described the difference between **andragogy**, the education of adults, and **pedagogy**, the education of children. Knowles's concepts are timeless and form the foundation for educating adults even today. His four andragogical assumptions are that adults:

1. Move from dependency to self-directedness.
2. Draw on their reservoir of experience for learning.
3. Are ready to learn when they assume new roles.
4. Want to solve problems and apply new knowledge immediately.

Keeping these assumptions in mind is helpful when planning any educational intervention for promoting the health of the adult, whether an individual, a spouse/partner, or the parent of a child. Accordingly, nurses teaching adults should follow these guidelines:

- Include the patient in the learning plan.
- Arrange for a diagnosis of learner needs and interests.

TABLE 5-5 Pedagogy and Andragogy: A Comparison

ASSUMPTIONS (KNOWLES)			DESIGN FOR TEACHING (KNOWLES)		
	PEDAGOGY	**ANDRAGOGY**		**PEDAGOGY**	**ANDRAGOGY**
Self-concept	Dependent	Self-directed	*Climate for learning*	Authority oriented, formal, competitive	Mutuality, respectful, collaborative, informal
Experience	Builds with age	A resource for learning	*Planning*	Nurse	Mutual between patient and nurse
Readiness	Depends on biological development and social pressures	Depends on developmental task of social roles (parent, spouse, employee, etc.)	*Diagnosis of needs*	Nurse	Mutual between patient and nurse
Time perspective	Postponed application	Immediate application	*Formulation of objectives*	Nurse	Negotiated by patient and nurse
Orientation to learning	Subject-centered	Problem-centered	*Design*	Focus on subject and content	Developed in terms of patient preference and need to problem-solve
			Evaluation	Nurse	Mutual evaluation by nurse and patient with rediagnosis of needs

Source: Adapted from Smith, M. K. (1996/1999). Andragogy. *The encyclopaedia of informal education,* http://www.infed.org/lifelonglearning/b-andra.htm last updated September 2, 2009.

- Identify the learning objectives based on the diagnosed needs.
- Build on learning from simple to complex components.
- Evaluate the quality of the learning as it is occurring.
- Rediagnose needs for further learning.

Table 5-5 compares these assumptions and teaching design considerations in the context of pedagogy to andragogy. This comparison provides valuable information to be considered when developing the health-promotion plan.

THE LEARNING ENVIRONMENT

Creating a supportive, nonthreatening environment for learning can greatly enhance the communication process in teaching. First, the nurse needs to recognize that learning can take place at any time or any place as long as the patient feels comfortable. Sometimes learning is best done informally on a one-to-one basis or perhaps in a group setting in the home where those with shared interests can gather. Proper lighting, room temperature, and seating should be considered, whether in a clinic, hospital setting, or community gathering.

In the role of educator, the nurse can personally influence the learning environment. The nurse must be knowledgeable about the subject being communicated. Being open to listening to what the patient wants to say creates an atmosphere of acceptance and encouragement.

RESEARCH NOTE

Patient-Centered Communication for Women of Families with *BRCA1/2* Mutation

STUDY PROBLEM/PURPOSE
The early identification of inherited breast cancer risk using genetic testing for the breast cancer gene *BRCA1* or *BRCA2* (*BRCA1/2*) is advantageous for determining primary risk status for surveillance purposes and secondary risk status for determining treatment based on the possibility of developing breast cancer. Those who seek genetic testing receive counseling regarding the communication of results to at-risk healthy family members, which can be complicated in terms of family dynamics and the members' understanding of cancer genetics. This study was conducted to create a better understanding of the experience of communicating the results of *BRCA1/2* testing to at-risk young and middle-aged female family members.

METHOD

The methodology for this study was Heideggerian hermeneutics to obtain the lived experience of 19 women age 18–50 years who received communication of *BRCA1/2* mutation testing from a biologic relative. Purposive and network sampling was used to recruit participants who had received news of the genetic mutation from a family member. In-depth interviews were conducted to obtain reflections on insight into helpful and unhelpful communication from family and health care providers. Following the Interpretive Phenomenology Seven-Step Process, transcripts were analyzed by a team for dependability and conformability of findings.

FINDINGS

Five themes and two constitutive patterns were identified that revealed both fear and empowerment in the communication of *BRCA1/2* genetic test results. The themes were (1) situating the story, (2) receiving the message, (3) responding to receipt of the message, (4) impacting family communication, and (5) advice for communicating risk. The two patterns identified were communicating risk as a message of fear and empowerment and integrating the message by taking one step at a time.

IMPLICATIONS

The role of health care providers is important in providing anticipatory guidance through therapeutic communication for successful adaptation after a family member receives news of breast cancer risk. It is vital that nurses and other health care providers understand that communication with patients must take into consideration their culture, history, and communication patterns.

Source: Crotser, C. B., & Dickerson, S. S. (2010). Women receiving news of a family *BRCA1/2* mutation: Messages of fear and empowerment. *Journal of Nursing Scolarship, 42*(4), 367–378.

TECHNOLOGY AND COMMUNICATION

The major influence of technology on communication in contemporary health care cannot be disputed or overemphasized. Technology has become an integral part of how nurses function. For example, the use of computerized charting and medication administration is becoming routine in a majority of health care institutions.

Patient information, such as health histories, signs and symptoms, laboratory tests, medications, and treatment plans, can be obtained and shared among health care professionals via email and the Internet (Estes, 2006). The U.S. Department of Health and Human Services has advocated for a national network of health information that can be accessed by all health care organizations. Electronic records of patients' care, based on data standards that make health information uniform and understandable to all, will facilitate the exchange of information among providers and patients (U.S. Department of Health and Human Services, 2011b). Although using technology to facilitate communication has great benefits for patients and health care providers, nurses need to be aware of associated legal issues.

Technological advances in communication, including the Internet, computer programs, videos, teleconference capabilities, email, and even cellular phones with picture and text messaging, have changed how people interact, store and retrieve information, and learn. Nurses work to promote the health of patients of all ages and backgrounds, and they have a wide range of technological abilities and capabilities. Therefore, choosing the appropriate technology to achieve the purpose intended, whether the patient is an individual, a group, or a community, is important for the success of any health-promotion endeavor.

GLOBAL HIGHLIGHTS IN HEALTH PROMOTION
Promoting Digital Health Communication in Kenya

The National Center for Health Marketing's Global Health Communication (GHC) Team, along with the Centers for Disease Control and Prevention (CDC), has teamed with the Kenya Ministry of Health, CDC-Kenya Global Disease Detection Division (GDD), and the Kenya Health Workforce Project to promote the use of information and communication technology (ICT) for improved health communications.

Using satellite technology, hardware and software has been installed in provincial medical offices in all seven of Kenya's provinces where there was previously no Internet access. Through this communicative technology, Webinars and mentored guidance for hands-on experience for government health workers became possible.

Most health workers in Kenya have never experienced using a computer for individualized learning and can use this new information for immediate application. Cell phone use is common in Kenya, and further efforts are underway to unite Internet technology with mobile phone communication, especially for the management of tuberculosis.

Source: Centers for Disease Control and Prevention, Department of Health and Human Services. (2009). *Global health communication: Spotlight: Promoting digital health communication in Kenya.* Retrieved from http://www.cdc.gov/HealthMarketing/SpotLight/Archive/KenyaApril09/

SUMMARY

Nurses have a responsibility to promote the health of patients whether they are individuals, families, groups, or communities. This responsibility requires verbal and nonverbal therapeutic communication with patients. It requires much skill to do this on different levels with children, adolescents, and adults and with consideration of the various domains (biological, psychological, sociocultural, spiritual, and environmental). To be effective in promoting the health of patients, nurses must develop and exercise effective communication skills.

This chapter presented the elements of communication, the types of communication, and the use of therapeutic communication skills for health promotion. Promoting health without communication is impossible. Communication is a cornerstone for health promotion.

KEY CONCEPTS

1. Communication is the process of conveying ideas, thoughts, opinions, or facts from one person to another.
2. The six elements of communication include message, encoder, channel, decoder, feedback, and context.
3. The two types of communication are verbal (the use of words to convey messages) and nonverbal (the conveyance of messages without the use of words).
4. Communication is inevitable even though we are not using words because we are constantly conveying messages in nonverbal ways as well.
5. The nurse characteristics that promote effective communication are unconditional positive regard, empathy, authenticity, caring, and active listening.
6. Nurses use therapeutic techniques of communication to gain information about patients and their perceptions, and they provide information to patients in order to assist them to change health-related behaviors and to foster behaviors that promote health.
7. Teaching is a major role of the nurse in health promotion. Whether teaching occurs informally when a need arises or more formally in a care plan, the nurse must understand the differences in teaching adults and children. Knowledge of the teaching environment, what to teach, when to teach, and how to teach are vital to effective teaching.
8. Technology is an important adjunct to teaching patients and promoting health. Nurses can be facilitators in using and teaching the use of the appropriate technology for information exchange and for educating patients.

CHAPTER REVIEW

Learning Activities

1. With the assistance of your instructor, arrange to observe a health care professional in communication with a patient. Identify the various types of therapeutic techniques you observe, nurse characteristics that promote communication, and how personal space is used.
2. Under the direction of your nursing instructor, select an actual patient and interview this person about what she or he does to stay healthy. Include attention to the biological, psychological, sociocultural, spiritual, and environmental domains.
3. Explain the difference between the encoder and the decoder of a message.
4. What part does context play in communicating a message?

Multiple Choice

1. Mr. George is looking out the window, with his back to the door. A nurse opens the door and says, "You will not be able to eat or drink after supper because of tests tomorrow." Then the nurse leaves. Did communication take place?
   a. No. There was no feedback.
   b. No. There was no eye contact.
   c. Yes. Mr. George had to hear the message.
   d. Yes. There was a sender, receiver, and message.

2. What is the best way to communicate?
   a. It depends on the message.
   b. Nonverbally
   c. Verbally
   d. Verbally and nonverbally together

3. When performing a nursing procedure on a patient the nurse should:
   a. always have someone witness the procedure.
   b. avoid eye contact to reduce embarrassment.
   c. be aware of his or her own nonverbal messages.
   d. listen to only what the patient says.

4. The nurse is aware that most nursing procedures are performed in which spatial comfort zone?
   a. Intimate
   b. Personal
   c. Public
   d. Social

5. Adult patients would most typically want to learn about health promotion when they:
   a. admit that they do not know enough.
   b. are told by the nurse that they need to know more.
   c. feel a social pressure to learn.
   d. feel the information relates directly to them.

6. Which of the following terms refers to adults as learners?
   a. Alogia
   b. Andragogy
   c. Pedagogy
   d. Proxemics

7. A nurse says to a new patient, "You say you popped your knee. Can you tell me more about this?" This is a therapeutic communication technique intended to:
   a. clarify what the patient has stated that is otherwise not clear.
   b. allow the nurse to interpret what he or she heard from the patient.
   c. offer assurance of understanding or validation of what the patient said.
   d. provide a broad opening in which the patient can select the topic.

8. Paralanguage is a form of communication that does which of the following?
   a. Alters the meaning or quality of verbal messages
   b. Offers hearing impaired individuals a means of communication
   c. Uses personal presentation, proxemics, kinesics, and touch for communication
   d. Validates the understanding of messages

ORGANIZATIONS AND WEBSITES

American Speech-Language-Hearing Association (ASHA): The professional, scientific, and credentialing association for speech-language pathologists, audiologists, and speech, language, and hearing scientists in the United States and internationally: **http://www.asha.org**

Handspeak™: A subscription-based Website consisting of the American Sign Language (ASL) online dictionary, lessons, and resources, including Baby Sign, International Sign Language, Emoticon + Bodicon (facial expression + body language), gestures, manual alphabet (fingerspelling) and numerals, sign stories, and arts: **http://www.handspeak.com**

The Human Face: How factual cues are connected to emotions, identity, attractiveness and other characteristics of communication. Retrieved from **http://nonverbal.ucsc.edu/facerev.html**

The Human Voice: Focuses on language and vocal paralanguage, that is, what can be inferred about a speaker from spoken language. Retrieved from **http://nonverbal.ucsc.edu/voice.html**

IPT and IPT-15: Offers two video self-tests that enable viewers to see how accurately they can decode nonverbal cues and interpersonal behavior: **http://nonverbal.ucsc.edu/index.html**

U.S. Department of Education: Provides an exploration of information literacy as it relates to schools, workplaces, individuals, and society: **http://www.ed.gov**

University of California Extension Center for Media: Offers a series of videos including the following: **http://nonverbal.ucsc.edu/index.html**

A World of Differences: Examines verbal and nonverbal ways that people from two different cultures can experience communication failures and conflict. Retrieved from **http://ucmedia.berkeley.edu/brochures/brochuregif/diversity9899.pdf**

A World of Gestures: Reveals cultural and national differences in gestures, cross-cultural misunderstandings, etc. Retrieved from **http://nonverbal.ucsc.edu/gest.html**

REFERENCES

Alligood, M. R., & Marriner-Tomey, A. (2010). *Nursing theory: Utilization and application.* St. Louis, MO: Mosby.

Barnett, S., McKee, M., Smith, S. R., & Pearson, T. A. (2011). Deaf sign language users, health inequities, and public health: Opportunity for social justice. *Preventing Chronic Disease, 8*(2). Retrieved from http://www.cdc.gov/pcd/issues/2011/mar/10_0065.htm

Bastable, S. (2007). *Nurse as educator: Principles of teaching and learning for nursing practice.* Sudbury, MA: Jones & Bartlett.

Centers for Disease Control and Prevention, U.S. Department of Health and Human Services. (2009). *Global health communication: Spotlight: Promoting digital health communication in Kenya. Retrieved from* http://www.cdc.gov/HealthMarketing/SpotLight/Archive/KenyaApril09/

Estes, M. E. Z. (2009). *Health assessment & physical examination* (4th ed.). Clifton Park, NY: Delmar Cengage Learning.

Hall, E. T. (1966). *The hidden dimension.* Garden City, NY: Doubleday.

Knowles. M. (1970). *The modern practice of adult education: Andragogy versus pedagogy:* Chicago, IL: Follet.

National Academies: Advisors to the Nation on Science, Engineering and Medicine. (2003, November 20). *Reducing medical errors requires national computerized information systems; Data standards are crucial to improving patient safety.* Retrieved from http://www8.nationalacademies.org/onpinews/newsitem.aspx?RecordID=10863

Parker, M. E. & Smith, M. C. (2010). *Nursing theories and nursing practice* (3rd ed.). Philadelphia, PA: F. A. Davis.

Pender, N. J., Murdaugh, C. L., & Parsons, M. A. (2010). *Health promotion in nursing practice.* Upper Saddle River, NJ: Pearson Education.

Peplau, H. E. (1952). *Interpersonal relations in nursing.* New York, NY: G. P. Putnam's Sons.

Rogers, C. R. (1942). *Counseling and psychotherapy: Newer concepts in practice.* Boston, MA: Houghton Mifflin.

Smith, M. K. (1996, 1999). Andragogy. *The Encyclopedia of Informal Education.* Retrieved from http://www.infed.org/lifelonglearning/b-andra.htm

U.S. Department of Health and Human Services. (2011a). *Healthy people 2020 framework.* Retrieved from http://healthypeople.gov/2020/Consortium/HP2020Framework.pdf

U.S. Department of Health and Human Services. (2011b). *Nationwide health information network: Overview.* Retrieved from http://healthit.hhs.gov/portal/server.pt?open=512&mode=2&cached=true&objID=1142

CHAPTER 6
Cultural Considerations

M. Sandra [Sandy] Sánchez, PhD, RN

KEY TERMS

acculturation
cultural competence
cultural tapestry
culture
emic knowledge

ethnicity
ethnocentrism
etic knowledge
folk health sector
lay/popular health sector

medicocentrism
nationality
professional health sector
race
worldview

OBJECTIVES

Upon completion of this chapter, the reader should be able to:

- Discuss the concept of culture, including its components.
- Differentiate among the concepts of culture, race, ethnicity, and nationality.
- Explain how culture is holistic.
- Describe how culture impacts each metaparadigm concept.
- Identify examples of bigotry, discrimination, prejudice, racism, and ethnocentrism.
- Describe how cultural assessment relates to the nursing process.
- Complete a cultural assessment of yourself and others.
- Become aware of your own culture and how it permeates your life.
- Describe how culture is interwoven with wellness and illness.
- Differentiate among cultural awareness, cultural sensitivity, and cultural competence.
- Specify ways of culturally advocating for patients.

INTRODUCTION

This chapter is not intended to serve as a comprehensive survey of culture. Rather, it is intended to provide a very basic introduction to concepts of culture. The more people understand about themselves and others, the better they may understand one another. That is how bridges are built instead of walls, and health promotion is all about building bridges. Understanding your own unique culture and those of others creates an awareness that is fundamental to providing culturally competent patient care.

THE CONCEPT OF CULTURE

Culture is holistic. It is more than the sum of its parts. It affects everything, including thoughts and behaviors. But what is culture? It is sometimes hard to talk about culture because it is all-encompassing. Entire books and journals are written about it. Undergraduate and graduate courses are devoted to it. Students major in it. Research focuses on it. Theories are developed about it. Yet a concrete definition remains elusive to many people, probably because much of culture is intangible. Culture is probably something most people do not think about until they are confronted with something or someone from a different culture. The natural reaction then is to say, "He's different."

WHAT IS CULTURE?

Culture is a buzzword that is commonly thrown around today, and yet most people, even anthropologists, have slightly different ideas about it. So what is culture? It is certainly more than ethnicity or religion, although those affect culture. It is much more than race, itself a superfluous label.

Culture is defined in various ways. Leininger, a recognized nurse leader and theorist on transcultural nursing, defined culture as the "learned, shared, and transmitted knowledge of values, beliefs, and lifeways of a particular group that are transmitted intergenerationally and influence thinking, decisions, and actions in patterns or certain ways" (Leininger & McFarland, 2002, p. 47). Other definitions, including those listed in Box 6-1, are also relevant, with each offering something to the concept of human culture. They may be incorporated into a meaningful understanding of human culture when viewed simply as "the act or process of cultivating living material in prepared nutrient media" (Mish, 2007, p. 304). In other words, culture is the expert cultivation of a human being in a nurturing milieu. As such, human growth and development begin in a rich womb and continue throughout life to foster an ingrained pattern of attitudes, beliefs, values, morals, knowledge, and behaviors that are unique to *each* individual. Of course, the reverse may be true as well.

In this chapter, **culture** is defined as dynamic adaptation, a learned way of life that includes interrelated attitudes, morals, beliefs, values, ideals, knowledge, symbols, artifacts, customs, traditions, and norms of a particular group that guide behavior, make life meaningful, and are transmitted intergenerationally. Individuals live in the larger society and absorb "culture" through their daily activities. Culture represents a particular group's overarching lifeways *as well as* each individual's worldview and way of life. Culture affects what is seen and thought. It is the lens for each person's view of the world. And what is seen, consciously or not, often determines behavior. Box 6-2 lists attributes of culture.

BOX 6-1
CULTURE DEFINITIONS

Here are some interesting and thought-provoking definitions. As a noun, culture is defined as:

- Cultivation, tillage
- The act of developing the intellectual and moral faculties, especially by means of education
- Expert care and training
- Enlightenment and excellence of taste acquired by intellectual and aesthetic training
- Acquaintance with and taste in fine arts, humanities, and broad aspects of science as distinguished from vocational and technical skills
- The integrated pattern of human knowledge, belief, and behavior that depends on the human capacity for learning and transmitting knowledge to succeeding generations
- The customary beliefs, social forms, and material traits of a racial, religious, or social group; also, the characteristic features of everyday existence shared by people in a place or time

- The set of shared attitudes, values, goals, and practices that characterizes an institution or organization
- The set of values, conventions, or social practices associated with a particular field, activity, or societal characteristic
- The act or process of cultivating living material in prepared nutrient media; also, a product of such cultivation. (In other words, culture is what you are prepared in _and_ what you are!)

As a verb, to culture means to:

- Cultivate (i.e., to foster the growth of)
- To grow in a prepared medium
- To start a culture from

As an adjective, cultured means:

- Cultivated

BOX 6-2
ATTRIBUTES OF CULTURE

- Dynamic adaptation
- Learned, shared, transmitted intergenerationally
- Integrated and interrelated attitudes, values, ideals, morals, beliefs, knowledge, symbols, artifacts, customs, norms of a particular group that guide behaviors
- Interwoven intellectual, moral, aesthetic, religious, social aspects
- Way of life
- Meaningful
- Unique

ASK YOURSELF

What Are Your Customs?

Customs can include foods, holidays, clothing, art, music, dance, communication, childrearing, wellness-illness routines and rituals, rites of passage, celebrations, prayers, roles, and language. What are your customs?

WORLDVIEWS

There are many worldviews. **Worldview** is the way individuals perceive the world, including the inherent nature of its inhabitants. No two people, regardless of culture, are exactly alike or share the same worldview, not even people in the same family. Why? Recall that each person has his or her own unique

culture derived from the overarching culture. Certainly, siblings may possess many cultural similarities that are transmitted from their parents and families, but they also have unique differences. Some of those differences might be attributed to variations in age, personal preferences, and/or individual history. That is why it is critical to realize that although culture is pervasive, discerning a person's culture is difficult without knowing or talking to that person.

PARTICULAR GROUP

Cultural traditions are passed down from generation to generation within a particular group. The group might be a tiny clan living in an isolated part of the world or a large collection of people in the United States. It could be made up of believers in Catholicism or Hinduism. It could be composed of Northerners or Southerners. The group could consist of Californians or Texans, Irish Americans or Mexican Americans. It could represent black or white, and so forth.

The number of possible groups is virtually limitless. Some of the more common particular groups include those bound by race, ethnicity, religion, and/or nationality, with each of those having its own subgroupings. Box 6-3 lists other particular groups.

RACE

Race is a misunderstood term. It is not uncommon to hear people referring to the British race, the Jewish race, or the white race. This may result from the various definitions of **race** as "a family, tribe, people, or nation belonging to the same stock" or "a category of humankind that shares certain distinctive physical traits" (Mish, 2007, p. 1024). Although these definitions offer value, for the most part, the last definition is used in this chapter. Ideally, there would be one simple overarching term—the *human* race.

Anthropologically, race refers to physical characteristics that a particular group of people share. These shared characteristics, initially due to a common geography, include head shape, facial features, bone structure, hair texture, and skin color. Throughout history, however, certain physical characteristics attributed to racial differences have been used as a basis

BOX 6-3
EXAMPLES OF PARTICULAR GROUPS

In addition to race, ethnicity, religion, and nationality, other particular groups that share traditions include those delineated by:

- Regions of the country (East Coast, West Coast, North, South, Southwest)
- States (Alabama, Delaware, Florida, Maine, Oregon, Texas, etc.)
- Agencies (Apple, 3M)
- Professions (nursing, medicine, pharmacy, teaching)
- Clubs (sororities, fraternities, Girl Scouts, Boy Scouts, 4-H)
- Gangs

- Prisons
- Gender (female, male)
- Socioeconomic status (upper, middle, lower; rich, poor)
- Universities (students, alumni, faculty, staff)
- Athletics (basketball, tennis, cycling, soccer)
- Acting (film, stage)
- Degree major (art, business, engineering, journalism, math, nursing)
- Homelessness
- Sexual orientation (heterosexual, homosexual, bisexual)
- Physical ability (able-bodied, disabled)

SPOTLIGHT **ON**

Forgetful Foreigners

With few exceptions, the United States is made up of foreigners of one sort or another. Some came willingly, such as the Pilgrims or Ellis Island immigrants. Others, such as many Africans, were not so willing, and their struggle to become full U.S. citizens. has been difficult. Some foreigners mistreated the residents, such as Native Americans, Alaska Natives, Mexicans, and so forth, by taking their land and resources, often brutally.

TABLE 6-1 Demographic Profile of the U.S. Population by Race

RACE	PERCENTAGE OF POPULATION (%)
1. White	72.4
2. Black, African-American, Negro	12.6
3. American Indian and Alaska Native	0.9
4. Asian (collapsed)	4.8
5. Native Hawaiian and other Pacific Islander (collapsed)	0.2
6. Some other race	6.2
7. Two or more races	2.9

Source: United States Census 2010, U.S. Census Bureau Random Samplings, 2010. Retrieved from http://blogs.census.gov/

for social discrimination and oppression. Interestingly, the least important characteristic is skin color, as it is the one with the most variation within racial classifications. Yet, ironically, it is the one characteristic to which most people steadfastly cling and begs the question "do blind people see race?" (Obasogie, 2010, p. 585).

Many anthropologists point out that categorizing people according to race is "virtually meaningless" (Wali, 1992, p. 7) because there is at least as much variation within racial groups as among them. Furthermore, *race* is often misused as a political term. The American Anthropological Association (AAA) states that race is no longer "a real, natural phenomenon" and laments that "the concept of race has become thoroughly—and perniciously—woven into the cultural and political fabric" of the United States, leading the AAA to advocate using "specific, social categories such as 'ethnicity'" because less negativism is associated with them (AAA, 1997, p. 6).

Further blurring the value of race as a criterion, the 2010 U.S. census form included 15 different self-identification response categories that "generally reflect a social definition of race recognized in this country, and not an attempt to define race biologically, anthropologically or genetically" (U.S. Department of Commerce Bureau of the Census, 2010, p. 27). Seven of the response categories were Asian *ethnicities,* and four were Native Hawaiian or other Pacific Islander groups. The 15 response categories are:

- White
- Black, African-American, or Negro
- American Indian or Alaska Native (with a space for the name of the enrolled or principal tribe)
- Asian Indian
- Chinese
- Filipino
- Japanese
- Korean
- Vietnamese
- Other Asian (with a space for the name of the race)
- Native Hawaiian
- Guamanian or Chamorro
- Samoan

- Other Pacific Islander (with a space the for the name of the race)
- Some other race (with a space for the name of the race)

Even with these extra categories, some of which are more precisely ethnicities, race is an extremely broad category, providing only general information at best. In addition, a person may be a product of a biracial or multiracial union. For example, a person's mother might be white and the father Asian. Fortunately, the U.S. Office of Management and Budget (OMB) now allows people to check more than one race on census and other federal forms, a move that ideally will provide more precise statistics. Table 6-1 presents the most current profile of the U.S. population according to race.

Note that *Hispanic* describes not a race but an ethnicity. Hispanics may belong to any of the designated races. (See the Ethnicity section in this chapter.) Nonetheless, numerous people in government, education, industry, politics, and the press continue to refer to Hispanics as a race. Such usage is erroneous. If, however, someone has to be identified as Hispanic, the proper reference is Hispanic white, Hispanic black, non-Hispanic white, non-Hispanic black, and so on.

Similar notes should be made about the various ethnicities listed as races on the census form. Although members of the black race are commonly referred to as African American, the term itself most precisely refers to an

GLOBAL HIGHLIGHTS IN HEALTH PROMOTION

Cultural Health Promotion via Cultural Awareness

Go to this fascinating Website for a virtual tour of the history, human variation, and lived experience of "race": http://www.understandingrace.org/home.html

ethnicity because Africans can be of any race. Nonetheless, that common usage resulted in the incorrect listing of African American as a race starting with the 1990 census form. The ethnic Asian and Pacific Islander designations that first appeared on the 2010 census form are further perplexities. Will the race categories be replaced with selected ethnicities on upcoming census forms?

ETHNICITY

Ethnicity is more of a social term than a term pertaining to physical traits. Ethnicity comes from the word *ethnos,* meaning nation and people, or "a shared sense of peoplehood" (Clinton, 1986, p. 571). In general, **ethnicity** refers to a large group of people classified according to common national, tribal, linguistic, or cultural origin or background *and* who feel a sense of shared identity. Examples of ethnicity are Cuban, English (usually termed Anglo), Filipino, French, German, Haitian, (East) Indian, Irish, Italian, Jamaican, Mexican, Polish, Scottish, Spanish, Thai, Turkish, and so on. Although African may be considered an ethnicity, it is more precise to state the national origin within that continent, such as Algerian, Egyptian, Ethiopian, Kenyan, Libyan, Nigerian, and so on. Do not presume to know a person's ethnicity or what that person wishes to be called based on physical appearance. Ask, because that person may offer some other ethnic designation or multiple ethnicities.

Although *Hispanic* is a popular ethnic designation, it is probably too broad to be useful. The term, first used on the 1980 U.S. census forms, refers to people of Mexican, Puerto Rican, Cuban, South or Central American, or other Spanish culture or origin, regardless of race (U.S. Department of Commerce Bureau of the Census, 2010). Because a multitude of ethnicities are subsumed under that heading, expecting that such a wide variety of people would share exactly the same culture is unrealistic. Consequently, it is preferable to cite a specific ethnicity, such as Cuban, instead of the overarching term *Hispanic.* Furthermore, note that not all Hispanics appreciate the term because many believe it to be a political label of convenience that blurs cultural identity. Despite ongoing movements to change the term, it is probably here to stay, unfortunately, because the government has latched onto it. Nonetheless, as with any label, the health professional must go beyond terminology and interact with each unique person in order to determine culturally congruent care.

SPOTLIGHT ON

A World without Race

"Within 200 years, the very concept of race will be meaningless. There will be more and more mixing of races, until the time comes when people stop defining themselves and other people on the basis of race."

"But if that really does happen—if race ceases to mean anything—then who will people hate?" "Hopefully, no one," Maharidge said (Greene, 1996).

NURSING ALERT

Understanding Hispanic Ethnicities

Hispanic ethnicities include Argentinean, Colombian, Costa Rican, Cuban, Dominican, Ecuadoran, Guatemalan, Honduran, Mexican, Nicaraguan, Peruvian, Puerto Rican, Salvadoran, and Spanish, among many others. Knowing that your patient is Hispanic is only part of his or her uniqueness.

African American is also an ethnic designation; however, do not automatically assign that term to black people because it too is imprecise. For example, not all Africans are black, and not all black people are from Africa. Therefore, some may prefer another qualifier that best addresses their own cultural ancestry.

Race and ethnicity are not mutually exclusive terms. For example, a person may be of the black race and of Haitian ethnicity. Or a person may be white and of Mexican ancestry. Although *ethnicity* is not as broad a term as *race,* it is still somewhat of an umbrella term. As a result, keep in mind that, although people of the same ethnic origin may share many similarities, there are wide intraethnic variations. No two people within the same ethnic group behave exactly the same—nor should they be expected to do so. It is incumbent on health care professionals to recognize each person's uniqueness in order to avoid falling into the trap of stereotyping. Consider the child pictured in Figure 6-1 who could be erroneously stereotyped as one race or ethnicity although she is uniquely multiracial and multiethnic.

RELIGION

Religion can be interpreted as a belief in a higher power. However, it often refers to being affiliated with an organized religion, of which there are many.

Sometimes people list a religion on health forms, but they do not practice that religion. Conversely, some people are quite spiritual but have no religious affiliation. That is why a nurse should find out what religious or spiritual practices are relevant for each of every patient. Often, spiritual needs can be addressed simply by asking what brings comfort to the person.

NATIONALITY

Although the word **nationality** has various connotations, in general, it refers to the country of origin, such as Canada, France, Mexico, or the United States of America. For example, a child who is born in Canada and does not change citizenship is Canadian.

In the United States, people often identify themselves with a larger ethnic group. Examples are Chinese American, Irish American, Italian American, Mexican American, Polish American, and so forth. (See the section on Ethnicity.) When identifying self, those qualifiers can signify cultural pride. When identifying others, those same qualifiers can signify cultural discrimination. It depends on the tone.

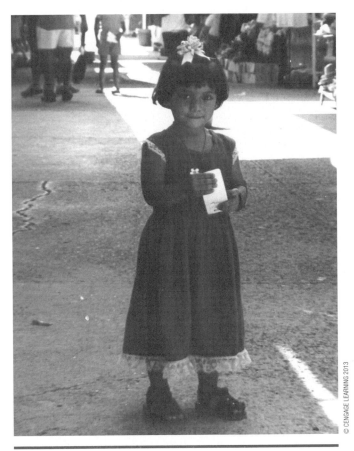

© CENGAGE LEARNING 2013

FIGURE 6-1 This child represents the unique multicultural, multiracial tapestry of which we are all a part.

Equally important, some U.S. citizens want to be identified only as nonhyphenated Americans. Supporters of this stance indicate that the past is in the past, and it is time to build a better future. Their attitude is, "How long do we have to be here in order to just be called 'American'?" Given such varying attitudes, individuals must be asked what they want to be called.

NURSING **ALERT**

Effect of Socioeconomic Status

People who share the same socioeconomic status (e.g., income, education) probably have more in common than those who do not, regardless of ethnicity.

LABELS

The bottom line is that these descriptors are all just labels. The problem with labels is that they rarely serve any useful purpose other than convenience. Additionally, the use of labels when referring to people tends to depersonalize and/or dehumanize them. In many respects, labels reflect a caste system mentality that effectively categorizes and rank-orders people. As such, the use of labels sometimes serves to create artificial boundaries, reinforce territoriality, and aggravate social discrimination.

SPOTLIGHT **ON**

Don't Call Me That

The gifted actor Morgan Freeman says, "If you want to give me an adjective, call me black . . . But don't call me African. I'm an American. Long, long bloody history . . . just like every other American. When I was a kid, we were colored . . . Then we became Negro . . . Then we became Afro, in the '60s, Afro-American ... So this quest for identity—it's like, number 1, misguided . . . This latest one, it just sets my teeth on edge. I think it's another one of those attempts to separate yourself . . . I'm walking around with this one-man crusade saying, 'DON'T CALL ME THAT [African American]!' " (Rowe, 1997).

- How can you use this information to provide culturally competent care?
- What do *you* want to be called?

NURSING **ALERT**

Using Correct Labels

Getting away from the use of labels is an uphill battle. Using precise labels is an even steeper climb (even among people who should know better). For example, white is not an ethnicity. It is a race. Hispanic is not a race. It is an ethnicity, albeit a broad term. America is not a country. It is a continent. So, if you must use a label for whatever reason, make sure you use a correct one.

Nonetheless, if labels are to be used for whatever reason, they must be used precisely. For example, when talking about race, the nurse should use one of the accepted racial classifications. Often, people use incorrect terms due to ignorance, not malicious intent; however, puzzlingly, some people continue to use incorrect terms even when the distinctions among the various terms are known. Is it habit or bigotry? Is it an easy way for an insecure ego to feel superior? In any case, the motivation for the continued use of incorrect terms should be suspect.

CULTURAL PRIDE

For a long time, the United States was referred to as a melting pot where all cultural groups were supposed to be melted, blended, or homogenized into one culture. Instead of being proud of family legacies, people were made to feel ashamed if they were different in appearance, speech, dress, faith, or custom. Names were Americanized, native languages were banned, accents were silenced, family traditions were abandoned, and ethnic jokes were encouraged. Although the melting pot mentality seemingly prevailed, some proudly held on to their cultural gifts. Slowly but surely, the word got out that cultural differences should be sources of pride, not embarrassment and that having differences does not preclude having similarities as well. Health care professionals need to learn about similarities so that they may be used to build bridges to provide culturally congruent care.

CULTURAL COMPETENCE

Everyone—and just about every life event—is influenced by culture, and the impact of culture extends into the health arenas (lay/popular, folk, professional). A person's culture serves to assign meaning to various health experiences. If nurses are to provide culturally congruent care, they should be culturally competent. To become so, they must realize that culture affects them as well as their patients. Such cultural competence requires nurses' self-awareness of their *own* culture and its myriad influences on their daily live (Anderson & McFarlane, 2011) in order to fully appreciate their patients' culture.

? ASK YOURSELF

What Does Your Cultural Heritage Look Like?

Does a **cultural tapestry**, woven with intricate yet distinctive strands that form a beautiful textured pattern, represent your unique cultural heritage? How about a meticulously pieced-together patchwork quilt? What about an intricate sculpture? Or is a bland piece of assembly-line fabric more representative? Which symbol would you choose if you could?

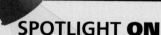

SPOTLIGHT ON

Build a Bridge

An old saying goes, "Build bridges instead of walls, and you will find a friend." When people focus only on differences, they build walls of fear and resentment instead of bridges of appreciation and joy. Don't waste energy building impenetrable walls. Walk across that bridge. Enjoy what you find there.

? ASK YOURSELF

Hospitalization and Culture Shock

People suddenly thrown into a strange environment can experience culture shock, causing them to feel lost and helpless. Similarly, sometimes hospitalized people can experience culture shock. Can you imagine how they may feel? Can you think of ways to alleviate their disorientation?

To become culturally competent, health care professionals must first become culturally aware and learn what is culturally relevant not only for themselves but also for the people in their care. Essentially, **cultural competence** is being able to incorporate *emic* and *etic* cultural knowledge into holistic and culturally congruent patient care. *Emic* **knowledge** is an insider's viewpoint of a culture, whereas *etic* **knowledge** is an outsider's viewpoint. Cultural competence also includes appreciating, respecting, and accepting people's cultural influences as well as incorporating them into appropriate wellness and illness patient care. By enhancing communication, cultural competence facilitates positive health outcomes. Cultural competence is, indeed, a worthwhile goal. Box 6-4 offers tips for enhancing communication for cultural competence.

BOX 6-4
COMMUNICATION TIPS

- Be aware of your verbal and nonverbal communication and your patient's.
- Provide a pleasant ambiance.
- Introduce yourself.
- Explain the purpose of the cultural assessment and the projected time to complete it. (It may take more than one visit to complete.)
- Convey your earnestness to learn as much as you can about your patient's culture.
- Keep your manner calm and unhurried, your tone nonthreatening, and your mind open.
- Use eye contact appropriately.
- If the other person is unsure of what you are asking, offer examples but do not lead patient responses.
- Listen carefully, letting the patient talk with as few interruptions as possible.
- Ask for clarification or feedback as needed.
- To avoid framing the patient's responses into your own views, periodically summarize what you have heard and ask for patient validation.
- Focus on patient strengths, not weaknesses.
- Remember that the cultural assessment is holistic.

SPOTLIGHT ON

Cultural Competence

Cultural competence involves being culturally aware and learning what is culturally relevant for each individual person. Cultural competence also includes appreciating, respecting, and accepting those cultural influences as well as incorporating them into appropriate wellness and illness patient care. By enhancing communication, cultural competence facilitates positive health outcomes.

CULTURAL ASSESSMENT

Because knowing everything there is to know about all cultures is impossible, a nurse's mission is to ask patients what is culturally relevant for them. Many caregivers conduct cultural assessments on their patients so that they may plan culturally appropriate care.

CULTURAL ASSESSMENT TOOLS

There are many cultural assessment tools, frameworks, and models (Andrews & Boyle, 2008; Giger & Davidhizar, 2008; Leininger, 1978; Leininger & McFarland, 2002). Most involve systematically collecting information about a person's particular group(s), spiritual beliefs, communication styles, interpersonal relationships, diet, wellness-illness practices, and lifestyles, in the hope of deriving that person's cultural attitudes, values, beliefs, knowledge, norms, customs, and so on. Because these assessment tools are designed to elicit so much cultural information via interviewing and observing, they take a considerable

HEALTH PROMOTION THEORY LINK

Process of Cultural Competence in the Delivery of Health Care Services Model

Dr. Josepha Campinha-Bacote's model is a culturally conscious model that describes cultural competence as a "process of becoming" rather than of "being" able to work effectively within the client's cultural context. Her model includes the constructs of cultural awareness, cultural knowledge, cultural skill, cultural encounters, and cultural desire (transculturalcare.net). She describes her model as a "volcano. At the base, there must be a true desire to be culturally competent. Once this desire is developed, it wells up and finally erupts, pervading all decisions made as a healthcare provider" (medscape.com).

Sources: http://www.medscape.com/viewarticle/513607, retrieved April 3, 2011; http://www.transculturalcare.net/Cultural_Competence_Model.htm, retrieved April 3, 2011

amount of time to complete and are best done in the patient's home and community over several visits. Even so, the cultural assessment is simply one source of patient data, which should be placed in perspective and updated as needed. Box 6-5 presents a sample framework for cultural assessment, including demographics, based on Leininger's (1978) Cultural Domains.

Cultural assessment, like any other assessment, is the first step of the nursing process. What is done with the cultural information determines cultural competence—that is, how well the nurse incorporates culturally relevant information into culturally congruent patient care. If the cultural assessment is

---

BOX 6-5

SAMPLE CULTURAL ASSESSMENT FRAMEWORK

Demographics

Name _____ Gender _____ Religion _____

Race(s) _____ Ethnicity(ies) _____

Date of Birth _____ Birthplace _____ Where Raised _____

Marital Status _____ Generation in U.S.A. _____ Years in U.S.A. _____

Language(s) Spoken _____ Primary Language _____

Preferred Language _____ Education _____ Occupation _____

Source: *Cultural Domains* (as identified by M. Leininger, 1978)

- General cultural life patterns or lifestyle
- Cultural values, norms, and expressions of an individual or a cultural group
- Cultural taboos and myths
- Worldview and ethnocentric tendencies
- Life-caring rituals and rites of passage

- Lay, folk, and professional wellness-illness cultural systems
- Specific caring behaviors and health care values, beliefs, and practices
- Cultural diversities, similarities, and variations
- Cultural changes and acculturation aspects

Source: Adapted from M. Leininger's *Cultural Domains* (1978).

done well, it is holistic insofar as the domains are interrelated, with each affecting the other; the product is more than the mere sum of its domains.

DEMOGRAPHICS/INDIVIDUAL PROFILE/IDENTIFYING INFORMATION

Demographic data is much more than filled-in information on a form; it provides personal connections to patients and must not be taken for granted. When viewed as a whole, an individual's demographic data provides essential information to derive a cultural profile that may effectively be incorporated into relevant wellness-illness care. For example, learning a woman's birthplace, age, marital status, years in the United States, and educational level tells you much more about her than simply knowing her generation in the United States.

For the most part, demographic information indicates each person's preferred designation(s) regarding self-identity. Sometimes nurses may need to provide examples or probe to uncover the relevant information, but they should not impose answers. For example, if a person's mother is French and his father is Irish, then that person should be allowed to claim both ethnicities. To claim only one is to disclaim the other. To claim only one is to conform to external expectations and is not an accurate representation of that person's identity.

NAME

A name is part of a person's cultural identity, and, as such, it should be treated with respect because it is part of who that person is. Often a name is part of a family's culture as well. For example, a child is often named after a favored aunt or a grandfather. Or patients may have hyphenated surnames passed on by their fathers. Hyphenated names also occur when individuals add a spouse's surname onto their own. Hyphenated names are fitting tributes to the families they proclaim. Whether or not a name reflects family traditions, it is still a big part of each individual. Ask what the person wants to be called, and then pronounce it properly.

GENDER

Gender is part of a person's cultural identity because many cultural components are related to gender, such as norms, roles, self-worth, and body image. So note an individual's gender, and then follow up with what cultural matters are gender based. For example, do the husband and wife, father and mother, have different roles? Are different chores assigned to sons and daughters? Are there different rites of passage? Household rules? Behaviors? Expectations? Are sons and daughters treated equally regarding dating practices, curfews, use of the family car, outside jobs, and so on? Are family attitudes about premarital sex the same for both the sons and the daughters? Are communication styles different for each gender? Are there rules about interacting with members of the opposite gender? Are male infants more prestigious than female infants?

RELIGION/SPIRITUALITY/FAITH

Religious or spiritual beliefs are integral to culture and extend into all aspects of life, such as attitudes about a higher authority, birth, death, good, evil, food, drink, sex, marriage, wellness, illness, health practices, choice, destiny, fate, afterlife, interconnectedness, and so on. A nurse should be very careful when discussing religious or spiritual beliefs with patients so as not to inadvertently denigrate their views.

When asking about an individual's religious or spiritual beliefs, merely listing a person's religion on a form is not enough. Not all people from a given religion have the same spiritual beliefs or needs. Some people may list a given religion on their health records even though they have not practiced the religion in a long time. Others may not list a religion at all or may not even believe in a supreme being, but they may be spiritual. For that reason, a health care provider should ask what religious or spiritual factors are important to each patient. Besides religion, these factors may include inner strength, life's purpose or meaning, or sources of comfort. A nurse should not presume to know what the patient believes or needs. For example, it could be rather unnerving for some people to see a religious leader walking into their hospital room.

RACE(S)

Race impacts a person's culture by how the race is viewed, not only by the self but also by society at large. Refer to the discussion on race earlier in this chapter. When nurses talk to patients, they should use only the five minimum race groups as outlined by the U.S. Census (white, black, American Indian or Alaska Native [including the principal tribe or nation], Asian, or Native Hawaiian or other Pacific Islander). Hispanic should not be listed as a race.

ETHNICITY

Ethnicity, as a social concept, has a strong connection to a person's culture. (Refer to the earlier discussion on ethnicity in this chapter.) Bear in mind that people may be multiethnic, so a nurse should not force them to list only one ethnicity. Also, race should not be confused with ethnicity. For example, white or black are not ethnicities. And, when people answer that they are Hispanic, you might ask them to specify which their ethnicity (e.g., Cuban, Mexican, Puerto Rican) because Hispanic is a very broad term.

DATE OF BIRTH/AGE

Age has a bearing on culture in several ways, but mainly in terms of the personal history lived by each individual. For example, a 5-year-old may have never experienced anything beyond the family's culture, whereas a 50-year-old might have been exposed to a variety of cultures, picking and choosing what is best for him. A teenager might feel quite differently about death than a centenarian. A school-age child might be much more in tune with the culture of computers than a 70-year-old, and so on.

❋ NURSING ALERT

Respecting People's Names

People should be called by their preferred name and with the correct pronunciation. If you do not know how to pronounce the name, ask.

It is disrespectful to use only people's surnames, to call them by their first name without permission, to mispronounce their name, or to address them with familiar names such as Grandma, Sweetie, Honey, Pop, Tía (aunt), or Bro. Such presumptions can very well be considered rude or impolite, as is referring to patients by their diagnoses, surgical procedures, or room numbers.

BIRTHPLACE/WHERE RAISED

Because culture tends to vary with geography, finding out a person's birthplace is helpful. More important, however, might be learning where the person grew up and the length of time spent in that location. A nurse should elicit the names of the city, state, and country.

MARITAL STATUS

In conducting a cultural assessment, a nurse should indicate whether the person is single (never married), separated, married, divorced, or widowed. Also helpful is knowing how long that person has been in the specific marital category. That information may provide added cultural insight into the person's present situation and hence in planning culturally congruent care.

ASK YOURSELF

Generation Determination

He was born in the United States. His mother immigrated here, so she is first-generation. His father and his family have lived here for five generations. What is he: first-generation, second-generation, third-generation, or mixed?

GENERATION IN THE UNITED STATES

To a large extent, generational status affects cultural identity, affiliation, beliefs, attitudes, practices, and so on because more recent immigrants generally cling to the culture of their homeland. However, much depends on the person's reason for immigrating as well as the length of time in the United States.

Determining generational status may be complex. Strictly speaking, an immigrant is considered to be a first-generation resident. An immigrant's child who is born in the United States is considered second-generation. An immigrant's grandchild is considered third-generation, and so forth. The complexity occurs when there is a difference between the immigration status of a child's parents or grandparents.

YEARS IN THE UNITED STATES

The length of time a person has lived in the United States affects that person's culture. For example, a person who has lived in New York for 40 years is more likely to have acculturated to the U.S. culture than someone who has lived there six months. That is not always the case, however, because much depends on the circumstances of each person's life.

All things being equal, how long a person has lived in the United States is probably more culturally influential than generational status. Consider the following examples of two 30-year-old people. The first person was born here but has lived the bulk of her life elsewhere. The second person has lived here since being brought over by his parents when he was 6 months old. Who is more likely to be "American"?

SPOTLIGHT ON

The Meanings of Language

Language conveys meaning that might be unique to a culture, vary among members of the same culture, or be shared among cultures. Sometimes, even when people speak the same language, one word can mean something entirely different to those who use it and to those who hear it, and its meaning might vary situationally. For example, *shot* might have different meanings depending on the context.

LANGUAGE(S) SPOKEN, PRIMARY LANGUAGE, AND PREFERRED LANGUAGE

Language and culture are intertwined. Language is one of the main means by which culture is transmitted. Language is also integral to both intracultural and intercultural communication. A shared language is a godsend, a welcomed familiarity, especially when two seeming strangers meet.

Primary language is the first language a person learns. It is sometimes also called native language. Occasionally, people may not have *one* primary language because they were taught two or more simultaneously. Preferred language is simply the language preferred by an individual. It may or may not be the same as the primary language. When possible, a nurse should use a patient's preferred language to enhance interpersonal communication, especially during times of stress. A multilingual person may not have a preference.

Practically all languages change after intermingling with other cultures. Dialects (regional language variations) may emerge. These frequently possess subtle yet significant differences from the main language. Cajun is an excellent example. Sometimes dialects reflect a combination of two or more languages (code switching, word borrowing, or word coining).

In the United States, speaking a language other than English has elicited both positive and negative responses. Throughout the twentieth century, some immigrants made a concerted effort to learn English and even encouraged their children to speak only English. Some did so in an attempt to adapt to the homogeneous melting pot mind-set. Others did so out of shame due to the stigma of being different. They wanted to blend in with the rest, so diversity was not valued in either case. Consequently, entire generations of people grew up without learning their culture's native tongue (e.g., German, Hebrew, Italian, Polish, Spanish, etc.). Recently, people have realized that being multilingual is a gift because the world is not monolingual. As a result, there has been renewed interest—and pride—in learning and being able to speak more than one language.

EDUCATION

When conducting a cultural assessment, a nurse should specify the number of years of formal education because that may affect the person's culture (or vice versa). However, the nurse should never confuse a lack of formal education with ignorance or diminished mental ability. A limited formal education does not mean that an individual is incapable of comprehending directions.

OCCUPATION

A nurse conducting an assessment needs to determine the patient's job, not only to determine health influences but also because occupations often have their own culture. As with education, the health care provider should not presume that a blue-collar worker or unemployed person lacks intelligence.

CULTURAL DOMAINS

In addition to factors such as marital status, birthplace, and years in the United States, a nurse must address several other areas during a cultural assessment. These include values, taboos, rituals, and more. Throughout the various domains, solicit information about the person's foods and celebrations, two things that often intertwine. Inquire not only about *what* is celebrated but *how* it is.

GENERAL CULTURAL LIFE PATTERNS OR LIFESTYLE

Describe your life, focusing on what you do during a typical day. If your days vary due to work or school, then describe each day. It is also a good idea to compare weekdays to weekends. Think about your lifestyle, that is, what you do on a typical day and with whom, including what you eat and where you eat it, who prepares your food, where you go, how long you sleep, and so on.

CULTURAL VALUES, NORMS, AND EXPRESSIONS OF AN INDIVIDUAL OR CULTURAL GROUP

Value is to the relative worth of a person, idea, thing, and so on. A value may be good or bad, desirable or not. For example, life might be valued above all costs, or it might be considered worthless unless a person is productive. A male child might be valued over a female. Although some values may be easily determined by watching or listening, others might be revealed only after questioning or inferring from behavior.

A norm is a cultural standard or rule that guides behavior. Norms are related to cultural values because they usually stem from whatever is valued. For instance, if a culture values virginity, then the norm might be to remain a virgin until marriage. If a culture values the elderly, then old people will be treated with respect and dignity. Families might have their own norms, such as which university to attend, which major to select, or which club to join. Norms may also have ages associated with them, such as getting married by age 21 or having children by age 25.

Reflecting both cultural values and norms, expressions may be verbal or nonverbal, tangible or not. Expressions may include prayer, meditation, songs, music, art, food, dance, exercise, gifts, eye contact, language, voice tone or pitch, personal space, celebrations, smiles, laughter, crying, visits with loved ones, hugs, kisses, attire, makeup, and other symbols.

CULTURAL TABOOS AND MYTHS

Taboos and myths are intertwined and related to cultural values, norms, and expressions. A taboo is something that is forbidden, such as a dangerous thought or unacceptable behavior. For example, in cultures where honesty is valued, cheating on tests or stealing might be taboo. Many taboos pertain to life, marriage, or sex, such as abortion, adultery, divorce, incest, or murder. Some taboos have become laws that prohibit or limit certain actions. A patient's taboos may also have profound implications in nursing care. For example, Jehovah's Witnesses consider it taboo to accept blood—even in cases of life and death.

A myth is a popular historical belief, tradition, or story that is unverifiable or unfounded but that may be hard to disprove. Because a myth makes sense to particular groups, it often serves to reveal a person's cultural worldview as well as explain beliefs and behavior. Myths may also highlight taboos and their consequences. For instance, if a taboo forbids a pregnant woman from viewing an eclipse, the corresponding myth might reveal that, if she does view it, her child will be born with a cleft lip. Numerous myths about health exist, while others revolve around sexual situations.

A superstition is a belief or practice resulting from ignorance, fear of the unknown, trust in magic or chance, or a false conception of causation. A superstition may also be defined as an irrational idea or as a notion maintained despite evidence to the contrary. The nurse must find out about people's superstitions because they may have evolved from cultural taboos, myths, or even rituals and may affect health practices. Although taboos and myths might be considered mere superstition by those who do not share similar cultural worldviews, keep in mind that people's beliefs usually guide their actions. It does not matter whether anyone else considers those beliefs to be myths, superstitions, or fact.

SPOTLIGHT **ON**

Worldview and Behavior

Consider how these various worldviews might affect behavior.

- People are good.
- The world is magical.
- Trust no one.
- If you do not take care of yourself, no one else will.
- The human body is a machine.
- Humans have souls. There is life after death.
- Human beings are physical creatures. Once you die, there is nothing more.
- God looks after you.
- Health care professionals are cold and impersonal.

WORLDVIEW AND ETHNOCENTRIC TENDENCIES

A person's worldview reflects values, norms, expressions, taboos, myths, rituals, rites, and so forth. It refers to how a person perceives the world, including issues of health, wellness, illness, sickness, death, human nature, and the like. Because culture affects worldview, and worldview usually affects actions, it is essential to understand how people see the world and what they think about it.

Ethnocentrism is the belief that one's cultural beliefs, worldview, and way of life are better than another's. It is rare to find a person who is not ethnocentric to at least a small degree. The important thing is to recognize internalized ethnocentrism so that it may be kept in rein.

Medicocentrism is the belief that professional health care practices are superior to any others, such as lay/popular or folk. Some people are reluctant to reveal their health care practices to health professionals for fear of being ridiculed. Nurses' success as health care professionals is enhanced if they truly appreciate, respect, and remain open to learning about other people's cultures.

LIFE-CARING RITUALS AND RITES OF PASSAGE

Rituals and rites of passage are intimately related to values, norms, expressions, worldview, taboos, health systems, and caring behaviors. Rituals and rites of passage are themselves intricately interwoven. A ritual is defined as a repeated act or series of acts. A rite of passage, on the other hand, signifies a transition associated with a crisis or a person's change of status, such as the first school day, obtaining a driver's license, the debutante ball/*quinceañera*, marriage, parenthood, widowhood, and other key events. Not all rituals signify rites of passage, but rites of passage usually involve rituals of sorts, often related to how the particular passage is carried out or celebrated. Although some religious practices are considered rituals, some are also rites of passage (e.g., receiving religious sacraments). Additionally, practices that deal with dying and death can be both rituals and rites of passage. For example, some people commemorate the dead by honoring them on special days (birthdays, Memorial Day, All Souls' Day/*Día de los Muertos*), by placing flowers or food at their graves, homes, or death sites, or by dedicating memorials (altars, statues, plaques, pictures, plants, trees, etc.) to them. (Figure 6-2 shows an altar commemorating *Día de los Muertos*/All Souls' Day.)

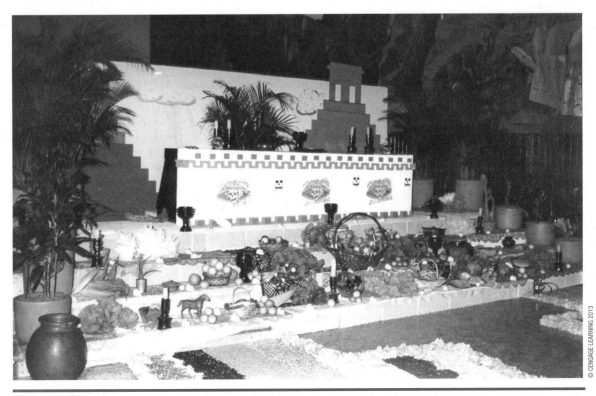

© CENGAGE LEARNING 2013

FIGURE 6-2 An altar in celebration of *Dia de los Muertos*/Day of the Dead/All Souls' Day.

LAY, FOLK, AND PROFESSIONAL WELLNESS-ILLNESS CULTURAL SYSTEMS

Cultural health systems are related to values, norms, caring behaviors, rituals, and taboos. According to Kleinman (1980), the overarching health care system in most societies is made up of three overlapping cultural health care arenas or sectors: lay/popular, folk, and professional. As health care professionals, nurses must recognize the existence of these arenas. To ignore even one of them is to miss out on the holistic nature of an individual's health care experience.

Both the lay/popular and folk health care arenas are nonprofessional in nature. The **lay/popular health sector** is made up of the individual along with family and friends. (Either term may be used, that is, *lay* or *popular*.) An example of lay health care is a mother feeding her child hot oatmeal on a cold morning to keep him well. The **folk health sector** consists of unlicensed, nonprofessional specialists who are usually members of the local community. A *curandero* (Mexican healer) is an excellent example of a folk specialist who uses mental, spiritual, and physical levels in providing health care. The **professional health sector**, by contrast, represents the formally organized, modern, scientific health community of licensed providers. Professional health care encompasses much more than medical care, which is, for the most part, provided by physicians. A registered nurse is an example of a professional health care provider. Table 6-2 presents other examples of health care providers within the various sectors.

No health care sector is necessarily better than another, although some are used more frequently. It has been estimated that most health care takes place in the nonprofessional sectors, with the bulk of that being wellness care in the lay/popular arena. Furthermore, both formal and informal research has documented that people tend to use the health care sectors simultaneously rather than unilaterally, picking and choosing what they want or need to stay well or to get well again.

Although numerous terms in the literature convey the notion that both nonprofessional and professional aspects of health care are practiced, perhaps the best are *complementary* and *integrative*. Complementary or integrative health care suggests that people enhance or complement their health by simultaneously engaging in multiple health care approaches from various nonprofessional and professional providers within the three overlapping sectors, which blend into a unified whole. The word *alternative*, on the other hand, suggests "instead of" rather than "together with," so avoid it. Think holism. *Complementary* or *integrative* is a much more realistic term because health care rarely exists in isolation, that is, in only one sector or with only one approach being used at a time. Health care professionals must therefore recognize that reality and ask about nonprofessional care in a nonthreatening way in order to provide holistic and culturally congruent care. For example, in a Navajo reservation hospital, there is a special room for conducting traditional healing ceremonies by the shaman or various other healers. Thus, both nonprofessional and professional types of health care are provided, and culturally congruent care is facilitated.

? ASK YOURSELF

What Are Your Health Beliefs?

As a budding health care professional, you probably now include aspects of the professional health care system in your culture. Are they in concert with your prior beliefs, or do they conflict? How will you handle these new influences? Will they become part of your culture? Will you accept them and discard others? Will you modify the new influences so that they fit with your previous values? Or will you compartmentalize your values as much as possible to reduce dissonance? Are you embarrassed about any of your (or your family's) health beliefs or behaviors?

TABLE 6-2 Health Care Arenas and Examples of Providers	
ARENA	**PROVIDERS**
Lay/ Popular	Yourself (the most important provider!)
	Parents, grandparents
	Siblings, children
	Spouse
	Friends, roommates
Folk	Health food store employee
	Spiritual healer
	"Barefoot" doctor
	Intuitive nutritionist
	"Granny" midwife
	Spa worker
Professional	Registered nurse
	Certified nurse-midwife
	Registered pharmacist
	Registered massage therapist
	Licensed dentist
	Licensed physician

© Cengage Learning 2013

Certain approaches are not limited to one health care arena. Instead, an approach may be used by providers from each arena. For example, an individual may choose to use ylang-ylang in a bath for its calming effect (lay), a folk herbalist may recommend arnica for a sore ankle, and nurses may incorporate the scent of lavender to create a healing environment. These essential oils are used throughout the various health care arenas (lay/popular, folk, and professional).

SPECIFIC CARING BEHAVIORS AND HEALTH CARE VALUES, BELIEFS, AND PRACTICES

Caring behaviors are intimately tied to values, norms, expressions, worldview, ethnocentrism, rituals, lay/popular, folk, and professional health cultural systems. Knowing how people view other people, wellness, illness, and healing can often help a nurse understand which health care values, beliefs, practices, and providers the patients will accept. Examples of these views about health include various health definitions, philosophies, meanings, expectations, or explanatory models (EMs). For instance, a person might define health as wellness, with wellness being the harmonious balance of mind, body, and spirit. Another person may believe that you are well as long as you can get your work done. To yet another, health may mean being disease-free.

Nurses need to understand their own and their patient's cultural health views because caring behaviors usually stem from health beliefs and reflect cultural expectations or norms. For instance, cultural traditions may designate the recipient of care, the health care provider(s) (e.g., women, men, nonprofessionals, professionals), and the type of care, which should be congruent with EMs, or explanations of the cause of the illness. Cultural health practices may include getting acupressure, preparing special food, administering medications, the laying on of hands, lighting candles, making *promesas* (promises), caring for the body after death, and so forth. There may also be forbidden health practices, such as blood transfusions, surgery, or being cared for by the opposite gender.

CULTURAL DIVERSITIES, SIMILARITIES, AND VARIATIONS (NONFAMILY)

Consider how your culture compares to those around you—your classmates, coworkers, friends, neighbors, and others—regarding each of the other domains, such as values, norms, taboos, expressions, rites of passage, and so forth. What is the same, and what is different? Think about your religion/spirituality, language(s), food, eating style, clothes, physical appearance, hygiene, recreation, music, parenting practices, job, income, degree major, lifestyle, worldview, health, symbolic objects, and so on. Appreciate both your similarities and differences!

CULTURAL CHANGES AND ACCULTURATION (FAMILY)

Acculturation refers to the process of adapting to or adopting aspects of another culture. Although something may be gained in the process, something is also usually lost. It is beneficial to reflect on your acculturation in comparison to your close family members, especially your parents, grandparents (both sets), brothers, sisters, children, and others. This comparison is especially striking when it involves generations. It is also interesting to compare yourself to your siblings who are either much older or younger than you. In essence, this domain integrates all the others—values, norms, expressions, taboos, worldviews, rituals, rites of passage, celebrations, and the like—as you compare yourself to your other family members regarding each domain.

ASK YOURSELF

Eclectic Healing: So What, If It Works?

Wellness-illness cultural systems can include music, art, dance, aromas, crystals, prayer, and so forth. What would you do if you found one of your patients (or friends):

- Being healed by a shaman in the hospital?
- Rubbing an herbal poultice on her body?
- Wearing an amulet to ward off the Evil Eye?
- Praying to be well?
- Fasting in observance of a cultural event?
- Listening to what he calls healing music?
- Burning sandalwood incense for its calming effects?
- Giving chamomile (*manzanilla*) tea to her baby to treat colic?

Just as you compared yourself to your friends, classmates, neighbors, coworkers, and others in Cultural Diversities, Similarities, and Variations (Nonfamily), do the same with your family. Consider how you and your family members have been acculturated, including similarities and differences. Think about your religion/spirituality, language(s), food, eating styles, physical appearance, hygiene, clothes, recreation, music, job, income, lifestyle, worldview, parenting practices, health conditions, symbolic objects, and so on.

CULTURAL COMPETENCE IN A MULTICULTURAL SOCIETY

Culture permeates life. For that reason, nurses must become culturally conscious so that they may acknowledge when their attitudes, values, norms, taboos, and so forth may affect those around them, including patients. Although expecting nurses or other health care professionals to always reconcile cultural differences is unrealistic, they still need to recognize and respect those differences in order to incorporate them into culturally realistic care.

There is no way to reduce cultural considerations to a simple formula that may be memorized and used as needed. There are no key words providing ready-made answers to real-life situations. There are also no books with titles like *Culture for Dummies, Ten Steps to Cultural Competence,* or *All You Ever Wanted to Know about Culture But Were Afraid to Ask.* Efforts

NURSING ALERT

Go to the Source

In most instances, patients are the most valuable and reliable resource about what is culturally relevant to and for them. So just ask them.

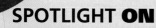

SPOTLIGHT ON

Cross-Generational Communication

Different generations commonly speak different languages. For example, a grandmother talks to her grandson in German. He talks to her in English. Yet, amazingly, both understand exactly what the other person says.

How do you think he learned to understand that other language even though he cannot speak it? Many children have admitted that they learned their family's non-English language by deciphering it whenever their parents started speaking it—out of curiosity to know what they were saying.

to do so have failed abysmally, resulting in mere cultural cataloging, misguided messages, and inevitably stereotyping.

But all is not lost. A nurse may provide culturally competent care by realizing that, although everybody has a culture, what is culturally relevant varies from person to person. When possible, a health care professional should willingly seek what is culturally relevant for each individual. That endeavor can be facilitated simply by being tuned into and responsive to each person's unique culture.

CULTURAL CATALOGING

A nurse cannot know everything about everyone else's culture. Not all Catholics want to see a priest. Not all Californians surf. The best way a nurse can find out what is culturally relevant to any one person is to ask. A nurse should not make decisions impacting health care based on cultural cataloging found in a handbook of highlights about various cultural groups. Stereotyping and negative prejudices may be inadvertently reinforced, resulting in cultural incongruence and distancing between the nurse and patient. Information from a cultural catalog should be validated with a patient before implementing it.

SUMMARY

Nurses are the logical mediators, teachers, enablers, and patient advocates. They ensure that a patient's cultural health rights and fundamental human rights are understood and respected in the professional health care arena. Accordingly, nurses must recognize both their own beliefs and those of their patients. By striving for cultural competence, they may promote positive health behaviors *outside* the professional health care arena as well as deliver culturally competent care *within* it.

KEY CONCEPTS

1. The concept of culture is composed of an interrelated set of attitudes, morals, beliefs, values, ideals, knowledge, symbols, artifacts, customs, traditions, and norms of a particular group that are transmitted intergenerationally and reflected in the perceptions, cognitions, and behaviors that are *unique* to every individual, group, organization, and community.

2. Culture is holistic in that it is all-encompassing: It is pervasive in the life of every individual; integral to groups, organizations, and communities; reflected in thoughts, feelings, behaviors, and lifestyles; and, thus, greater than the sum of its parts.

3. Because the interrelated concepts of culture, race, ethnicity, and nationality are not mutually exclusive, care must be taken to avoid confusion concerning them.

4. Although often equated only with environment, in truth, culture impacts each of the four concepts of nursing's metaparadigm: person, health, nursing, environment.

5. Bigotry, discrimination, prejudice, racism, and ethnocentrism take many forms, including labeling others, being judgmental, and even committing hate crimes.

6. Cultural assessment, as any other assessment, is the first step of the nursing process; as such, it is vital to the analysis, planning, implementation, and evaluation phases of the nursing process.

7. Culturally competent care begins with completing a cultural self-assessment.

8. Performing a cultural self-assessment creates a keen sense of awareness of your cultural heritage and its evidence in all aspects of your life. Knowing how your culture influences how you think, feel, and act increases your appreciation of the influence that culture has in the lives of your patients.

9. Values, beliefs, customs, norms, and rituals are parts of culture that manifest themselves in how we strive to attain, maintain, enhance, or regain our wellness.

10. Cultural competence incorporates *emic* and *etic* cultural knowledge into holistic and culturally congruent patient care; cultural competence involves cultural awareness, appreciation, sensitivity, and responsiveness.

11. Being a cultural advocate for your patients involves promoting positive health behaviors outside the professional health care arena, as well as delivering culturally competent care within it to ensure that your patient's culture is recognized, understood, and respected as a human right.

12. Aim for the highest and the best: Practice safe, holistic, culturally competent patient care.

CHAPTER REVIEW

Learning Activities

1. Complete a cultural self-assessment.

2. How did you feel when you first enrolled in nursing school? Was your reaction in any way akin to culture shock? Were any of your beliefs, attitudes, values, and the like in conflict with those held by members of the professional health care system? Did you share those conflicts with your teachers and classmates? If not, why not? If so, what was their reaction?

3. Arrange a cultural celebration with your classmates. Bring in favorite foods, music, knickknacks, pictures, videos, clothing, and other things that reflect your culture. After each of you has discussed the cultural significance of your items, you can feast on the foods and browse through the wares. You can learn a lot and have fun in the process.

4. What is meant by the culture of professional nursing? What components are involved? Language? Values? Norms? Expressions? Myths? Taboos? Superstitions? Rituals? Rites of passage? Foods? Caring behaviors? Celebrations? Ethnocentrism/medicocentrism? Acculturation?

5. At the end of each clinical day, do you reflect on the culturally congruent care you provided—or should have provided—to your patients?

6. If you still think you do not have a culture, read Miner's (1956) classic article on the Nacirema.

Multiple Choice

1. A mother is observed breast-feeding her 4-year-old son, who is a patient in the pediatrics wing of the hospital. A nurse is overheard talking in the nursing station about the "weird" way the mother has continued to breast-feed a 4-year-old. She comments that the "American" way is the best. The nurse is guilty of:
   a. ethnocentrism.
   b. failing to teach the mother about her child's nutrition.
   c. stereotyping.
   d. unusual break behavior.

2. Which of these patients would most likely refuse a blood transfusion, even if his or her life were in jeopardy?
   a. Hindu
   b. Jehovah's Witness
   c. Jew
   d. Mormon

3. The nurse must know the patient's religion in order to:
   a. chart it on his record.
   b. meet his physical needs.
   c. pray for him.
   d. provide holistic care.

4. A characteristic of culture is that it is:
   a. biologically inherited.
   b. individually determined.
   c. learned.
   d. stagnant.

5. *Hispanic* refers to:
   a. a homogeneous population.
   b. an ethnicity.
   c. a race.
   d. Spanish speakers.

6. When a patient says to the nurse, "I need to pray with my pastor in order to get well," the most appropriate response from the nurse is:
   a. "May I call your pastor and ask him to visit you?"
   b. "The medicine you take will make you well."
   c. "When you are released from the hospital, you can go to church and pray."
   d. "Why do you think prayer will make you well?"

7. The nurse should be aware of cultural aspects of health because:
   a. cultural groups assign various meanings to health.
   b. differences in health outcomes are based on culture.
   c. reimbursement is related to ethnicity.
   d. some cultural groups are represented in greater numbers than others.

8. Multiple health care approaches from various professional and nonprofessional practitioners are best termed:
   a. alternative.
   b. complementary.
   c. integrative.
   d. Both b and c

9. A patient's perspective or viewpoint is best referred to as:
   a. emic.
   b. etic.
   c. personal.
   d. worldview.

10. Cultural competence begins when the nurse:
    a. and patient are of the same culture.
    b. and patient speak the same language.
    c. is aware of the patient's culture.
    d. is aware of her or his own culture.

ORGANIZATIONS AND WEBSITES

Agency for Healthcare Research and Quality (AHRQ): The AHRQ mission is to improve the quality, safety, efficiency, and effectiveness of health care for all Americans: **http://www.ahrq.gov/**
 U.S. Department of Health & Human Services
 540 Gaither Road
 Rockville, MD 20850
 Phone: (301) 427-1364

American Anthropological Association (AAA): Founded in 1902, the AAA is the world's largest organization of individuals interested in anthropology: **http://aaanet.org/**
 2200 Wilson Boulevard; Suite 600
 Arlington, VA 22201
 Phone: (703) 528-1902/ Fax: (703) 528-3546

American Association of Colleges of Nursing (AACN): The AACN is the national voice for baccalaureate-and higher-degree nursing education programs. See "Toolkit for Cultural Competent Education" for BSN curricula:
http://www.aacn.nche.edu/Education/cultural.htm

The Center for Cross-Cultural Health: The vision is to achieve a state of health equity for all people. Its early mission was to integrate culture into health:

    34 Thirteenth Avenue NE; Suite 2002B
    Minneapolis, MN 55413
    Phone: (612) 331-3311/Fax: (612) 331-3337

National Center for Complementary and Alternative Medicine (NCCAM) (National Institutes of Health): The federal government's lead agency for scientific research on complementary and alternative medicine (CAM):

    9000 Rockville Pike
    Bethesda, MD 20892
    Phone: (888) 644-6226
    TTY: (866) 464-3615 (For hearing impaired)
    Fax: 866-464-3616
    http://nccam.nih.gov/

National Center for Cultural Competence (NCCC): The NCCC provides national leadership and contributes to the body of knowledge on cultural and linguistic competency within systems and organizations:

    Georgetown University Center for Child & Human Development
    Box 571485
    Washington, D.C. 20057-1485
    (202) 687-5387 or (800) 788-2066; TTY:(202) 687-5503
    Fax (202) 687-8899
    http://nccc.georgetown.edu/

National Center for Cultural Healing: Provides education in cultural diversity:

    2331 Archdale Road
    Reston, VA 20191
    Phone: (703) 626-1619
    http://www.culturalhealing.com

*The Office of Minority Health (OMH) (U.S. Department of Health & Human Services
National Standards on Culturally and Linguistically Appropriate Services [CLAS]):* The OMH is dedicated to improving the health of racial and ethnic minority populations through the development of health policies and programs that will help eliminate health disparities. OMH was reauthorized by the Patient Protection and Affordable Care Act of 2010 (P.L. 111-148):

    Resource Center
    PO Box 37337
    Washington, D.C. 20013-7337
    Phone: (800) 444-6472
    Fax: (301) 251-2160
    info@minorityhealth.hhs.gov
    http://minorityhealth.hhs.gov/assets/pdf/checked/finalreport.pdf

RACE: Are We So Different? A public education project funded by the American Anthropological Association: http://www.understandingrace.org/home.html and
http://www.aaanet.org/resources/A-Public-Education-Program.cfm

Resources for Cross Cultural Health Care: A national network of individuals and organizations in ethnic communities and health care organized to offer technical assistance and information on linguistic and cultural competence in health care:

    8915 Sudbury Road
    Silver Spring, MD 20901
    Phone: (301) 588-6051
    http://www.DiversityRX.org

Transcultural Nursing Society: Transcultural Nursing Society's mission is to enhance the quality of culturally congruent, competent, and equitable care that results in improved health and well-being for people worldwide: **http://www.tcns.org/index.html**

REFERENCES

American Anthropological Association. (1997, September). *Response to OMB directive 15: Race and ethnic standards for federal statistics and administrative reporting*. Retrieved from http://www.aaanet.org/

Anderson, E. T., & McFarlane, J. (2011). *Community as partner: Theory and practice in nursing* (6th ed.). Philadelphia, PA: Wolters Kluwer Health/Lippincott Williams & Wilkins.

Andrews, M. M., & Boyle, J. S. (2008). *Transcultural concepts in nursing care* (5th ed.). Philadelphia, PA: Wolters Kluwer Health/Lippincott Williams & Wilkins.

Clinton, J. (1986). Sociocultural issues relevant to health. In C. Edelman & C. L. Mandle (eds.), *Health promotion throughout the life span*. St. Louis, MO: Mosby, 570–583.

Giger, J. N., & Davidhizar, R. E. (2008). *Transcultural nursing: Assessment and intervention* (5th ed.). St. Louis, MO: Mosby.

Greene, B. (1996, November 10). United States with a white minority will be a significant change for the country. *The Monitor,* 7F.

Hall, E. T. (1990). *The hidden dimension*. New York, NY: Anchor Books.

Kleinman, A. (1980). *Patients and healers in the context of culture: An exploration of the borderland between anthropology, medicine, and psychiatry*. Berkeley, CA: University of California Press.

Leininger, M. M. (ed.). (1978). *Transcultural nursing: Concepts, theories, and practices*. New York, NY: Wiley.

Leininger, M. M., & McFarland, M. (2002). *Transcultural nursing: Concepts, theories, research, and practice* (3rd ed.). New York, NY: McGraw-Hill.

Miner, H. (1956). Body ritual among the Nacirema. *American Anthropologist, 58*(3), 503–507.

Mish, F. C. (ed.). (2007). *Merriam-Webster's collegiate dictionary* (11th ed.). Springfield, MA: Merriam-Webster.

Obasogie, O. K. (2010). Do blind people see race? Social, legal, & theoretical considerations. *Law & Society Review, 44*(3-4), 585–616.

Rowe, D. J. (1997, October 28). Morgan Freeman: The hardest part of acting is "getting jobs." *The Monitor,* 7B.

U.S. Census 2010. (2010). U.S. *census bureau random samplings*. Retrieved from http://blogs.census.gov/

U.S. Department of Commerce Bureau of the Census. (2010). *United States census 2010 questionnaire reference book* (D-1210). Retrieved, from http://2010.census.gov/partners/pdf/langfiles/qrb_English.pdf.

Wali, A. (1992). Multiculturalism: An anthropological perspective. *Report from the Institute for Philosophy and Public Policy* (University of Maryland at College Park), *12*(1), 6–8.

CHAPTER 7
Environmental Factors

JANICE A. MAVILLE, EdD, MSN, RN

KEY TERMS

anosmia
biomonitoring
building-related illness
carcinogens
chemical sensitivity
chi
chromotherapy
disease cluster
dose response
environmental health hazard
environmental health risk

ergonomics
feng shui
mutagens
noise
outgassing
particulate matter
posttraumatic stress disorder
   (PTSD)
SAD syndrome
sha
sick building syndrome

simultaneous perception
tao
teratogens
terrorism
toxins
utter watchfulness
volatile organic compounds
   (VOCs)
weapons of mass destruction
   (WMDs)
weapons of mass effect (WMEs)

OBJECTIVES

Upon completion of this chapter, the reader should be able to:

- Identify factors influencing environmental health.
- Distinguish between the attributes of a supportive versus a threatening environment.
- Recognize common symptoms resulting from occupational and environmental pollutants.
- Describe the process of chemical sensitization.
- Discuss the nurse's role in promoting environmental health.
- Assess a variety of environments for sources of toxins.
- Select interventions to improve environmental health.
- Explain the relationship between natural, technological, or terror-related disasters and posttraumatic stress disorder.
- Discuss ways to empower citizens to protect a community's environmental health.

INTRODUCTION

Promoting a healthy environment is essential for people all over the world. No matter where nurses practice, they are involved with all that affects individuals—the air they breathe, the water they drink, the food they eat, the homes they inhabit, and the political and economic factors that influence their quality of life.

Creating an entirely pollution-free environment is virtually impossible. It is therefore critical to understand how human bodies respond to the environment. If health is to prevail or healing is to occur, nurses must focus on total health, including environmental surroundings. They can take steps to minimize the effects of environmental toxins, and all health professionals share the responsibility of promoting a healthy, supportive environment.

Interventions for air, water, and land pollution are well-known. On a macro level, many of the changes needed to improve air, water, and land quality are expensive and complex, and they require the involvement of many people. At the same time, interventions for promoting a healthy *personal* environment are often overlooked. These approaches are generally easy, inexpensive, and individually controlled.

This chapter is a guide through the maze of environmental hazards. It provides an integrated view of the body and how it interacts with the environment. Identification of pollutants, environmental assessment, and methods to prevent or minimize the effects of toxins are discussed. Other environmental factors (e.g., noise and color) are also included. Suggested interventions are critical, as both preventative and curative measures. Environmental disasters and terrorism are given special attention.

PROBLEM IDENTIFICATION

The environment encompasses all conditions, circumstances, and influences that may affect individuals and populations. The immediate environment includes home, school, or workplace. These are surroundings that an individual may encounter moving through normal daily activities. Factors affecting the local community, the global community, and its atmosphere are a larger part of everyone's environment.

Health is affected by complex and interrelated factors in the environment. Environmental health and threats cannot be viewed in isolation. If an ecosystem is healthy, then individuals in that ecosystem are healthier. As an ecosystem deteriorates, so does human health. Deterioration may be immediate (e.g., toxic chemicals, contaminated groundwater), or they may accumulate over time (e.g., destruction of the ozone layer).

It has been estimated that some 3000 chemicals are produced in the United States and available in the marketplace that have not undergone any testing for toxicity, yet they are in materials used to furnish, clean, build, and insulate our homes, schools, public buildings, and workplaces. The Centers for Disease Control and Prevention (CDC) has measured 219 chemicals in the blood and urine of participants in the National Health and Nutrition Examination Survey (Centers for Disease Control and Prevention, 2009); however, the agency is monitoring only exposure, not health effects. The CDC is just one of many federal agencies that exist for the health of the people of the United States. Another major agency is the Environmental Protection Agency (EPA), created in 1970, whose mission is to protect human health and the environment (EPA,

2011a). The EPA leads the nation's environmental science, research, education, and assessment efforts. These efforts are accomplished through enforcing regulations, providing grant funding for research and environmental education projects, and promoting education to enhance the public's consciousness in caring for the environment. Conserving water and energy, minimizing outdoor air pollution, controlling indoor air pollution, and eliminating pesticide risks are a few of the focus areas for education and research by the EPA.

Such agencies are instrumental in identifying environmental problems or diseases or both. Epidemiology is the study of the distribution and determinants of disease in a population as well as the occurrence and causes of health effects in humans (Gordis, 2008). Using the epidemiological approach, agencies may link environmental health hazards and risks to the problem.

A substance or agent with the ability to cause any type of adverse health effect is an **environmental health hazard**. The effect can range from a minor illness, to a serious illness, to death. An **environmental health risk** is defined as the probability that there will be actual consequences from the potential danger of the hazard. For example, asbestos-containing materials (such as ceiling tile) are usually considered relatively harmless (a *risk*). Ceiling tile, however, may release asbestos fibers if disturbed. These asbestos fibers, once airborne, can be inhaled and become a *hazard*.

Environmental hazards are toxins, carcinogens, mutagens, or teratogens with specific consequences. **Toxins** cause harm or may be fatal to humans in low doses. **Carcinogens** promote the growth of or cause cancer. **Mutagens** change genetic material found in chromosomes. **Teratogens** cause birth defects.

A **disease cluster** is defined as a group of individuals experiencing the same disease in greater numbers than would otherwise be expected. An abnormally high level of colon cancer in a community is an example of a disease cluster. When a disease cluster is identified, biological and environmental factors are generally suspected (e.g., microorganisms or pollutants). Epidemiologists study disease clusters, identifying and studying patterns of health and illness in populations.

THE EPA MODEL OF RISK ASSESSMENT

The model used by the EPA, depicted in Figure 7-1, involves four major steps to assess risk when a disease cluster is identified (EPA, 2010a). First, the potential environmental hazards are delineated. This includes identifying the type of agent, how it works in the human body, and the seriousness of the damage done.

Second, the **dose response** process is delineated. The amount that is toxic and the human response must be determined. The model of response may be linear or threshold. In the linear model, harmful effects coincide in proportion to the dose. In the threshold model, certain levels of the substance may not be harmful; however, once a threshold is reached, harm occurs.

Estimation of the exposure is the third step. This includes determining the amount of the pollutant in the environment and the amount likely to reach a target site in the body. The fourth and final step is to characterize the risk in terms of the seriousness of the harm and susceptibility of the population. When this process is completed, appropriate steps are taken to reduce risk to the public. Nurses are frequently among the first to recognize disease clusters and bring them to the attention of other individuals or agencies.

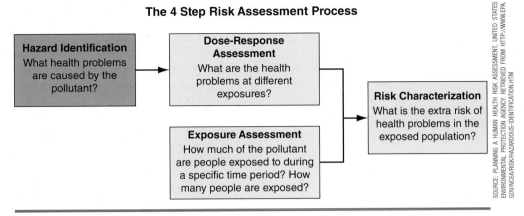

The 4 Step Risk Assessment Process

Hazard Identification	**Dose-Response Assessment**	**Risk Characterization**
What health problems are caused by the pollutant?	What are the health problems at different exposures?	What is the extra risk of health problems in the exposed population?

Exposure Assessment
How much of the pollutant are people exposed to during a specific time period? How many people are exposed?

SOURCE: PLANNING A HUMAN HEALTH RISK ASSESSMENT, UNITED STATES ENVIRONMENTAL PROTECTION AGENCY. RETRIEVED FROM HTTP://WWW.EPA. GOV/NCEA/RISK/HAZARDOUS-IDENTIFICATION.HTM

FIGURE 7-1 EPA model of risk assessment.

THE BODY'S RESPONSE TO ENVIRONMENTAL INFLUENCES

Nurses play a critical role in supporting individual health in a threatening environment. "Knowledge deficit related to risk of environmental hazards" and "potential for injury related to toxic exposure" are examples of nursing diagnoses related to environmental health. As disease entities are identified, the nursing plan of care can be expanded to include nursing diagnoses related to specific symptoms or illnesses.

The body produces internal toxins when under mental and emotional stresses. These toxins plus external pollutants significantly diminish the body's capacity to resist disease. Poor environmental conditions contribute either directly or indirectly to virtually all major chronic illnesses shown in a selected listing of adverse responses linked to known pollutants (see Table 7-1). No body system is safe from environmental harm. Fortunately, many of the physical illnesses and mental disturbances caused by environmental health hazards are reversible with the removal of the pollutant.

ACUTE AND CHRONIC EXPOSURE

Illness may result from acute or chronic exposure to pollutants. Acute exposure is described as exposure to high concentrations of a pollutant for a short period of time. Examples of acute exposure include smog or chemical emissions. Consequences from acute exposure range from mild symptoms (e.g., headaches and itchy eyes) to death from high concentrations of a particular substance (e.g., carbon monoxide). **Biomonitoring** is used in assessing human exposure to chemicals through the measurement of the chemicals or their metabolites in the body from such human specimens as blood or urine.

Exposure to low levels of a pollutant over an extended time is classified as chronic exposure. In the past this low-level but prolonged exposure was believed to be harmless. Definitive links have now been made between chronic exposure and the development of disease (Shi & Singh, 2011). Examples of chronic exposure are lead paint ingestion and the inhalation of asbestos fibers. Pregnant women need to be especially alert because chronic exposure is more likely to be embryotoxic (toxic to a developing fetus) than is acute exposure.

TABLE 7-1 Potential Adverse Responses Linked to Pollutants

PHYSIOLOGICAL	ADVERSE RESPONSES
Gastrointestinal	Nausea, vomiting, diarrhea, cancer
Central nervous system	Headaches, sinus pain, sensory disturbances (auditory, visual, olfactory), dizziness and vertigo, blackouts, impaired mental functioning
Musculoskeletal	Weakness, muscle cramps, tremors
Respiratory	Nasal congestion, coughing, wheezing, asthma, emphysema, cancer
Genitourinary	Infertility, urine color changes, pain on urination, difficulty urinating or decreased urination
Integumentary	Rash, itching, hair loss
Immune responses	Irritated eyes, fever, chills, fatigue, chemical sensitivity
Psychological	Irritability, depression, loss of concentration, nervous breakdowns, short-term memory loss, mental confusion, personality changes, hyperactivity, learning disabilities, belligerence, temper outbursts, social withdrawal, criminal behavior, attention deficit disorder
Syndromes	Chronic fatigue syndrome, Epstein-Barr syndrome, Gulf War syndrome, severe acute respiratory syndrome (SARS)

Sources: Peiris, J. S., & Poon, L. L. (2011). Detection of SARS coronavirus, *Methods in Molecular Biology, 665,* 369–382; Caravati, E. M., & McGuigan, M. A. (2004). *Medical Toxicology.* Philadelphia: Lippincott Williams & Wilkins; Colls, J. F., & Tiwary, A. (2010). *Air Pollution,* New York: Routledge.

Often, the accumulation and combination of environmental threats cause disease. One or two environmental stressors may be tolerated well. However, when another stressor is added, the biological system fails.

Pollutant sensitivity varies with the individual. Adverse reactions may be suffered by one individual while another remains symptom free. A formerly symptom-free individual may develop **chemical sensitivity** as a result of chronic exposure. Chemical sensitivity is the physiological response to a toxic substance following long-term exposure to low-level chemicals that were not recognized as harmful in the past. Following chemical sensitization, an individual develops a severe response with minimal exposure to the pollutant. Box 7-1 lists sample questions to ask when pollutants are suspected of causing physical symptoms.

SOURCES OF POLLUTION EXPOSURE

Common sources of widespread pollution exposure include the air, water, and soil. Other sources that are more localized are sound, light, and place. Disasters, not usually considered sources of pollution, cause both immediate and long-term devastating effects on the environment and its inhabitants.

AIR POLLUTION

A contaminated atmosphere contributes to the full spectrum of physical ills. Fortunately, the environment has a very efficient cleaning system (e.g., wind, rain, temperature change) that purges the outside atmosphere periodically. Nevertheless, the body wages a constant battle for survival against inhaled pollutants from the atmosphere. Nasal hairs, called cilia, in the upper airway passages serve as filters. Coughs or sneezes are reflexes that expel many substances that get past the filtering system. Residual particles remain in the body to be fought by the immune system.

INDOOR AIR

The Environmental Protection Agency (2011a) estimates that indoor levels of many pollutants may range from 2 to 5 times and sometimes even 100 times higher than outdoor levels,

making indoor air pollution among the top five environmental risks to public health. With people spending on average about 90% of their time inside a building, indoor air quality has become a distinct field of study for environmental health.

NURSING ALERT

Sensing Pollutants

The sense of smell can perceive between 2000 and 4000 odors and is 10,000 times more sensitive than the sense of taste. Nonetheless, smell is not an accurate tool for detecting pollutants because it begins to dull and adapt to odors during exposure. Even though an odor may be pleasing to an individual, such as that of perfumes, air deodorants, or scented candles, it may not be harmless.

The current air quality issue began in the early 1980s with building designs to conserve energy. Consequently, many buildings were constructed or remodeled to be airtight, with fresh air vents either plugged or omitted in the planning for air handling systems. As a result, rather than circulating fresh air, stale air was recycled. One report suggested that up to 30% of new and remodeled buildings worldwide were responsible for excessive complaints related to indoor air quality (EPA, 2010b).

The term **sick building syndrome** was coined to describe situations in which building occupants experienced acute health and comfort effects that appeared to be linked to time spent in a building, regardless of the building's location, without having a specific illness or cause identified (EPA, 2010c). In contrast, the term **building-related illness** describes a diagnosable illness that can be directly linked to airborne building contaminants (EPA, 2010c). An example is hypersensitivity pneumonitis, a nonallergic, immunologic pulmonary disease caused by the inhalation of dusts from contaminated humidifiers, moldy organic debris, animal proteins, and certain chemicals. Table 7-2 compares indicators for each of these terms. As seen in Table 7-3, the symptoms from various sources of indoor

---

BOX 7-1
CONNECTING POLLUTANTS WITH SYMPTOMS

The following is a selected sample of questions that may be used when pollutants are suspected.

- Do you think your symptoms can be associated with exposure to pollutants?
- When and where do your symptoms occur or worsen?
- Do others in the same setting experience the same symptoms and pattern of occurrence?
- Do symptoms diminish when you are away from the suspected setting for any length of time?
- Have you traveled or vacationed recently? Where?

- Have you flown on an airplane lately?
- Have you been swimming in rivers or lakes that might be contaminated?
- What cleaning supplies, fertilizers, herbicides, and other substances are being used near you?
- Do you use any substances at work or in hobbies that may contain harmful chemicals?
- Have there been alterations in the growth patterns of your indoor plants? Signs that the inside air is heavy with unhealthy chemicals are stems growing in strange, unnatural directions; abnormal growth rates; leaf tips that are curled or discolored.

TABLE 7-2 Sick Building Syndrome versus Building-Related Illness: A Comparison of Indicators

INDICATOR	SICK BUILDING SYNDROME	BUILDING-RELATED ILLNESS
Building occupant complaints	Headache; eye, nose, or throat irritation; dry cough; dry or itchy skin; dizziness and nausea; difficulty in concentrating; fatigue; and/or sensitivity to odors	Cough; chest tightness; fever; chills; muscle aches
Cause of the symptoms	Unknown	Clinically defined and clearly identifiable
Relief from symptoms	Soon after leaving the building	Prolonged recovery times after leaving the building

Source: U.S. Environmental Protection Agency (EPA) (2010c). "Indoor Air Facts No. 4 (revised): Sick Building Syndrome (SBS)." Retrieved from http://www.epa.gov/iaq/pubs/sbs.html.

TABLE 7-3 Checklist for Possible Symptoms and Related Indoor Air Pollutants

SYMPTOMS	ENVIRONMENTAL TOBACCO SMOKE	OTHER COMBUSTION PRODUCTS	BIOLOGICAL POLLUTANTS	VOLATILE ORGANICS	HEAVY METALS	SICK BUILDING SYNDROME
Respiratory						
Rhinitis, nasal congestion	✓	✓	✓	✓		✓
Epistaxis				✓[1]		
Pharyngitis, cough	✓	✓	✓	✓		✓
Wheezing, worsening Asthma	✓	✓		✓		✓
Dyspnea	✓[2]		✓			✓
Severe lung disease						✓[3]
Other	✓	✓	✓	✓		✓
Conjunctival irritation	✓	✓	✓	✓		✓
Headache or dizziness	✓	✓	✓	✓	✓	✓
Lethargy, fatigue, malaise		✓[4]	✓[5]	✓	✓	✓
Nausea, vomiting, anorexia		✓[4]	✓	✓	✓	
Cognitive impairment, personality change		✓[4]		✓	✓	
Rashes			✓	✓	✓	
Fever, chills			✓[6]		✓	
Tachycardia		✓[4]			✓	
Retinal hemorrhage		✓[4]				
Myalgia (muscle aches)				✓[5]		✓
Hearing loss				✓		

1. Associated especially with formaldehyde.
2. In asthma.
3. Hypersensitivity pneumonitis, Legionnaires' disease.
4. Particularly associated with high CO levels.
5. Hypersensitivity pneumonitis, humidifier fever.
6. With marked hypersensitivity reactions and Legionnaires' disease.

Source: U.S. Environmental Protection Agency (EPA). (2010d), "Indoor Air Pollution: An Introduction for Health Professionals." Retrieved from http://www.epa.gov/iaq/pubs/hpguide.html

air pollutants vary. Therefore, determining whether the individual is suffering from sick building syndrome, building-related illness, or another cause can be difficult. For example, psychological factors (job or school stress, coworker conflict, work dissatisfaction, etc.) or health conditions (asthma, eczema, etc.) may be *caused* by or *exacerbated* by indoor air quality problems. Figure 7-2 depicts an example of internal and external sources of air pollution that may be found in schools.

Common sources for indoor pollutants are tobacco smoke, unvented gas appliances, chemically treated building materials, foam insulation, synthetic carpeting, particle board furniture, aerosol products, cleaning products, cooking fumes, and naturally emitted radon gas. These examples, along with other indoor air pollutants, can be categorized into three major areas:

- Particulate matter (e.g., environmental tobacco smoke, asbestos, dust)
- Biological contaminants (e.g., animal dander, fungal spores, bacteria, pollens, viruses)
- Gases and vapors (e.g., carbon monoxide, formaldehyde, radon, pesticides) (EPA, 2010e)

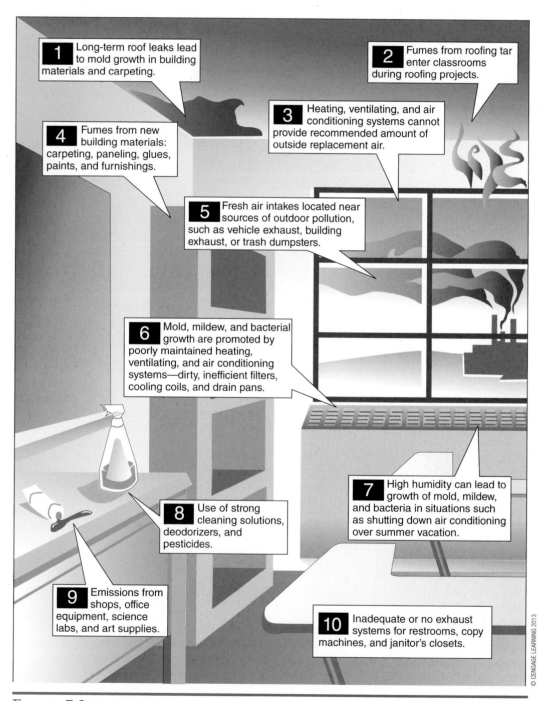

© CENGAGE LEARNING 2013

FIGURE 7-2 **Ten sources of air pollutants in schools. Internal and external factors can influence air quality in schools.**

Particulate Matter

Particulate matter consists of small particles or liquid droplets that can be suspended in the air. The amounts and sources of particulate matter in the air vary. The biggest sources of indoor particulates are windblown dust, house dust, and tobacco smoke. Other sources are woodstoves and appliances like furnaces and nonelectric heaters. The health effects of particulate matter vary in severity and may include:

- Coughing, wheezing, shortness of breath.
- Aggravated asthma.
- Lung damage (including decreased lung function and life-long respiratory disease).
- Premature death in individuals with existing heart or lung diseases ("What is particulate matter?" n.d.).

Environmental tobacco smoke (ETS), also known as secondhand tobacco smoke, contains a mixture of over 4000 chemical compounds and is the single most preventable indoor air pollutant (EPA, 2010f). The EPA estimates that exposure to secondhand smoke causes over 3000 lung cancer deaths per year in nonsmokers. Infants and children are especially affected by the damaging effects of ETS, which include asthma, middle ear infections, pneumonia, bronchitis, and sudden infant death syndrome.

Asbestos is a source of particulate matter that is known to cause cancer. Asbestos was once commonly used in construction for insulation, fireproofing, soundproofing, and roofing, as well as in other industrial work. It was even used in household products such as ironing board covers, hot pads, and oven mitts. Workers and their clothes would become covered with the white powder of asbestos. Years later, many of those exposed to asbestos powder and fibers were found to have developed gastrointestinal and lung cancers. A certain type of deadly cancer called mesothelioma is a direct result of asbestos exposure (National Heart Lung and Blood Institute, 2011; Mesolink, 2010). Because the substance was not known to be hazardous, asbestos-containing products were not labeled. Over time, materials containing asbestos disintegrate and, if disturbed, release microscopic fibers into the air to be inhaled. The removal of materials known to contain asbestos is recommended only as a last resort because this increases exposure; sealing or encapsulating the asbestos is recommended (EPA, 2010c; Mesolink, 2010). Buildings constructed before 1978 are considered suspicious for asbestos and should be inspected by construction professionals or local environmental agencies.

Biological Contaminants

Biological contaminants include bacteria, viruses, molds, mildew, animal dander and cat saliva, house dust, mites, cockroaches, and pollen (EPA, 2010b). Even protein in urine from rats and mice is a potent allergen when it dries and becomes airborne. Biological contaminants are found everywhere—in schools, offices, workplaces, stores, and homes. Contaminated central air-handling systems can become breeding grounds for mold, mildew, and other sources of biological contaminants that can be spread throughout a building (EPA, 2010b). For example, Legionnaires' disease, a potentially fatal bacterial pneumonia, and its lesser form, Pontiac fever, were found to be spread indoors via moisture from contaminated air conditioning systems.

Three types of human disease can be attributed to biological contaminants in the air: (1) infections, where pathogens invade human tissues; (2) hypersensitivity diseases, where specific activation of the immune system causes disease; and (3) toxicosis, where biologically produced chemical toxins cause direct toxic effects (EPA, 2010c). Action to protect against biological contaminants is directed at eliminating the sources as much as possible. Efforts should be taken to repair leaks; dry areas where moisture has collected; keep the relative humidity at 30–50%; vent areas where moisture can collect, such as bathrooms and kitchens; maintain clean filters in air conditioning systems; wash bedding and soft toys frequently in water at a temperature above 130° F to kill dust mites; and vacuum carpets and upholstered furniture regularly (EPA, 2010c). Sensitive individuals should avoid contact with pets and dust and use a commercially available HEPA (high-efficiency particulate air) filtered vacuum.

✹ NURSING **ALERT**

Efforts to Reduce Biological Contaminants

- Repair leaks.
- Dry areas where moisture has collected.
- Keep relative humidity at 30–50%.
- Vent areas where moisture can collect, such as bathrooms and kitchens.
- Maintain clean filters in air conditioning systems.
- Wash bedding and soft toys often in water temperature above 130° to kill dust mites.
- Vacuum carpets and upholstered furniture regularly.
- Sensitive individuals should avoid contact with pets and use a HEPA (high-efficiency particulate air) filtered vacuum.

Gases

Gaseous pollutants can be emitted from a variety of indoor sources due to malfunction or improper use: gas appliances, fireplaces, furnaces, wood or coal stoves, and kerosene stoves, heaters, or lights. In addition to natural gas emission, combustion sources can cause serious atmospheric pollution by releasing such gases as carbon monoxide (CO), nitrogen dioxide (NO_2), and sulfur dioxide (SO_2) (EPA, 2010d).

Radon is a tasteless, colorless, and odorless gas that is second only to cigarette smoking as the leading source of lung cancer, accounting for approximately 20,000 deaths each year in the United States (EPA, 2010c). Radon is a decay product of uranium and occurs naturally in soil and rock. It may also contaminate the water supply, especially in private wells. Radon has been identified in every state. It is estimated that 6% of U.S. homes, or one in 15, have elevated levels of radon. Radon enters the home from the ground through cracks in concrete floors and walls, space between the slab and the floor, and around pipes and drains (WHO, 2004). The most effective intervention for reducing radon levels in the home is depressurization of sub-slabs with vent pipes with exhaust fans in garages and attics (National Collaborating Centre, 2008). Moderately effective is increased ventilation and least effective is sealing or caulking problem areas (National Collaborating Centre, 2008). Box 7-2 highlights information on testing for radon.

Volatile organic compounds (VOCs) are gases released from certain solids or liquids and are found in thousands of products. Box 7-3 lists examples of VOC sources. Concentrations of many VOCs are up to 10 times higher indoors than outdoors (EPA, 2005c). The effects from exposure to these VOCs can be short or long term; nonetheless, they can contribute to the creation of an indoor chemical crisis for some individuals.

Formaldehyde is the most well-known of volatile organic compound (VOC) pollutants. It is a common ingredient in plywood, particle board, laminated lumber, vinyl panels, wallpaper, glue adhesives, and insulating materials. In high temperatures and humidity, formaldehyde breaks down into a toxic gas. This process is called **outgassing**. The strength of the odor is usually directly proportional to the degree of outgassing. That "new carpet smell" or "new car smell" and the haze on a car's windows result from formaldehyde outgassing. The outgassing process from plastics and upholstery in a new car may last a couple of years. Formaldehyde is also found in permanent press fabrics, rubber, and consumer products ranging from cosmetics to medicines. Certain occupations (such

---

BOX 7-2
TESTING FOR RADON

Low-cost radon test kits are available by mail order, in hardware stores, and through other retail outlets. Depending on whether a short-term or long-term test is used, it takes anywhere from 2 to 90 days for results. Long-term tests give a more accurate annual average radon level than do short-term tests because radon levels vary from day to day and season to season. Only home test kits labeled "meets EPA requirements" should be used.

BOX 7-3
SOURCES OF VOLATILE ORGANIC COMPOUNDS

Paints, paint strippers, varnishes, lacquers, waxes
Rug and oven cleaners
Dry-cleaned clothing
Pesticides
Building materials and furnishings
Office equipment such as copiers and printers
Correction fluids and carbonless copy paper
Graphics and craft materials, including glues and adhesives
Permanent markers
Photographic solutions

From An Introduction to Air Quality: Volatile Organic Compounds, *By Environmental Protection Agency (EPA), 2010g,* http://www.epa.gov/iaq/voc.html

---

GLOBAL HIGHLIGHTS IN HEALTH PROMOTION
World Health Organization's Global Focus on Indoor Air Quality

The World Health Organization has recognized that clean air is fundamental to life and that exposure to indoor air pollutants poses a major problem to global health, especially in developing countries. To address this global health problem, the organization has published a series of guidelines that focus on air pollution. The guidelines are intended to be used by public health professionals involved in preventing the health risks of environmental exposures and by those involved in the design and use of buildings, indoor materials, and products in all regions of the world. The guidelines on indoor air quality synthesize scientifically based evidence on nine selected pollutants and address the source, relationship to outdoor levels, kinetics and metabolism, health risks and effects from exposure, and recommendations to reduce the health risks.

World Health Organization (WHO). (2010). *WHO guidelines for indoor air quality: Selected pollutants.* Retrieved from http://www.euro.who.int/__data/assets/pdf_file/0009/128169/e94535.pdf

---

as morticians and pathologists) are exposed to high levels of formaldehyde. Formaldehyde monitors are available. Monitors may be hung in a room and then submitted to a laboratory for analysis. Symptoms of exposure include eye irritation, heart palpitation, coughing, chest tightness, and headache.

It is important to note that some common household cleaners may be extremely toxic when combined. For example, when chlorine-based cleaners are mixed with ammonia, a deadly gas called chloramine is formed. Reading and following instructions and warning labels on all products is essential for safe use and for avoiding exposure to harmful pollutants. Box 7-4 lists questions that could be used in assessing for risks from indoor air pollutants.

WORKSITE AIR QUALITY MANAGEMENT

One of the many roles of occupational health nurses is indoor air quality management at the worksite. These nurses work as facilitators or team leaders to improve workplace environmental conditions, including air quality.

Indoor air quality problems at the worksite arise from various sources, as shown in Box 7-5. An interdisciplinary group of professionals may be required to assess the situation and to develop a plan to minimize or eliminate the problem. The team may be composed of an occupational health nurse, a physician, an industrial hygienist (environmental hygienist), a microbiologist, an epidemiologist, a toxicologist, and/or a professional engineer. The complexity and seriousness of the identified problem determine the size and membership of the team.

A team should investigate a situation if at least 20% of the employees report a similar problem. Individual, nonrecurring problems can be addressed by the occupational health nurse. Once the problem is identified and resolved, employees enjoy better health, leading to improved efficiency, decreased absenteeism, and increased worker satisfaction.

OUTDOOR AIR

One of the most pressing worldwide problems in the new century is outdoor, or ambient, air pollution. Contributors to ambient air pollution are factories releasing particulate matter,

---

BOX 7-4

RISK ASSESSMENT FOR INDOOR AIR POLLUTANT EXPOSURE

Sick Building Syndrome

- Are problems temporally related to time spent in a particular building or part of a building?
- Do symptoms resolve when the individual is not in the building?
- Do symptoms correspond to the need for heat or air conditioning?
- Have coworkers' peers had similar complaints?

Biological Contaminants

- Are symptoms related to the workplace, home, or other location?
- What are possible sources of contaminants in the suspected location?
- Is the relative humidity in the home or work place consistently above 50%?
- Are humidifiers or other water-spray systems in use? How often are they cleaned?
- Are they cleaned appropriately?
- Has there been flooding or leaks?
- Is there evidence of mold growth (visible growth or odors)?
- Are organic materials handled in the workplace?
- Is carpet installed on unventilated concrete (e.g., slab-on-grade) floors?
- Are pets in the home?
- Are there problems with cockroaches or rodents?
- Is adequate outdoor air being provided?
- Are foul odors present (fishy or locker room smells)?

Sources of Combustion (Stoves, Heaters, Fireplaces, etc.)

- What types of combustion equipment are present, including gas furnaces or water heaters, stoves, unvented gas or kerosene space heaters, clothes dryers, fireplaces? Are fuel-burning appliances, such as gas stoves and fireplaces, properly vented to the outside?
- Are household members exhibiting influenza-like symptoms during the heating season?
- Are they complaining of nausea, watery eyes, coughing, headaches?
- Is a gas oven or range used as a home heating source?

- Is the individual aware of odor when a heat source is in use?
- Is heating equipment in disrepair or misused? When was it last professionally inspected?
- Does the structure have an attached or underground garage where motor vehicles may idle?
- Is charcoal being burned indoors in a hibachi, grill, or fireplace?

Heavy Metals (Airborne Lead and Mercury)

- Does the family reside in old or restored housing?
- Has renovation work been conducted in the home, workplace, school, or day care facility?
- Is the home located near a busy highway or industrial area?
- Does the individual work with lead materials, such as solder or automobile radiators?
- Does the child have a sibling, friend, or classmate recently diagnosed with lead poisoning?
- Has the individual engaged in art, craft, or workshop projects?
- Does the individual regularly handle firearms?
- Has the home interior recently been painted with latex paint that may contain mercury?
- Does the individual use mercury in religious or cultural activities?

Volatile Organic Compounds (Formaldehyde, Pesticides, Solvents, Cleaning Agents)

- Does the individual reside in a mobile home or new conventional home containing large amounts of pressed wood products?
- Has the individual recently acquired new pressed wood furniture?
- Does the individual's job or a vocational pursuit include clerical, craft, graphics, or photographic materials?
- Are chemical cleaners used extensively in the home, school, or workplace?
- Has remodeling recently been done in the home, school, or workplace?
- Has the individual recently used pesticides, paints, or solvents?

Source: U.S. Environmental Protection Agency (EPA). (2010d). "Indoor Air Pollution: An Introduction for Health Professionals." http://www.epa.gov/iaq/pubs/hpguide.html

---

BOX 7-5

SOURCES OF WORKSITE AIR POLLUTION

Indoor Sources

Housekeeping and maintenance—some cleansers, dusting, vacuuming, disinfectants, pesticides, and adhesives

Occupant—tobacco products, office equipment (printers, copiers), microwaves, cooking appliances, art supplies, marking pens, personal products, tracked-in dirt/pollens

Shared space—dry cleaners, pet stores, laboratories (chemicals, moisture), print shops, art stores, beauty salons, restaurants, cafeterias, medical offices

Building—construction materials and adhesives, asbestos, insulation, wall/floor coverings, wet building products, upholstered furniture, renovation materials, and transformers

HVAC (heating, ventilation, and air conditioning) system—filters, ducts, humidifiers, drain pans, mechanical rooms, lubricants, combustion appliances, refrigerants

Vehicles—underground/attached garage

Outdoor Sources

Vehicles—traffic, loading docks

Commercial/manufacturing—dry cleaners, restaurants, automotive shops, gas stations, paint shops, electronics manufacturers

Utilities/public works—utilities/power plants, incinerators, water treatment plants

Agriculture—pesticide use, processing plants, ponds

Birds/rodents—droppings, nests

Building maintenance—painting, roofing, sanding, pesticides, trash, refuse

Water—pools of water on roofs, cooling tower mist

Ground/underground—soil, water, sewer gas, underground storage tanks

Sources: U.S. Environmental Protection Agency (EPA) (2010e). "An Office Building Occupant's Guide to Indoor Air Quality." Retrieved from http://www.epa.gov/iaq/pubs/occupgd.html, Rom, W. N. (2012). *Environmental policy and public health: Air pollution, global climate change, and wilderness.* Hoboken, NJ: Wiley.

---

nitrogen, and sulfur oxides; vehicles emitting carbon monoxide; and natural phenomena diffusing particulate matter (i.e., volcanic eruptions and geysers). Diesel exhaust contains 20–100 times more particles than gasoline exhaust, along with dangerous gases, including nitrous oxide, nitrogen dioxide, formaldehyde, benzene, sulfur dioxide, hydrogen sulfide, carbon dioxide, and carbon monoxide (American Federation of State, County, and Municipal Employees, n.d.). Not surprisingly, diesel exhaust from common sources, such as trucks, buses, and trains, is linked to increases in asthma, bronchitis, emphysema, and cancer. Landfills can also be a source of outdoor air pollution by outgassing methane and buried toxic chemical fumes.

Under normal conditions, warm air rises, dispersing pollutants and carrying them away from Earth. Wind also dilutes pollutants. When a temperature inversion occurs, pollutants are trapped as the warm air settles to Earth.

Atmospheric airflows, however, contribute to the global transportation of pollutants. For example, the continental airflow across the United States distributes air pollution from the Midwest throughout the Northeast, contributing to high levels of air pollution in the New England states (Kleim & Rock, n.d.). In fact, the New England states have been referred to as the tailpipe of the United States as the airflow moves polluted air eastward across the Atlantic Ocean and on into Europe.

In the past, the term *smog* was used to describe smoke, ashes, soot, and other particulate matter and substances in the air. Today the term also includes photochemical smog resulting from the sun's reaction with chemicals in the air. Ozone is one of the largest components of photochemical smog. Ozone in the upper atmosphere acts as a protective shield to Earth's inhabitants, but ozone in the lower layer of the atmosphere is associated with adverse health effects.

Another form of outdoor pollution is acid rain, which forms when emissions of sulfur dioxide and nitrogen dioxide combine with other chemicals high in the atmosphere. As a result, droplets are carried by winds, perhaps far from the pollutant-producing area, and fall to Earth as either dry or wet (rain, snow, fog) acid-contaminated droplets. Acid rain threatens ecology and defaces monuments and buildings.

Conflicting research reports create uncertainty about the effects of electromagnetic radiation. Radio, television, household wiring, and household appliances, have low levels of electromagnetic transmission. Higher levels (e.g., coming from high-voltage power lines, the heavy usage of computers, and microwave ovens) have been implicated in neurological damage and cataracts. The World Health Organization has classified cellular or mobile phone use and other radiofrequency electromagnetic fields as possibly carcinogenic (National Cancer Institute, 2011). Although research on the use of devices emitting electromagnetic radiation is ongoing and inconclusive, it is recommended that exposure be kept to a minimum

HEALTH PROMOTION AND NURSING INTERVENTIONS FOR AIR QUALITY

Strides have been made in developed countries to address the issues of indoor air quality. New issues, however, continue to emerge. Issues of concern relate to synthetic organic compounds, intentionally introduced viruses and other infectious organisms (addressed later in this chapter), and engineering and design factors in the workplace. The role of the nurse continues to be of great importance in current and emerging issues related to indoor air quality. The first step in this role is to identify problems and then to determine the need for professional assistance. Improving outdoor air quality is more difficult and requires cooperation among individuals, communities, and industries.

Prevention is the key to air quality problems. Not all air pollutants, however, can be prevented. Table 7-4 summarizes the major threats to indoor air quality and presents a health-promotion guide for the nurse to use with clients to prevent adverse effects.

TABLE 7-4 Health-Promotion Guide to Indoor Air Quality Management

POLLUTANT	SOURCE	POSSIBLE ADVERSE HEALTH EFFECTS	HEALTH PROMOTION GUIDE
Environmental tobacco smoke (ETS)	Cigarettes Cigars Pipes	Respiratory irritation Bronchitis SIDS in infants Pneumonia in children Emphysema Cancers (lung, brain, leukemia, lymphoma) Heart disease	Do not smoke. Do not smoke in your home or permit others to do so. Seek nonsmoking restaurants and other public social venues. Do not smoke if children are present, particularly infants and toddlers. If smoking indoors cannot be avoided, increase ventilation in the area where smoking takes place. Open windows or use exhaust fans.
Carbon Monoxide	Unvented or malfunctioning gas appliances Woodstoves Indoor vehicle work Tobacco smoke	Headache Nausea Angina Impaired vision Impaired mental functioning Death at high concentrations	Keep gas appliances properly adjusted. Consider purchasing a vented space heater when replacing an unvented one. Use proper fuel in kerosene space heaters. Install and use an exhaust fan vented to outdoors over gas stoves. Open flues when fireplaces are in use. Choose properly sized woodstoves that are certified to meet EPA emission standards. Make certain that doors on all woodstoves fit tightly. Have a trained professional inspect, clean, and tune up the central heating system (furnaces, flues, and chimneys) annually. Repair any leaks promptly. Do not idle vehicles inside garage.
Nitrogen oxide	Unvented or malfunctioning gas or kerosene appliances Ice resurfacing equipment	Eye, nose, and throat irritation Respiratory infections	Refer to steps for Carbon Monoxide
VOCs (formaldehyde, chemical solvents, pesticides)	Aerosol sprays Solvents Glues, hobby products Cleaning agents Pesticides Paints Moth repellents Air fresheners Dry-cleaned clothes Environmental tabacco smoke Cosmetics Pressed wood (plywood, particleboard) Furnishings (carpet, draperies, furniture) Wallpaper Durable press fabrics	Eye, nose, and throat irritation Allergic reaction Headaches Loss of coordination Liver, brain, and kidney damage Cancer, leukemia Pulmonary edema	Use household products according to manufacturer's directions. Make sure you provide plenty of fresh air when using these products. Throw away unused or little-used containers safely; buy in quantities that you will use soon. Keep out of reach of children and pets. Never mix household care products unless directed on the label. Use "exterior-grade" pressed wood products (lower-emitting because they contain phenol resins, not urea resins). Use air conditioners and dehumidifiers to maintain moderate temperature and reduce humidity levels. Increase ventilation, particularly after bringing new sources of formaldehyde into the home.

(continues)

TABLE 7-4   Health-Promotion Guide to Indoor Air Quality Management (continued)

POLLUTANT	SOURCE	POSSIBLE ADVERSE HEALTH EFFECTS	HEALTH PROMOTION GUIDE
Respirable particles	Cigarettes Woodstoves Fireplaces Aerosol sprays House dust	Eye, nose, and throat irritation Respiratory infections and bronchitis Lung cancer	Have a trained professional inspect, clean, and tune up central heating system (furnace, flues, and chimneys) annually. Repair any leaks promptly. Change filters on central heating and cooling systems and air cleaners according to manufacturer's directions.
Bioaerosols (bacteria, viruses, fungi, animal dander, mites)	House dust Pets Bedding Poorly maintained air conditioners, humidifiers, and dehumidifiers Wet or moist structures Furnishings	Allergic reaction Asthma Eye, nose, and throat irritation Fever Influenza and other infectious diseases (i.e., Legionnaires' disease, bird flu)	Install and use fans vented to outdoors in kitchens and bathrooms. Vent clothes dryers to outdoors. Clean cool mist and ultrasonic humidifiers in accordance with manufacturer's instructions and refill with clean water daily. Empty water trays in air conditioners, dehumidifiers, and refrigerators frequently. Clean and dry or remove water-damaged carpets. Use basements as living areas only if they are leak-proof and have adequate ventilation. Use dehumidifiers, if necessary, to maintain humidity between 30 and 50 percent.
Asbestos	Damaged or deteriorating insulation Fireproofing and acoustical materials	Asbestosis Mesothelioma, lung cancer, and other cancers	Do not disturb. Use trained and qualified contractors for control measures that may disturb asbestos and for clean-up. Follow proper procedures in replacing woodstove door gaskets that may contain asbestos.
Lead	Sanding or open-flame burning of lead paint. House dust	Nerve and brain damage, particularly in children Anemia Kidney damage Growth retardation	Keep areas where children play as clean and dust-free as possible. Leave lead-based paint undisturbed if it is in good condition; do not sand or burn off paint that may contain lead. Do not remove lead paint yourself. Do not bring lead dust into the home. If your work or hobby involves lead, change clothes and use doormats before entering your home. Eat a balanced diet that is rich in calcium and iron.
Radon	Soil under buildings Some earth-derived construction materials Well water	Lung cancer	Test the home for radon. Fix the home if radon level is 4 picocuries per liter (pCi/L) or higher. Radon levels less than 4 p Ci/L still pose a risk, and in many cases may be reduced.

Source: Canadian Centre for Occupational Health and Safety." Indoor Air Quality—General." retrieved from http://www.ccohs.ca/oshanswers/chemicals/iaq_intro.html; U.S. Environmental Protection Agency. Office of Radiation and Indoor Air. "The Inside Story: A Guide to Indoor Air Quality" (EPA Document # 402-K-93-007), retrieved from http://www.epa.gov/iaq/pubs/insidestory.html

Individuals with respiratory sensitivity can minimize their responses to outdoor air pollutants by remaining indoors when pollen and mold counts are high and during smog and ozone alerts. Print and electronic media provide information regarding smog and ozone alerts as well as pollen counts. Sun-sensitive individuals should pay particular attention to ultraviolet light level reports as well.

Individuals who have developed chemical sensitivity may be diagnosed as having environmental illness or multiple chemical sensitivities. Although such diagnoses are controversial among medical professionals, individuals who suffer health consequences from chemicals in their environment also suffer from the accompanying stresses, including strained or lost relationships with family and friends and reduced access to public places. A safe environment is imperative for the well-being of chemically sensitive individuals.

A safe environment is one that is, as nearly as possible, void of chemical pollutants. Protective steps must be taken for the individual to survive. These individuals spend a great deal of time in a chemically free environment and lead an isolated existence. Care must be taken so that pollutants are not reintroduced into the controlled environment. Creating a chemical-free living space has been rated the highest of all treatment methods for chemically sensitive individuals (Larson, 2010). Box 7-6 provides a nursing checklist for creating a safe haven for the chemically sensitized individual.

WATER AND SOIL POLLUTION

Pure water is essential to life. Surface water is the water source for most large metropolitan areas and comes from lakes, rivers, reservoirs, and streams. Organic contaminants from naturally decaying animal and vegetable materials pose a threat to surface water. Other sources of contamination are acid rain, urban storm water runoff, pesticide runoff, industrial waste, and synthetic chemicals.

Groundwater comes from underground aquifers. Underground aquifers are long stretches of underground rock formations filled with water. Wells, which are more commonly found in rural areas, tap into these aquifers. Sources of groundwater pollution include pesticides, herbicides, and fertilizers; hazardous industrial wastes; leaking underground gasoline storage tanks; discarded household chemicals; and other synthetic chemicals. Industries can work to prevent groundwater pollution and provide safe water recreation areas.

Contaminated soil affects people's surroundings and food and water supplies. Some workers, such as those working in landfills or at chemical dumps, may face exposure to high levels of soil-carried toxins. Most individuals are affected to a lesser extent. Gardeners and constructions workers may be exposed by digging in it. Children may be exposed by playing in it. Anyone may inhale dust from it or eat food grown in it.

Soil pollution may result from fertilizers and pesticides that leach into the ground, and from leaking gas tanks or chemical barrels. Soil may be contaminated from refuse brought to the surface with mining. Other sources include chemicals from chemical spills, disposal ponds, and landfills, and even leaks that wash off parking lots and highways.

Each year, millions of tons of waste are labeled as hazardous. Oil refineries and chemical manufacturers generate at least half of this total toxic waste. Materials must be biologically or chemically treated to remove toxins prior to disposal. Guidelines for toxic waste disposal have increased in stringency over the years. Special sites are designated as toxic waste dumps. Soil structure or special linings prevent the leakage of toxins into the ground and into underground water sources.

HEALTH PROMOTION AND NURSING INTERVENTIONS FOR WATER AND SOIL QUALITY

Individuals contribute significantly to the reduction of health risks caused by water and soil contamination. Nurses may assist in reducing risks for individuals by encouraging them to use nontoxic cleaning materials, such as vinegar and baking soda; substitute organic insecticides and compost for toxic chemicals and fertilizers; and select consumer products with minimal packaging to reduce waste. Home gardeners and do-it-yourself pest controllers must be made aware of the long-lasting dangers of pesticides and herbicides.

BOX 7-6

NURSING CHECKLIST FOR CREATING A SAFE HAVEN FOR THE CHEMICALLY SENSITIZED INDIVIDUAL

1. Remove fabrics and synthetic items such as stuffed toy animals, curtains, tablecloths, upholstered furniture, and the like.
2. Clean air conditioning vents and ducts and replace filters often.
3. Wash walls, windows, blinds, and other objects with water and unscented cleaner, such as baking soda, vinegar, or hydrogen peroxide.
4. Replace carpet with untreated hardwood or terrazzo tile.
5. Encase pillows and mattresses in hypoallergenic material.
6. Use natural-fiber fabrics such as cotton.
7. Keep paper products at a minimum (chemicals, inks, and dyes may produce a reaction).
8. Do not use scented candles or air fresheners.
9. Use a room-size air purifier, and replace the filter frequently.
10. Assess grooming items for toxins.
11. Replace furniture made of particleboard.
12. Use electric appliances.
13. Do not use pesticides, exterminators, or lawn care companies.
14. Introduce new items individually to test tolerability and add other items after a four-day wait.

On a larger scale, nurses and nursing organizations may work to influence the agricultural industry's development of more insect-resistant crops and the use of fewer pesticides. Many nurses have become involved with environmental groups and have paired with communities to sponsor massive cleanup campaigns and to organize beach, waterway, and roadside pickups of litter. Long-term recycling programs, including organic and nonorganic materials, should be encouraged. Many communities sponsor composting classes and furnish compost bins to participants in order to encourage recycling of organic materials. Newspapers, glass, plastic, and aluminum are commonly recycled household wastes. Automotive repair shops recycle tires, batteries, and oil. Artificial reefs for water wildlife have been created from old tires and metal wastes.

Even though water looks, tastes, and smells fine, it may still be hazardous. In fact, waterborne microorganisms can be lethal. Coliform, a harmless microbe, serves as an indicator organism in the coliform test. It usually coexists with disease-causing organisms such as *Escherichia coli* and *Klebsiella*. Water in public systems goes through a series of treatments, including filtering, treating, and aerating, which provide consumers a high level of protection. Those using private wells must test their water annually for contaminants to ensure the same protection. Adequate water testing and treatment must be enforced to ensure the safety of water supply to the population.

Improved landfill technology confines current hazardous wastes more effectively than in years past. Waste sites and dumps that have been filled or covered prior to the availability of improved technology must be identified and tested for toxicity. Consumer education regarding the identification and proper disposal of toxic materials (e.g., leftover insecticides, paint, and batteries) reduces improper disposal practices. The development of alternative waste technology and stricter guidelines for industrial and commercial emissions will reduce future risks.

SOUND POLLUTION

Silence, the absence of sound, is something most people today experience all too infrequently. The ears remain open and working whether people are awake or asleep. Silence can be deafening if stimulation is needed or restorative if a period of relaxation is needed. Silence provides a shift or break from the usual sounds.

Conversely, sound or noise can become an environmental pollutant when it is extremely annoying and potentially harmful to hearing when individuals are exposed to noise at high levels. Sound pollution has a long history. Indeed, the Romans went so far as to ban chariots on cobblestone streets at night. Today, sound pollution is growing to epidemic proportions. People are almost constantly barraged with sounds, such as office noises; voices in a crowded room; urban noise from vehicles and church bells; airport noise; recreational noise, including rock music and sports; and heating and air conditioning gusts. Hearing becomes diminished as a result of prolonged exposure to loud sounds.

Nearly 300 million people in the world have impaired hearing (World Health Organization, 2010). Hearing impairment can result from a variety of causes, including diseases such as measles, mumps, meningitis, and chronic ear infections; trauma; the use of ototoxic drugs; or exposure to noise. Whether it is referred to as a disability, a disorder, or impairment, hearing loss is one of the most common chronic health conditions affecting all age groups, ethnicities, and genders.

RESEARCH NOTE

Hearing Protection and Farmers

STUDY PROBLEM/PURPOSE

Noise-induced hearing loss (NIHL) is permanent and progressive with continued exposure to noise. The impact of NIHL has a negative effect on the quality of life through impaired communication, reduced self-esteem, impaired ability to interact with the environment, disruption of intimacy, and tinnitus. The incidence of NIHL is higher in farmers than in workers in most other industries, and there is evidence of a lower use of hearing protective devices (HPD) among this group.

METHODS

With use of HPD as the dependent variable, the Health-Promotion Model was used to create a model to identify the influence from independent variables of (a) the perceived barriers to the use of HPDs, (b) the perceived benefits of using HPDs; (c) the self-efficacy of using HPDs; (d) the access/availability of HPDs; (e) interpersonal influences, specifically perceptions of norms, modeling, and support for using HPDs by other farmers and family members; (f) age, and (g) gender. Data collectors telephoned 1173 farm households from the population of 171,064 farmers in the upper Midwest four-state database. The data collectors administered a 65-question survey to those who agreed to participate.

FINDINGS

There were 532 participants in the study, with 69% male and 31% female. The majority were white Caucasian non-Hispanic. Results indicated that barriers to using hearing protection (e.g., difficulty communicating) were negatively related to use. Having greater access/availability of hearing protectors and male gender were positively related to use. The model correctly predicted the use of hearing protection for 74% of the cases. In general, the use of HPD among the participants was low and similar to those from previous studies of non-farm workers. The hypothesized higher use of HPDs among women farmers was not supported in the study participants. The model correctly predicted a large proportion of cases, but, noting that not all of the components of the model were significant, the researchers suggested the potential for model revision. It was suggested that findings from this study will be useful in designing interventions to increase farmers' use of HPD and to decrease their rates of NIHL.

IMPLICATION

Knowledge from this study can be integrated into care by nurses in agricultural areas in expanding their assessment of patients who are exposed to high levels of noise associated with farm work. Teaching about the risk of NIHL and the use of HPD should be incorporated into the plan of care.

McCullagh, M. C., Ronis, D. L., & Lusk, S. L. (2010). Predictors of use of hearing protection among a representative sample of farmers. *Research in Nursing & Health, 33*(6), 528–538.

The Hearing Foundation of Canada (2010) reports that hearing impairment is one of that country's most prevalent and fastest growing health conditions. Box 7-7 provides some general demographic facts about hearing loss in the U.S. population.

All cells in the body act as sound receptors, eliciting physiological and psychological responses. Some individuals are particularly sound sensitive. The body reacts adversely to strong sounds. Behaviors are amplified. Tension develops, and energy is depleted. In contrast, welcome sounds trigger a relaxation response and create energy.

Noise is any loud, discordant, or disagreeable sound or sounds that may decrease body energy or cause auditory damage. Potential harm from a sound is determined by several characteristics: sound pressure level (loudness, intensity), frequency (pitch), rhythm, and duration. Even good music becomes noise if played so loudly that distortion occurs. Certain repetitive rhythms may be depressing. The damaging effects of noise are cumulative.

Exposure to noise is responsible for the majority of hearing loss (Danielson, n.d.). After exposure to loud noises, a person's hearing grows dull, causing a temporary hearing threshold shift. Hearing returns to its normal sharpness with cessation of the noise. A sudden, extremely loud noise, such as an explosion, creates pressure waves with enough intensity to cause actual physical trauma to the inner ear.

Sound loudness is measured in decibels (dB) with 0 dB being the lowest possible audible sound for a person with normal hearing. Standards set by the Occupational Safety and Health Administration (OSHA) indicate that hearing impairment can occur with continued exposure to noise over 85 decibels averaged over an 8-hour day (OSHA, 2008). Table 7-5 presents examples of common sounds and their decibel measurements.

BOX 7-7
HEARING LOSS DEMOGRAPHICS

Hearing loss occurs in:

- 1 out of 10 Americans in general.
- 3 out of 1000 newborns.
- 1 out of 20 people ages 12–19.
- 1 out of 12 people age 30–50.
- 1 out of 8 people age 50.

Sources: Berke, J. (2010). "Hearing loss demographics: Statistically how many are deaf and hard of hearing?" retrieved from http://deafness.about.com/cs/earbasics/a/demographics.htm; Kochkin, S. (2009). "MarkeTrak VIII: 25-year trends in the hearing health market." Hearingreview.com, retrieved from http://www.betterhearing.org/pdfs/Kochkin_MarkeTrak8_OctHR09_hr.pdf

---

TABLE 7-5 How Loud Is Too Loud? Average Decibel Levels for Everyday Sounds and Their Categories of Loudness:

PAINFUL:
150 dB = fireworks at 3 ft
140 dB = firearms, jet engine
130 dB = jackhammer
120 dB = jet plane takeoff, siren

EXTREMELY LOUD:
110 dB = maximum output of some MP3 players, model airplane, chain saw
106 dB = gas lawn mower, snowblower
100 dB = hand drill, pneumatic drill
90 dB = subway, passing motorcycle

VERY LOUD:
80–90 dB = blow-dryer, kitchen blender, food processor
70 dB = busy traffic, vacuum cleaner, alarm clock

MODERATE:
60 dB = typical conversation, dishwasher, clothes dryer
50 dB = moderate rainfall
40 dB = quiet room

FAINT:
30 dB = whisper, quiet library

Source: Adapted from How loud is too loud; how long is too long? (2009). Retrieved on September 24, 2009, from http://www.noisyplanet.nidcd.nih.gov/info/pages/howloud.aspx and www.lhh.org/noise/facts/environment.html

---

NURSING **ALERT**

Potential Hearing Loss

Any of the following symptoms could be a danger sign of permanent hearing loss:

- Tinnitus (ringing in the ears)
- Sensation of "stuffiness" or fullness in the ear
- Dullness of hearing (even if temporary)
- Need to lip-read in order to "hear"

Noise is probably the most common occupational hazard facing people today. It is estimated that as many as 30 million Americans are exposed to potentially harmful sounds at work. Even away from the workplace, many people participate in recreational activities that can produce harmful noise (musical concerts, the use of power tools, etc.). Sixty million Americans own firearms, and many people do not use appropriate hearing protection devices.

Although it is 100 percent preventable, noise-induced hearing loss is permanent. Other effects of long-term, low-intensity noise include tension headaches, a lack of concentration, anxiety, hypertension, and insomnia. The warning signs of dangerous noise levels demand immediate action to preserve hearing.

Throughout life, from birth to death, individuals are able to adapt to noise. Adaptation occurs as the body diminishes its awareness of continuous or repetitive sounds. However, the body continues to respond to the noise even though awareness has decreased. Therefore, adaptation places us at risk for the continuing physiological and psychological effects of sounds as well as auditory damage. Recovery rates and quality of life can be improved through the control of a client's auditory environment. Sensory messages are transmitted during sleep, even during deep anesthesia-induced sleep. The unconscious client may be able to hear, though other sensory stimuli are blocked. Hearing is believed to be the last sense lost during the dying process.

HEALTH PROMOTION AND NURSING INTERVENTIONS RELATED TO SOUND

The body can discriminate between beneficial and detrimental sounds, responding physiologically and psychologically. Good music and most natural sounds have a therapeutic effect, strengthening the body.

Music is an integral part of behavioral kinesiology. Behavioral kinesiology suggests that each gesture or movement a person makes is the body's response to a need to tonify or to correct an imbalance in a certain body system. Muscle tension and relaxation in response to sounds can be measured. Music elicits body movement (e.g., swaying or dancing to music). Orchestra conductors move with the music, experiencing the healing qualities of music while vigorously tonifying the body. Observe music conductors. Most are trim, healthy, and relaxed, and they live for many years.

Rhythm in music can stimulate or depress. Individuals tend to breathe with the rhythm of music. A 4/4 tempo corresponds to the normal heart rate, eliciting a relaxation response. Rapid, even drumbeats are highly stimulating, and progressively slower rhythms lead to relaxation and sleep. Commercially produced intrauterine sounds, for example, quiet newborns within 30 seconds.

A decrease in hearing can be a part of the normal aging process. In the presence of biological symptoms, however, nurses must consider not only physiological causes but environmental causes as well. The nurse must work to achieve a balance between sensory deprivation and sensory overload. Taking research into the practice arena, nurses should minimize the sources of loud sounds (e.g., conversations, radios, telephones, incubators, respirators, cardiac monitors, and other equipment). Routine nursing interventions— suctioning, inserting various tubes, and personal care (e.g., changing diapers on the preterm infant)—must be evaluated for frequency and necessity.

Nurses in many ways have used music as an environmental intervention. Music can help clients increase movement, mobility, and positive self-expression. Music can significantly decrease a client's awareness of pain. For agitated clients or hyperactive children, music can reduce activity level. For the developmentally disabled child, the

? ASK **YOURSELF**

Sound Awareness

Sit quietly for at least 5 minutes. Really listen. Jot down the sounds in your environment.

- Which sounds were already in your awareness?
- Which sounds came into awareness only with real concentration?
- What subtle changes occur in your body in response to these sounds?
- Are there sounds that irritate you, make you tense, and drain your energy?
- Which sounds are soothing and help to energize you?
- How can you diminish the unwelcome sounds? Increase the welcome ones?

rhythmic drive of music can aid in mental, emotional, and social maturation. It can help bring a sense of wholeness to scattered individuals and bring about positive interactions (Morris, 2009).

What sounds make us whole? The sounds of nature bring pleasure to the listener. Remember some of your favorite natural sounds. Maybe it was the rustle of fall leaves beneath your feet, the crunch of fresh snow, or rain splashing against the window. In some countries, nature's sounds are built into homes and temples. Bamboo steps in homes in Thailand produce sounds similar to those made by a bamboo musical instrument. Wind chimes are used in the garden to create outside music and to extend the defensive sound zone beyond the confines of the home. A trickling waterfall and the rustling sounds created by breezes blowing through trees and other garden greenery help to create an environment of renewal. Fountains and waterfalls are becoming more popular as a part of interior decoration. The soothing and invigorating sounds of running water and birds are incorporated into many relaxation audiotapes.

Upholstered furniture, curtains, and carpet soften sounds. Acoustical consultants have identified approaches to reduce noise in the workplace, including substituting quieter processes or equipment, separating employees from noisy equipment, altering the direction of the noise, and absorbing the noise with specially designed noise dampeners. Noise from building construction (e.g., jackhammers, riveting) can be baffled by hanging steel-mesh blankets.

Ear protection should be worn to prevent hearing loss. An informal test of noise level can be done. If you have to shout above noise to be heard an arm's length away from another person, the noise level is approximately 90 dBA, a level that can cause permanent hearing loss. Protective equipment is needed. Earplugs or over-the-ear muffs offer protection. Attention should be paid to the noise-reduction rating of these protective devices. Using both plugs and muffs simultaneously may be needed in extremely noisy environments.

SPOTLIGHT ON

Effects of Light Intensity on Hormones

The endocrine glands are sensitive to daily and seasonal cycles of light intensity and duration. The hormone melatonin is generally overproduced by the endocrine system during prolonged dark periods or in dim light, causing sleepiness, melancholia, and depression. On the other hand, another endocrine hormone, serotonin, provides the opposite effect.

NURSING ALERT

Retinopathy of Prematurity

A disease called retinopathy of prematurity (ROP) causes an estimated 600 premature babies to go blind annually. Countless others suffer from lesser eye damage. Immaturity of the eyes' blood vessels and underdeveloped retinas place preterm infants at risk. The excessively high levels of oxygen given to premature babies were identified initially as the cause of ROP. Monitoring of oxygen levels has reduced but not eliminated the occurrence of ROP, and other factors are being examined.

ROP came into existence with the introduction and widespread use of fluorescent lighting in nurseries about 50 years ago. One father, whose premature infant became blind, noticed that workers in factories were exposed to fluorescent lighting, which was considered a blue light hazard. Workers wore protective eyewear to prevent retinal damage from prolonged exposure to this blue light. Animal studies had shown that retinal blood vessel damage could result from blue-violet rays. A connection was made. Premature infants have underdeveloped eyes and are continuously exposed to concentrated blue-violet rays from the fluorescent lighting in intensive care nurseries. Parents urged hospitals to stop using fluorescent lighting or to use filters.

Hearing screenings can be highly important in identifying individuals with hearing loss at any age. Most hospitals test the hearing of newborns, and schools have ongoing hearing testing for children. Adults, however, may not have their hearing disorder identified until it is well advanced. It has been found that only 14.6% of physicians and nurses include a hearing screen as part of a routine physical exam (Kochkin, 2009). Health care providers need to include this screening as part of a comprehensive assessment.

LIGHT AND HEALTH

The human response to light lies on a continuum. One individual may be more sensitive to a particular level and length of exposure to light than another person. Disturbances caused by lighting level may occur because of inadequate exposure, overexposure, or adequate amounts at the wrong time of day (e.g., jet lag). Exposure or the lack of exposure to both natural sunlight and artificial light have an effect on health.

As winter days get shorter and darker, humans tend to feel apathetic and depressed. Decreased daylight in the middle of winter can cause seasonal affective disorder, or **SAD syndrome**, believed to be related to increased melatonin levels. The symptoms associated with SAD syndrome include fatigue, increased craving for carbohydrates in the diet, weight gain, lethargy, and severe clinical depression. Physiological problems such as infertility, alterations in menstrual cycles, and premenstrual syndrome may also occur. Suicides occur most frequently during the late winter months. People with depression feel worse, and alcohol-related problems increase. Interestingly, those born in areas of prolonged darkness do not suffer from SAD to the same extent as those transplanted from other parts of the country (Mayo Clinic, 2008).

High levels of light from sunlight or prolonged exposure to fluorescent lighting may cause eyestrain, headaches, increased stress, and hyperactivity. Retinal damage may occur from fluorescent lighting in neonatal intensive care units. Biochemical and physiological changes in the retina may lead to later problems with visual acuity and color vision for those infants.

Adequate lighting in nurseries plays a significant role in the early detection of skin color changes indicative of complications such as jaundice or lack of oxygen. Signs of seizures might be overlooked in lowered lighting.

LIGHT-RELATED HEALTH PROMOTION AND NURSING INTERVENTIONS

Provide as much natural lighting in a space as possible. Rooms flooded with daylight and the longer and brighter days of spring and summer increase serotonin production, resulting in more positive attitudes and higher energy levels. SAD sufferers sit in bright-light boxes for about 2 hours a day. The light in these boxes is 5 to 10 times brighter than a normal room's lighting. Phototherapy (light therapy) has been successful in treating severe cases of SAD (Miller, 2005).

When adding light, a word of caution is necessary. Light from both natural and artificial sources can create a glare. In offices, a computer monitor acts like a mirror. To identify the source of glare or reflections, turn off the screen and use it as a mirror to locate the source. Antiglare screens are recommended. Dust accumulated on computer screens adds to glare (Mayo Clinic, 2006). Screens should be cleaned each day using treated screen wipes. This dust is electromagnetically charged and may cause skin problems if hands are used to clean the screens and then touched to the face.

Designers plan lighting to influence mood. The interplay of shafts of bright daylight, darkness, and shadows is called visual acoustics by some architects. Dim lighting (i.e., candlelight, fireplace fire) is romantic and relaxing. Brighter lighting and spotlights focus attention. Adequate lighting is a safety consideration in the home and in the workplace.

HEALTH PROMOTION THEORY LINK

Florence Nightingale's Theory of Environmental Manipulation

Florence Nightingale (1820–1910) is known as the founder of modern nursing. Her contributions to nursing have had a tremendous impact on the philosophy and practice of the profession. One of her major contributions is her Theory of Environmental Manipulation. The fundamental premise for her theory is that environment is important for good health and for healing to occur and that healthy surroundings were necessary for proper nursing care. Her theory, developed in 1850, included five essential components of environmental health: pure air, pure water, efficient drainage, cleanliness, and light. In caring for patients, she instructed nurses to manipulate their environment by keeping the air pure with open windows for ventilation; to move patients to allow for exposure to direct sunlight; to bath themselves and patients daily, along with frequent handwashing, to prevent contamination; and to assess the need for and provide quiet and the avoidance of noise. In her writings she emphasized the role of the nurse in controlling the environment of patients, both physically and administratively, to protect the patient from stress and to promote rest for healing to occur. Through her Theory of Environmental Manipulation, Florence Nightingale fostered her belief that nursing was to assist nature in healing patients.

Source: Pfettscher, S. A. (2010). Modern nursing. In M. A. Alligood & A. M. Tomey (eds.), *Nursing theorists and their work*. Maryland Heights, MO: Mosby Elsevier, pp. 71–90.

Nurses need to bear these suggestions in mind in order to promote health in their personal and work environments. When working with clients through infancy and old age, lighting practices that protect health and promote well-being should be integrated into care.

SPACE AND HEALTH

Generally speaking, an individual's living space is harmonized with his or her lifestyle. Individuals interact with the environment through all their senses. People are significantly influenced by these sensory interactions with the environment. The musculature of the body adjusts as a person experiences the surrounding space, whether it is expansive or cramped. The balancing mechanisms of the inner ear also become involved as someone moves through the space, climbing stairs and turning corners. The body's reaction to space is referred to as the body's reading a building. Architects use knowledge about these kinesthetic responses when planning and designing space in a building.

Dwellings reflect social and societal needs. Consider the cultural and environmental influences of homes around the world. Construction reflects materials readily available in the environment: log cabins, grass/reed or mud huts, caves, adobe pueblos, igloos, brick or stone houses. Culture and class determine the home's size. The organization and meaning of spaces and rooms within a home evolve from social patterns of a culture. Interior spaces need to be in harmony with the environment, ecology, and the people who live and work there.

Culture and building site determine not only the orientation of the house to the land but also the level of security. Security needs are less for primitive tribes who have few possessions and whose goods are freely shared with others in the group. Huts are built close together. There are no doors or locks or fences. As societies grow larger, possessions multiply. The potential for trouble escalates. The need for security increases.

A place must feel safe in order for simultaneous perception to occur. **Simultaneous perception** allows responses from each of our senses to be combined. In this secure setting, a person can pay equal attention to everything at once, a characteristic called **utter watchfulness**. No incoming stimuli are eliminated or emphasized. A sudden change in stimuli, such as a loud noise or a sudden movement, diminishes or eliminates utter watchfulness. Incoming stimuli are no longer experienced as equal. That specific sensory stimulus takes precedence over all others. A potential threat has been identified. Utter watchfulness returns as the threat is dismissed or diminished (Hiss, 1990).

The site or setting of a home or workplace influences the sense of well-being. If settings and personal preferences are in synchrony, a person experiences a sense of ease. For example, in a rural environment, change is gradual and periodic. Space is open and expansive. The pace is slow and relaxed. The urban environment is characterized by quick and continuous change with multiple and intense stimuli. Space is crowded. The pace is rapid, often frantic. A country dweller may become tense, stressed, and ill at ease in the city. A city dweller may experience similar feelings when placed in the country.

Crowding has been blamed for crime and violence. An individual's typical negative or positive reactions to a given situation intensify in crowding. Exposure to high-density situations is usually brief (e.g., heavy traffic, a crowded subway or elevator). Generally, crowding is tolerated well.

Close physical proximity to other people almost forces some kind of interaction. Factors influencing the response to close proximity are individual personal characteristics, the relationship between those involved, the formality of the situation, and ethnicity. For example, close proximity is better tolerated with friends than with strangers. Social withdrawal is a coping strategy used to handle unwanted social demands that typically accompany prolonged crowding.

Dealing with others becomes increasingly difficult and stressful when resources and crowding are insufficient. Competition for resources intensifies and produces negative effects, such as increased tension and aggressiveness. High crime rates and poverty often coexist. In contrast, crime rates may be low in highly populated parts of the world if food, transportation, housing, energy, and other resources are adequate.

Architects work with design elements to reduce the sense of environmental crowding. Rooms with more light are perceived as less crowded than rooms with less natural light.

SPOTLIGHT ON

Dejunking for Lifetime Saving

Have you ever spent 10 minutes looking for an item in your home or at work? Multiply that by the number of items you look for each day. If you spend just 30 minutes each day shuffling through clutter, that adds up to a week of time each year lost to clutter. Think about the amount of time you could save over a lifetime by organizing clutter and eliminating items that are no longer needed.

ASK YOURSELF

Environmental Self-Image Color Analysis

1. Which colors give you a pleasant, relaxed feeling?
2. What colors strengthen you (make you feel strong, that everything around you is supporting you)?
3. What colors make you feel the most secure (totally fulfilled, want nothing, have it all)?
4. Which colors portray the image you desire?
5. Which colors in a favorite painting appeal to you?
6. What colors make you restless or uncomfortable?

Your "feeling" colors (1, 2, 3), when used in your environment, will support you.

If you are not comfortable with these colors, others portraying your desired image (4) or those in a favorite painting (5) may be better. Avoid any colors that you identified as making you feel uncomfortable (Mella, 1988).

Spaces that are subdivided decrease the perception of crowding, improve socialization, and decrease social withdrawal. The layout of a home's floor plan influences interaction patterns within the home.

At the work site, the overall office design (e.g., how enclosed, how noisy) has an effect on job performance, job satisfaction, interoffice communication, and satisfaction with the surroundings. Personal health, safety, and productivity depend on how furniture and workstations are laid out. Reportedly, people generate most of their ideas from face-to-face contact but are reluctant to move from their work area to exchange thoughts and ideas with other.

Clutter has a potential physiological and psychological effect on health and safety. Clutter and disorganization in a room encourage frenetic and chaotic lives. Clutter junks up the environment, harboring dust and other unmentionables that degrade our environment. A disorganized desk may indicate a disorganized life. Cluttered spaces suggest confused or nonspecific goals, inefficient work methods, and an inability to complete projects.

Clutter interferes with our most important resource: time. Shuffling through clutter makes every job harder and takes more time. Dejunking is a cheap, fast, and effective way to improve the quality of your life by altering your environment (Ware, 2010). The ability to focus improves. Productivity increases. Time management improves.

SPACE-RELATED HEALTH PROMOTION AND NURSING INTERVENTIONS

Changing the usual indoor or outdoor environment may have restorative benefits. When someone moves from the high-tech, high-stress level of a crowded work setting and takes a short walk in a nearby park, the internal gears shift. The body responds by relaxing, and a sense of balance is restored. A mix of short- and long-term restorative experiences maintains inner balance. The following sections describe how manipulating the senses through color and smell and developing a sense of safety within our environmental space have health-promoting effects. The Asian philosophy of feng shui is also introduced as an integrative approach for a healthy environment.

COLOR AND HEALTH

People respond to colors. Color expresses personality. The same color may have different influences on people. If an individual sees a color and likes it, the whole body system relaxes. Outlook becomes more optimistic. Therefore, a color that brings about a favorable response should be incorporated into that individual's surroundings. Because biological and psychological changes can be attributed to color, the nurse needs to be attentive to individual color preferences and their effects.

The goal is to achieve balance while avoiding monotony of color and overstimulation by color. Visualize a color. Place it along a continuum ranging from the lightest to the darkest shade. Limit the use of the color at either extreme of the continuum or combine the extremes to achieve balance. Staying in the color midrange on the continuum also provides balance. Colors that are too bright or too dramatic can be distracting and cause discomfort. Adjustments can be made by increasing or reducing the intensity, the amount, or the purity of a color. Adding white to a color reduces its brightness and changes its tint to a soothing pastel.

Variety is achieved by using contrasts between bright colors that stimulate and dark colors that relax. Variety is also achieved by using warm colors that excite and cool colors that soothe. For example, the blue (cool) end of the spectrum decreases arousal. Blue, violet, and green are cool, passive, and calming. Colors on the red end of the spectrum (warm) cause increased arousal. Red and its analogous hues are warm, active, and exciting. Contrary to the theory of warm colors being stimulating, certain pink hues have a tranquilizing effect. Bubble gum pink, called passive pink, creates an almost immediate reduction in aggressive behavior, making it particularly useful with agitated clients or prisoners (Schweitzer, Gilpin, & Frampton, 2004). Short-term exposure to a color does not necessarily have an effect.

Colors must be pleasing to be psychologically or physically therapeutic. The use of color can improve the way the body functions, deals with crises, and interacts with the environment. **Chromotherapy**, or photobiology, is the use of color to treat disease. Acceptance of chromotherapy as a means of healing and of maintaining a high level of wellness is growing.

In manipulating the environment through color, consider who will be affected and for how long, where it will be used, and why it is being used. For example, color in educational environments can affect children's performance. It was found that children with attention deficit hyperactivity disorder (ADHD) had better handwriting when writing on colored paper—an effect not found in children without ADHD (Imhof, 2004).

Visitors are affected in a hospital lobby. The surroundings there should be pleasant and cheerful. A variety of both warm and cool colors is appropriate. In a maternity unit, where the client is not seriously ill, peach or rose provides a comfortable environment. The cool tones of blues, greens, and grays create a restful environment for chronically ill clients. Relaxation of the surgical client could be accomplished with the use of greens and blue-greens. Certain colors should be avoided in health care institutions such as those that cast unfavorable reflections on the human complexion—yellow-greens, yellow, and lavender.

When at home, people rest, relax, rejuvenate, and create. While on the job, the focus is on work. People produce, serve, and solve job-related problems, resting little if at all. Energy is therefore consumed more at work than at home. Using favorite colors can enhance a work environment. The benefit from personal favorite colors is maximized if they are placed within 3 ft of a working space: on a table, a desk, or a chair; in a piece of art; or as an accent color. Colors can act as strong energizers, improving mood and increasing productivity. The use of color for holistic health is further discussed in Chapter 19.

SCENT AND HEALTH

People see only when there is enough light, touch only when contact is made with someone or something, and hear only sounds that are loud enough. But with every breath, the sense of smell is active. Smell is the mute sense, one without words. Smells are usually described in terms of other things such as smoke, fruit, flowers, and citrus or by the feelings they inspire—disgusted, delighted, sickened, hypnotized, or intoxicated.

The sense of smell brings pleasure, and it is also a protective device. Odors can elicit reactions of fear or a flight response (e.g., gas, ammonia, insecticides), alerting us to danger in our environment. The smells of spoiled food, smoke, and gas spell danger for those with a sense of smell. This protective device is missing for those with anosmia, placing them at risk. **Anosmia** is the absence of the sense of smell.

Aromas form a direct link to emotions and memories. With the tripwire of smell, memories explode and complex visions are elicited by certain odors. When a scent enters the body, a message is sent to the cerebral cortex and into the limbic system, the emotional portion of the brain. The fragrance of roses may trigger the memory of a romantic moment or a special garden. What about the smell of fresh-baked cookies or bread? Evergreens,

bayberry, and cinnamon? These aromas may elicit a relaxation response as they bring back memories of very special times. The smell of wood smoke may serve as a reminder of a fun-filled experience around a campfire or a devastating home fire.

The goals of aromatherapy include relaxation and healing. A therapeutically scented environment uses aromas that are associated with good past experiences. Although research to support the use of aromatherapy in nursing practice other than for relaxation is inconclusive, mounting evidence suggests its benefits especially for symptom management and the creation of feelings of well-being (Potts, 2009). Nurses who intend to incorporate aromatherapy in their plan of care should complete formal education in aromatherapy to obtain basic knowledge of the chemical and physical properties of essential oils as well as their safe application and evaluation of effects.

WORKPLACE SAFETY AND HEALTH

A person's workplace is like a second home. Many employees spend 8–12 hours at work each day. The air, sound, space, and light in the work environment are therefore vital to employee job satisfaction, productivity, and safety. Smoke, noise, vibrations, crowded quarters, poor ventilation, and improper lighting can create undue stress. Temperature and humidity can cause physical uneasiness. Posture, reaching, and lifting all affect how the employee works.

Employers are required by law to provide training about potential exposure to hazardous materials. The prevention and control of exposures ensure a safe and healthy workplace. Controls fall into four major categories:

1. *Substitution controls* replace a hazardous substance or work process with a less hazardous one (e.g., substituting steam for gas sterilization or water-based paint for oil-based paint).

2. *Engineering controls* literally reengineer the work process or equipment to reduce the possibility of exposure or injury (e.g., installing an exhaust system to remove fumes or acoustic tiles to reduce noise levels).

3. *Administrative controls* reduce exposure through education, implementing safe work practices, and rotating jobs.

4. *Equipment control* provides personal protective equipment (e.g., goggles, gloves, or safety shoes) (OSHA, n.d.).

SPOTLIGHT **ON**

Using Controls for Workplace Safety

A client is admitted to your unit with a contagious condition that is spread by direct contact. Which of the four controls can be used to increase employee safety? What measures related to these controls can decrease the possibility of contamination to others?

A combination of controls may be needed to control exposure and to improve safety. For example, while using solvents to clean silkscreen, a woman became lightheaded and noticed a rash on her hands. The installation of an exhaust fan to remove fumes (engineering control) and the use of gloves and a respirator (equipment control) would reduce her exposure to the pollutants.

Ergonomics is the science of the relationships of furniture and tools to the human body. Poor ergonomics can be connected to nonspecific aches, pains, and stresses. More specifically, ergonomic problems contribute to the following:

- Lowered production and reduced quality of work
- Increased lost time/absenteeism/turnover
- Increased medical costs due to injuries and strains
- Increased probability of errors and accidents
- Increased workers' compensation costs

The two major goals of improving ergonomics are to provide a more effective workplace and to improve work conditions. Meeting these goals satisfies the needs of both employees and employers. The benefits of an ergonomics program include greater comfort and higher morale, improved quality of work with fewer errors, greater efficiency, improved productivity with fewer errors, lower turnover, greater safety with fewer injuries, and reduced absenteeism.

An ergonomic specialist or team conducts a worksite analysis, recognizing, identifying, and prioritizing ergonomic hazards. More and more nurses are becoming ergonomic specialists. Information is gathered through observation, anthropometric data (human body measurements), an ergonomic checklist, videotapes, and analysis of the tasks performed. The ergonomic checklist covers issues that relate to the use of hands, the use of force, upper and lower body stress, work area, tool design, the pace of activity, and the number of repetitions. Findings are analyzed. Actions to reduce the number of repetitions, reduce the force required, and eliminate awkward positions are prioritized. A plan is developed and approved by management. Immediate actions usually include education and quick fixes. Many solutions are no cost or low cost (e.g., height adjustments, supports, training) and are highly visible to employees. Larger and more expensive design issues follow. Once the plan is in effect, a work site team monitors progress, identifying continuing and new problems, taking necessary corrective action, and consulting with the ergonomic specialist as needed.

An ergonomic audit may take 2–4 weeks, depending on the complexity and the work area's size. Cost depends on the complexity of the area. Often the cost of doing nothing exceeds the cost of an extensive audit. An ergonomic audit often has a positive impact on employee morale simply because it proves that the company cares. Management often lacks information about ergonomic issues. Some managers believe that ergonomics assessments are not important because audits do not add value to their product. Therefore, there is a lack of interest and funding for ergonomic assessments.

Ergonomic interventions are the most successful if the affected individuals are included in discussions of action, prioritizing different available solutions, and making small improvements. People are motivated to make changes when presented with examples of similar situations in which improvements were successful.

Overall, workplace injuries have decreased. However, the incidence of repetitive strain injury (RSI), or cumulative

SPOTLIGHT **ON**

Preventing Back Injuries in Health Care

Back injuries are the most common of work-related injuries for health care workers. Pain and injuries to muscles, tendons, discs, and other parts of the back occur mostly in nonprofessional employees whose jobs involve moving clients. Nurse's aides, orderlies, and attendants are noted to have the highest rates of back injuries. Those with jobs in laundries, kitchens, environmental services, and others who must lift, push, and pull objects are also at risk.

Ergonomics involves changing jobs to fit the abilities and needs of the workers rather than trying to fit the worker to the job. An ergonomics program in the workplace helps to reduce injuries of various types, including back injuries. The use of back belts and training on techniques have not been shown to be effective in preventing back injuries. A better approach is to eliminate tasks that require heavy lifting if possible, using equipment designed to perform lifts, having sufficient staff to form lifting teams that use lifting equipment, and prohibiting single-person lifts. Reviewing injury logs, incident reports, sick leave usage, and workers' compensation can be helpful in identifying and taking steps to reduce commonly occurring injuries. Employers and employees can both benefit from early reporting of injuries and early injury intervention to reduce the overall costs, financially and in terms of human productivity.

trauma, continues to rise. RSI is an umbrella term for several cumulative trauma disorders caused by low-intensity forces applied over a long period. Repetitive motions irritate specific anatomical structures. Tendons, tendon sheaths, muscles, ligaments, joints, and nerves are commonly affected. Microscopic damage, called microtrauma, occurs. Normally, healing of microtrauma occurs overnight, but the healing process cannot keep pace with ongoing injury. Over time, tissues become inflamed and damaged, causing pain and limiting function. Carpal tunnel syndrome is an RSI resulting from the overuse of the hands and arms, common among computer users. Tissues in the hand, arm, neck, and shoulders are involved.

Fatigue and sustained awkward posture may be as damaging as repetitive motion. Improper posture while working can bring the head position forward, increasing pressure on the muscles and nerves of the neck. Shoulders become stressed and fatigued, resulting in a nagging discomfort. Prolonged inappropriate posture can result in permanent physiological changes. Preventive and corrective measures reduce the risk of RSI. Work site health can be improved using the ergonomic approaches summarized in Box 7-8.

BOX 7-8

TIPS TO PREVENT BACK, NECK, AND JOINT INJURIES

Lifting

1. Objects:
   - Test weight first. Get help if needed.
   - Move close to object. Don't extend arms.
   - Form solid support by spreading feet apart to width of shoulders, bend your knees, and lift the object with the strength of your legs, not your back.
   - Never lift higher than your chest.
   - Break up heavy loads into smaller loads, use small steps, move slowly, and take frequent breaks from lifting.

2. Clients from bed:
   - Raise bed to your level.
   - Ask for help if needed.
   - Safeguard transfers with use of a trapeze, sliding board, lateral assist device, transfer chair, or powered lift.

Ergonomics

1. Sitting:
   - Get a quality desk chair with height adjuster.
   - Knees should be level with hips, feet flat on floor.
   - Sit up straight. Use chair back for support (extra support with pillows if needed).
   - Hold in stomach muscles.
   - Balance head over shoulders, and avoid leaning forward.

2. Standing:
   - Place one foot slightly in front of the other.
   - Wear low-heeled shoes with good arch supports.

3. Using computers:
   - Place keyboard and mouse close to you.
   - Adjust top of computer screen to eye level.
   - Type with elbows at your side and forearms parallel to the floor.
   - Use armrests.
   - Relax shoulders and hands.
   - Vary work tasks.
   - Use wrist rest at base of keyboard.
   - Look away from screen every 10 minutes to avoid eyestrain.

Preventive Measures

- Stretch before you start. Keep muscles limber and warm.
- Exercise regularly and actively to keep fit, flexible, and strong.
- Wear properly fitting shoes allowing for toe wiggle.
- Invest in a high-quality mattress (firm with numerous coils and thick padding), replace it every 10 years, and rotate it 180 degrees at least four times a year to prolong its life.

Sources: Santulli, E. (2004). No strain? No pain! *Hospital Nursing, 34*(3).7–8; Meinhart, P. L. (n.d.) Ergonomic injury prevention in healthcare *Ergonomics in Healthcare*, retrieved from http://ergonomicsinhealthcare.org; Waters, T., Collins, J., Galinsky, T. L., & Caruso, C. (2006). NIOSH research efforts to prevent musculoskeletal disorders in the healthcare industry. *Orthopaedic Nursing, 25*, 380–389

FENG SHUI

Eastern and Western philosophies differ on the subject of human coexistence with the environment. To generalize, the Eastern philosophy believes nothing happens without consequence to something else. Western countries, by contrast, approach life and the environment with a philosophy of "I came, I saw, I conquered." The fundamental premise of feng shui is that *where we are* is as important as *who we are*. **Feng shui** (pronounced "fung shway") is an ancient Chinese practice of configuring one's environment to promote a healthy flow of chi, or vital energy, for health, happiness, and prosperity (Elioupoulis, 2010).

Feng shui is being used as an antidote to modern life, providing peace and serenity in a complex time of change, confusion, and stress. The Chinese believe that manipulating the environment can change fate. Feng shui teaches that a keen awareness of space can greatly improve circumstances.

Feng shui is a cross between art and science. Its roots are in ecology, aesthetics, philosophy, astrology, and interior design. It involves the use of geometric lines, colors, numbers, animal symbols, and the elements of fire, earth, metal, water, and wood to align furnishings, buildings, and the landscape. Though it transcends the confines of rational thought and the realm of logic, feng shui is firmly grounded in common sense and scientific observations.

✳ NURSING **ALERT**

Reducing Risk for Carpal Tunnel Syndrome for Computer Users

- Maintain neutral position at a computer keyboard: wrist straight, middle knuckle aligned with center of the wrist.
- Keep fingers curved.
- Avoid stretching fingers to reach keys.
- Use the arm to move hand over keyboard.
- Don't rest wrists on edge of desk while typing.
- Schedule frequent breaks from the keyboard.
- Do exercises to strengthen the fingers, wrists, arms, and shoulders.
- Stretch and use exercises to relax muscles affected by typing.
- Don't rush. Work at a comfortable pace.

In China, Indonesia, and other parts of Southeast Asia, feng shui is used in selecting building sites and in placing buildings and furnishings. Building sites are selected to harmonize with the energies of the land. This is believed to attract good luck, health, and fortune. The totality of the location of the building, the arrangement of its furniture and accessories, and the use of color within each room make for an environment that can be balanced, energizing, and positive or one that is unbalanced, enervating, and negative. When inhabitants, buildings, and furnishings are in harmony with nature, good feng shui exists; serenity is evident.

The benefits of feng shui are being recognized in the West. Feng shui specialists were brought in to reorient parts of the Denver airport that had experienced many malfunctions during construction, costing millions of dollars.

Many homeowners and businesspeople alike would not consider beginning construction without consulting a geomancer, an expert who uses lines, figures, and geographic features in design. Working with the principles of feng shui, the geomancer assesses the geology and topography of a building's location. Land should not include harmful mineral deposits and should support vegetation but not be overgrown. There should not be stagnant water. The outdoor environment and view from the structure are also considered. An environment with a view of nature supports health if the scene contains healthy vegetation.

The traditional concepts of Asian life (Tao, chi, yin, and yang) are incorporated into feng shui. **Tao** means to be connected. Each part of life is dependent on another to create a whole. Plants, pictures, and colors similar to outdoors provide a sense of connectedness with nature when used indoors. A connectedness should permeate the home as one moves from room to room.

Chi is invisible energy, or vitality. All living things are interrelated by cosmic chi that circulates through the earth and sky. In feng shui, efforts are made to encourage the flow of chi, echoing the gentle curves of nature in the environment. Poison arrows of straight lines and sharp edges or angles cause chi to move too swiftly or to be easily blocked. Straight lines can be broken by curves created by adding plants. Too much chi results in chaos; too little results in lifelessness.

Sha is bad chi and is believed to bring bad luck and poor health as well as family and business difficulties. Architectural elements and accessories in the home or office can be used to enhance or inhibit chi. Table 7-6 lists the enhancers and inhibitors of chi that affect environmental balance.

As discussed in Chapter 1, yin and yang represent opposites, and the goal is to bring them into balance. Without balance, there is the danger of poor physical and mental health. An individual with a yin personality is quiet, reflective, introspective, and down to earth. An individual with a yang personality is outgoing and talkative, an extrovert, and always on the go. Each needs the other to maintain balance in their lives. The environment also contains the elements of yin and yang. Enhancers of yin and yang as related to elements in our environment are listed Table 7-7.

The exterior and the interior of a home work together. The exterior is like the shell of a crab, protecting the soft interior. The appearance of the exterior is a reflection of the interior, an indicator of the health and success of its inhabitants. Feng shui interventions include the following (Kennedy, 2011; Tchi, 2011):

1. Repositioning the furniture to change how the living space is experienced.
2. Working with light and air (e.g., focusing on having good-quality light and air with open windows, full-spectrum lighting, air-purifying plants).

TABLE 7-6 The Environment and Chi

	CHI ENHANCERS	CHI INHIBITORS
Architecture:	Curving pathways, open windows	Straight walls, closed doors
Space:	Uncluttered, open space	Clutter
Light:	Brightness and light	Darkness
Temperature:	Comfortable	Extremes
Shape:	Curves, undulating lines, rounded	Sharp angles
Movement:	Swaying plants, wind chimes, prisms, fans	Stillness

Adapted from The Feng Shui Bible: The Definitive Guide to Improving Your Life, Home, Health, and Finances, by S. Brown, 2005, New York: Sterling; and Chic Living with Feng Shui: Stylish Designs for Harmonious Living, by S. Stasney, 2004, New York: Sterling.

TABLE 7-7 The Environment and Yin/Yang

	YIN ENHANCERS	YANG ENHANCERS
Light	Muted light: less wattage, candles, closed drapes	Brighter lights, open drapes
Sound	Create silence	Add music, ticking clocks, etc.
Color	Muted, dark colors; monochromatic themes; cool, subdued, muted vibrant patterns	Bright, primary, contrasting colors; patterns
Humidity	Increase with fountains	Decrease with dehumidifier
Fabrics	Soft, silky, velvety	Solid colors, vertical stripes, shiny
Air movement	Decrease	Increase with fans, wind chimes
Furnishings	Low, heavy, solid furniture and accessories	Tall, thin, clear, light, firm, delicate, irregular shapes
Space	Increase flow of chi by removing clutter, opening space	Decrease flow of chi by filling space with form (plants, friends)
Social	Solitude	Company

Sources: From Ash, S. (2003). *The Healing Home: Practical Ways to Harmonize Your Home and Energize Your Spirit.* New York: Sterling; Brown, S. (2005). *The Feng Shui Bible: The Definitive Guide to Improving Your Life, Home, Health, and Finances,* New York: Sterling; Chissell, H. G. (2004). "Feng Shui Tips for Your Workspace," *Lilipoh, 9*(38), 17.

3. Using color to alter the mood of persons entering a space.

4. Adding different colors, shapes, and textures of plants to unite people with outdoors and instill a sense of being connected.

5. Incorporating and maintaining a balance of movement (e.g., adding objects that initiate action, such as fans, chimes, cuckoo clocks).

6. Attending to the placement of reflective surfaces (mirrors, metal) and heavy objects (tables, sofas, sculptures).

7. Incorporating sounds, both artificial (music) and natural (rustle of vegetation, water, rain, wind, critters).

8. Adding water, believed to be central to our existence.

9. Maintaining an uncluttered environment in the belief that cleaning up areas in your home can be a first step toward cleaning up parts of your life.

ENVIRONMENTAL DISASTERS

Environmental disasters can result from either natural, technological, or terrorist sources. Whatever the cause, environmental disasters unleash devastating forces. They are never expected. No community is immune to actual or potential threats to its health. In a world filled with technological advances, systems fail and exposure to toxic materials happens. Box 7-9 identifies the major causes of disasters facing the world today.

The causes, occurrences of, and results from natural, technological, and terror-related disasters vary, but the effects of any disaster can cause acute stress followed by extended periods of uncertainty. Universally key to any disaster situation is that language barriers put people at even greater risk if they do not understand the warnings given in a language unfamiliar to them.

The physical and psychological health of those involved can be altered for many years and sometimes for life. The following sections discuss major natural, technological, and terror-related disasters and associated health-promotion aspects.

BOX 7-9

CAUSES OF DISASTERS

- Broken or breached dams
- Earthquakes
- Extreme heat
- Fires
- Floods
- Hazardous materials
- Hurricanes
- Landslides
- Multihazard accidents
- Nuclear accidents
- Terrorism
- Thunderstorms
- Tornadoes
- Tsunamis
- Volcanoes
- Wildfires
- Winter storms

NATURAL DISASTERS

Individuals, communities, and health care systems are all affected by natural disasters. People living in areas prone to natural disasters may be lulled into a sense of complacency, suppressing the fact that these events often occur without warning. Discussing the causes of all natural disaster is beyond the scope of this chapter. Those most recently experienced by the world, and those considered the most devastating, are discussed here.

EARTHQUAKES

An earthquake is a sudden and rapid shaking of the ground caused by shifting rock plates beneath the Earth's surface. Fault lines are areas where plates meet and have the potential to break free and cause an earthquake, although earthquakes can occur in the middle of a plate as well. On average, about 70–75 earthquakes occur in the world each year. Injury and death from an earthquake come not from the actual ground movement but from collapsing buildings, flying debris and glass, and panic.

Earthquakes are responsible for some of the worst natural disasters in the history of the world. In December 2004, an earthquake far out in the Indian Ocean produced a devastating tsunami that caused an estimated 223,000 deaths in India, Indonesia, Malaysia, Thailand, and other smaller countries (Wilder-Smith & Steffen, 2005; Van-Rooyen & Leaning, 2005). Haiti suffered a 7.0-magnitude earthquake in January 2010, leaving thousands dead and injured and nearly 1 million homeless. Even more devastating was Japan's 9.0-magnitude earthquake in March 2011; the following tsunami resulted in more than 23,000 dead or missing persons and thousands of survivors who will need long-term mental health care to prevent debilitating conditions that could lead to suicide or long-term health issues ("Japan Earthquake," 2011). Even as Japan struggled with a post-earthquake rescue effort, it also faced the worst nuclear emergency since Chernobyl, as nuclear reactors at the Fukushima Daiichi Nuclear Power Station suffered partial meltdowns and fires that released radioactive material directly into the atmosphere and water supply (New York Times, 2011). The effects of contamination in the food supply and the population will have long-term consequences.

Tsunamis are ocean waves produced by earthquakes and by volcanic eruptions. Tsunamis are often incorrectly referred to as tidal waves, which is actually a misnomer. A tidal wave is an enormous and destructive ocean wave caused by extremely strong winds or earthquakes. *Tsunami* is a Japanese word for any large wave caused by an earthquake. Not all earthquakes produce tsunamis, but when they do, the waves may sweep ashore causing damage locally and at places thousands of miles from the earthquake epicenter.

In the United States, California experiences the most frequent damaging earthquakes, and Alaska experiences the greatest number of large earthquakes—mostly in uninhabited areas. For populated earthquake-prone areas, earthquake preparedness has become a way of life. In the event of a major earthquake, freeways and surface streets may be impassable, and public services could be interrupted or taxed beyond their limits. Therefore, everyone must know how to provide for personal needs over an extended period of time, whether at work, at home, or on the road. Knowing how to prepare yourself for an earthquake in various areas is important to avoid serious injury. The following tips will help you be better prepared should an earthquake strike (American Red Cross, 2009).

- *High-rise building*—Move against an interior wall, drop and cover, and hold on. Move as little as possible. Protect your head with your arms. Do not use the elevators. Do not be surprised if the alarm or sprinkler systems come on. Stay indoors to avoid falling debris and broken glass.
- *Outdoors*—Move to a clear area away from trees, signs, buildings, electrical wires, and poles, and drop down.
- *Sidewalk near buildings*—Duck into a doorway to protect yourself from falling bricks, glass, plaster, and other debris.
- *Driving*—Pull over to the side of the road and stop. Avoid overpasses, power lines, and other hazards. Stay inside the vehicle until the shaking is over. If a powerline falls on the vehicle, wait for assistance; do not get out.
- *Crowded public place*—Do not rush for exits. Move away from display shelves containing objects that could fall.
- *Wheelchair*—Stay in it, and move to a place of cover. If possible, lock your wheels, and protect your head with your arms.
- *Kitchen*—Move away from the refrigerator, stove, and overhead cupboards. (Appliances should have been prepared with anchors, and security latches should have been placed on cupboard doors.)
- *Stadium or theater*—Stay in your seat and protect your head with your arms. Do not try to leave until the shaking is over, and then leave calmly and in an orderly manner without rushing.

After an earthquake has passed, be prepared for aftershocks, and plan to continue the tips just listed. Check for injuries, avoid broken glass, and watch for fires, gas leaks, and live electric wires. Communication is vital, and having access to a radio or television for emergency broadcasts is essential. Above all, remain calm and reassure others.

HURRICANES

Floyd, Ivan, Jeanne, Katrina, and Rita are all innocent-sounding names, but people who were in the paths of these devastating hurricanes can attest to their fury. According to the Federal Emergency Management Administration (FEMA, 2010a), a hurricane is a tropical storm with winds that have reached a constant speed of 74 mph or more. Hurricane winds blow in a large spiral around a relatively calm center known as the eye. The eye is generally 20 to 30 mi wide, and the storm may extend outward 400 mi. As a hurricane approaches, the skies begin to darken, and winds grow in strength. As a hurricane nears land, it can bring torrential rains, high winds, and storm surges. A single hurricane can last for more than 2 weeks over open waters and can run a path across the entire length of the Eastern seaboard. August and September are peak months during the hurricane season, which lasts from June 1 through November 30.

Advanced meteorological science has enabled the prediction and tracking of hurricanes for days and often weeks in advance. A hurricane watch is issued when there is a threat of hurricane conditions within 24 to 36 hours, and a warning is issued when the winds are 74 mph or greater or when dangerously high water and rough seas are expected in 24 hours or less. This system usually allows for adequate preparation

and evacuation as needed. Even so, as seen with Hurricane Katrina, which struck the Gulf Coast of the United States in 2005, there can be catastrophic loss of life, injuries, exposure to toxins, widespread property damage, disease, and despair ("Norovirus Outbreak," 2005; "Surveillance for Illness," 2005). The cultural, psychological, social, economic, and political effects of the displacement of people from New Orleans to areas throughout the United States are still being felt.

TORNADOES

A tornado is a violently rotating column of air extending from a thunderstorm to the ground. The National Oceanic and Atmospheric Association (NOAA) has estimated that approximately 1200 tornadoes occur each year in the United States (NOAA, 2011). Box 7-10 provides additional facts about tornadoes, and Box 7-11 highlights important tornado terms.

BOX 7-10
TORNADO FACTS

- In the United States, tornadoes occur most frequently east of the Rocky Mountains during the spring and summer months.
- On average, 800 tornadoes are reported nationwide, resulting in 80 deaths and over 1500 injuries.
- The most violent tornadoes are capable of tremendous destruction with wind speeds of 250 mph or more.
- Damage paths can be larger than 1 mi wide and 50 m long.

Source: Federal Emergency Management Administration (FEMA). (2010b, August). *Tornadoes*. Retrieved from http://www.fema.gov/hazard/tornado/index.shtm

---

BOX 7-11
IMPORTANT TORNADO TERMS

Tornado watch: Tornadoes are possible in your area. Remain alert for approaching storms.
Tornado warning: A tornado has been sighted or indicated by weather radar. If a tornado warning is issued for your area and the sky becomes threatening, move to your predesignated place of safety.
Severe thunderstorm watch: Severe thunderstorms are possible in your area.
Severe thunderstorm warning: Severe thunderstorms are occurring.

Source: Federal Emergency Management Administration (FEMA). (2010b, August). *Tornadoes*. Retrieved from http://www.fema.gov/hazard/tornado/index.shtm

Despite advanced warning, many people are killed or seriously injured by tornadoes. Those most at risk during a tornado are people in vehicles, the elderly, infants and children, people with disabilities, and mobile home dwellers.

TECHNOLOGICAL DISASTERS

With technological disasters, the threat of potential exposure precedes the threat created by actual exposure. Long-term uncertainty, chronic stress, and mental health problems are more likely to occur as a result of the psychophysiological processes associated with these disasters. Psychological processes may add to or exacerbate the physiological effects on the body.

A most recent example of technical disaster is the oil spill in the Gulf of Mexico that resulted from the explosion at a Billups Petroleum offshore drilling rig. Even though the human death count of 11 is low in comparison to other disasters, the event is quickly becoming the biggest ecological disaster the United States has ever experienced. During a 4-month period in 2010, oil spilled continuously into the Gulf, having immediate effects and laying the foundation for long-term effects that will affect generations to come.

Many long-term consequences have been projected from this catastrophe (Donovan, 2010). The families of the persons who lost their lives will be affected in countless ways. The assault on the environment will continue to affect wildlife, sealife, and surrounding sandy beaches not only from the oil itself but also from the millions of gallons of dispersants used to contain the oil. In humans, exposure to volatile chemicals in the oil, including benzene, ethylbenzine, and xylene, have been associated with skin conditions, respiratory disease, miscarriages, and cancer. In addition, stress on individuals and families from previous technological disasters have shown increases in the rates of alcoholism, suicide, violence, and divorce. The extent of the impact on the seafood industry is yet to be seen, as well as the effect on the once thriving business of tourism. If any good is to come from such a disaster, there is hope for legislation addressing offshore drilling, environment protection, and the push for clean sources of energy.

TERROR-RELATED DISASTERS

In recent years, the world has experienced terror-related disasters unparalleled in history. No country in the world is immune to terroristic threats or acts.

On September 11, 2001, terrorists attacked the United States by flying two hijacked planes into the Twin Towers of the World Trade Center in New York City, resulting in 2752 deaths, while a third plane flown into the Pentagon killed 189 people, and another 44 were killed when a fourth hijacked jet crashed into a field in Pennsylvania. On July 7, 2005, a series of coordinated suicide bombings struck London's public transport system during the morning rush hour. The bombings killed 52 civilians and injured over 700 people.

According to the U.S. Federal Bureau of Investigation (FBI), **terrorism** is the "unlawful use of force and violence against persons or property to intimidate or coerce a government, the civilian population, or any segment thereof, in furtherance of political or social objectives" (Code of Federal Regulations Title 28). Although thousands of people have lost their lives in terrorist attacks, the goal of terrorism is to destroy the sense of well-being and trust in government. Terrorist-related disasters can result from the use of biological, chemical, or radiological (nuclear) weapons from national or international sources (Shi & Singh, 2011). These weapons, intended to cause death or serious bodily harm to a significant number of people, were deemed to be **weapons of mass destruction (WMDs)** by the U.S. Congress in 1996 (Mothershead, 2004). The U.S. Department of Homeland Security has recently used the term **weapons of mass effect (WMEs)**, which more clearly denotes the motives of terrorists to cause widespread chaos and despair by whatever method is used (Mothershead, 2004).

A detailed discussion of WMEs is beyond the scope of this chapter. However, it is important to have an awareness of what to expect following a terrorist attack. The following was learned from the events of September 11, 2001:

- There can be significant numbers of casualties, damage to buildings and the infrastructure, or both. Employers need up-to-date information about any medical needs you may have and about how to contact your family or significant others.
- Heavy law enforcement involvement at local, state, and federal levels follows a terrorist attack due to the event's criminal nature.
- Health and mental health resources in the affected communities can be strained to their limits, perhaps even overwhelmed.
- Extensive media coverage, strong public fear, and international implications and consequences can continue for a prolonged period.
- Workplaces and schools may be closed, and there may be restrictions on domestic and international travel.
- You and your family or household may have to evacuate an area, avoiding roads blocked for your safety.
- Recovery may take many months.

The successes of recent terrorist attacks have generated greater preparedness by government agencies. Nations, individual states, and local governments have more responsibility than ever in providing public health protection. Because of its multifaceted nature, the issue and incidence of terrorism require multiple approaches, including political, military, technologic, scientific, and economic (North Atlantic Treaty Organization, 2011). Nurses are vital to the response to and management of any disaster. After the September 11 attacks, state boards of nursing required that nurses complete continuing education on bioterrorism. Box 7-12 describes the nurse's role in bioterrorism preparedness. Sources for completing continuing education on bioterrorism are listed at the end of this chapter. Regardless of cause, all disasters involve risk assessment, preparedness, responsiveness, and recovery—the key principles in disaster planning and management.

POSTTRAUMATIC STRESS DISORDER

Victims of trauma are at risk for development of **posttraumatic stress disorder (PTSD)**. PTSD is a constellation of continuing, long-term detrimental effects, including flashbacks, nightmares, insomnia, and concentration difficulties, resulting from exposure to trauma. The traumatic event may be a natural disaster (e.g., tornado, hurricane, flood, fire, earthquake,

BOX 7-12
THE NURSE'S ROLE IN BIOTERRORISM

1. Recognize cases and clusters of cases that could result from biological terrorism or from naturally occurring outbreaks.

2. Provide prompt evaluation and medical management.

3. Initiate and coordinate prompt communication with public health officials from local to state and national levels as needed.

4. Create a culture of safety and confidence.

Sources: Adapted from *Bioterrorism Basics for Nurses* (2005). Columbus, OH: The Bioterrorism Institute; Coyle, A. J. (2005). "Nursing Management Models for Response to Bioterrorism." *Pulsepage*, 24–27

TABLE 7-8 Responses to Trauma

Early symptoms of acute stress	Fear, shock, anxiety, anger, irritability, insomnia, difficulty making decisions, inability to think creatively, forgetfulness, uncomfortable being alone, hyperalert, easily startled, jumpiness, flashbacks, feeling loss of control, helplessness, loss of feeling secure in the world, sadness, increased use of alcohol and/or drugs, social withdrawal, headaches, nausea, chest pain, change in appetite, "emotional numbing," exhaustion
Symptoms of PTSD	
1. Hyperarousal	Heightened startle response, irritability, insomnia, strong emotions rekindled by reminders of the trauma
2. Intrusion	Intrusive recollections, obsessing, flashbacks, nightmares
3. Constriction	Physical withdrawal, social isolation, avoidance of reminders, emotional numbing, depression, substance abuse

Sources: Lee, H. A., Gabriel, R., & Bale, A. J. (2006). "Clinical Outcomes of Gulf Veterans' Medical Assessment Programme Referrals to Specialized Centers for Gulf Veterans with Post-traumatic Stress Disorder," *Military Medicine, 170*(5), 400–405; "Tips for recovering from disasters and other traumatic events." (2011). *American Psychological Association*, retrieved from http://www.apa.org/helpcenter/recovering-disasters.aspx; Hudek, C, (2007). "Dealing with Vicarious Traumatization in the Context of Global Fear." *The Folio*, 95–101.

volcanic eruption), a technological or manmade disaster (e.g., massive toxic contamination from chemicals or radiation), a dramatic change in a work environment (e.g., restructuring, downsizing, reengineering), physical assault, or many other causes. Nearly all 3700 survivors of the World Trade Center terrorist attack in 2001 continue to have at least one symptom of PTSD, and about 15% of them have been diagnosed with the full-symptom profile of PTSD (Carter, 2011).

Responses to trauma, including specific symptoms of PTSD, are listed in Table 7-8.

Individuals experiencing PTSD may experience increased health problems, a decline in work or school performance, and a deterioration of family life. Symptoms of PTSD tend to decrease over the first several years. Interestingly, PTSD from natural disasters tends to disappear within 2 years of the event. However, the effects of technological disasters seem to be more prolonged, lasting years (Hyams, Murphy, & Wessely, 2002).

Much of the PTSD research centers on combat veterans. The findings of these research studies correlate with those of victims of natural or technological disasters. The severity of the traumatizing event affects the development, extent, and duration of PTSD. The number of lives lost, the amount of property damage, and the effect on normal routines (e.g., school and work attendance) enter into the equation.

The effects of a disaster may last for years. Symptoms may develop months, even years later, after a period of no apparent symptoms. Many clients go undiscovered. A link is not made between the event and the current symptoms. Health care professionals are also at risk because of the nature of their work. They may experience vicarious traumatization even though they may not have been directly involved with the incident (Hudek, 2007).

Comorbidity, or coexisting disease, has been examined in stress research, with particular attention to the coexistence of psychiatric disorders and PTSD. The most frequent comorbid disorders are substance abuse, depression, generalized anxiety disorders, panic disorders and phobias, somatization disorders characterized by physical suffering, psychotic disorders, and personality disorders. Comorbid disorders may precede or create vulnerability to PTSD and may not be truly separate from PTSD (Schnurr & Green, 2004).

NURSING ALERT

Steps to Minimize the Psychological Effects of a Disaster

1. Provide precise instructions about dealing with an anticipated disaster.

2. Identify sources of accurate information.

3. Minimize exposure to death and injury.

4. Protect family members from unnecessary exposure to body parts, grotesque bodies, or the dead.

5. Initiate public education to normalize early stress responses.

6. Mobilize support systems and cross-linkages among professionals.

7. Participate in developing disaster-specific support systems.

HEALTH PROMOTION AND NURSING INTERVENTIONS FOR ENVIRONMENTAL DISASTERS

The important role of health care professionals cannot be overemphasized in caring for the sick and injured as a result of natural, technological, or terror-related disasters. Emergency and trauma care typically focuses on physical health. Little or no attention is given to preventing long-term psychological effects.

Promoting both physical and psychological health for disaster victims is possible. Nurse therapists and clinical nurse specialists may fill key roles, especially in preventing PTSD, in working with people experiencing PTSD, and in educating others about the problem. The simplest approach to intervention should be used. Crisis intervention should be early, brief, and problem focused. Box 7-13 lists actions for emotional first aid for trauma victims.

Certain individuals are at high risk for PTSD following a disaster. Elderly, psychologically disturbed, or mentally retarded persons or people with disabilities are dependent on a psychosocial stability. Turmoil surrounding a disaster places them at high risk. Others in high-risk categories are traumatized survivors; children, particularly if separated from their parents; close relatives of those who died suddenly or traumatically; those responsible for removing the bodies of those who died; and those living in devastated communities. At-risk groups must be identified as well as risk behaviors, symptoms, or signs that PTSD is developing.

Particular attention should be paid to young victims of traumatic stress, such as the thousands of children directly affected by the events of September 11, 2001, and the hundreds of thousands more who were affected indirectly by the massive media coverage. One report identified the following factors as important in understanding children's response to disaster (Hagan, 2005):

1. Parental awareness of their reactions on their children—how parents respond affects how children respond.
2. Stages of children's response to disaster—stage one is fright and disbelief, followed by a desire to help, reflecting the resilience of children. Stage two manifests as regression with heightened emotional distress and other behaviors, including depression, sleep disturbances, play themes related to disaster, and others.
3. Developmental stage of children—infants, toddlers, young children, and older children all respond differently according to their unique developmental stage.
4. Gender and ethnicity of children—boys act out behaviorally, whereas girls internalize reactions but are more vocal regarding their feelings.
5. Other factors—poor social support, a history of psychological problems, introverted personality, and level of exposure to losses from a disaster are additional factors to consider.

PREPARATION FOR DISASTERS

Nurses have been and will be committed to being on the front lines as caregivers and managers in natural, technological, and terror-related disasters. The completion of continuing education programs and participation in mock disaster drills can increase the efficiency and effectiveness of response to disaster in the community, hospital, or clinic setting. Nurses caring for families can help them prepare for a disaster using the Family Disaster Planning Guide in Box 7-14. Recommended contents for a disaster supply kit can be found in Box 7-15.

Nurses also play key roles in environmental health through the use of assessment, collaborative, and political skills. Depending on the issue at hand and entities involved, processes in which nurses are involved can range from simple to complex, from inexpensive to expensive, from traditional to nontraditional, and from short-term to long-range.

Nurses are important in identifying hazards, planning remedial or removal interventions, and educating the public. Community education is crucial. Methods of involvement include participating in community forums, giving or attending speeches at meetings of community organizations or events, making written and audiovisual materials available, and collaborating with mass media. Communicating problems, needs, and possible solutions to political representatives is also a responsibility that nurses have as professionals and as citizens. Public opinion and communication have a tremendous influence on policy development for a healthier environment.

BOX 7-13

EMOTIONAL FIRST AID

Nurses can promote psychological health by helping the disaster victim to:

- Recognize symptoms of stress.
- Identify resources and activities.
- Recognize psychologically painful situations.
- Accept the reality of the situation.
- Develop an optimistic attitude.
- Avoid placing blame on others.
- Accept help and support.
- Resume the activities of daily life.
- Connect with religious beliefs.

Source: Fairbrother, G. (2004) "Unmet Need for Counseling Services by Children in New York City After the September 11th Attacks on the World Trade Center: Implications for Pediatricians." *Pediatrics, 113*, 1367–1374; Meisenhelder, J. B. (2002). "Terrorism, Posttraumatic Stress and Religious Coping." *Mental Health Nursing, 23*(8), 771–782; Schnurr, P. P., & Green, B. L. (2004). "Understanding Relationships Among Trauma, Post-Traumatic Stress Disorder, and Health Outcomes," *Advances in Mind-Body Medicine, 20*(1), 18–29.

BOX 7-14
FAMILY DISASTER PLANNING GUIDE

1. *Gather information about hazards.* Contact your local National Weather Service office, emergency management or civil defense office, and American Red Cross chapter. Find out what types of disasters could occur and how you should respond. Learn your community's warning signals and evacuation plans.

2. *Meet with your family to create a plan.* Discuss the information you have gathered. Pick two places to meet: (1) a spot outside your home for an emergency such as fire and (2) a place away from your neighborhood in case you cannot return home. Choose an out-of-state friend as your "family check-in contact" for everyone to call if the family gets separated. Discuss what you would do if advised to evacuate. Don't forget the special needs of the elderly and handicapped.

3. *Implement your plan.* Use the following steps in implementing your plan:
   a. Post emergency telephone numbers by phones.
   b. Install safety features in your house, such as smoke detectors and fire extinguishers.
   c. Inspect your home for potential hazards (such as items that can move, fall, break, or catch fire) and correct them.
   d. Have your family learn basic safety measures, such as CPR and first aid; how to use a fire extinguisher; and how and when to turn off water, gas, and electricity in your home.
   e. Teach children how and when to call 911 or your local emergency medical services number.
   f. Keep enough supplies in your home to meet your needs for at least three days. Assemble a disaster kit (see Box 7-15) with items you may need in case of an evacuation or to take with you to a shelter. Store these supplies in sturdy, easy-to-carry containers, such as backpacks or duffel bags. Keep important family documents in a waterproof container. Keep a smaller disaster supply kit in the trunk of your car.
   g. Plan for the care of pets. Shelters do not usually accept pets, nor do many hotels.

4. *Practice and maintain your plan.* Ask questions to make sure your family remembers meeting places, phone numbers, and safety rules. Conduct drills. Test your smoke detectors monthly, and change the batteries at least once a year. Test and recharge your fire extinguisher(s) according to the manufacturer's instructions. Replace stored water and food every 6 months.

Source: American Red Cross. (2001), "Terrorism—Preparing for the unexpected." Retrieved from http://www.redcross.org/www-files/Documents/pdf/Preparedness/AreYouReady/Terrorism.pdf; Federal Emergency Management Administration (FEMA). (2005, December). "Hazards: Hurricanes," retrieved from http://www.fema.gov/hazard/hurricane/index.shtml; Federal Emergency Management Administration (FEMA). (2006, July). "Are you ready? An in-depth guide to citizen preparedness," retrieved from www.fema.gov/areyouready/

BOX 7-15
DISASTER SUPPLY KIT ESSENTIALS

- A 3-day supply of water (1 gal per person per day) and food that will not spoil
- Kitchen supplies, such as disposable utensils, plates, and cups
- One change of clothing and footwear per person
- Sanitation and hygiene items
- One blanket or sleeping bag per person
- A first-aid kit, including prescription medicines
- Emergency tools, including a battery-powered AA Weather Radio, a portable radio, a flashlight, and plenty of extra batteries
- An extra set of car keys and a credit card or cash
- Entertainment such as games, puzzles, books, toys
- Special items for infants and family members who are elderly or disabled

Sources: American Red Cross, (2006.). Disaster supplies kit, retrieved from http://www.redcross.org/preparedness/cdc_english/kit.asp; Federal Emergency Management Administration (FEMA). (2010a). Hazards: Hurricanes, retrieved from http://www.fema.gov/hazard/hurricane/hu_hazard.shtml; Federal Emergency Management Administration (FEMA). (2006, July). Are you ready? An in-depth guide to citizen preparedness, retrieved from www.fema.gov/areyouready/

SUMMARY

Promoting environmental health is a complex, challenging task. Citizens and health care workers must continue to work together in the fight against environmental pollution. Researchers must continue to expand the knowledge base about the biological and psychosocial effects of environmental pollution.

Community and environmental groups and legislatures must work together toward reducing risk from environmental hazards and hold accountable those who place the environment at risk. Individuals and industries must be responsible in the use and disposal of potentially toxic products.

KEY CONCEPTS

1. Air, water, soil, sound, light, and space, as well as environmental disasters, influence environmental health.

2. The goals in environmental health are to minimize or eliminate pollutants in a threatening environment and to create an environment supportive of good health.

3. Psychological and physiological symptoms in every body system have been linked to occupational and environmental pollutants; however, determining the exact cause is difficult.

4. The reduction of or removal of pollutants is important to prevent chemical sensitization even in the absence of symptoms.

5. The nurse, using the nursing process and leadership skills, plays a key role in assisting individuals and communities to improve environmental health through personal and political action.

6. The alert nurse evaluates for potential environmental pollutants during assessments of individuals and their living and working areas.

7. Nursing interventions to improve environmental health may be simple or complex, inexpensive or expensive, traditional or nontraditional.

8. Natural, technological, or terror-related disasters create environmental risks and are associated with posttraumatic stress disorder.

9. All disasters involve risk assessment, preparedness, responsiveness, and recovery components.

10. Citizen groups have been successful in protecting their community's health. The nurse may be instrumental in forming and guiding these groups.

CHAPTER REVIEW

Learning Activities

1. Go to http://www.epa.gov/myenvironment/ and enter your zip code to see a map of your region. Find out what emissions are being released into the air, where polluted waters exist, and what is being done (tracking, restoring, protecting) to aid the environment in your area.

2. Develop a family disaster plan for your family.

3. Participate in a mock disaster drill conducted by your educational facility, local hospital, or community organization, and write down your experiences in a journal.

Multiple Choice

1. A patient presents to the local clinic complaining of respiratory symptoms, which she feels are a result of chemicals in her office building. The nurse knows that a diagnosable illness that can be directly linked to airborne building contaminants is known as:
   a. building-related illness.
   b. environmental health hazard.
   c. SAD syndrome.
   d. sick building syndrome.

2. A nurse is conducting a presentation on home safely to parents at a school health fair. In discussing air pollution, the nurse should emphasize that the single most preventable source of indoor air pollution is:
   a. carbon monoxide.
   b. natural gas.
   c. radon gas.
   d. tobacco smoke.

3. A new employee working in a noisy factory is concerned about a decrease in hearing since starting work 2 weeks ago. As the occupational health nurse, you know that standards set by the Occupational Safety and Health Administration (OSHA) indicate that hearing impairment can occur with continued exposure to noise that is:
   a. 55 decibels or higher over 5 hours.
   b. 65 decibels or higher over 6 hours.
   c. 85 decibels or higher over 8 hours.
   d. 95 decibels or higher over 10 hours.

4. A charge nurse of a medical floor has submitted a proposal to administration for changes in the nurses' station focusing on ergonomic concepts. His proposal would define the term *ergonomics* as the:
   a. conservation of human energy.
   b. science of relationships of furniture and tools to the human body.
   c. study of work-related injury and disease.
   d. work involved with colors and sounds for improved work production.

5. Nurses living in earthquake-prone areas need to know how to promote safety for themselves, their families, friends, and patients. Which of the following actions to be taken during an earthquake is appropriate advice to follow and provide to others?
   a. If driving, keep driving and pull under an overpass for protection.
   b. If in a high-rise building, move against an interior wall.
   c. If in a stadium, leave your seat and move quickly to the nearest exit.
   d. If outdoors, move to the nearest tree for shelter and support.

6. A patient voices concern about the possibility of radon gas in her home. As her nurse, you inform her that the detection of radon gas is:
   a. by its bluish tint and pungent odor.
   b. difficult due to its colorless and odorless properties.
   c. found only in air samples.
   d. tested for only by qualified environmental professionals.

7. A community health nurse is attending a town hall meeting where public health officials are discussing an environmental health issue specifically referred to as outgassing. The nurse is aware that outgassing occurs when:
   a. atmospheric airflow of contaminants flows from the United States to Europe.
   b. emissions of sulfur dioxide and nitrogen dioxide combine, resulting in acid rain.
   c. formaldehyde becomes a toxic gas in high temperature and humidity.
   d. vents are installed in bathrooms and kitchens to remove biological contaminants.

8. A patient has been diagnosed with noise-induced hearing loss from sound pollution. Nursing support for this patient is based on the knowledge that this diagnosis is a major health concern due to the following reason:
   a. It cannot be reversed by surgery.
   b. Recovery from hearing loss surgery is lengthy.
   c. The return of hearing takes many years.
   d. Those affected suffer intractable pain.

9. A nurse is providing discharge instructions to parents whose 3-year-old daughter has recovered from lead toxicity. They have two other children, ages 1 and 4 years. With regard to lead toxicity, which of the following is an appropriate instruction for the health of this child and her siblings?
   a. Ensure a balanced diet that is rich in calcium and iron.
   b. Remove all doormats from outside entrances.
   c. Sand or burn off lead-based painted surfaces.
   d. Use a strong solvent to remove paint that contains lead.

10. Ted, 13 years old, has been diagnosed with multiple chemical sensitivities. Which of the following is important to include in a teaching plan for Ted and his parents to facilitate the creation of a safe haven for him?
    a. Introduce new items in the environment at 24-hour intervals.
    b. Substitute human-made polyester for all cloth items made of cotton.
    c. Replace natural wood furniture with items made of particleboard.
    d. Wash wall, windows, and blinds with water and baking soda, vinegar, or hydrogen peroxide.

ORGANIZATIONS AND WEBSITES

American Association of Poison Control Centers (AAPCC): Lists poison control centers. Sources for continuing education on bioterrorism: **http://www.aapcc.org**

Centers for Disease Control and Prevention Training and Education: **http://www.bt.cdc.gov**

The CE Solutions Group: **http://www.healthceonline.com**

Environmental Protection Agency (EPA): Contains an overview of the agency's mission, structure, strategic plan, budget, offices, and staff. Provides data on environmental laws, regulations, research, standards, compliance, and enforcement. Contains maps of specific regions accessible by zip code. Tells what facilities in the region release emissions into the air or if there are any polluted waters, among other information. Also tells what is being done (tracking, restoring, and protecting) to aid the environment in that area: **http://www.epa.gov**

Hotline: Operates 24 hours a day, seven days a week. Callers may order an information package and/or speak to an information specialist: (800) 424-LEAD (5323).

Indoor Air Quality Information Clearinghouse: Distributes EPA publications, answers questions on the phone, and makes referrals to other nonprofit and governmental organizations: **http://www.healthfinder.gov/orgs/HR3287.htm**

Lead Poisoning Prevention Branch of the Centers for Disease Control and Prevention: Resource for information on lead poisoning detection, prevention, and management. Hotline: (800) 488-7330; **http://www.cdc.gov/nceh/lead**

National Pesticide Information Center (NPIC): Sponsored by the Environmental Protection Agency, this center provides information about pesticides to the general public and the medical, veterinary, and professional communities, Hotline: (800) 858-PEST/(800) 858-7378: **http://www.npic.orst.edu/**

National Radon Hotlines: Information recording on radon; operates 24 hours a day. Hotline: (800) SOS-RADON/(800) 767-7236: **http://sosradon.org/national-radon-hotlines**

Nurses' Study Resource: **http://www.westernschools.com**

Occupational Safety and Health Administration (OSHA): Provides information and takes complaints on work site health and safety issues, standards, and regulations: **http://osha.gov**

Office on Smoking and Health of the Centers for Disease Control and Prevention: Resource for information on smoking-related issues: **http://www.cdc.gov/tobacco/osh/index.htm**

Online Continuing Education for Nursing and Nursing Professionals: **http://www.ceregistration.com**

Safe Drinking Water Hotline: Provides information on regulations under the Safe Drinking Water Act and on lead and radon in drinking water, filter information, and a list of state drinking water offices. Hotline: (800) 426-4791: **http://water.epa.gov/drink/contact.cfm**

Texas Statewide Bioterrorism Continuing Education Project: Operates Monday to Friday, 9 a.m. to 5 p.m. Eastern Standard Time (EST): **http://www.son.utmb.edu**

Toxic Substances Control Act (TSCA) Assistance Information Service: Provides information on regulations under the Toxic Substances Control Act and on the EPA's asbestos program. Phone: (202) 554-1404: **http://www.epa.gov/oecaagct/lsca.html**

U.S. Consumer Product Safety Commission (CPSC): Teletypewriter for the hearing impaired (outside Maryland): (800) 638-8270. Takes complaints and answers questions about product safety. Product safety hotline: (800) 638-CPSC: **http://www.cpsc.gov**

U.S. Public Health Service: Provides indoor air quality consultative services to federal agency managers: **http://www.usphs.gov**

Division of Federal Occupational Health
Office of Environmental Hygiene, Region III, Room 1310

REFERENCES

American Federation of State, County, and Municipal Employees (AFSCME). (n.d.). *Health and safety fact sheet: Diesel exhaust.* Retrieved from http://www.afscme.org/news/publications/workplace-health-and-safety/fact-sheets/diesel-exhaust

American Federation of State, County, and Municipal Employees (AFSCME). (2002, March). *Preventing back injuries in health care workers.* Retrieved June 5, 2006, from http://www.afscme.org/news/publications/workplace-health-and-safety/fact-sheets/preventing-back-injuries-in-health care

American Psychological Association. (2011). *Tips for recovering from disasters and other traumatic events.* Retrieved from http://www.apa.org/helpcenter/recovering-disasters.aspx

American Red Cross. (2009). *Be Red Cross ready: Earthquake safety checklist.* Retrieved from http://www.nehrp.gov/pdf/redcrosschecklist.pdf

American Red Cross. (n.d.). *Terrorism: Preparing for the unexpected.* Retrieved from http://www.redcross.org/services/disaster/0,1082,0_589_,00.html

Ash, S. (2003). *The healing home: Practical ways to harmonize your home and energize your spirit.* New York, NY: Sterling.

Berke, J. (2010, September). *Hearing loss demographics: Statistically how many are deaf and hard of hearing?* Retrieved from http://deafness.about.com/cs/earbasics/a/demographics.htm

Brown, S. (2005). *The feng shui bible: The definitive guide to improving your life, home, health, and finances.* New York, NY: Sterling.

Caravati, E. M., & McGuigan, M. A. (2004). *Medical toxicology.* Philadelphia, PA: Lippincott Williams & Wilkins.

Carter, S. (2011, January 9). *Victims of the World Trade Center attack still experiencing symptoms.* Retrieved from http://www.examiner.com/health-in-dallas/victims-of-the-world-trade-center-attack-still-experiencing-symptoms

Centers for Disease Control and Prevention (CDC). (2009). *Fourth national report on human exposure to environmental chemicals.* Retrieved from http://www.cdc.gov/exposurereport/

Chissell, H. G. (2004, Winter). Feng shui tips for your workspace. *Lilipoh, 9*(38), 17.

Code of Federal Regulations Title 28, *Judicial administration,* Chapter I. Department of Justice, Part O, Subpart P, Federal Bureau of Investigation, Section 0.85, general functions.

Colls, J. F., & Tiwary, A. (2010). *Air pollution.* London: Spon Press.

Coyle, A. J. (2005, February). Nursing management models for response to bioterrorism. *Pulsepage,* 24–27.

Danielson, R. W. (n.d.). *Hearing loss prevention* Retrieved from http://betterhearing.org/hearing_loss_prevention/index.cfm

Donovan, T. W. (2010, May). *7 long-term effects of the Gulf oil spill.* Retrieved from http://www.huffingtonpost.com/2010/05/10/7-long-term-effects-of-th_n_562947.html#s87715&title=Families_Of_The

Elioupoulis, C. (2010). *Invitation to holistic health: A guide to living a balanced life.* Sudbury, MA: Jones & Bartlett.

Environmental Protection Agency (EPA). (2010a). Planning a human health risk assessment, Retrieved from http://www.epa.gov/ncea/risk/hazardous-identification.htm

Environmental Protection Agency (EPA). (2010b). Sources of indoor air pollution: Biological pollutants. Retrieved, from http://www.epa.gov/iaq/biologic.html

Environmental Protection Agency (EPA). (2010c). Indoor air facts no. 4 (revised): Sick building syndrome (SBS). Retrieved from http://www.epa.gov/iaq/pubs/sbs.html

Environmental Protection Agency (EPA). (2010d). Indoor air pollution: An introduction for health professionals. Retrieved from http://www.epa.gov/iaq/pubs/hpguide.html

Environmental Protection Agency (EPA). (2010e). An office building occupant's guide to indoor air quality. Retrieved from http://www.epa.gov/iaq/pubs/occupgd.html

Environmental Protection Agency (EPA). (2010f). Health effects of exposure to secondhand smoke. Retrieved from http://www.epa.gov/smokefree/healtheffects.html

Environmental Protection Agency (EPA). (2010g). An introduction to air quality: Volatile organic compounds. Retrieved from http://www.epa.gov/iaq/voc.html

Environmental Protection Agency (EPA). (20011a). The origins of EPA. Retrieved from http://www.epa.gov/aboutepa/history/origins.html

Environmental Protection Agency (EPA). (20011b). An introduction to indoor air quality: Volatile organic compounds(VOCs). Retrieved from http://www.epa.gov/iaq/voc.html

Fairbrother, G. (2004, May). Unmet need for counseling services by children in New York City after the September 11th attacks on the World Trade Center: Implications for pediatricians. *Pediatrics, 113,* 1367–1374.

Federal Emergency Management Administration (FEMA). (2010a, August). Hazards: Hurricanes. Retrieved from http://www.fema.gov/business/guide/section3d.shtm

Federal Emergency Management Administration (FEMA). (2010b, August). Tornado. Retrieved from http://www.fema.gov/hazard/tornado/index.shtm

Federal Emergency Management Administration (FEMA). (2006, July). Are you ready? An in-depth guide to citizen preparedness. Retrieved from http://www.fema.gov/areyouready/

Gordis, L. (2008). *Epidemiology*. Philadelphia: W. B. Saunders.

Guzzetta, C. E., & Morris, D. (2005, 2009). Music therapy: Hearing the melody of the soul, In B. Dossey, L. Keegan, & C. Guzzetta (eds.). *Holistic nursing: A handbook for practice* (4th ed., pp. 617–640). Sudbury, MA: Jones and Bartlett, pp. 617–640.

Hagan, J. F. (2005). Psychosocial implication of disaster or terrorism on children: A guide for the pediatrician. *Pediatrics, 116*(3), 787–795.

Hearing Foundation of Canada. (2010). Statistics. Retrieved from http://www.thfc.ca/cms/en/KeyStatistics/KeyStatistics.aspx?menuid=87

Hiss, T. (1990). *The experience of place*. New York, NY: Alfred A. Knopf.

How loud is too loud; how long is too long? (2009). Retrieved from www.noisyplanet.nidcd.nih.gov/parents/athome.htm

Hudek, C. (2007). Dealing with vicarious traumatization in the context of global fear. *The Folio*, 95–101.

Imhof, M. (2004). Effects of color stimulation on handwriting performance of children with ADHD without and with additional learning disabilities. *European Child & Adolescent Psychiatry, 13*(3), 191–198.

Japan earthquake survivors at risk for suicide. (2011, June). *KWTS. COM.* Retrieved from http://www.kwtx.com/nationalnews/headlines/Japan_Earthquake_Survivors_At_Risk_Of_Suicide_123634834.html

Kennedy, D. D. (2011). *Feng shui for dummies.* Indianapolis, IN: Wiley Publishing, Inc

Kleim, B., & Rock, B. (n.d.). *The New England region's changing climate.* Retrieved from http://www.necci.sr.unh.edu/necci-report/NERAch2.pdf

Kochkin, S. (2009, October). MarkeTrak VIII: 25-year trends in the hearing health market. *Hearing review.com.* Retrieved from http://www.betterhearing.org/pdfs/Kochkin_MarkeTrak8_OctHR09_hr.pdf

Larson, L. (2010). *Environmental health sourcebook.* Detroit, MI: Omnigraphics.

Laskoski, J. (2010, January). Is bright light therapy effective for improving depressive symptoms in adults with Seasonal Affective Disorder (SAD)? *Internet Journal of Academic Physician Assistants*, 7(2).

Lee, H. A., Gabriel, R., & Bale, A. J. (2005, May). Clinical outcomes of Gulf Veterans' Medical Assessment Programme referrals to specialized centers for Gulf veterans with post-traumatic stress disorder. *Military Medicine, 170*(5), 400–405.

Mayo Clinic. (2006, July 24). Eyestrain and your computer screen: Tips for getting relief. Retrieved from http://www.cosc.canterbury.ac.nz/policy/health+safety/oos/mayo/eyestrain.htm

Mayo Clinic. (2008). *Seasonal affective disorder treatment: choosing a light therapy box.* Retrieved from www.mayoclinic.com/health/seasonal-affective-disorder-treatment/dn00013.

McCullagh, M.C., Ronis, D. L., & Lusk, S. L. (2010). Predictors of use of hearing protection among a representative sample of farmers. Research in Nursing & Health, *33*(6), 528–538.

Meisenhelder, J. B. (2002, December). Terrorism, posttraumatic stress and religious coping. *Issues in Mental Health Nursing, 23*(8): 771–782.

Mella, D. L. (1988). *Language of color.* New York, NY: Warner Books, Inc.

Mesolink. (2010). Retrieved from http://www.mesolink.org

Miller, A. (2005). Epidemiology, etiology, and natural treatment of seasonal affective disorder. *Alternative Medicine Review, 10*(1), 5–13.

Moran, E. (2002). *The complete idiot's guide to Feng Shui.* Indianapolis, IN: Alpha Books.

Mothershead, J. L. (2004). The new threat: Weapons of mass effect. In K. J. McGlown (Ed.), *Terrorism and disaster management* (pp. 27–49). Chicago, IL: Health Administration Press.

National Cancer Institute (NCI). (2011, May). *NCI statement: International Agency for Research on Cancer classification of cell phones as "possible carcinogen".* Retrieved from http://www.cancer.gov/newscenter/pressreleases/2011/IARCcellphoneMay2011

National Collaborating Centre. (2008, December). Effective interventions for reducing indoor radon exposure. Retrieved from http://www.ncceh.ca/sites/default/files/Radon_Interventions_Dec_2008.pdf

National Heart Lung and Blood Institute. (2011, May). What are asbestos-related lung diseases? Retrieved from http://www.nhlbi.nih.gov/health/dci/Diseases/asb/asb_whatare.html

National Oceanic and Atmospheric Association (NOAA). (2011, April). Tornados 101: Stay alert and stay alive. Retrieved from http://www.noaa.gov/features/03_protecting/tornadoes101c.html

Norovirus outbreak among evacuees from Hurricane Katrina—Houston, Texas, September 2005. (2005, October). *Mortality and Morbidity Weekly Report, 54,* 1016–1018.

North Atlantic Treaty Organization (NATO) (2011, March). NATO and the fight against terrorism. Retrieved from http://www.nato.int/cps/en/natolive/topics_48801.htm

New York Times. (2011, August 27). Japan—Earthquake, tsunami and nuclear crisis. Retrieved from http://topics.nytimes.com/top/news/international/countriesandterritories/japan/index.html

Occupational Safety and Health Administration (OSHA). (n.d.). Diesel exhaust. Retrieved from http://www.osha.gov/SLTC/dieselexhaust/index.html

Occupational *Safety and Health Administration (OSHA).* (2008). Hearing conservation program. Retrieved from http://http://www.osha.gov/pls/oshaweb/owadisp.show_document?p_table=DIRECTIVES&p_id=4007

Peiris, J. S., & Poon, L. L. (2011). Detection of SARS coronavirus. *Methods in Molecular Biology, 665,* 369–382.

Pfettscher, S. A. (2010). Modern nursing. In M. A. Alligood & A. M. Tomey (eds.), *Nursing theorists and their work.* Maryland Heights, MO: Mosby Elsevier, (pp. 71–90)

Potts, J. (2009). Aromatherapy in nursing practice. *Australian Nursing Journal, 16*(2), 2.

Rom, W. N. (2011). *Environmental Policy and Public Health: Air Pollution, Global Climate Change, and Wilderness.* San Francisco, CA: Jossey-Bass.

Santulli, E. (2004). No strain? No pain! *Hospital Nursing, 34*(3), 7–8.

Schnurr, P. P., & Green, B. L. (2004). Understanding relationships among trauma, post-traumatic stress disorder, and health outcomes. *Advances in Mind-Body Medicine, 20*(1), 18–29.

Schweitzer, M., Gilpin, L., & Frampton, S. (2004). Healing spaces: Elements of environmental design that make an impact on health. *Journal of Alternative and Complementary Medicine, 10*(1), 71–83.

Shi, L. & Singh, D.A. (2011). *The nation's health.* Sudbury, MA: Jones & Bartlett.

Stasney, S. (2004). *Chic living with feng shui: Stylish designs for harmonious living.* New York, NY: Sterling.

Surveillance for illness and injury after Hurricane Katrina—New Orleans, Louisiana. *Mortality and Morbidity Weekly Report, 54,* 1018–1021.

Tchi, R. (2011). *Feng sjui 2011 tips and updates—Good feng shui in 2011.* Retrieved from http://fengshui.about.com/od/thebasics/p/2007fengshui.htm

VanRooyen, M., & Leaning, J. (2005). After the tsunami: Facing the public health challenges. *New England Journal of Medicine, 353*(5), 435–438.

Ware, C. (2010). Declutter your life: Tossing things we don't need can free up more than closet space. *AARP The Magazine.* Retrieved from http://www.aarp.org/home-garden/housing/info-01-2010/declutter-your-life.html

Waters, T., Collins, J., Galinsky, T. L., Caruso, C. (2006). NIOSH research efforts to prevent musculoskeletal disorders in the healthcare industry. *Orthopaedic Nursing, 25,* 380–389.

"What is particulate matter?" (n.d.). Retrieved from http://www.airinfonow.org/html/ed_particulate.html

Wilder-Smith, A., & Steffen, R. (2005, May 1). Tsunami and the role of the international travel health community. *Journal of Travel Medicine, 12*(3), 117–119.

World Health Organization (WHO). (2004). Radon and health. Retrieved from http:/www.who.int/phe/radiation/en/2004Radon.pdf

World Health Organization (WHO). (2010, April). Deaf and hearing impaired. Retrieved from http://www.who.int/mediacentre/factsheets/fs300/en

BIBLIOGRAPHY

Barrett, J., Coolidge, J., & Steenburger, M. (2003). *Feng shui your life.* New York, NY: Sterling.

Bower, L. M. (2000). *The healthy house : How to buy one, how to build one, how to cure a sick one.* Bloomington, IN: Healthy House Institute.

Gibson, P. R. (2002). *Understanding and accommodating people with multiple chemical sensitivity in independent living.* Houston, TX: UIRU Publications.

Scaief, K. (2004). Womb pollution? *The Environmental Magazine, 15*(6), 12.

World Health Organization (WHO). (2010). *WHO guidelines for indoor air quality: Selected pollutants.* Retrieved from http://www.euro.who.int/en/what-we-publish/abstracts/who-guidelines-for-indoor-air-quality-selected-pollutants

Simonsen, C. E., & Spindlove, J. R. (2009). *Terrorism today: The past, the players, the future.* Upper Saddle River, NJ : Prentice Hall.

CHAPTER 8
The Mind-Body-Spirit Connection

JANICE A. MAVILLE, EdD, MSN, RN

KEY TERMS

coping strategies
crisis
general adaptation syndrome
 (GAS)
holistic medicine
hypnosis
immune modulation

immunoenhancement
mind-body dualism
perceptions
prospective studies
psychoneuroimmunology (PNI)
relaxation techniques
retrospective studies

social support
spirituality
stress
stressor
stress response

OBJECTIVES

Upon completion of this chapter, the reader should be able to:

- Describe how the neural and endocrine systems modulate the immune function.
- List the outcome measurements used to determine changes in immune status.
- List five chemicals involved in the communication among the neural, endocrine, and immune systems.
- Describe how stress impacts the neural, endocrine, and immune systems.
- Discuss research findings on psychoneuroimmunology, stress, and illness.
- Identify normal lifetime stressors, emotional states, and diseases that can negatively impact the immune function.
- Describe at least three nursing interventions useful in promoting immunoenhancement.

INTRODUCTION

Behavioral scientists have long been aware of the impact of the mind on the development of and recovery from certain physical complaints such as headache, pain, and allergies. In fact, the belief in the interrelatedness of psychological states and illness can be traced to ancient times. The health beliefs of American Indians, such as the Navajo, include the need for harmony with nature and an integrated relationship with the earth and sky (Flowers, 2005). The physician Galen, about CE 200, noted that, compared to sanguine women, the more melancholy women had a higher susceptibility to breast cancer; current research supports this ancient connection (Mailoo & Williams, 2004; Douglas, 2007).

In spite of these ancient beliefs, modern medicine has functioned mainly on a Cartesian **mind-body dualism** philosophy. This separateness view of the mind and body, which has existed in medicine at least since the time of Descartes in 1619 (Harrington, 2008), has allowed investigation and treatment to focus on the illness of the body, with only a few diseases being regarded as having a primary cause related to the mind. This view, however, has not been without criticism. Sir William Osler, the father of modern medicine, noted over 100 years ago that the patient's belief and the physician's belief are more important than what the physician actually does (Osler, 1913/2006). Belief in the integration of the mind with the physical body developed into the concept of **holistic medicine**, which uses social, psychological, and spiritual means to bring about wellness. Even though there are many clinical descriptions and cultural beliefs reflecting the mind-body connection, the development of health care standards for practice must be based on rigorous experimental research.

The touting of numerous unproven therapies that were later shown to be ineffective has caused many health care workers to be cautious of all mind-body treatments. During the last decade or two, however, the other half of the dualistic paradigm, the mind, has received more scientific attention and research.

Coming from the more recent research is an expanding body of knowledge about the influence of psychological factors on disease development, severity, and recovery. A model developed by Borysenko and Dveirin (2005) postulates that three factors influence disease susceptibility: genetic predisposition, the environment, and the behavioral or psychological component. In this model, any one of the three components can be the primary cause of disease or the components can interact with one another. So genetics alone may be the cause of the disease, as in hemophilia A; an environmental exposure may interact with a genetic predisposition, as with smoking and emphysema; or a psychological stressor may interact with a genetic predisposition or environmental factor or both. This model fits very well with the belief that disease etiology is multifactorial. In addition, the model explains why some people get diseases and others do not even with apparently the same environmental exposures or the same genetic predisposition or both.

Although the study of the mind-body interrelationship has gone under several names in previous years, this field of study is now being called **psychoneuroimmunology (PNI)**. PNI is concerned with the bidirectional communication between the brain and the immune system. Inherent in PNI is the information about how psychological factors may inhibit or enhance immune function. Psychological factors that suppress the immune system may result in disease. On the positive side, changes in the mind that enhance the immune system may reduce the symptoms of disease even if they do not cure it. Development of the PNI body of knowledge has many implications for nursing practice. It provides the scientific foundation for many current and proposed nursing interventions in the areas of disease prevention, symptom modification, and health promotion. Nurses are responsible for assessing patients' emotional status, perceived stressors, and **coping strategies**, including **social support**.

Through PNI research, nursing will gain the knowledge needed to be able to give more holistic care and to support patients and their families in using effective coping strategies. Nurses can help diminish the negative effects of illness on patients and their families by including biological-psychological-social-spiritual aspects in their care.

SPOTLIGHT ON

Genetics and Disease

Even when research has shown a strong hereditary factor for a disease, such as rheumatoid arthritis, not all siblings with the same gene pool develop the disease. Some individuals inherit only a predisposition to the disorder with the disorder remaining dormant until some noxious stimulus (stress) triggers it. If that is so, then the disorder might be preventable by reducing the stimulus.

ASK YOURSELF

Attitude and Disease

Have you ever noticed that people with a pessimistic attitude about the future seem to have more problems and greater difficulty dealing with an illness than those with a positive attitude? Does the negative attitude affect their perception of the stressors and the coping strategies that they use?

THE PHYSIOLOGICAL BASIS

To understand the research on the mind-body interaction, a basic understanding of key systems is required. The nervous, endocrine, and immune systems can interact with one another in many unexpected ways to influence health.

THE NERVOUS SYSTEM

The nervous system (Figure 8-1) is divided into the central nervous system (CNS) and peripheral nervous system (PNS). These two major sections are further divided, with the CNS being composed of the brain and spinal cord and the PNS

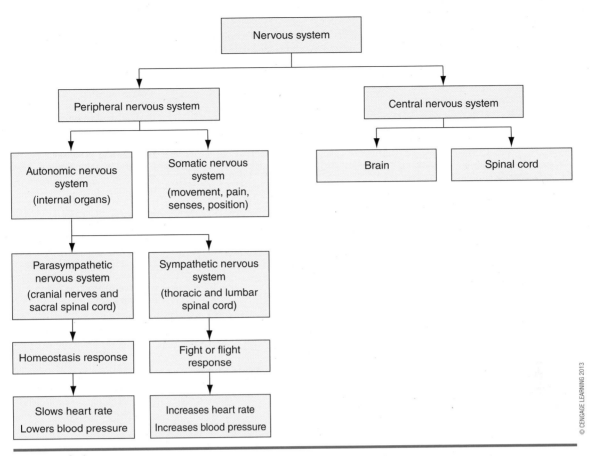

FIGURE 8-1 Divisions of the nervous system.

consisting of the somatic nervous system and the autonomic nervous system (ANS). The somatic nervous system assists in interactions with the environment by controlling body movements and sending sensory messages related to pain, temperature, touch, sense of body position, vision, taste, hearing, and smell. The ANS helps regulate the internal organs through its two branches: sympathetic and parasympathetic nervous systems. The sympathetic branch is connected to the CNS along the thoracic and lumbar regions of the spinal cord. Its main function is to prepare the body for stress through the fight-or-flight response, and it innervates all the major parts of the immune system. The chief messengers of the sympathetic nervous system are the two catecholamines: epinephrine and norepinephrine. The parasympathetic branch is connected through the cranial nerves and the sacral portion of the spinal cord and functions to maintain homeostasis and to prepare the body for functions such as digestion and elimination.

Neurons are the specialized cells of the nervous system that transmit electrical impulses from their dendrite along their axon. These electrical impulses are then sent across the synapses to other neurons or cells of the organ systems by neurotransmitters.

THE NEUROPEPTIDES

Over 100 molecules of amino acid called neuropeptides have been identified that carry messages between the brain, the endocrine system, and the immune system. Neuropeptides, therefore, act as a type of informational connective tissue that unites and coordinates all the cells, tissues, glands, organs, and systems of the body. Their unique ability to modulate chemical

and physical responses in the body has earned them the title "healing molecule" (Glassey, n.d.). Two examples of skin wound healing provide an illustration. One study reported that neuropeptides were found to increase a substance in the skin called activin, which causes pain and thereby protects the skin from further injury (Cruise, Xu, & Hall, 2004). In another study, diminished neuropeptide levels were found to contribute to the impaired skin healing response associated with diabetes mellitus (Gibran et al., 2002).

Although neuropeptides play a major role in effecting responses in cells and tissues, they are generally considered to be mood specific. Components of the limbic system (the seat of the emotions), which include the thalamus, hypothalamus, hippocampus, amygdala, and parts of the basal ganglia, are concentration areas for neuropeptides. The hormone serotonin, which is responsible for our mood and feelings of well-being, is produced in the basal ganglia and projected into the hypothalamus from the brain stem, where it is also produced. The emotions, or feelings, that are produced are the result of a biochemical process between neuropeptides and receptor sites on cell membranes. Feelings are important pieces of information and, like the information received from our sense of smell or touch, allow our bodies to make physiologic changes affecting the status of our health. The location of neuropeptide receptor sites on immune cells leads to the conclusion that they also influence healing.

THE ENDOCRINE SYSTEM

The endocrine system is composed of glands that produce and secrete hormones that help the body maintain and regulate

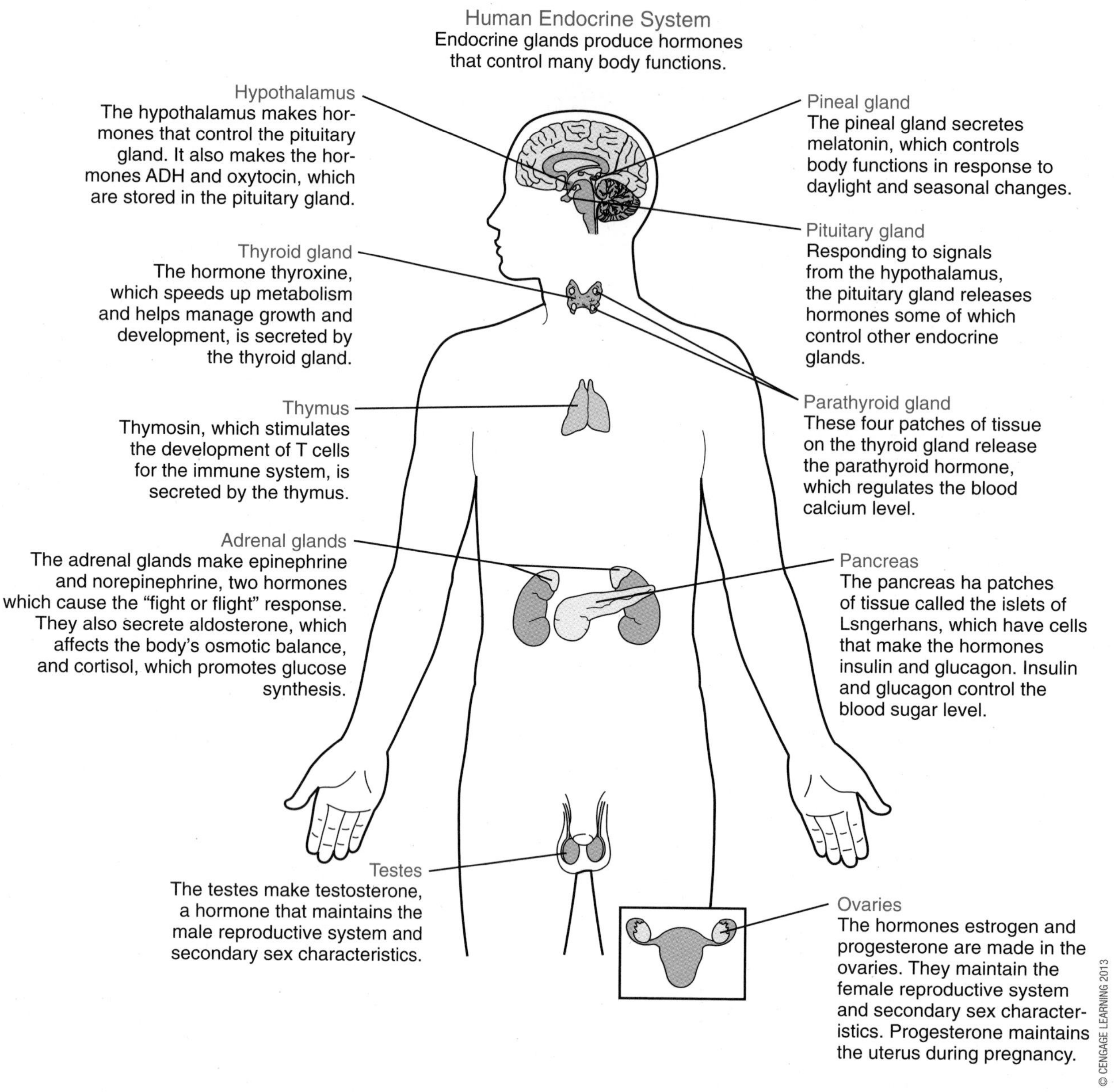

Human Endocrine System
Endocrine glands produce hormones
that control many body functions.

Hypothalamus
The hypothalamus makes hormones that control the pituitary gland. It also makes the hormones ADH and oxytocin, which are stored in the pituitary gland.

Pineal gland
The pineal gland secretes melatonin, which controls body functions in response to daylight and seasonal changes.

Pituitary gland
Responding to signals from the hypothalamus, the pituitary gland releases hormones some of which control other endocrine glands.

Thyroid gland
The hormone thyroxine, which speeds up metabolism and helps manage growth and development, is secreted by the thyroid gland.

Parathyroid gland
These four patches of tissue on the thyroid gland release the parathyroid hormone, which regulates the blood calcium level.

Thymus
Thymosin, which stimulates the development of T cells for the immune system, is secreted by the thymus.

Adrenal glands
The adrenal glands make epinephrine and norepinephrine, two hormones which cause the "fight or flight" response. They also secrete aldosterone, which affects the body's osmotic balance, and cortisol, which promotes glucose synthesis.

Pancreas
The pancreas ha patches of tissue called the islets of Lsngerhans, which have cells that make the hormones insulin and glucagon. Insulin and glucagon control the blood sugar level.

Testes
The testes make testosterone, a hormone that maintains the male reproductive system and secondary sex characteristics.

Ovaries
The hormones estrogen and progesterone are made in the ovaries. They maintain the female reproductive system and secondary sex characteristics. Progesterone maintains the uterus during pregnancy.

© CENGAGE LEARNING 2013

FIGURE 8-2 The endocrine system structure and function.

vital functions. At one time, the endocrine system was thought to consist of the pituitary, gonads, adrenal glands, thyroid, parathyroid, and pancreas. Other organs, however, have been identified as producers of hormones, such as the kidney, liver, gastrointestinal tract, and salivary glands. Chiefly through the hypothalamic-pituitary-adrenal (HPA) axis, the endocrine system assists the body in response to stress, in growth and development, and in reproduction. In addition, the endocrine system maintains the electrolyte and acid-base balance and regulates energy metabolism. Figure 8-2 demonstrates the connection between the endocrine system structure and vital body functions such as growth and reproduction.

In the HPA axis, neurotransmitters such as serotonin, acetylcholine, and norepinephrine regulate the release of corticotropin-releasing factor (CRF) from the hypothalamus.

CRF causes the pituitary to secrete adrenocorticotropin hormone (ACTH) which stimulates the adrenal gland to release glucocorticoids. The level of glucocorticoids in the bloodstream serves as a negative feedback loop to inhibit the release of further CRF. The glucocorticoids have a biphasic effect on the immune system. At low levels, the immune system is activated, with the T lymphocytes being their most aggressive against antigens, and at high levels, like those released in response to stress, the T lymphocytes are damaged or destroyed.

THE IMMUNE SYSTEM

The immune system operates as a surveillance system that is designed to protect the body from foreign substances.

Responses to a foreign substance are either nonspecific or specific. Nonspecific responses result from phagocytosis, which is the body's first line of defense against viruses and bacteria. Phagocytic cells include monocytes and neutrophils, which circulate in the blood, and macrophages located in the tissues. The phagocytic cells engulf the foreign substance and, through the activation of chemicals, destroy it. These chemicals from the phagocytic cell also initiate the inflammatory process.

Specific responses are humoral (involving the B lymphocytes) and cell mediated (involving the T lymphocytes). T lymphocytes and B lymphocytes represent the two broad classes of lymphocytes, and they differ in their function. B lymphocytes, when activated by a pathogen, form plasma cells that produce antibodies or immunoglobulins: IgG, IgM, IgA, IgE, and IgD. Each immunoglobulin is designed to attack the specific pathogen that stimulated its production. The antibodies function by combining with the antigen, activating the complement system, and stimulating phagocytosis, or pathogen cell destruction. The presence of antigens also stimulates the production of anti-idiotypic antibodies that interfere with the production and function of the immunoglobulin and help maintain the balance of the immune system.

T lymphocytes come in a variety of cells. Helper T cells produce lymphokines, which facilitate the production of antibody from the B lymphocytes and produce interleukin-2, which stimulates the production of cytotoxic T cells and suppressor T cells. Cytotoxic T cells directly attack tumor cells and secrete cytokines that regulate other cells of the immune system. Suppressor T cells regulate the immune response by blocking the activation of B lymphocytes. Activation of both B and T lymphocytes produces some memory cells that can be activated rapidly in the future. Memory cells result in a more efficient system with the next exposure and can produce antibodies within 48 to 72 hours of exposure to the specific antigen.

Natural killer (NK) cells, another set of lymphocytes, have the ability to kill tumor cells and cells infected with microbes. In contrast to other lymphocytes, these lymphocytes are a major component of the body's natural immune system and fight tumors and viruses; their activity is inhibited by glucocorticoids and enhanced from other hormones. NK cells do not require prior exposure to the antigen for activation.

The protection of the body against pathogens is facilitated by both fever and sleep. Because of the importance of these two processes, the immune system is capable of initiating these responses. Fever can be produced by the effect of the cytokine interleukin-1 (IL-1) on the anterior hypothalamus. The resultant increase in temperature is lethal to many microorganisms and enhances most aspects of the immune system. In addition, IL-1 induces slow-wave sleep. Growth hormone is produced during this stage of sleep and further augments the immune system.

Laboratory methods used to measure immune response have improved over the years. Early studies have identified abnormalities in peripheral blood smears. Levels of antibody production are used as a measure of whether the first-line defenses have failed or whether a dormant infection has progressed to an active form, as in reactivation of tuberculosis, Epstein-Barr virus, herpes virus, or cytomegalovirus infections. Conversely, high levels of antibody titer following immunization are a reflection of a functioning immune system. Many studies measure lymphocyte activation by stimulating lymphocytes with mitogens. More recently, studies have added NK cell activity

against tumor cells as a quantitative measure of the immune system's responsiveness.

MODULATION BETWEEN THE NEUROENDOCRINE AND IMMUNE SYSTEMS

Through PNI research, various pathways by which the nervous and endocrine systems impact the immune system have been identified. Table 8-1 shows the chemical responses of specific hormones. A physical, emotional, or treatment variable facilitates the enhancement or suppression of immune functioning. This process is called **immune modulation**.

Support for the interaction between the brain and the immune system comes from a variety of studies involving immune modulation. Examples of such studies are those demonstrating that immune responses can be conditioned (Shealy, Norris, & Fahrion, 2002); that stress and low autonomy in workers alters the immune responses and the increases development of the metabolic syndrome—a precursor to heart disease and diabetes (Chandola, Brunner, & Marmot, 2006); and that a correlation exists between depressive symptoms and the immune system (Irwin & Miller, 2007).

There is much evidence showing that innervation of the immune system can arise from glucocorticoids, catecholamines, neuropeptides, and hormones. The neuropeptides are endorphins, substance P, vasoactive intestinal polypeptide (VIP), and neuropeptide Y. Current studies indicate that the hormones may include prolactin and growth hormone (GH). A major communication pathway between the immune system and the brain is through cytokines such as interleukins, interferons, tumor necrosis factors, and growth-stimulating factors. These cytokines act on a number of organ systems to produce the many physiological and behavioral responses to infection such as anorexia, fever, and sleepiness. The actions of these chemicals on the brain, endocrine system, and immune system indicate a much more complex process of bidirectional communication between the systems than was previously thought.

TABLE 8-1 The Chemical Effects of Hormones on the Immune System

HORMONE	CHEMICAL EFFECTS
ACTH	Suppresses T lymphocyte response
	Enhances natural killer (NK) cell activity
Glucocorticoids	Suppresses T lymphocyte response
Norepinephrine	Suppresses T lymphocyte response
	Enhances NK cell activity
Growth hormone	Augments T lymphocyte cell activity
	Augments NK cell cytolytic activity
Thyroxin	May increase NK cell activity

© Cengage Learning 2013

Evidence also exists that the immune system impacts the other bodily systems. The activation of the immune system produces a decrease in norepinephrine that decreases the sympathetic stimulation. The exact mechanism for this effect, however, has not been demonstrated. The hormones secreted by the immune cells include ACTH, endogenous opioids, thyrotropin, VIP, GH, and luteinizing hormone. Leukocytes produce chemicals similar to pituitary hormones that stimulate the neuroendocrine systems. Monocytes secrete IL-1, which can increase ACTH and corticosterone levels.

THE ROLE OF STRESS

Stress is an emotional and physiological response to a stressor. In the 1940s, Hans Selye (1976) recognized the impact of stress on the body. A **stressor** was defined as a factor that places a demand on the body, necessitating an adaptational response. Three phases of the **general adaptation syndrome (GAS)** were noted: alarm reaction, resistance or adaptation phase, and exhaustion phase. The alarm reaction phase is initiated by an event or situation that requires some type of adaptive response by the individual. In response, the pituitary gland and the sympathetic branch of the autonomic nervous system are activated, sending a message to the central nervous system via epinephrine or norepinephrine that elicits the fight-or-flight reaction, otherwise known as the stress response, to the stressor. The resistance or adaptation phase is a coping mode whereby the body allows itself to return to a more normal state of functioning. Exhaustion occurs when the individual is exposed to long-term stress or stressors without adaptation.

GAS theory includes the impact of modulators such as social support and coping ability. Outcomes of the stress could be psychological growth, no change, or an adverse health change. Selye's work identified the subjectivity of stress with the individualized reactions of different people and different reactions at different times in the same person. However, the responses to similar stressors shared many common features. These features, called the **stress response** and sometimes the fight-or-flight response, formed a set of physical changes that the human body makes in response to a stressor or threat. The immediate and prolonged effects of the stress response on selected body organs are identified in Table 8-2. Documented physiological responses to stress are the activation of the sympathetic nervous system, causing increased circulating catecholamines, and the stimulation of the HPA system with increased secretion of glucocorticoids and endorphins.

The chemicals released in response to stress have numerous effects on the immune system. T lymphocyte response is reduced by ACTH, glucocorticoids, epinephrine, and norepinephrine. These hormones are released into the bloodstream, making their way to the various target cells throughout the body. Varying changes occur in the NK cell. Growth hormone, which enhances both T lymphocyte and NK cell activity, may either increase or decrease in response to stress. In addition, neurohormones diminish the function of macrophages against tumor cells.

Factors that have been documented through research as impacting the individual's response to stressors are genetics, **perceptions**, environmental factors including socioecomonic status, and the type of stressor (McEwen & Gianaros, 2010). The genetic factors are predisposition to disease, gender, and prior exposure with its physiological conditioning. A person's positive or negative perception about the stressor influences the impact on the body. Often, if a person views a stressor as negative, then any positive aspects of the stressor are totally ignored (Segerstrom, 2010). Coping strategies are part of the perception factor and allow individuals to be trained to deal with stressors and to overcome the negative perceptions. Environmental stressors have been shown to alter the immune status. Some of these factors are trauma, irradiation, malnutrition, drug and alcohol usage, temperature, and aging.

GLOBAL HIGHLIGHTS IN HEALTH PROMOTION

Prolonged Stress and Victims of Natural Disaster

Disasters have occurred with alarming frequency in countries around the world. On average, for example, 17 major earthquakes of a magnitude 7.0–7.9 and 1 earthquake of magnitude 8.0 or above occur around the world each year.

The victims of natural disasters, such as those surviving devastating earthquakes, hurricanes, tornadoes, tsunamis, fires, and floods, face stressors that begin as short-term challenges that, for many, evolve into long-term, life-altering conditions. Research across the countries affected by the 2004 Sri Lanka earthquake and tsunami found high levels of posttraumatic stress disorder (PTSD) 15 months afterward; the loss of work and income were related to mental health symptoms, especially among females. In Thailand, the relatives of tsunami victims who were never found worried that the spirits of their family members were not at rest. After an explosion at a fireworks storage depot in the Netherlands, it was found that at least 30% of those affected experienced serious physical and mental health problems. Research on victims of Hurricane Katrina, which devastated the United States Gulf Coast in 2005, revealed a high rate of hurricane-related mental health problems, including PTSD, in the residents of the affected area two years following the event. The extent of the long-term effects on the earthquake victims of the 2010 Japanese earthquake are yet to be discovered.

The types of disasters share many common effects, but each disaster is unique, with varying effects on survivors. Continuing aftershocks following an earthquake, displacement, loss of income or employment, life threat, or cultural beliefs are but a few of the factors that can contribute to mental and physical health problems in disaster survivors all over the world. Nurse responders, whether providing care for such victims immediately or much later, need to be aware that any or all of the categories of stress identified in Table 8-3 could be apparent.

Source: National Center for PTSD, Department of Veterans Affairs (2010). Traumatic effects of certain types of disasters. Retrieved from www.ptsd.va.gov/PTSD/professional/pages/traumatic-effects-disasters.asp;

TABLE 8-2 Immediate and Prolonged Effects of the Stress Response on Selected Body Organs, Systems, and Tissues

BODY ORGAN, SYSTEM, OR TISSUE	RESPONSE TO STRESS	IMMEDIATE RESPONSE/ BENEFICIAL EFFECT	PROLONGED RESPONSE/ADVERSE EFFECT
Eyes	Pupils dilate	Greater acuity to see danger and escape routes	Unknown
Brain	Increased blood flow, increased metabolism of glucose	Greater focus and increased thought processes	"Thought" fatigue
Cardiovascular system	Increased heart rate and force of contractions	Increased cardiac output for more blood supply to muscles	Vasospasm leading to stroke or infarction
Pulmonary system	Increased respiratory rate and dilation of bronchi	Increased oxygen supply for energy	Fatigue; carbon dioxide retention and respiratory acidosis
Liver	Increased glucose production; increased gluconeogenesis; decreased glycogen synthesis	Increased energy	Depletion of energy reserve
Muscles	Increased breakdown of glycogen to glucose (gluconeogenesis) and increased muscle tension	Immediate energy	Nervous behavior, irritability, and discomfort
Fat tissue	Increased breakdown of stored fat (lipolysis); more fatty acids in the bloodstream	Immediate energy	Increased risk for heart disease and stroke
Stomach	Increased acidity and decreased motility	Conserves energy for use by muscles and brain	Discomfort, nausea, ulceration
Salivary glands	Decreased flow of saliva	Conserves energy	Thickened or lack of saliva, dry mouth, "cotton mouth"
Pancreas	Increased glucose production	Immediate energy	Stress-induced diabetes
Excretory system	Neuron stimulation of the bladder	Reduced urine flow and intestinal motility	Urge to urinate in spite of the fact that urine flow is reduced; possible constipation followed by diarrhea
Lymph tissue	Increased release of T cells and natural killer cells	Heightened immune function	Reserve depletion; decreased immune function
Skin	Decreased blood flow	Conserves blood supply for use by muscles and brain	Cold hands/feet
Sweat glands	Increased sympathetic nervous system response	Temperature regulation	Excessive sweating; blood plasma volume depletion; decreased blood pressure; weakness; fainting

Source: Based on McCance, K. L., & Huether, S. E. (2010). *Pathophysiology: The biologic basis for disease in adults and children* (6th ed.). St. Louis, MO: Mosby-Elsevier.

TABLE 8-3 Categories of Stressors

STRESSOR	EXAMPLES
1. Acute time-limited stressor	Public speaking, mental arithmetic
2. Brief naturalistic stressor	Academic exams, real-life short-term challenges
3. Stressful event sequences	Loss of a loved one, major natural disaster
4. Chronic stressors	Debilitating health condition, caregiver, refugee
5. Distant past stressors	Sexual assault in younger years, witness to traumatic event, prisoner of war

Source: Based on Segerstrom, S. C., & Miller, G. E. (2004). psychological stress and the human immune system: A meta-analytical study of 30 years of inquiry. *Psychological Bulletin, 130*(4), 601–630.

The impact of the stressor is also influenced by its severity, by timing (chronic, repetitive, or acute), by its escapability, and by its controllability. Stressful experiences can be both helpful and harmful to the body and brain. As seen in the Research Note, short-term, acute stressful experiences can enhance adaptive changes in physiology and behavior that help to meet the challenges of environmental, social, or medically invasive events and protect against threats to internal homeostasis. Long-term stress, however, can lead to maladaptive changes in physiology and behavior that adversely affect health, cognition, mood, and longevity (Gianaros et al., 2007)

Five categories of stressors, as shown in Table 8-3, have been identified and are distinguished according to duration and course (Segerstrom & Miller, 2004). (See also Figure 8-3.)

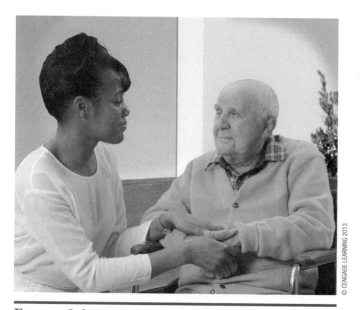

FIGURE 8-3 Clasping the client's hand is one way to communicate through touch. What messages do you think are communicated by the nurse to the client in this situation?

RESEARCH NOTE

Fight or Flight Stress Response and Recovery from Surgery

STUDY PROBLEM/PURPOSE

Each year, 1.3 million Americans undergo knee surgery, and how quickly they recover depends on many factors, including their age, the severity and location of the injury, and preexisting conditions, such as arthritis. Having knee surgery induces a short-term, fight-or-flight physiological stress response. Knowing that immune response at the site of surgery enhances tissue repair, researchers were curious as to how well the surgical stress-induced immune cell redistribution profiles from blood samples served as predictors and potential mediators of short- and long-term postoperative recovery from knee surgery.

METHODS

This prospective longitudinal study involved 57 patients undergoing meniscectomy knee surgery. Blood tests for levels of lymphocytes, monocytes, and neutrophils were taken on three occasions: several days prior to the surgery to establish a baseline count; the morning of surgery prior to patients' being anesthetized to assess for an effect from anxiety; and then 30 minutes after surgery based on prior knowledge that blood-borne immune cells exit the circulation and enter tissues at the site of surgery for healing to begin.

Using the clinically validated Lysholm scale, mechanical function, pain, mobility, and the ability to perform daily activities were used to assess knee function preoperatively and at 1, 3, 8, 16, 24, and 48 weeks postoperatively.

FINDINGS

It was found that patients whose immune systems responded to the stress of surgery with increased numbers of lymphocytes, monocytes, and neutrophils recovered more quickly and completely than patients whose immune cell count before surgery was unresponsive during the short-term stress. Another interesting finding was that women were less likely than men to respond with an adaptive stress response, leading to a delayed recovery time of 48 weeks compared to 16 weeks for men. It was concluded that immune cell redistribution induced by the stress of undergoing surgery can predict postoperative healing and recovery and may even be a mediator in the recovery process.

IMPLICATIONS

These findings could be used in predicting which patients could benefit from pharmacologic and behavioral interventions that would enhance their immediate and long-term recovery from surgery. The results of this

© CENGAGE LEARNING 2013

study suggest that the activation of fight-or-flight stress responses might enhance immune system protection in other situations and conditions.

Source: Rosenberger, P. H., Ickovics, J. R., Epel, E., Nadler, E., Jokl, P., Fulkerson, J. P., Tillie, J. M., & Dhabhar, F. S. (2009). Surgical stress-induced immune cell redistribution profiles predict short-term and long-term postsurgical recovery: A prospective study. *Journal of Bone & Joint Surgery, 9,* :2783–2794. DOI:10.2106/JBJS.H.00989.

BOX 8-1
PNI RESEARCH FOCUS AREAS

The effect of negative stressors
The effect of stress on diseases
The effect of various stress management techniques

PSYCHONEUROIMMUNOLOGY RESEARCH

The PNI literature includes much animal and human research. In the field of PNI, it is more difficult and sometimes unethical to conduct the needed, tightly controlled, prospective studies on humans. **Prospective studies** are research studies that follow subjects without the disease (or outcome of interest) forward in time. Animal subjects are followed for enough person-years to establish incidence, morbidity, or mortality rates. Therefore, there is currently much more animal than human research. Stress in animals has been induced through such measures as overcrowding, noise, and electric shock. In general, the results of these studies have shown decreased immune function with increased susceptibility to cancer and infectious diseases. The evidence validating a direct relationship between environmental stress and the development of cancer in rodents is inconclusive. Research in mice has indicated, however, that stress can affect tumor growth and spread, but the exact biological mechanisms underlying these effects are not well understood (Thaker et al., 2006). The major problem with these studies is the unknown generalizability of the results to humans.

Much of the research on humans is done using **retrospective studies** after the stressor or disease has occurred, preventing the researcher from controlling or manipulating the stressor. As highlighted in Box 8-1, human research in PNI has three areas of focus: (1) the effect of negative stressors such as examinations, bereavement, childbirth, depression, loneliness, and hopelessness; (2) the effect of stress on diseases such as tuberculosis, rheumatoid arthritis, acquired immunodeficiency syndrome (AIDS), and herpes virus; and (3) the effect of various stress management techniques on **immunoenhancement**, such as social support, **relaxation techniques**, biofeedback, and **hypnosis**. Because of the volume of research studies, only samples of the studies will be presented to illustrate the mind-body connection related to each of the three areas of PNI research. Chapter 19 provides a more in-depth discussion on various stress management techniques.

THE EFFECT OF NEGATIVE LIFE STRESSORS

Psychoneuroimmunology research has evaluated the changes in the immune function that occur with normal lifetime stressors such as academic examinations, bereavement over the loss of a significant other, and childbirth. In addition, the effects of various emotional states like depression, loneliness, and hopelessness, and various types of stress like controllable and predictable stress have been evaluated.

EXAMINATION STRESS

Stress is an emotional and physiological response to a stressor that triggers the sympathetic division of the autonomic nervous and endocrine systems into preparation for change or adaptation. For students, an impending examination could be identified as a stressor invoking emotional and physiological changes that could be described as examination stress. Research has documented the various emotional and immunological effects associated with students in academia. For example, one recent study found that college students have increased circulating monocytes, decreased CD4 and CD8 cells, and higher cortisol levels on exam days, as well as increased antibody titers to latent viruses such as herpes simplex, Epstein-Barr virus, and cytomegalovirus (Segerstrom & Miller, 2004). Lower levels of T cells and higher self-reported incidences of health problems such as upper respiratory infections also have been found among students during exam times (Höglund et al., 2006).

Research studies such as this one are significant in psychoneuroimmunology. However, inherent in such research is the possibility of confounding factors that cannot be eliminated from influencing the subjects' health. As an example, researchers studying college freshmen found that a lack of social support is a risk factor for depression in college students that is compounded by social isolation and feelings of loneliness resulting in weakened immunity (Pressman, Cohen, Miller,

SPOTLIGHT **ON**

Perceptions Alter Stress

Our everyday lives are often filled with stressors, and many of these we believe are beyond our control. Projects or assignments may have been put off because of previous difficulties with similar tasks. As the due date for the project approaches, the stress level increases. Some of the problem may be in our thinking that we have to approach the task in the same manner that it was done the last time. Opening up our minds to other alternatives—changing our perceptions—gives us more control over the stressor. Perhaps it would be better to start writing a paper on a section that is known well rather than beginning with the introduction, or perhaps to make a game out of a nasty household chore. Without such measures, we could be increasing our own stress through our own negative perceptions.

Barkin, Rabin, & Treanor, 2005). Nonetheless, regardless of its source, a clear connection is evident among stress, decreased immunity, and higher risk for alterations in the health of college students.

The examination stress model provides for understanding individual responses to other brief naturalistic stressors that result in stress. For example, preparing for a speech or presentation to a group or organization may produce pressures similar to students' feelings of stress and anxiety as they prepare for exams.

ASK **YOURSELF**

Stress and Disease

Have you or any of your friends ever gotten sick during or immediately after a highly stressful time such as when a major paper was due or around final examinations? Did the stressful situation precipitate the illness or perhaps increase the severity of the illness?

Many instruments have been developed to assess stress. One in particular was developed especially to measure students' stress. It is the Hassles Assessment Scale for Students in College (HASS/COL) developed by Sarafino and Ewing (1999). The original scale listed 54 hassles, later revised to 57, with each to be rated according to frequency and unpleasantness in the past month and the degree to which it was dwelt upon (Pitt, 2005). Using valid instruments such as this one is important for college counselors and health professionals when determining interventions for stress reduction. Helping students manage stress early on may influence how they deal with stressful events in their adult lives. Box 8-2 offers some helpful tips to ease mental stress.

BOX 8-2

TIPS TO EASE MENTAL STRESS

- Take time out regularly, ideally outdoors, to improve circulation and the delivery of nutrients and oxygen to the brain.
- Breathe. Deep breathing increases oxygen delivery to the brain.
- Keep away from stimulants. Avoid relying on stimulants such as caffeine, cigarettes, and drugs.
- Drink plenty of water (6–8 glasses a day). Dehydration negatively affects brain function.
- Eat healthy small meals regularly. This stabilizes blood sugar (glucose) levels, which is fuel for the brain.
- Use social support. Communicate with family members and friends who can be supportive.

BEREAVEMENT

Bereavement is an indeterminate time of grieving the loss of a loved one, most likely through death, but it can also accompany the separation or the severance of a relationship. Bereavement is a highly stressful event related to a variety of physical problems, including physical exhaustion, sleep disturbance, heart palpitations, shortness of breath, headaches, recurrent infections, high blood pressure, changes in weight and eating patterns, stomach upsets, hair loss, disruption of the menstrual cycle, irritability, worsening of any chronic condition such as diabetes or eczema, and susceptibility to opportunistic infections such as influenza.

The death of a spouse has been rated as the most stressful life event across all ages and cultural backgrounds (Holmes & Rahe, 1967). Research continues to support the stressful effect of widowhood and the death rates of surviving spouses (Boyle, Feng, & Raab, 2011). The loss of a loved one activates the stress response mechanism of the autonomic nervous system and immune system. Much research on bereavement and immune function, focused mainly on the elderly, has documented that individuals undergoing bereavement show reduced indicators of immune function, including suppression of lymphocyte stimulation, reduction of NK cell activity, T cell suppression, increased plasma cortisol levels, and altered response to antibody production (Segerstrom & Miller, 2004; Phillips, Carroll, Burns, Ring, Macleod, & Drayson, 2006).

Preexisting or chronic conditions often become worse, explaining, in part, why people are at higher risk of dying during the first year after the loss of a loved one. Several studies related to the mortality risk of the surviving spouse noted that survivors were at increased risk of death from any cause with an even greater risk for men (Boyle, Feng, & Raab, 2011). The length of time in providing care for a dying spouse has been found to have a beneficial effect on the surviving spouse, with longer periods of caregiving related to lower depressive symptoms (Keene & Prokos, 2008). A study on caregivers found that those with few symptoms of depression before bereavement tended to maintain these states afterward, but emotionally distressed caregivers tended to become more distressed, indicating that self-esteem and socioemotional support play protective roles (Vitaliano & Katon, 2006).

Researchers have identified the existence of an immune system pathway that links caregiver stress to serious health problems (Vitaliano & Katon, (2006). It has been reported that spousal caregivers have higher levels of interleukin-6 (IL-6), a compound that circulates in the blood and helps regulate the immune system. Excess IL-6 contributes to muscle atrophy and several diseases of aging. It also promotes the production of CReactive protein (CRP), a risk factor for cardiovascular disease. Both IL-6 and CRP are implicated in Type 2 diabetes, osteoporosis, and arthritis. The IL-6 and CRP effects continued in caregivers for several years after the spouse had died, suggesting that chronic stress may have a lasting impact on the immune system. The unhealthy habits that people develop in response to stress, such as smoking, overeating, sleeping too little, and not exercising, are also linked to higher IL-6 levels.

CHRONIC STRESS

Stress is useful to promote the adaptation of our bodies to events and conditions. Prolonged stress, however, results in

SPOTLIGHT **ON**

Patients' Expectations of Disease Outcomes

Negative expectations about the potential outcome of a disease have been found to have an impact on the actual outcome. Therefore, when taking a health history, include the patient's explanation of the problem, ideas on care that will help, and expectations about prognosis. This information could be used in providing more individualized care.

BOX 8-3
SOURCES OF CHRONIC STRESS

Anger	Electromagnetic fields
Fear	Radiation
Worry	Geophysical stressors
Anxiety	Malabsorption
Depression	Low blood sugar
Guilt	Poor diet
Overwork	Nutritional deficiencies
Excessive exercise	Food allergies
Sleep deprivation	Inhalant allergies
Lifecycle disruption	Noise pollution
Late hours	Poor digestion
Surgery	Traumas (mental, emotional, physical)
Gluten intolerance	Cortisol imbalance
Injury	Adult attention deficit disorder (AADD)
Whiplash	
Inflammation	Seasonal affective disorder (SAD)
Pain	
Temperature extremes	Electromagnetic sensitivity (from extensive computer use)
Toxic chemical exposures	
	Toxic personal relationships
Infections (chronic/ acute)	Perfectionism
Heavy metals	

Sources: Garrish, M. (2005). Stress: The mind-body connection. WebMed Live Events Transcript (October 6, 2005); Sergerstrom, S. C. (2010). Stress, energy, and immunity. *Annals of Behavioral Medicine, 40*(1), 114–125; Scott, E. (2010). Stress and metabolic syndrome: Chronic job stress is a risk factor for heart disease. About.com Stress Management, retrieved from stress.about.com/od/stresshealth/a/jobstress.htm

---

wear and tear on the body. Box 8-3 lists many of the sources of chronic stress. The chronic activation of cortisol and adrenaline, the body's response to stress, overactivates the body's fight-or-flight response, possibly can produce unhealthy physiological outcomes. Some of the results of chronic stress include the following:

- Aging.
- Hypertension.
- Diabetes.
- Atherosclerosis.
- Obesity.
- Immune suppression.
- Osteoporosis.
- Muscle atrophy.
- Brain atrophy.
- Depression.
- Skin disorders.
- Cardiovascular disease (Thoma, 2011; Robles, Glaser, & Kiecolt-Glaser, 2005).

CRISIS

Any stressful event has the potential to become overwhelming, resulting in crisis. A **crisis** is a situation of severe disorganization resulting when an individual's coping mechanisms are not effective, or when usual resources are lacking, or when a combination of both occurs (Schwecke, 2007). Crises are not limited to individuals' they can occur within families, groups, and communities. This discussion focuses on crisis in the individual patient but is applicable to families, groups, and communities.

Many patients seen by nurses are in some form of crisis. Crises may arise from events ranging from relatively minor ones, such as being late for an appointment or stuck in traffic, to major ones, such as the death of a loved one. The stressor or event is not the crisis; the crisis is the resulting lack of effective coping skills. The ineffective ability to cope results in a state of distress often leading to panic. What results in crisis for one person may not have the same effect on another. The effects of crisis may be physical, psychological, cognitive, or relational distress. A person in crisis may become physically ill

with nausea or vomiting, adopt dysfunctional coping patterns such as taking drugs, have irrational thoughts or ideas including suicide, or lose the ability to relate to others.

Crises are affected by culture, both that of the person or group experiencing the crisis and that of those intervening. Culture influences how situations are perceived and how they are responded to; perceptions and reactions vary according to how individuals and communities view and appraise their own responses (Dykeman, 2005). Understanding the cultural context of the crisis is paramount to its resolution.

It is important to note that crises create an opportunity for growth and development as well as for negative outcomes. Once individuals learn how to cope with crisis situations they gain stability and self-confidence from learning new ways to cope or from garnering new resources (Schwecke, 2007). Research to support a crisis theory might establish a cause-effect relationship.

Crisis intervention requires immediate attention. It is a type of emotional first-aid (Rosenbluh, 2002). Basic intervention strategies for individuals or groups experiencing crisis are addressed in Box 8-4.

THE EFFECT OF STRESS ON DISEASE

Extensive research literature has shown a relationship between psychosocial stress and immune dysfunction in autoimmune diseases. Many other diseases have been studied with implications of similar psychological reactions, including the common cold, malignant melanoma, asthma, AIDS, and hypertension. However, there is still much variability in the individual's response to stress and perception of what is stressful. Additional factors considered in the stress reaction that may alter the response of an individual's immune function are personality and emotions, vulnerability, and perceptions of the stressful event, among others (Segerstrom & Miller, 2004). The effect of stress on disease has been extensively documented in the literature; therefore, examples related to depression, psychocutaneous disease, and cancer have been selected for a brief discussion in the following sections.

NURSING ALERT

Destressing after Crisis Intervention

Helping a patient through a crisis situation can be stressful on the nurse. The nurse must be able to relieve personal tension through a debriefing with a trusted colleague or other professional and to practice a relaxation technique of choice, even if only for a few minutes.

DEPRESSION FACTORS

Patients with depression have been evaluated for response to mitogens and NK cell activity, which indicate decreased immune function. Depression frequently exists with other disease conditions. It is a potential risk factor for poor health and even death among individuals with numerous medical conditions, such as heart disease and AIDS. There is strong evidence that depression is an independent risk factor for patients with congestive heart failure and coronary artery disease. There is no research, however, showing that treating depression, either with therapy or antidepressant drugs, makes a difference in heart disease prognosis (European Society of Cardiology, 2008).

The impact of depression on AIDS has been the focus of many studies. One study found that improvements in the diagnostic status of major depression were related to increases in NK cell activity among HIV-seropositive women (Cruess et al., 2005). Another study positively correlated depressive symptoms with viral load in patients with HIV infection (Lampe et al., 2010).

Because of its effect on disrupting the anti-inflammatory process of the immune system, depression can influence several conditions associated with aging, including cardiovascular disease, osteoporosis, arthritis, Type 2 diabetes, certain cancers, periodontal disease, frailty and functional decline, prolonged infection, and delayed wound healing (Haddad, 2010; Shen et al., 2010; Christian et al., 2007).

ASK YOURSELF

Relaxation Techniques and Disease

Relaxation techniques have been shown to help treat existing psoriasis. What other conditions might be helped in this manner? Could these relaxation techniques be used in genetically predisposed individuals to prevent disease?

PSYCHOCUTANEOUS DISEASE

For many decades, psychological factors, including stress, have been implicated in the development and exacerbation of many skin disorders. Even some skin diseases have been noted to occur in certain personality types. However, because of the retrospective nature of such research, it is unclear whether the psychological factors or the skin changes occur first. Some researchers have hypothesized that the emotional stressors occur first, reducing the time the person has to tend to the skin disease, and the result is an exacerbation of the disease.

Most clinicians and researchers agree that stress affects the course of dermatologic conditions such as psoriasis. Treating the condition should therefore include therapies aimed at reducing psychophysiological stress. Biofeedback training, psychotherapy, and hypnosis are examples of adjuncts to traditional medical treatment that can reduce stress levels and that have been shown to have a positive effect on the course of psoriasis.

Many individuals with psoriasis use complementary and alternative modalities (CAM) as an adjunct to conventional treatment. One study found that as many as 62% of psoriasis patients used CAM (Ben-Arye et al., 2003). The National Psoriasis Foundation (2011) endorses the supplemental use of practices that promote relaxation and stress reduction to manage stress and to gain a sense of control over the disease, including massage, meditation, yoga, aromatherapy, guided imagery, progressive relaxation, tai chi, and reflexology.

CANCER

The relationship between stress and cancer has been demonstrated in animal studies with highly stressed mice having a higher incidence of cancer and faster growing tumors. In human studies, controlling individual patient variables and the type of stress is more difficult. Therefore, the results have been less consistent in humans.

The National Cancer Institute (NCI, n.d.) recognizes that, although studies have shown that stress factors (such as the death of a spouse, social isolation, and medical school examinations) alter immune system functions, they have not provided definitive evidence of a direct cause-effect relationship between these immune system changes and the development of cancer. The NCI (n.d.) recommends more research to find whether there is a relationship between psychological stress and the transformation of normal cells into cancerous ones.

> ### ? ASK **YOURSELF**
>
> #### Use of Distraction
>
> Getting involved with enjoyable activities has been found to be effective in relieving the negative symptoms of illness. Have you ever had a bad headache or pain from an injury that you "forgot about" while doing other fun activities?

For the past four decades, researchers have been evaluating the cancer personality. However, most of these studies have been retrospective with information about the prior personality based on the cancer patient's recall. The major weakness in these designs is that patients' current emotional states may be altering their perceptions of prior functioning. In addition, cancer has long latency periods during which the biological changes from the tumor could have been altering the patient's emotional state long before the cancer was detected or diagnosed. Therefore, the best study design is a long-term prospective approach following healthy subjects.

However, some studies have provided meaningful information regarding psychological factors reflecting the perceptions and life events of individuals with cancer. One such study examined the perceived threat to life of the stage of cancer (stages are 1 to 4, with 1 being a small tumor with no lymph node involvement and 4 being cancer spread to other organs). The researchers found that, more than the stage of the cancer, the perception of the threat to life was significantly related to psychological distress and quality of life (Laubmeier & Zakowski, 2004). In another study, stressful life events, perceptions of global stress, and perceptions of cancer-related traumatic stress were studied in women with breast cancer (Golden-Kreutz & Andersen, 2004). The researchers found that each of these variables increased the risk for depressive symptoms and recommended the assessment of multiple sources of stress in order to promote health and well-being.

SPIRITUALITY AND PSYCHONEUROIMMUNOLOGY

Spirituality is often confused as being synonymous with religion. Simply put and in a broader perspective, **spirituality** encompasses a belief in a universal power greater than oneself, a sense of interconnectedness with all living creatures, and promotes feelings of hope, comfort, and peace. The subjects of faith or spirituality and of health and healing has become of great interest to researchers of complementary or alternative medicine (CAM) practice. In fact, the National Center for Complementary and Alternative Medicine (NCCAM) was created by the National Institutes of Health (NIH) to use rigorous research in CAM practices, to train CAM researchers, and to provide authoritative information to the public and professionals (NCCAM, 2005).

The NCCAM sponsored a large and comprehensive survey on Americans' use of complementary and alternative medicine. Surveying more than 31,000 adults, this study found that within the preceding 12 months of the survey, 36% of those surveyed had used CAM, exclusive of prayer as part of the definition; when prayer was included in the definition of CAM, 62% had used CAM (Barnes et al., 2004). Among all complementary methods used (massage, chiropractic, yoga, etc.), praying for health was the method used most often. A subsequent survey showed an even greater use of CAM, with 38.3% of adults over age 18 and 11.8% of children under age 17 reporting use of some form of CAM (Barnes, Bloom, & Nahin, 2008). The latter survey, however, did not include prayer, specifically noting that many CAM methods incorporate spirituality

A growing body of research supports the possibility that spirituality affects physical health via the neuroendocrine and immune mechanisms (Koenig & Cohen, 2002; Koenig, 2008; Boerner, 2009). Studies have credited spirituality with lowering blood pressure, lowering mortality rates from heart disease, reducing stress, increasing the sense of well-being, prolonging life, and reducing costs through shorter hospital stays (Etnyer et al., 2005; Koenig & Cohen, 2002; NCCAM, 2005). Such research is problematic in that there is lack of consensus on how to quantify spirituality or spiritual well-being in order for rigorous research to occur (Burkhardt & Nagai-Jacobson, 2005). In general, researchers are consistent on two points: (1) Religiosity/spirituality is linked to health-related physiological processes, including cardiovascular, neuroendocrine, and immune function. (2) More solid evidence is needed. Nonetheless, recognizing the importance of spirituality in the lives of patients is important because nurses provide holistic care. Understanding the relevance of spirituality for both the nurse and the patient enhances the compassion that is fundamental to the practice of nursing.

A recent review of literature from North America and Europe summarized that, in the last two decades, there has been a positive association between spirituality and health care outcomes but that the integration and implementation of spirituality in nursing practice has not kept pace. This failure to keep pace is associated with a lack of a shared understanding of spirituality, the insufficient emphasis on spirituality in nursing education, attitudes, organizational and cultural factors, and individuality (Tiew & Creedy, 2010).

CONTROVERSIES RELATED TO PNI RESEARCH

Even given the volumes of PNI research, the findings are still considered controversial. In general, the issues concerning the studies are related to the use of animals for study, the retrospective nature of human studies, the multifactorial nature of stress and illness, and measurement problems. This is all in addition to the problem with interpreting animal and retrospective studies.

Multiple factors are related to stress and contribute to illness, making it difficult to pull out one factor for study. The multifactorial aspects include the many different types of stress, different perceptions about the stressor, different genetic predispositions, and different coping strategies. Added to these are different psychological functioning, age, nutritional status, sleep patterns, physical activity, use of alcohol or medications, and menstrual phases. With all these factors involved, the sample sizes need to be much larger to be able to statistically evaluate the variables.

Measurement has been a problem in relation to immune function, stress, and symptomology of disease. The use of only one measurement of immune function has been known to miss important existing relationships. The use of peripheral blood for samples may be inaccurate because cortisol may result in changes in the migration of the peripheral cells. Also, stress and personality variables have been included in some instruments to assess disease. This is especially true of diseases that are thought to have a psychological factor and diseases that have fatigue and pain as symptoms, such as AIDS, chronic fatigue syndrome, and cancer.

NURSING IMPLICATIONS

Even Florence Nightingale recognized the importance of nursing's role in producing a state of body and mind that is conducive to healing (Hood & Leddy, 2009). Nightingale noted that healing could be promoted by paying attention to promoting comfort, hygiene, nutrition, and sleep. Recommended changes in the environment that were important in promoting adequate sleep were to reduce noise and patient anxiety. The current PNI research gives further support to these beliefs of Nightingale and encourages further endeavors to reduce the negative effects of stress.

It is important for nurses to assess the patient's level of stress, type of stress, sources of stress, perception of the stress, and effectiveness of coping strategies. Attention must be directed toward assisting the patient in modulating the stress through measures like increasing social support, maintaining open communication in expressing emotions, using humor, and regaining control.

Many times when ill, people lose control over their environment. Regaining control, even if only in a limited way, can help ameliorate the stress. Patients need to be allowed to participate in their own care and to decide which parts they want control over, even if they are able to control only a small fraction of the care. For hospitalized patients who have been removed from their familiar home environment, nurses can still allow choices in the daily schedule, type of food within limits, type of music in the room, and the timing and amount of visiting hours for family.

Patient undergoing stressful situations can be offered complementary and alternative stress reduction therapies. Such alternative methods should not be used to replace the standard medical treatments, but they can be used to reduce anxiety and depression and to ameliorate the negative effects of stress. Interventions that can be tried include the following:

- Relaxation techniques, including progressive muscular relaxation, meditation, and yoga
- Selective awareness, including hypnosis and guided imagery
- Biofeedback
- Cognitive distraction involving hobbies or video games
- Movement, including exercise and dance
- Humor
- Prayer

Because the responses to these therapies vary with individuals, nurses should be able to guide patients in selecting an appropriate therapy or therapies. Further information about these interventions and how to use them is presented in Chapter 19.

HEALTH PROMOTION THEORY LINK

Jean Watson's Theory of Human Caring/Caring Science

Caring is the core of nursing. Practicing nursing with the art of caring has been compromised by multiple factors in health care delivery, such as challenges in working with high levels of technology, increasingly complex patient acuity, and greater demands from the public and employers. Watson's Theory of Human Caring is founded on the idea that love and care have therapeutic properties and that they can become major healing forces. In her theory, Watson embraces the mind-body-spirit connection through a transpersonal caring relationship with patients that includes so-called heart-centered/healing caring, based on practicing and honoring the wholeness of mind-body-spirit in the self and others. Many nurses, hospitals, and nursing schools have adopted Watson's Theory of Human Caring/Caring Science as their framework for nursing practice.

Source: Watson, J. (2008). *Nursing: The philosophy and science of caring* (rev. ed.), Boulder: University Press of Colorado.

SUMMARY

The nervous, immune, and endocrine systems are in constant biochemical communication using their chemical signals. These same chemical signals can also affect individual behavior and the response to stress. The disruption of this communication network in any way by factors related to the environment, existence of multiple diseases, or psychological state can exacerbate the infectious, inflammatory, autoimmune, and mood diseases that these systems guard against.

Health care professionals can no longer ignore current research in the field of psychoneuroimmunology associating the impact of the mind, the emotions, or the spirit on the health or well-being of the body or on the disease and healing processes. Even though the studies do not always have consistent results, there is enough evidence to support the use of complementary and alternative therapies by health care providers to reduce the negative effects of stress and to promote the health of the body and mind.

Nursing theorists such as Florence Nightingale (Environmental Theory of Nursing), Martha Rogers (Science of Unitary Human Beings), Madeleine Leininger (Cultural Care Diversity and Universality), Jean Watson (Theory of Human Caring), and others discussed in Chapter 2 reflect the rich tradition of nursing that incorporates a holistic philosophy of mind-body interconnectedness (Hood & Leddy, 2009). Disease and distress can be viewed as opportunities for the nurse, as a facilitator of healing, to apply the concepts of psychoneuorimmunology and mind-body-spirit connectedness, in the incorporation of caring-healing interventions to promote whole-person health.

CASE STUDY

Doug Cunningham: Managing Exam Stress

OBJECTIVES/GOALS: By participating in the discussion of this case study, participants will have the opportunity to:

1. Identify stressors and conditions that contribute to stressors.
2. Relate symptoms to the physiological effects of stress.
3. Apply the general adaptation syndrome theory.
4. Discuss measures to cope with stress.

HEALTH PROMOTION CONCERN, HISTORY AND PHYSICAL, PRESENT HEALTH STATUS, PAST HEALTH STATUS, FAMILY HISTORY, AND SOCIAL HISTORY

Doug Cunningham is a 38-year-old, white, non-Hispanic male returning to the university to study for a degree in architecture. He began college immediately after graduating from high school, completed 2 years, but dropped out after marrying his high school girlfriend. He is now a newly divorced father of 3 children aged 16, 12, and 7. He changed from working full-time to part-time at the construction company where he has been employed as a roofer for the past 8 years. Child support payments take most of his paycheck, and he struggles financially each month. He was an only child, and the recent death of his parents has left him with a very small inheritance that he is using to finance his return to school. He decided to return to school in order to become more financially secure and to reach his dream of becoming an architect.

Doug is 6 ft, 2 in. tall and weighs 190 lb. He had hepatitis during his sophomore year in high school and is at risk for hypertension because both his parents had it. His mother died after having a stroke, and his father passed away following a massive myocardial infarction. Doug lives in a small 3-room apartment and has his children with him every other weekend. He enjoys socializing with friends from work, eats out every day at fast-food restaurants, drinks one or two beers on the weekend, and has 6–8 cups of regular coffee per day. He stopped smoking after the birth of his first child but began again during his first semester back in college. He exercises daily by doing sit-ups and push-ups.

He studies every night for at least 5 hours and sleeps only 4–5 hours nightly compared to his usual 7 hours. He admits to feeling exhausted and "on edge." Although he says that he does his best when he pushes himself, he reveals that he feels extremely anxious about taking exams and feels pressured to make all As because he is the oldest in all his classes. He takes one multivitamin daily (7/week) and two full-strength aspirin for headaches (about 14/week). Doug is concerned about the effect that stress is having on him and wants to know how to better manage it.

(Continues)

CASE STUDY

(Continued)

REVIEW OF PERTINENT DOMAINS

Biological Domain

Physical examination reveals a well developed and generally physically healthy middle-aged male. Vital signs were blood pressure 126/74, pulse 88, respirations 18. A 2-in. healing abrasion (scratch) is noted behind his right ear.

NEUROLOGICAL: Experiences dull headaches about 3 times weekly, especially in the evening while studying.

GASTROINTESTINAL: Reports upset stomach usually 2 days prior to a major exam. Before an exam last week, he had two episodes of vomiting. He eats irregularly, and his diet is high in carbohydrates, sugars, and caffeine and is void of fruits.

CARDIOVASCULAR: Reports having a "pounding heart" several hours before an exam and during the night when he tries to sleep.

INTEGUMENTARY: Has been noticing a fine rash on his neck, face, and arms that goes away after an exam. The rash is accompanied by itching, and he finds himself unconsciously scratching behind his right ear.

NOSE AND THROAT: Complains of "always getting a cold" after an exam, with scratchy throat, cough, stuffy nose.

DIAGNOSTIC TESTING: All of Doug's blood tests are within normal range.

Psychological Domain

COGNITIVE: He has maintained a 4.0 grade point average during the first semester back in college. He is aware that he is experiencing stress, stating that he has trouble concentrating and that his mind seems to "jump from one thing to another."

PSYCHOLOGICAL: States that he feels "good" about himself and that he is trying to better himself to make life better for his children. He commented that he is "afraid to fail."

Social Domain

Doug is alert, oriented, and able to communicate verbally with appropriate affect. He enjoys being with his children and friends. He admits having a strained relationship with ex-wife.

Environmental Domain

Doug lives alone, interacting daily with fellow students or friends or both. He does not cook for himself and eats at fast-food restaurants.

QUESTIONS FOR DISCUSSION

1. Identify two major stressors in Doug's life. Identify at least five conditions contributing to the stressors.
2. Doug knows that his symptoms are connected to stress but wants to know how stress causes them. Explain this to him using the general adaptation syndrome theory and factors from psychoneuroimmunology.
3. Doug wants to know how he can manage stress. What are some ways that you can suggest?
4. What other risks to health are apparent in Doug's life that indicate a need for health promotion?

KEY CONCEPTS

1. The nervous system impacts the immune system through the neurotransmitter receptor sites on immune cells.
2. The sympathetic nervous system stimulates the secretion of catecholamines and encephalins from the adrenal glands, which modulate the immune system.
3. The HPA axis inhibits the immune function through the secretion of glucocorticoids.
4. Immune function can be measured through antibody levels, lymphocyte activation by mitogens, and NK cell activity against tumor cells.

5. Communication among the neural, endocrine, and immune systems is done through chemicals such as catecholamines, glucocorticoids, serotonin, interleukins, interferons, endorphins, and encephalins.

6. Stress activates the sympathetic nervous system, causing increased circulating catecholamines and stimulation of the HPA system with increased secretion of glucocorticoids and endorphins.

7. Normal life stressors that can have negative effects on the immune system include examinations, bereavement, childbirth, depression, loneliness, and hopelessness.

8. Immunoenhancement has been demonstrated through the use of social support, relaxation therapy, movement, biofeedback, guided imagery, cognitive distraction, humor, hypnosis, exercise, and prayer.

CHAPTER REVIEW

Learning Activities

1. Find three nursing research studies focusing on the influence of stress on illness, and identify their implications for nursing practice.

2. Reflect on stress management techniques you use to manage your personal stress. Make a list of them.

3. Share and compare your stress management strategies with fellow nursing students.

Multiple Choice

1. Mind-body dualism is:
   a. a harmonious blending of the mind and body, where one is affected by the other.
   b. a philosophy founded on the notion that the mind and the body conflict with one another.
   c. a result of the influence of spirituality on health and well-being.
   d. an asynchronous view of the mind and body where one is separate from the other.

2. The chief messengers of the sympathetic nervous system are the two catecholamines, identified as:
   a. ACTH and thyrotropin.
   b. adrenaline and interleukin-1.
   c. epinephrine and norepinephrine.
   d. monocytes and corticosterone.

3. Natural killer cells are:
   a. antibodies that interfere with the production of immunoglobin.
   b. lymphocytes that can destroy tumor cells.
   c. released after exposure to an antigen for activation.
   d. stimulated from the helper T cells in the immune system.

4. Which of the following nursing theorist embodies human caring with a focus on mind-body-spirit wholism?
   a. Florence Nightingale
   b. Jean Watson
   c. Madeleine Leininger
   d. Martha Rogers

5. Which of the following characterizes the alarm stage in Selye's general adaptation syndrome theory?
   a. Decreased cortisol levels in the circulatory system
   b. Decreased pituitary gland activity
   c. Increased parasympathetic nervous system activity
   d. Increased sympathetic nervous system activity

6. Which of the following is not a characteristic of the stress response?
   a. Increased urine flow
   b. Decreased pupil size
   c. Decreased muscle tone
   d. Increased gastric motility

7. Which one of the following is the amino acid that is responsible for major communication and that unites and coordinates all the cells, tissues, glands, organs, and systems of the body?
   a. Cortisol
   b. Epinephrine
   c. Neuropeptides
   d. T lymphocytes

8. Which of the following would be the most immediate nursing action for appropriate crisis intervention?
   a. Assisting in developing a plan of action and commitment to the plan
   b. Guiding rational thought processes
   c. Helping to identify personal coping skills, resources, and support systems
   d. Providing for physical and emotional safety

ORGANIZATIONS AND WEBSITES

American Holistic Nurses Association (AHNA): A nonprofit educational organization open to nurses and other individuals interested in holistically oriented health care practices throughout the United States and the world; supports the education of nurses, allied health practitioners, and the general public on health-related issues: **http://www.ahna.org/**

American Institute of Stress: A nonprofit organization established in 1978 at the request of Hans Selye to serve as a clearinghouse for information on all stress-related subjects; publishes a monthly newsletter, *Health and Stress:* **http:// www.stress.org**

Center for Mind-Body Medicine: Includes a list of online resources and training programs sponsored by the Center, including Mind-Body-Spirit Medicine: **http://www.cmbm.org**

HealthWorld Online: Offers a general overview of mind-body medicine, including articles such as "Introduction to Mind/Body Medicine," "Mind/Body Therapies," and "Mind/Body Approaches to Health Disorders." Includes links to interviews with Larry Dossey, MD, Deepak Chopra, MD, and James Gordon, MD: **http://www.healthy.net**

National Institute for Clinical Applications of Behavioral Medicine: Offers continuing education on mind-body topics for health care practitioners: **http://www.nicabm.com/**

VIDEOS

An Introduction to the Mind/Body Medical Institute (Herbert Benson, MD): Introduces the field of mind-body medicine and the work of the M/BMI: http://www.mbmi.org/shop/

The Biophysiology of Stress (Richard Friedman). Describes the psychological, behavioral, and biological consequences (acute and chronic) of exposure to stress. Emphasizes ways in which the perception of stress changes internal physiology and the way these changes can affect the development of physical illnesses. Tapes can be ordered online at http://www.mbmi.org/shop/.

Body, Mind and Soul (Deepak Chopra, MD): Provides an introduction to the practice of ayurveda, a system of health care that treats the whole person, operating on the guiding principle that the mind exerts the deepest influence on the body. Dr. Chopra addresses such questions as, "What are the mechanics of perception?" . . . "What is the body, and what is the mind?" . . . "Does the soul really exist?"

Energetics of Healing (Caroline Myss, PhD, Sounds True, Boulder, Colorado): Using computer graphics created especially for this program, Dr. Myss pulls back the body's energy anatomy and discusses the chakra centers and correlates them with daily practices for learning the physical language of the spirit—and the spiritual language of the body.

The Living Matrix (Greg Becker, director): Full-length film with dynamic graphic animation woven with interviews of leading researchers and health practitioners as they share their discoveries on the so-called miracle cures that traditional medicine cannot explain. Addresses energy and information fields as driving forces in human physiology and biochemistry, and it illustrates the benefits of integrating conventional and complementary health care.

Recovering the Soul: A Scientific and Spiritual Search (Larry Dossey, MD). Dr. Dossey details scientific data that suggest a spiritual dimension of the individual person and of the person in relation to others. He suggests ways in which we might honor our soul-based dimensions.

AUDIOTAPES AND CDs

Basic Relaxation/Mindfulness Meditation (Olivia Hoblitzelle): Reviews the relaxation response and key techniques such as breath awareness, body scan relaxation, and the use of a focus word. Provides breath and awareness as "primary tools" that enable relaxation response to be incorporated into daily activities. Tapes can be ordered online at http://www.mbmi.org/shop/

Nurturing Your Immune System (Lynn W. Brallier, RN, MSN, PhD): Addresses immune functioning and stress. Selections can be ordered by calling (888) 553–4010.

Self-Empathy/Nurturing Change (Peg Baim, RN, MS, NP): Uses peaceful and rhythmic music with guided meditation to counter anxiety, enhance self-awareness, and enhance total well-being. Tapes can be ordered online at http://www.mbmi.org.

Sound Body, Sound Mind (Andrew Weil, MD): One-hour tape that includes eight meditations for optimum health. Tapes can be ordered online at http://www.amazon.com or http://www.bn.com.

Why People Don't Heal: Spiritual Madness, Spiritual Power, Spiritual Practice (Caroline Myss, PhD): Discusses the connection between the mind, body, and healing. Audiotapes can be ordered online at http://www.amazon.com or http://www.amazon.ca.

REFERENCES

Barnes, P. M., Bloom, B., Nahin, R. (2008). National Center for Complementary and Alternative Medicine. CDC national health statistics report #12. Complementary and alternative medicine use among adults and children: United States, 2007. Retrieved from http://nccam.nih.gov/news/camstats/2007/

Barnes, P. M, Powell-Griner, E., McFann, K., & Nahin, R. L. (2004). National Center for Complementary and Alternative Medicine. Complementary and alternative medicine use among adults: United States, 2002. *CDC Advance Data Report #343.* Retrieved from http://www.nccam.nih.gov/news/report.pdf

Beaton, D. (2003, November). Effects of stress and psychological disorders on the immune system. Retrieved from http://www.personalityresearch.org/papers/beaton.html

Ben-Arye, E., Ziv, M., Frenkel, M., Lavi, I., & Rosenman, D. (2003). Complementary medicine and psoriasis: Linking the patient's outlook with evidence-based medicine. *Dermatology, 207*(3), 302–307.

Benight, C. C., Harper, M. L., Zimmer, D. L., Lowery, M., Sanger, J., & Laudenslager, M. L. (2004). Repression following a series of natural disasters: Immune and neuroendocrine correlates. *Psychology & Health, 19*, 337–352.

Boerner, H. (2009). Positively healing. *Yoga Journal, 220*, 39-40, 42.

Boyle, P. J., Feng, Z,. & Raab, M. (2011). Does widowhood increase mortality risk? Testing for selection effects by comparing causes of spousal death. E*pidemiology, 22*(1), 1–5.

Borysenko, J., & Dveirin, G. (2005). *Say yes to change*. Carlsbad, CA: Hay House.

Burkhardt, M. A., & Nagai-Jacobson, M. G. (2005). Spirituality and health. In B. M. Dossey, L. Keegan, & C. E. Guzzetta (eds.), *Holistic nursing: A handbook for practice* (4th ed.). Sudbury, MA: Jones & Bartlett.

Chandola T., Brunner, E., & Marmot, M. (2006) Chronic stress at work and the metabolic syndrome: Prospective study. *BMJ, 332*, 521–525.

Christian L. M., Graham, J. E., Padgett, D. A., Glaser. R., & Kiecolt-Glaser, J. K. (2007). Stress and wound healing. *Neuroimmunomodulation, 13*(5–6), 337–346. DOI: 10.1159/000104862.

Cruess, D. G., Douglas, S. D, Petitto, J. M., Have, T. T., Gettes. D., Dubé, B., Cary, M., & Evans D. L. (2005). Association of resolution of major depression with increased natural killer cell activity among HIV-seropositive women. *American Journal of Psychiatry, 162*(11), 2125–2130.

Cruise, B. A., Xu, P., & Hall, A. K. (2004). Wounds increase activin in skin and a vasoactive neuropeptide in sensory ganglia. *Developmental Biology, 271*(1), 1–10.

Douglas, D. (2007). Depression might influence breast cancer risk. Retrieved from http://www.breastcancer.org/risk/new_research/20071219b.jsp

Dykeman, B. F. (2005). Cultural implications of crisis intervention. *Journal of Instructional Psychology, 32*(1), 45–48.

Etnyer, A., Rauschhuber, M., Gilliland, I., Cook, J., Mahon, M., Allwein, D., et al. (2005). Cardiovascular risk among older Hispanic women. *American Association of Occupational Health Nurses Journal, 54*(3), 120–128.

European Society of Cardiology (ESC) (2008, September 1). Does treatment of depression improve prognosis after heart attack? Retrieved from http://www.sciencedaily.com/releases/2008/09/080901090117.htm

Flowers, D. L. (2005). Culturally competent nursing care for American Indian patients in a critical care setting. *Critical Care Nursing, 25*(1), 45–50.

Garrish, M. (2005). Stress: The mind-body connection. *WebMed Live Events Transcript (October 6, 2005)*.

Gianaros, P. J., Jennings, J. R., Sheu, L. K., Greer, P. J., Kuller, L. H., & Matthews K. A. (2007). Prospective reports of chronic life stress predict decreased grey matter volume in the hippocampus. *Neuroimage. 35*(2), 795–803.

Gibran, J. S., Jang, Y. C., Isik, F. F., Greenhalgh, D. G., Muffley, L. A., Underwood, R. A., Usui, M. L., Larsen, J., Smith, D. G., Bunnett, N., Ansel, J. C., Olerud, J. E. (2002). Diminished neuropeptide levels contribute to the impaired cutaneous healing response associated with diabetes mellitus. *Journal of Surgical Research, 108*(1), 122–128.

Glaser, R., & Kiecolt-Glaser, J. (2005). Stress damages immune system and health. *Discovery Medicine, 5*(26), 165–169.

Glassey, D. J. (n.d.). Body work and neuropeptides: The molecules of healing. Retrieved from http://www.healtouch.com/csft/bodywork.html

Golden-Kreutz, D. M., & Andersen, B. L. (2004). Depressive symptoms after breast cancer surgery: Relationships with global, cancer-related, and life event stress. *Psycho-Oncology, 13*, 211–220.

Haddad, M. (2010). Caring for patients with long-term conditions and depression. *Nursing Standard, 24*(24), 40–50.

Harrington, A. (2008). *The cure within: A history of mind-body medicine*. New York, NY: W.W. Norton.

Höglund, C. O., Axén, J., Kemi, C., Jernelöv, S., Grunewald, J., Müller-Suur, … Lekander, M. (2006). Changes in immune regulation in response to examination stress in atopic and healthy individuals. *Clinical & Experimental Allergy, 36*, 982–992. DOI: 10.1111/j.1365-2222.2006.02529.x.

Holmes, T. H., & Rahe, R. H. (1967). The social readjustment rating scale. *Journal of Psychosomatic Research, 11*(2), 213–218.

Hood, L., & Leddy, S. (2009). *Leddy and Pepper's conceptual bases of professional nursing*. Philadelphia, PA: Lippincott Williams & Wilkins.

Irwin, M. R., & Miller, A. H. (2007). Depressive disorders and immunity: 20 years of progress and discovery. *Brain, behavior, and immunity, 21*(4), 374–383.

Jones, J. (2003). Stress responses, pressure ulcer development and adaptation. *British Journal of Nursing, 12*, 17–23.

Kanel, K. (2006). *Guide to crisis intervention*. Belmont, CA: Wadsworth.

Keene, J. R., & Prokos, A. H. (2008). Widowhood and the end of spousal care-giving: Relief or wear and tear? *Aging & Society*. 551–570. DOI:10.1017/So144668X076654.

Koenig, H. G. (2008). M*edicine, religion & health: Where science and spirituality meet*. West Conshohocken, PA: Templeton Foundation Press.

Koenig, H. G., & Cohen, H. J. (eds.). (2002). *The link between religion and health: Psychoneuroimmunology and the faith factor*. Oxford: Oxford University Press.

Lampe, F. C., Harding, R., Smith, C. J., Phillips, A.N., Johnson, M., Sherr, L. (2010). Physical and psychological symptoms and risk of virologic rebound among patients with virologic suppression on antiretroviral therapy. *Journal of Acquired Immune Deficiency Syndrome, 54*(5), 500–505. Retrieved from http://www.ncbi.nlm.nih.gov/pubmed/20150819

Laubmeier, K. K., & Zakowski, S. G. (2004). The role of objective versus perceived life threat in the psychological adjustment to cancer. *Psychology and Health, 19*(4), 425–437.

Mailoo, V. J., & Williams, C. J. (2004). Psychoneuroimmunology: A theoretical basis for occupational therapy in oncology? *International Journal of Therapy & Rehabilitation, 11*(1), 7–12.

McCance, K. L., & Huether, S. E. (2010). *Pathophysiology: The biologic basis for disease in adults and children* (6th ed.). St. Louis, MO: Mosby-Elsevier.

McEwen, B. (2004). Protection and damage from acute and chronic stress: Allostasis and allostatic overload and relevance to the pathophysiology of psychiatric disorders. *Annals of the New York Academy of Sciences, 1032*, 1–7. Retrieved from http://onlinelibrary.wiley.com/doi/10.1111/j.1749-6632.2009.05331.x/pdf

McEwen, B. S., & Gianaros, P. J. (2010). Central role of the brain in stress and adaptation: Links to socioeconomic status, health, and disease. *Annals of the New York Academy of Sciences, 1186*, 190–222. DOI: 10.1111/j.1749-6632.2009.05331.x.

National Cancer Institute (NCI) (n.d.). National Cancer Institute Fact Sheet. Psychological stress and cancer. Retrieved from http://www.cancer.gov/cancertopics/factsheet/Risk/stress

National Center for Complementary and Alternative Medicine (NCCAM). (2005). *Prayer and spirituality in health: Ancient practices, modern science, 12*(1). Retrieved from http://www.nccam.nih.gov

National Center for PTSD Department of Veterans Affairs. (2010). Traumatic effects of certain types of disasters. Retrieved from www.ptsd.va.gov/PTSD/professional/pages/traumatic-effects-disasters.asp;

National Psoriasis Foundation (2011). Mind-body medicine. Retrieved from http://www.psoriasis.org/about-psoriasis/treatments/alternative/mind-body.

Osler, W. (1913/2006). The evolution of modern medicine. Retrieved from http://www.gutenberg.org/files/1566/1566-h/1566-h.htm

Phillips, A. C., Carroll, D., Burns, V. E., Ring, C., Macleod, J., and Drayson, M. (2006). Bereavement and marriage are associated with antibody response to influenza vaccination in the elderly. *Brain, Behavior, and Immunity, 20*(3), 279–289.

Pitt, M. A. (2005). Development and psychometric evaluation of the revised university student hassles scale. *Educational and Psychological Measurement, 65*(6), 984–1010.

Pressman, S. D., Cohen, S., Miller, G. E., Barkin, A., Rabin, B. S., & Treanor, J. J. (2005). Loneliness, social network size and immune response to influenza vaccination in college freshmen. *Health Psychology, 24*(3), 297–306.

Research reveals biology of harmful stress. (2003). *Harvard Women's Health Watch, 11*(1), 1.

Robles, G. F., Glaser, R., & Kiecolt-Glaser, J. K. (2005). Out of balance: A new look at chronic stress, depression, and immunity. *Current Directions in Psychological Science, 14*(2), 111–115.

Rosenbluh, E. (2002). Emotional first aid. Retrieved from http://www.emotionalfirstaid.com

Sarafino, E. P., & Ewing, M. (1999). The hassles assessment scale for students in college: Measuring the frequency and unpleasantness of and dwelling on stressful events. *Journal of American College Health, 48*(2), 75–83.

Schwecke, L. H. (2007). Anxiety, coping, and crisis. In N. L. Keltner, L. H. C. E. Bostrom, & T. McGuinness (eds.), *Psychiatric nursing*. St. Louis, MO: Mosby, pp. 120–129.

Scott, E. (2010). Stress and metabolic syndrome: Chronic job stress is a risk factor for heart disease. *About.com Stress Management*. Retrieved from stress.about.com/od/stresshealth/a/jobstress.htm

Sergerstrom, S. C. (2010). Stress, energy, and immunity. *Annals of Behavioral Medicine, 40*(1), 114–125.

Segerstrom, S. C., & Miller, G. E. (2004). Psychological stress and the human immune system: A meta-analytical study of 30 years of inquiry. *Psychological Bulletin, 130*(4), 601–630.

Selye, H. (1976). *Stress in health and disease*. Boston, MA: Butterworth-Heinemann, Ltd.

Shealy, N. C., Norris, P. A., & Fahrion, S. L. (2002). *Mind-body medicines*. Retrieved from www.amsa.org/AMSA/Libraries/Committee_Docs/EDCAM_C2.sflb.ashx

Shen, C., Findley, P., Banerjea, R., & Sambamoorthi, U. (2010). Depressive disorders among cohorts of women veterans with diabetes, heart disease, and hypertension. *Journal of Women's Health, 19* (8): 1475–1486.

Shor-Posner, G., Miguez, M. J., Hernandez-Reif, M., Perez-Then, E., & Fletcher, M. 2004, *The Journal of Alternative and Complementary Medicine, 10*(6), 1093–1095.

Tafet, G. E., & Bernardini, R. (2003). Psychoneuroendocrinological links between chronic stress and depression. *Progress in Neuropsychopharmacology, Biology, and Psychiatry, 27*(6), 893–903.

Thaker, P. H, Han L. Y, Kamat, A. A, Arevalo, J. M., Takahashi, R. Lu, C. Jennings, N. B., Armaiz-Pena, G., Bankson, J. A., Ravoori, M., Merritt, W. M., Lin, Y. G., Mangala, L. S., Kim, T., J., Coleman, R. L., Landen, C. N., Li, Y., Felix, E., Sanguino, A. M., Newman, R. A., Lloyd, M., Gershenson, D. M., Kundra, V., Lopez-Berestein, G. Lutgendorf, S. K., Cole, S. W., & Sood, A. K. (2006). Chronic stress promotes tumor growth and angiogenesis in a mouse model of ovarian carcinoma. *Nature Medicine, 12*(8), 939–944.

Thoma, A. G. (2011). Immune system impairment in response to chronic anxiety. *Integrative Medicine: A Clinician's Journal, 10*(1), 20–24

Tiew L. H., & Creedy, D. K. (2010). Integration of spirituality in nursing practice: a literature review. *Singapore Nursing Journal, 37*(1): 15–20. Retrieved from http://web.ebscohost.com/ehost/pdfviewer/pdfviewer?vid=5&hid=108&sid=482aed21-8ca7-4b39-a82c-9d0cd903b667%40sessionmgr113

Varcarolis, E. M. (2011). *Manual of psychiatric nursing care planning: Assessment guides, diagnosis, and psychopharmacology*. St. Louis, MO: Saunders.

Vitaliano, P. P., & Katon, W. J. (2006). Effects of stress on family caregivers: Recognition and management. *Psychiatric Times, 23*(7). Retrieved from http://www.psychiatrictimes.com/display/article/10168/51416?verify=0

Watson, J. (2008). *Nursing: The philosophy and science of caring* (rev. ed.). Boulder, CO: University Press of Colorado.

Yehuda, R., & McEwen, B. (eds.). (2004). *Biobehavioral stress response: Protective and damaging effects*. New York, NY: New York Academy of Science.

BIBLIOGRAPHY

Benson, H. (1975). *The relaxation response*. New York, NY: Avon.

Block, S., & Block, C. B. (2005). *Come to your senses: Demystifying the mind-body connection*. Hillsboro, OR: Beyond Words Publishing.

Carlini, H. (2007). *The mind body connection to healing*. Retrieved from http://carliniinstitute.com/mindbody_connection

Koenig, H. G. (2007). *Spirituality in patient care: Why, how, when, and what*. West Conshohocken, PA: Templeton Foundation Press.

Mailis-Gagnon, A., & Israelson, D. (2005). *Beyond pain: Making the mind-body connection*. Ann Arbor, MI: University of Michigan Press.

O'Brien, M. E. (2003). *Prayer in nursing: The spirituality of compassionate caregiving*. Sudbury, MA: Jones & Bartlett.

Roberts, A. (2005). *Crisis intervention handbook: Assessment, treatment, and research* (3rd ed.). Oxford, UK: Oxford University Press.

Seeman, T. E., Dubin, L. F., & Seeman, M. (2003). Religiosity/spirituality and health: A critical review of the evidence for biological pathways. *American Psychologist, 58*(1), 53–63.

Sorajjakool, S., & Lamberton, H. H. (2004). *Spirituality, health, and wholeness: An introductory guide for the health care professional*. New York, NY: Hawthorne Press.

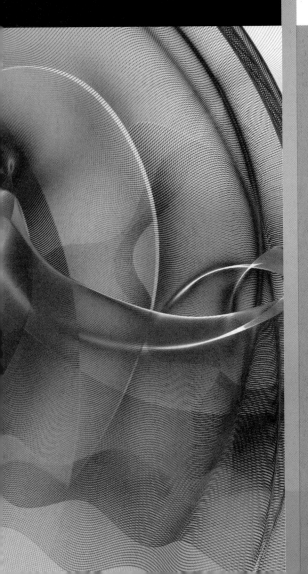

Section III

Promoting Health throughout the Life Cycle

CHAPTER 9
Promoting Mother, Infant, and Toddler Health

PATRICIA BOWDEN, MSN, RN

KEY TERMS

amenorrhea	diarrhea	mortality
amniocentesis	embryo	pica
attachment	fetus	postpartum
bruising	gestational diabetes	screening
congenital	infant	sexuality
constipation	isoimmunization	teratogens
couvade	morbidity	urinary incontinence

OBJECTIVES

Upon completion of this chapter, the reader should be able to:

- Examine preconception health-promotion strategies in the biological domain for women and their partners.
- Examine health-promotion strategies in the biological domain for mothers, infants, and toddlers.
- Identify nursing responsibilities for screening to promote the health of mothers, infants, and toddlers.
- Relate theories of cognitive and emotional development to health-promotion strategies in infants and toddlers.
- Identify social networks and their importance in maternal and infant health.
- Describe incidence, signs and symptoms, and nursing responsibilities related to child abuse and neglect.
- Identify legislative actions designed to improve the health of mothers and infants.
- Describe parental and nursing responsibilities for promoting infant and toddler safety.
- Relate normal sexual development to strategies designed to promote sexual health in infants.
- Describe spiritual influences on health promotion in pregnant women, infants, and toddlers.

INTRODUCTION

Improving the well-being of mothers, infants, and children is an important health-promotion goal for the United States. Ideally, health promotion for the mother and infant should begin prior to conception. As the focus of health care moves from a disease focus to a preventive and health-promotion focus, preconception education and screening provide the opportunity to promote a healthy beginning for the infant and the mother. Health-promotion teaching is a way of having a lasting effect on the health practices of a family. Health education should specifically transmit information, motivate the inner resource of the person, and help people adopt and maintain healthy practices and lifestyles. Health care providers cannot make decisions for patients, but patients should be given sufficient information so that they can make educated choices to promote health and engage in healthy behavior.

The impact of preconception health-promotion strategies on maternal and fetal **morbidity** (illness rate) and **mortality** (death rate) can be significant in terms decreased pregnancy-related complications, healthy birth outcomes, and the early identification and treatment of fetal and newborn disorders. The goal of preconception health promotion is to improve the health of women and increase the likelihood of a good pregnancy outcome by encouraging positive behaviors and controlling or preventing health problems before pregnancy. An important aspect of preconception health promotion is to begin education during adolescence for both females and males. This education should include information about the physiology of conception, maternal changes during pregnancy, fetal growth and development, and psychological preparation for parenthood. Information about promoting a healthy fetus should include proper nutrition and avoidance of substance abuse and of anything that can lead to the abnormal development of embryonic structures (**teratogens**). Appropriate preconception counseling promotes physically and emotionally healthy parents, resulting in optimal prenatal, intrapartum, and postpartum maternal and fetal health and ultimately in a healthy child and family.

Preconception education can enable sexually active adolescents to make informed choices that can result in the avoidance of an unintended pregnancy. According to a report from the Centers for Disease Control and Prevention (CDC), approximately 414,870 teenage births occurred in the United States in 2009 (Hamilton, Martin, & Ventura, 2010). This recorded data reflects that 3 in every 100 teenage girls in the United States become pregnant and give birth. An adolescent, also referred to as a teenager, is defined by the World Health Organization (WHO) as a person between 10 and 19 years of age (World Health Organization [WHO], 2011).

The majority of teenage pregnancies are unplanned. The rate of unintended pregnancies among adult women in the United States is approximately 50%. The rate of unintended teenage pregnancies is estimated to be over 61% (Teen Births, 2011). A delay in initiating prenatal care and the late recognition of pregnancy are both factors related to unintended pregnancy (Ayoola et al., 2010). In addition, negative maternal and fetal outcomes have been found to be associated with an unintended pregnancy (Ayoola et al., 2010). This is why preconception counseling and education are so important for both teenage and adult women. Health care providers must take advantage of every health care visit to discuss the potential for pregnancy and how women can protect their own health and the health of their fetus if pregnancy does occur.

The fetus is the most vulnerable to insult during the first 8 weeks postconception because the major organ systems begin to develop during this period. Preconception education and early prenatal care present a crucial opportunity to include information about promoting the healthy development of the fetus during this most vulnerable period of development. Once a pregnancy is established, some health-promotion interventions may not be as effective. Preconception education should include information to promote healthy maternal behaviors and lifestyle. A healthy lifestyle involves optimal nutrition, regular physical activity, maintaining a healthy weight, and avoiding any substances that may cause harm to the developing fetus. Healthy maternal behaviors include abstinence from cigarette smoking, alcohol consumption, and illegal or addictive drug use. In addition, avoiding exposure to infections that pose a risk to the fetus is important.

The incidence rate of a host of conditions affecting maternal and infant health has not changed significantly. Some of these conditions are congenital anomalies, preterm births, low birth weight, and complications with pregnancy or delivery leading to maternal mortality. Women who receive preconception counseling and education enter pregnancy with a higher level of wellness and are more likely to initiate early prenatal care. Health promotion prior to conception can have a significant impact on increased rates of planned pregnancies and on better pregnancy outcomes, as well as the long-term well-being of the mother and the infant. A healthy start in life for an infant maximizes the potential for growth and development throughout childhood and into adulthood.

This chapter covers health promotion for the mother, the infant, and the toddler. The biological, psychological, social, political, environmental, and sexual domains serve as a guiding framework.

THE MOTHER

A woman's health status, lifestyle, and family health history are important determinants of a healthy pregnancy outcome. Maternal health-promotion strategies for preconception, pregnancy, and postpartum are discussed in the following sections.

BIOLOGICAL DOMAIN

Knowledge of the biologic factors and physiologic processes involved in the functioning of the body before, during, and after pregnancy are of primary importance. Nutrition, screening, immunizations, and physical activity are covered in this domain.

Preconception

Prior to conception, access to safe and effective birth control and knowledge of the availability and safety of emergency contraception are critical to reducing the incidence of unplanned pregnancies. Table 9-1 discusses available birth control methods, choices, their effectiveness, and use. When educating others about birth control methods, make it clear that both females and males can obtain emergency contraception without a prescription at the pharmacy counter if they are 17 years of age or older (Davidoff & Trussell, 2006). The emergency contraception (EC) pill, also called the morning after pill, does not require a prescription, is approximately 72–89% effective, and should be taken as soon as possible after contraception failure or unprotected sexual intercourse; however, it can be effective if within 5 days or 120 hours (Rifampin, 2011). An important note is that EC does not protect against sexually transmitted infections.

TABLE 9-1 Birth Control Methods

METHOD	CHOICES	EFFECTIVENESS	HOW TO USE
Hormonal contraceptives prevent pregnancy by: • Preventing the ovary from releasing an egg into a fallopian tube • Thickening cervical mucus, making it difficult for sperm to enter the uterus to fertilize the egg • Thinning the lining of the endometrium to prevent implantation	Transdermal patch	99%	Applied once a week for 3 weeks in a row; week 4 without patch
	Oral contraceptive (the pill)	99%	Taken daily, at approximately the same time
	Contraceptive injection	99%	Injected monthly or every 3 months
	Progestin-releasing device (IUD)	99%	Inserted by health care provider into the uterus
	Vaginal ring	99%	Worn in vagina for 3 weeks in a row; week 4 without ring
Nonhormonal contraceptives prevent pregnancy by: • Providing a barrier against sperm • Interfering with sperm movement • Creating a difficult environment for sperm to travel or survive	Male condom	97%	New one used every time before sex
	Female condom	95%	New one used every time before sex
	Intrauterine device (IUD)	99%	Inserted by health care provider into the uterus
	Spermicidal foams, gels, creams or vaginal suppositories	94%	Inserted no more than 1 hour before sex Use with vaginal barrier increases effectiveness.
	Diaphragm	94%	Inserted up to 6–8 hours before sex Spermicide applied each time
	Cervical cap	84–91%	Inserted up to 48 hours before sex Spermicide applied each time
	Rhythm method	75%	Keeping track of changes in body temperature and vaginal discharge (fluid from the vagina) to pinpoint which days you are fertile. Sexual intercourse is prohibited then.
Nonhormonal permanent methods to prevent pregnancy: • Providing a barrier against sperm • Interfering with sperm movement	Microinsert	99%	Placed into each fallopian tube
	Female surgical sterilization	99%	Surgical interruption of fallopian tubes
	Male surgical sterilization: Vasectomy	99%	Surgical interruption of vas deferens

Preconception education regarding birth control should be provided to both males and females and should include adequate information about the variety of available contraceptive methods. The antibiotic Rifampin alters the effectiveness of oral contraceptives, and individuals should use another method of birth control while taking this medication (Rifampin . . ., 2011). Other antibiotics have also been found to affect the effectiveness of oral contraceptives; thus, sexually active females should consult with a pharmacist to see whether any prescribed medications affect the effectiveness of contraceptives. In addition, education should include how to correctly use each method and that the male/female condom (barrier method) is the only form of contraception that protects against sexually transmitted diseases. Most pregnancies among contraceptive users in the United States result from inconsistent or incorrect use, not from failure of the contraceptive method (Mosher & Jones, 2010). Health care providers have the opportunity to provide preconception counseling for women at every contact, such as visits for their own personal health care and annual exams and visits for the health care of their children at well child visits.

The evaluation of current dietary habits and preferences is an important part of preconception nutritional counseling. Education about a healthy well-balanced diet should be included in preconception counseling. Provide information about specific food sources and nutrients that should be in the diet of all women capable of becoming pregnant: good sources of iron, calcium, and B vitamins. The diet should be low in fat, but have sufficient calories to maintain a healthy weight. The diet should include lean meats, dairy products, dried beans, whole grain cereals and breads, as well as, folic acid-rich fortified grains and dark green leafy vegetables. The United States Preventive Task Force (USPTF) currently recommends that all women planning or capable of pregnancy take a daily dietary supplement of 0.4–0.8 mg (400–800 mcg) folic acid to prevent neural tube defects in the fetus (U.S. Preventive Services Task Force, 2009). Folic acid supplementation should be started at least 1 month before conception and continued through the first 2–3 months of pregnancy (U.S. Preventive Services Task Force, 2009). Women with a history of neural tube defects are recommended to take 4 mg of folic acid daily (Wolff et al., 2009). Folic acid supplementation is recommended, in addition to a diet rich in folic acid food sources, such as fortified grains and dark green, leafy vegetables. Neural tube defects, resulting from a malformation of the embryo's central nervous system (neural tube), affect approximately 1 in every 1000 pregnancies in the United States and can lead to a serious birth defect such as spina bifida or anencephaly.

Encouraging women to maintain a healthy weight prior to conception is important. Behaviors that should be discouraged are excessive dieting, eating disorders, and extreme exercise because these may lead to irregular or anovulatory menstrual cycles, making it difficult to conceive. Underweight and overweight conditions can lead to risk factors affecting the pregnancy outcome and should be managed prior to attempts to become pregnant.

Preconception counseling should always include the father if possible. For men who might become fathers, providing information regarding a healthy diet and lifestyle is important to promote reproductive health. Negative lifestyle behaviors, such as smoking, poor diet, alcohol abuse, obesity, or psychological stress, have all been linked to adverse effects on sperm production and motility (Tremellen, 2008). Nutrition education should include maintaining a well-balanced diet that incorporates antioxidants such as zinc, selenium, folate, vitamin C, vitamin E, and lycopene because these nutrients have been found to support healthy sperm production and motility (Tremellen, 2008). They are found in foods such as whole grain breads and cereals, fruits, beans, broccoli, and lean meats.

The promotion of a healthy, well-balanced diet for both parents contributes to their reproductive health and a healthy pregnancy outcome, and it can ultimately help in establishing healthy eating habits in children and in the family as a whole.

Genetic history screening helps the prospective mother and father to make their decision to conceive or to prepare for a child with special needs. The genetic history should include a review for previous preterm or low-birth-weight babies and children with significant malformations. In addition, obtain a family history of sickle cell or thalassemic anemias, Tay-Sachs disease or cystic fibrosis, genetic syndromes or chromosomal abnormalities, and congenital hearing loss. Genetic counseling should be recommended when any of these conditions are present in the family background of either potential parent. Women who are 35 years of age and older should receive genetic counseling regarding the risk of the chromosomal abnormality in the fetus resulting in Down syndrome, which is also known as trisomy 21. This risk increases with every year of maternal age, primarily after 35 years of age (Down Syndrome Facts, 2011). Prenatal counseling for the pregnant women who is 35 years of age or older should include the availability of specific tests to confirm Down syndrome in the fetus. This confirmation can allow the parents' time to prepare for the special needs of the child.

The prospective mother should be screened for medical conditions that can potentially place her at risk for complications during pregnancy. These medical conditions can also place the fetus at risk from the disease itself and/or teratogenous medications used to treat the mother. Women with documented diabetes need preconception counseling because the most common anomalies in infants born to diabetic women are to the organs that develop in the first 7–8 weeks of gestation. Instituting prevention strategies to control blood glucose prior to conception and during the first months of pregnancy can dramatically reduce the incidence of birth defects in infants born to diabetic mothers. Women with phenylketonuria (PKU) need to begin dietary phenylalanine restrictions at least 3 months prior to conception. Dietary control in women with PKU is important because of the serious consequences to the developing fetus as a result of exposure to elevated levels of phenylalanine. All prescription and over-the-counter medications and supplements should be reviewed by the health care provider for potential teratogenic effects. Medications for seizure disorders have a potential for being teratogens. The potential mother and her health care provider should make the decision whether to continue or discontinue seizure medications after weighing the risks to the fetus versus the benefits to the mother. Dental work should be done prior to the initiation of the pregnancy to avoid unnecessary exposure to x-rays and medications.

Additional screening should include the evaluation of immunizations and infectious disease risk. Women planning pregnancy should be up-to-date on the measles, mumps and rubella (MMR) vaccine, as well as varicella and hepatitis B vaccinations. Contracting these infections while pregnant can have serious detrimental effects on the developing fetus. These viruses are known to infect the fetus through transplacental transmission, placing the fetus at risk for abnormalities resulting from the disease (Guidelines . . ., 2011). With the exception of the hepatitis B vaccine, immunization for these infections is contraindicated once the woman becomes pregnant because the vaccinations contain live components of the virus, which can cause damage to the fetus (Guidelines . . ., 2011).

A tetanus booster is necessary for all women every 10 years. Pregnant women who have previously been vaccinated for tetanus but who have not received the vaccination within the last 10 years should receive a booster dose after the first trimester (Guidelines . . ., 2011). The Advisory Committee on Immunization Practices (ACIP) recommends that new mother receive a pertussis vaccine in the immediate postpartum period and preferably prior to discharge (CDC, 2010). This protects mothers from the disease and reduces the risk of exposing their infant to pertussis. Pertussis is most severe in infants less than 12 months of age, and infants less than 6 months of age are at the highest risk for mortality due to respiratory complications from the disease (CDC, 2010). Pertussis immunization is also recommended for all adults and adolescents that anticipate being in contact with the newborn and throughout infancy (CDC, 2010). Women should also be screened for human immunodeficiency virus (HIV) and for syphilis to decrease the risk of transplacental transmission to the fetus or to reduce the severity of disease in the fetus by initiating early maternal treatment if pregnancy occurs.

Potential mothers-to-be should be encouraged to have an exercise program that can be continued during pregnancy. Aerobic and strength-conditioning exercises that produce a better state of fitness prior to conception reduces the risk of obesity, gestational diabetes, pregnancy-induced hypertension, and physical complaints during pregnancy.

Providing preconception counseling to both women and men about avoiding smoking, drinking alcohol, and the use of illegal drugs helps prevent detrimental effects on both fertility and fetal development. For the counseling to be the most effective, the dangers to the fetus from smoking, alcohol, and illegal drugs should be explained very clearly and in a nonjudgmental manner. These dangers should be emphasized at every contact with the potential mother or father.

Women who are planning to become pregnant or who are capable of becoming pregnant should avoid any amount of alcohol. Alcohol has been found to be a teratogen and can cause permanent damage to the developing fetus (Sayal et al., 2009). A safe amount of alcohol that does not cause damage to the fetus is not known (Sayal et al., 2009). Fetal exposure to alcohol can result in a range of lifelong physical, mental, behavioral, and learning disabilities. Alcohol also affects the absorption and utilization of folic acid, which is necessary to prevent neural tube defects.

Maternal cigarette smoking is known to be associated with impaired or restricted fetal growth and low birth weight. The nurse can discuss smoking cessation strategies, along with the benefits of quitting. Even reducing smoking as much as possible can be of benefit.

Cocaine, heroin, marijuana, and other illegal drugs have a negative impact on the developing fetus and the newborn. Pregnant women with drug addictions may suffer from poor nutrition or altered immunity and can expose their unborn babies to hepatitis B and HIV infection. Newborns of drug-addicted mothers are at risk for drug withdrawal, low birth weight, and other complications.

PREGNANCY

Pregnancy (gestation) normally lasts approximately 40 weeks, 9 calendar months, 10 lunar months, or 3 trimesters. **Gestational age** is calculated from the first day of the last normal menstrual period, assuming the woman has a 28-day cycle. The product of pregnancy from conception to the end of 8 weeks is

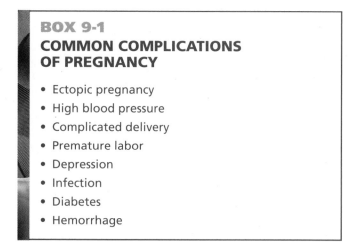

BOX 9-1

COMMON COMPLICATIONS OF PREGNANCY

- Ectopic pregnancy
- High blood pressure
- Complicated delivery
- Premature labor
- Depression
- Infection
- Diabetes
- Hemorrhage

termed an **embryo**. It is termed a **fetus** from the eighth week of pregnancy until the moment of birth. An **infant** is the live-born individual from the moment of birth until 1 year of life.

The diagnosis of pregnancy is usually made on the basis of a history of **amenorrhea** (cessation of menses), an enlarging uterus, and a positive pregnancy test. The estimated date of birth can be calculated by using Naegele's rule, which is counting back 90 days (3 months) from the first day of the last menstrual period, then adding 7 days and 1 year to that date. This calculation is for a woman with a 28-day menstrual cycle and assumes that pregnancy occurred on the 14th day of the cycle. Adjustments to this calculation formula are necessary if the cycle is longer or shorter than 28 days.

The number of pregnancies in the United States is approximately 6 million every year, and of these pregnancies, approximately 4,058,000 are live births, and 1,995,840 are pregnancy losses (Pregnancy Statistics, 2011). Pregnancy complications occur in approximately 875,000 pregnant women resulting in significant morbidity and mortality (Pregnancy Statistics, 2011). The 2008 maternal mortality rate in the United States was reported to be 12.7 deaths per 100,000 live births (Child Health USA, 2011). Unfortunately, this rate has not shown any significant decline since. Some of the leading causes of pregnancy-related deaths are hemorrhage, embolism, hypertension, and infection. Box 9-1 lists the most common complications of pregnancy. Better access to health care, better quality of prenatal care, and health and lifestyle changes can help prevent over half of these deaths. The following health-promotion interventions help reduce pregnancy-related complications and deaths.

Nutrition

Pregnant women should eat a well-balanced diet, including a variety of foods, with an increase of 350–450 kcal/day in the second and third trimesters. Adolescents need nutrition for both the pregnancy and their own physical growth. Adolescents and vegetarians may benefit from additional counseling by a registered dietitian. Women whose weight is in the healthy range, which is represented by a normal body mass index (BMI) of 18.5–24.9, before becoming pregnant should gain 25–35 lb while pregnant (Institute of Medicine [IOM], 2009). The current recommendation by the U.S. Institute of Medicine (IOM) is a weight gain of 1–4 lb total during the first 3 months (first trimester) and 2–4 lb per month during the fourth and ninth months (second and third trimester) (2009). Underweight pregnant women (BMI < 18.5) should gain a total of 28–40 lb throughout the pregnancy (IOM, 2009). The recommendation for weight gain in pregnant women who are overweight (BMI 25.0–29.9) should be a total of 15–25 lb (IOM, 2009). Weight gain of less than 25 lb has been associated with low birth weight and preterm birth, whereas greater weight gain has been associated with an increased risk of infants that are large for gestational age, birth trauma, cesarean delivery, and postpartum weight retention. Women who are obese (BMI > 30.0) should gain a recommended total of 11–20 lb during pregnancy (IOM, 2009).

A multivitamin is recommended for all pregnant adolescents and women. In addition, pregnant women should have a daily calcium intake of 1000 mg/day or 1300 mg/day for women under 19 years of age, 0.4–0.8 mg of folic acid, and 27–30 mg of iron (Dietary Guidelines, 2010). Some multivitamin supplements (prenatal vitamins) are especially formulated for pregnant women and meet all the preceding requirements. High levels of vitamin A from dietary sources or supplements should be avoided during pregnancy. Vitamin A deficiencies are not common in developed countries (Ross et al., 2009). Generally, pregnant women in non–vitamin A deficient areas have sufficient liver stores of vitamin A to provide for the added nutritional demand of pregnancy; therefore, supplementation is not recommended (Van de Brock et al., 2010). A high level of maternal vitamin A is teratogenic and is known to be associated with miscarriage and fetal malformations involving the central nervous system and the cardiac system (Van de Brock et al., 2010). In pregnancy, vitamin D deficiency has been found to be common among pregnant women in the United States (Asary et al., 2010). This deficiency can have detrimental effects primarily on the bone development of the fetus (Robyn et al., 2008). Women should be counseled and encouraged to take a vitamin D supplement during pregnancy. Although high levels of vitamin D have been thought to be associated with fetal malformations (Asary et al., 2010), the current literature indicates that high doses of vitamin D during pregnancy may reduce the risk of such pregnancy complications as gestational diabetes (Boyles, 2010). Women taking a vitamin D supplement should have levels monitored by their health care provider and receive nutritional counseling regarding fortified foods containing vitamin D.

Artificial sweeteners such as aspartame (Nutrasweet), sucralose (Splenda) are currently approved for consumption in moderation during pregnancy by the U.S. Food and Drug Administration (FDA). The artificial sweetener saccharin is approved for consumption by the general public; however, the FDA does not recommend the consumption of saccharin during pregnancy because it is known to cross the placenta and can remain in fetal tissue (Cleveland Clinic, 2011; Whitehouse, Boullata, McCauley, 2008). The World Health Organization (WHO) position on saccharin consumption during pregnancy is that it is safe when the amount ingested is within the acceptable daily intake (ADI) (for saccharin consumption during pregnancy, the ADI is 5 mg/kg/day) (Whitehouse, Boullata, McCauley, 2008).

Caffeine should be limited during pregnancy to 300 mg/day, which is equivalent to two 5-oz cups of coffee, three 5-oz cups of tea, and 12 oz of caffeinated soda (Cleveland Clinic, 2011). Limiting caffeine is recommended due to a potential association with spontaneous abortion and low-birth-weight infants.

Women should also be aware of food safety during pregnancy because of the risk of exposure to bacteria or parasites in certain foods (Cleveland Clinic, 2011). Foods that should be avoided are raw eggs, raw or rare meat, raw fish (sushi), unwashed fruits and vegetables; unpasteurized milk and milk products; and soft and blue-veined cheeses such as feta, brie,

and queso fresco or queso blanco (Cleveland Clinic, 2011). Other foods to avoid are hot dogs, luncheon/deli meats, rare beef, liver meat spreads, mayonnaise, and Caesar salad dressing (often prepared with raw egg) (Cleveland Clinic, 2011). All these foods should be avoided during pregnancy because of the risk of exposure to bacteria and parasites through hand-to-mouth transmission.

In addition, pregnant women can be exposed to parasites when handling a cat litter box. Maternal-acquired bacteria or parasites can be transmitted to the fetus. The fetal infection can cause spontaneous abortion, preterm delivery, or stillbirth (Cleveland Clinic, 2011). Some herbal products should also be avoided or used in moderation during pregnancy because they may contain substances that can cause serious adverse effects to the developing fetus (Khresheh, 2011). The National Center for Complementary and Alternative Medicine (NCCAM) has identified herbal teas containing chamomile, licorice, peppermint, and raspberry leaf as unsafe to consume during pregnancy (Badell, Ramin, & Smith, 2008). The FDA and the NCCAM urge caution with all herbal products during pregnancy and recommend that their use should be discussed with a health care provider.

Nausea and vomiting are common symptoms of pregnancy, affecting approximately 70–85% of pregnant women (Khresheh, 2011). The onset of these symptoms often begins between the fourth and seventh week after the first missed menstrual period and usually resolves by the 20th week of gestation. Nausea and vomiting without additional pathological symptoms indicating illness (fever, abdominal pain, jaundice, etc.) are usually associated with a positive pregnancy outcome. In addition, pregnant women commonly experience food and odor aversions or food cravings. Food cravings and food aversions are unlikely to have an adverse effect on the mother's nutritional status or weight as long as the overall diet is nutritionally balanced and sufficient.

The causes of nausea and vomiting during pregnancy are thought possibly to be due to changes in hormone levels, intestinal motility, dyspepsia (heartburn), and a heightened sensitivity of the sense of taste and smell (Khresheh, 2011). The first-line treatment for nausea and vomiting during pregnancy is a nonpharmacologic approach. Some pregnant women experience **hyperemesis gravidarum**, which is nausea and vomiting that do not improve or excessive and uncontrollable vomiting. These women usually require drug therapy (Badell, Ramin, & Smith, 2008). Ginger, an herbal product, is commonly used. The NCCAM recommends only the short-term use of ginger in moderate amounts to safely relieve symptoms during pregnancy (Ozgoli, Marjan, & Masoumeh, 2009). The FDA also considers ginger a safe herbal preparation for use in pregnancy (Ozgoli, Marjan, & Masoumeh, 2009). The recommended safe dose of ginger for use in pregnancy is 1000 mg/day (250 mg capsules 4 times a day) for no longer than 4 continuous days, and the dose can be repeated intermittently as long as it is not used for an extended period of time (Ozgoli, Marjan, & Masoumeh, 2009).

Besides nausea and vomiting, pregnant women experience numerous other discomforts, such as constipation, hemorrhoids, fatigue, backache, muscle cramps, edema, and heartburn. Table 9-2 lists recommendations to alleviate or reduce these common discomforts.

Pica is the practice of ingesting nonfood substances that have no nutritional value. Common examples of these substances are clay, chalk, laundry starch, paint chips, and soil. This practice is not unusual during pregnancy. Pica occurs in

TABLE 9-2 Common Complaints of Pregnancy

PROBLEM	RECOMMENDATIONS
Nausea/vomiting	Eat small, frequent, easily digested meals.
	Eat crackers upon arising.
	Drink fluids between meals, rather than with meals.
	Sip ginger tea or take ginger tablets.
	Take vitamin B_6 supplement 25 mg 3 times daily.
	Avoid sights and smells that trigger nausea.
	Use acupressure or acupuncture.
Constipation	Use bulk-forming, nonnutritive laxatives.
	Use a stool softener, such as docusate sodium.
	Exercise regularly.
	Drink 6–8 glasses of water daily.
Hemorrhoids	Avoid constipation.
	Apply topical anesthetics, witch hazel pads, and ice packs.
	Rest and sleep in side-lying position.
	Avoid straining while defecating.
Fatigue	Get adequate sleep and rest.
	Make sure diet is nutritionally adequate.
Backache	Practice the exercises of pregnancy (pelvic tilt, rocking back arch, etc).
	Avoid prolonged sitting or standing.
	Take warm tub baths.
	Use massage and relaxation techniques.
	Sleep on a firm, supportive mattress, in a side-lying position, and use pillows to support back and legs.
Calf/thigh/buttock muscle cramps	Avoid stretching legs, pointing toes, excessive walking.
	Do calf stretching exercises.
	Ensure adequate (not excessive) intake of dairy and calcium products.
Edema	Lie in a lateral recumbent position 1–2 hours/day.
	Avoid constrictive clothing on legs and arms.
	Get regular exercise.
Dyspepsia (heartburn)	Consume calcium carbonate, 1–2 tabs as needed.
	Avoid lying down, bending, or stooping for 2 hours after eating.
	Avoid restrictive clothing around waist.
	Avoid hot, spicy, fatty, gas-forming foods.
	Eat small, frequent meals.

© Cengage Learning 2013

approximately 25% of pregnant women in the United States (Corbiett, Ryan, & Weinrich, 2011). Contrary to popular myth, this practice is not derived from an actual physiologic craving or physiologic need. Pica is primarily attributed to cultural influence and folk customs; however, it does rarely occur in association with mental illness or psychological stress (Young, 2010). For example, among populations in areas of the southern United States, eating red clay is believed to protect the offspring from deformities (Murray, Zentner, & Yakimo, 2009, p. 220). The major concern with pica during pregnancy is that it may substitute nutritionless bulk for food containing good nutritional value. Another concern with pica during pregnancy is the risk of unknowingly consuming toxic or teratogenic substances, such as lead, that may be present in the ingested nonfood substances.

Substance Use

Alcohol is a known teratogen, and maternal intake at anytime during pregnancy can permanently damage fetal development (Sayla et al., 2009). A health-promotion strategy related to substance use is to screen all women of childbearing age for alcohol use or addiction and to provide them with education about the risks of alcohol use during pregnancy. In addition, health care providers should strongly urge pregnant women and women planning pregnancy to avoid alcohol. The adverse effects that can result from fetal exposure to alcohol are physical deformities, major cognitive impairment, growth restriction, and behavioral disorders (Perry, Hockenberry, Lowdermilk, & Wilson, 2010). Other problems associated with fetal alcohol exposure are attention deficit hyperactivity disorder (ADHD) and learning difficulty in childhood (Sayal, Hockenberry, Lowdermilk, & Wilson, 2009).

A safe amount of alcohol consumption during pregnancy is not currently known. Even small amounts of alcohol have the potential to result in permanent fetal damage. According to Murray et al. (2009), drinking as little as 3 oz of alcohol daily increases the risk of damage to fetal development and the risk of abruption placenta (p. 229). The maternal consumption of large amounts of alcohol at one time, also known as binge drinking, is thought to cause the greatest degree of permanent fetal damage (Sayal, Hockenberry, Lowdermilk, & Wilson, 2009). Many women develop an aversion to the taste and smell of alcoholic drinks during pregnancy and find it easy to avoid.

Another health-promotion strategy is counseling women that they should stop consuming alcohol at least 3 months before they plan to conceive. This can prevent the risk of fetal alcohol exposure before pregnancy is detected or confirmed. Health-promotion counseling regarding the avoidance of alcohol consumption during pregnancy should begin prior to conception and be reinforced throughout pregnancy. An important health-promotion strategy for pregnant women is to provide referrals for alcohol cessation programs and support, along with access to community support if needed.

Despite documented evidence that smoking cigarettes during pregnancy causes damage to a developing fetus, a substantial number of women continue to smoke throughout pregnancy. The prevalence of women in the United States who continue to smoke during pregnancy is approximately 12–15% of all pregnant women (Einarson & Riordan, 2009). These numbers are increasing annually, and the known significant fetal morbidity associated with maternal smoking demonstrates that this issue is a significant public health problem (Coleman, 2007). Cigarette smoke contains over 4000 toxic chemicals, including nicotine, and, of these chemicals, over 100 are known carcinogens. At least one of these carcinogens is known to cross the placenta (Oncken & Kranzler, 2009). Nicotine is also well-known to easily cross the placenta.

The nurse should advise smoking pregnant women that nicotine is not the only toxic chemical in cigarettes and that many other toxic chemicals can also be detrimental to fetal development. This information may have an impact on the maternal decision to quit smoking. The nurse should also inform pregnant women of the adverse effects of smoking during pregnancy that include "placenta previa, abruption placenta, spontaneous abortion, preterm birth, fetal growth restriction, low birth weight, sudden infant death syndrome (SIDS) as well as increase incidence of cleft palate and clubfoot in the newborn" (Einarson & Riordan, 2009, p. 326). In addition, specific cigarette toxic chemicals, such as carbon monoxide, nicotine, and lead, are well documented as fetal neurotoxines and detrimental to fetal growth (Oncken & Kranzler, 2009). According to a recent study by Lindbald & Hjern (2010), the incidence of ADHD in children born to mothers who smoked cigarettes during pregnancy is as high as four times greater than among children with mothers who did not smoke during pregnancy (p. 209).

The adverse effects of nicotine to the fetus are dose related: the greater the number of cigarettes consumed, the greater amount of nicotine that gets into the system. Because the effects of nicotine are dose related, even reducing the number of cigarettes to fewer than 10/day lowers the risks to the fetus. The nurse should provide information about available behavioral and pharmacologic smoking-cessation options. Behavioral counseling and techniques, including support groups for smoking cessation, are recommended as a first-line approach. The pharmacologic approach to smoking cessation in pregnancy commonly involves the drug bupropion (Zyban). Before making a decision for its use, pregnant women and the health care provider must consider a number of things about the drug. Bupropion has a high efficacy rate in smoking cessation, but it is categorized as an FDA pregnancy category C. A category C rating means that fetal risks cannot be ruled out. The decision must be based on whether the potential benefits of the drug outweigh the potential risks to the fetus from the drug compared to the risks from smoking. Nicotine patches or gums are not recommended during pregnancy because they contain nicotine, and nicotine is known to have adverse effects on the fetus. An additional method that may assist in smoking cessation is psychotherapy or group therapy.

The use of illegal drugs during pregnancy can lead to severe permanent damage to the developing fetus that can present as problems during infancy and that can continue into childhood. Cocaine use during pregnancy is associated with spontaneous abortion, abruption placenta, premature delivery, fetal growth retardation, and congenital defects. The use of heroin during pregnancy is associated with intrauterine growth restriction, infant hyperactivity, and severe withdrawal syndrome in the infant. Prematurity, low birth weight, and neurologic disturbances leading to tremors or jitteriness in the newborn may result from maternal use of marijuana (Murray, Zentner, & Yakimo, 2009). A health-promotion strategy is to screen all pregnant women for the use of illegal drugs. Pregnant women who are suspected or known to use illegal drugs should be referred to drug rehabilitation programs. The nurse should emphasize the adverse effects to the developing fetus of using illegal drugs during pregnancy. The nurse should be supportive and nonjudgmental, while offering access to community support groups and encouraging questions.

Screening

Couples should be screened for potential genetic disorders if they did not receive screening prior to conception. The areas to investigate are family history of genetic disorders, a previous fetus or child with a genetic disorder, or a history of recurrent miscarriage. Testing for neural tube defects and chromosomal abnormalities such as trisomy 21 (Down syndrome) and trisomy 18 (Edward syndrome) is available through serum triple-marker screening (human chorionic gonadotropin, unconjugated estriol, and alpha-fetoprotein [AFP] levels). These tests are usually performed at 16–18 weeks of gestation (Perry, Hockenberry, Lowdermilk, & Wilson, 2010, p. 204). Newer, less invasive screening for Down syndrome can be performed at 10–13 weeks of gestation. Women should be counseled that false positives and false negatives can occur with these tests. Pregnant women at increased risk for chromosomal abnormalities (Box 9-2) should be offered one of two tests: (1) an **amniocentesis**, which involves sampling the amniotic fluid through a transabdominal puncture with ultrasound guidance; (2) chorionic villus sampling (CVS), which involves obtaining a sample of the chorionic villi through the vagina. Amniocentesis can be performed after 15 weeks of gestation, and CVS is performed at 10–12 weeks of gestation. A definitive diagnosis of Down syndrome requires testing the amniotic fluid for AFP and chromosome analysis, combined with ultrasound

visualization of the fetus (Perry, Hockenberry, Lowdermilk, & Wilson, 2010). Each procedure carries a small risk of spontaneous abortion and maternal-fetal mixing of blood.

Health promotion during pregnancy requires early screening for asymptomatic bacteriuria, syphilis, rubella, hepatitis B, and HIV infection. Testing for gonorrhea, chlamydia, and bacterial vaginosis may also be indicated. A history of chicken pox and genital or orolabial herpes should be ascertained. All pregnant women should receive a vaginorectal swab for culture to screen for group B streptococcal infection. Screening for group B streptococcal infection should be done at 35–37 weeks of gestation. Each of these infectious diseases has a potential for severe and potentially fatal complications in the fetus or newborn.

As noted, one of the most effective means of preventing morbidity and mortality from infectious diseases among pregnant women and infants is immunization (Bruhn & Tillett, 2009). Because 50% of pregnancies in the United States are unintended, many pregnant women are not adequately immunized before they become pregnant. In general, live virus vaccines are contraindicated in pregnant women, and pregnancy should be delayed for 1 month after immunization with a live vaccine (CDC, 2011a). Inactivated vaccines contain killed organisms and are not contraindicated during pregnancy; however, vaccination should be delayed until the second trimester of pregnancy (CDC, 2011a). Immunization against polio is not recommended during pregnancy with either the live-virus or the inactivated-virus version (CDC, 2011a). Vaccination with inactivated influenza vaccine is recommended for all pregnant women during the influenza season (CDC, 2011a). All pregnant women should be tested for immunity to rubella, and women who are identified as nonimmune should be cautioned to avoid anyone with a rash or viral illness; they should also be immunized with the measles, mumps, and rubella (MMR) vaccine during the immediate postpartum period (Bruhn & Tillett, 2009). The varicella vaccine is also contraindicated during pregnancy; however, varicella-zoster immune globulin (VZIG) should be strongly considered for susceptible pregnant women who have been exposed (CDC, 2011a). If a pregnant woman contracts rubella, the rubella serum immunoglobulin will reduce her symptoms but will not alter the risk or the severity of congenital rubella syndrome in the newborn.

Pregnant women who have never been immunized for tetanus or diphtheria and those who have not received a booster within the last 10 years should be vaccinated. The vaccine for tetanus and diphtheria (Td) is made with toxoids and is considered safe during pregnancy. Immunization against polio with either the live-virus or the inactivated-virus version is not recommended during pregnancy. Pregnant women at risk of exposure to hepatitis B or hepatitis A can be given the vaccine or immune globulin. Rabies is a life-threatening disease, and the fatality rate is almost 100%. According to Wiwanitkit (2009), pregnant women who are at high risk for exposure to rabies or have been exposed to rabies are always vaccinated because the benefits of the vaccine greatly outweigh the potential risk of death (p. 1). The older version of the rabies vaccine is a live-virus vaccine. All currently available rabies vaccines are an inactivated form and are considered generally safe during pregnancy. "The current available immunoglobulin for rabies is highly purified and is known to be safe for use in pregnancy" (Wiwanitkit, 2009, p. 2).

All pregnant women should have blood type, Rh status, and atypical antibody titer screening early in pregnancy. Rh status refers to presence (Rh-positive) or absence (Rh-negative) of Rh antigen on the red blood cells. Rh-negative mothers can become sensitized (**isoimmunization**) as a result of exposure

---

BOX 9-2

RISK FACTORS FOR CHROMOSOMAL ABNORMALITIES

- Mother older than 35 with a singleton pregnancy
- Mother older than 32 with multiple fetus pregnancy
- Fetus with an identified structural anomaly
- Fetus with ultrasound showing increased fetal neck thickness (nuchal translucency)
- Mother with a previously affected pregnancy
- Couple with chromosomal abnormalities
- Mother with a positive maternal serum screen

to blood or blood products that contain an antigen not found on their own red blood cells. As a result, the mother's body produces antibodies to that antigen. If the fetus is Rh-positive and the mother is Rh-negative, maternal antibodies could be produced against fetal red blood cells. The effects can be the destruction of fetal red blood cells (hemolysis), resulting in severe anemia, liver failure, and ultimately fetal death. The incidence of isoimmunization of an Rh-negative mother to her Rh-positive fetus has significantly declined due to the administration of Rh immune globulin known as RhoGAM. The RhoGAM intramuscular injection is administered to nonsensitized Rh-negative women (1) during pregnancy at 28 weeks of gestation, (2) following any procedure where Rh-positive fetal blood might mix with Rh-negative maternal blood, and (3) within 72 hours after delivery of an Rh-positive newborn.

> **NURSING ALERT**
>
> ### Antihypertensive Medications during Pregnancy
>
> Pregnant women with chronic hypertension should not use angiotensin-converting enzyme inhibitors (ACEIs), angiotensin II receptor antagonists (ARBs), or thiazide diuretics during the first and second trimesters due to the possibility of birth defects. Methyldopa and calcium channel blockers can be safely used instead.

Pregnant women should be monitored for **gestational diabetes** (diabetes that occurs during pregnancy as a result of hormonal changes). Approximately 2–5% of women develop gestational diabetes. Increased rates of hypertensive disorders, large-for-gestational-age infants, and cesarean delivery are associated with this disorder. Women should be screened at 24–28 weeks of gestation using an oral glucose tolerance test. Treatment involves dietary intervention or intervention with insulin administration. The diabetes usually ceases with the end of the pregnancy; however, the mother is at increased risk to develop Type 2 diabetes later in life.

Pregnant women with chronic diseases require more frequent monitoring. Poorly controlled Type 1, insulin-dependent diabetes increases the rate of spontaneous abortion fetal anomalies and the incidence of stillbirth. Uncontrolled chronic hypertension increases the risk of preeclampsia, renal insufficiency, and intrauterine growth restriction of the fetus resulting from placental insufficiency.

Additional screening for pregnant women involves exploring the risk of exposure to hazards in the workplace or at home. Working pregnant women must be aware of any possible job-related exposure to hazardous substances or ionizing radiation. The prolonged exposure to pesticides and to solvents such as paint thinners and strippers must be avoided in the workplace and at home.

Exercise, Activity, and Sleep

Exercise recommendations during pregnancy have become less restrictive over the last decade. Physically fit women are encouraged to maintain a good fitness level throughout their pregnancy but to avoid trying to reach peak fitness or training for competition. Aerobic and strength-conditioning exercises with a low risk of loss of balance or fetal trauma are recommended. Previously inactive women are encouraged to start a program of moderate exercise. Pregnant women who do not participate in some form of exercise are at increased risk for loss of muscular and cardiovascular fitness, excessive weight gain, gestational diabetes, pregnancy-induced hypertension (PIH), the development of varicose veins, difficulty breathing, and low back pain. Table 9-3 lists other counseling issues during pregnancy.

> **NURSING ALERT**
>
> ### Important Precautions Against Maternal Infection
>
> Toxoplasmosis, cytomegalovirus (CMV), and parvovirus B19 (fifth disease) can infect the fetus if the mother becomes infected. Currently, there are no immunizations available for these viruses. The most effective prevention strategies to avoid contracting CMV or parvovirus B19 are good handwashing and avoiding exposure to infected individuals. Maternal infection of toxoplasmosis occurs through hand-to-mouth transmission of the parasite that causes the infection. The fetus becomes infected through transplacental transmission. To prevent contracting toxoplasmosis, avoid contact with cat feces in litter boxes, wear gloves while gardening, avoid handling raw or undercooked meat, wash fruits and vegetables thoroughly before eating them, and wash hands thoroughly following infant diaper changes.

Women may work during pregnancy as long as the pregnancy is uncomplicated and the workplace has no known hazards. Some modifications may need to be made, such as avoiding overtime hours, exhaustion, extreme temperatures, and noxious odors or fumes; taking breaks from long periods of standing or sitting; and avoiding strenuous work or lifting over 25 lb.

Sleep is important during pregnancy. Disturbed sleep occurs in approximately 78% of pregnant women. Problems sleeping can begin as early as 10 weeks of gestation, and by the third trimester some pregnant women report as little as 3–4 hours of sleep during the night due to increasing brief awakenings (Lee & Caughey, 2006). Awakenings during the night are often due to frequent urination and difficulty with positioning, especially in the third trimester. A study by Lee & Caughey (2006) found that "Pregnant women who sleep at least seven and a half hours with the majority of this time as undisturbed sleep are reported to have a shorter duration of labor" (p. 191). Lee & Caughey (2006) added that "Pregnant women that have frequent awakenings during sleep and increasing fewer hours of sleep are associated with a longer duration of labor and a higher incidence of cesarean section delivery compared to those women with adequate undisturbed sleep" (p. 191). A recent study found that an increase in the duration of labor that is associated with sleep deprivation can result from multiple factors, such as "mental and physical exhaustion, increased anxiety, increased stress hormone levels and elevated perception of pain" (Chang, Pien, Duntley, & Macones, 2010, p. 109).

TABLE 9-3 Counseling Issues During Pregnancy

CONCERN	TEACHING
Exercise	Get 30 minutes of moderate exercise daily.
	Avoid activities with risk of falls or abdominal injuries.
	Scuba diving is not recommended.
Workplace	Avoid prolonged standing or sitting.
	Avoid lifting more than 25 lb.
Travel	Air travel is generally safe until 4 weeks prior to the expected delivery.
	On lengthy trips, walk for 5–10 minutes every 2 hours; urinate every 2 hours.
	Have a list of obstetricians in the area and a copy of prenatal records.
	Avoid travel to high altitudes or in unpressurized airplanes.
	Discuss additional precautions for foreign travel with your health care provider.
Hot tubs, saunas	Avoid high temperatures due to the risk of fainting and risk of neural tube defects in the fetus during first trimester.
Hair treatments	Avoid hair dyes and treatments during the first trimester.
Medications, supplements, herbal remedies	Check with your health care provider before taking any medications (prescribed or over-the-counter), supplements, or herbal remedies.
Sex	Safe at any time during pregnancy except when membranes have ruptured or there is vaginal bleeding.
Constipation	Stool softeners may be needed to avoid constipation.

© Cengage Learning 2013

The increased stress hormones result in an altered physiological state with the onset of an "immunologically mediated process, altered glucose and fat metabolism, and an inflammatory process" (Chang, Pien, Duntley, & Macones, 2010, p. 109). All of these factors can have a detrimental effect on the labor process. Health-promotion strategies include encouraging women to schedule at least 8 hours in bed at night and reminding them that they are sleeping for two.

POSTPARTUM

The **postpartum** period is defined as the time between delivery and the return of a woman's reproductive organs to the nonpregnant state, generally about 6 weeks. Just as in pregnancy, the postpartum woman is faced with enormous physiological changes, which are necessary to accomplish physical restoration. Postpartum health-promotion strategies in the biological domain include nutrition, rest/sleep/activity, contraception, screening, and immunizations.

During the postpartum period, the mother's body begins to return to the nonpregnant state. The new mother should continue a well-balanced diet that includes protein, plenty of fruits and vegetables; dairy products, and a high fluid intake. A daily multivitamin supplement is also recommended during this period. Caloric intake should remain about the same as during pregnancy. High fluid intake is especially important if the mother is breast-feeding her infant. Lactation uses about 500 cal a day in the production of breast milk but should not be touted as a magic way to lose weight following childbirth. The more weight the mother gains during the pregnancy, the more she needs to lose after the pregnancy. Women who gain excessive weight during pregnancy are more likely to be overweight or obese following delivery.

Early ambulation following delivery provides a sense of well-being and promotes the return of the reproductive organs to their prepregnancy state. However, the new mother should not resume all of her previous activities immediately after delivery.

? ASK YOURSELF

Cesarean Section Trend

The rate of cesarean section delivery in the United States has continued to increase annually over approximately the last 15 years. According to the National Center for Health Statistics, cesarean section deliveries increased from 31.8% in 2007 to 32.3% in 2008. These rates continue to increase at a steady trend among all births including full-term, uncomplicated, and first-time births. This rising trend can be attributed to physician or maternal preference, decreased rates of vaginal births after a previous cesarean section (VBAC), and physician concerns regarding malpractice lawsuits in the occurrence of complications during a vaginal delivery. What is your opinion regarding this trend? What are the potential consequences for the mother and for the baby? What is the financial impact of having a cesarean section delivery compared to a vaginal delivery?

Rest is essential as the new mother adjusts to her new routine. Many new mothers do not get enough sleep during the night and should be encouraged to rest or nap when the infant is sleeping.

An exercise program to strengthen the muscles of the back, pelvic floor, and abdomen can be started within the first week postpartum; however, strenuous or excessive exercise should be postponed until approximately 3 weeks after delivery. New mothers can begin with a single exercise consisting of 5 repetitions done 3 times a day. Additional exercises can be added one at a time. Moderate exercise during lactation does not adversely affect breast milk production.

Pregnancy and childbirth are major risk factors for the development of **urinary incontinence** (the involuntary leakage of urine). Women with antenatal urinary incontinence, obesity, significant perineal trauma during delivery, delivery of large infants, and multiple pregnancies may be at increased risk for urinary incontinence. Urinary incontinence after childbirth is not uncommon and is usually temporary; however, many women continue to experience incontinence throughout their lives. Pelvic floor muscle exercises (also known as **Kegel exercises**) to strengthen the perivaginal and perianal musculature are recommended immediately postpartum to reduce or resolve urinary leakage.

A postpartum health-promotion strategy is to provide both parents with information regarding contraceptive methods prior to discharge from the hospital. New mothers should be informed that breast-feeding is not an effective birth control method and that a woman can become pregnant even if her menses has not resumed. The potential for pregnancy increases dramatically in breast-feeding women who have resumed their menstruation.

Postpartum women who are not immune to rubella should be immunized in the immediate postpartum period. Prior to discharge, new mothers should also receive a pertussis vaccination, which lowers the risk of exposure to the infant and protects the mother. All adults and adolescents who will have contact with the infant should also be immunized for pertussis to further decrease the risk of the infant's exposure. Infants younger than 12 months of age typically have the most severe clinical manifestation and morbidity related to pertussis (CDC, 2010). The risk of death from pertussis is highest among infants in the first 6 months of life and remains high until infants have received 1–2 doses of the pediatric pertussis vaccine (DTap) (CDC, 2010). The second dose of the DTap should occur by the time that the infant is 4 months old. Postpartum women who plan to breast-feed should be informed that breast-feeding is not contraindicated with maternal immunization against rubella or pertussis in the postpartum period (CDC, 2010).

PSYCHOLOGICAL AND SOCIOLOGICAL DOMAINS

The psychological domain involves individual feelings, behavior, and changes in behavior. The social domain encompasses social networks such as families, social groups, organizations, and communities.

A significant psychosocial development in the life of a woman is the decision to parent. In an ideal world, every pregnancy would be planned and wanted, resulting in a loved and wanted child. Pregnancy, whether planned or unplanned, brings with it enormous emotional upheavals, adjustments, and consequences. Having a child has a significant impact on the parents, on the family social networks, and on the individuals with whom the parents have bonded or maintained significant contact.

Preconception

Preconception care should include psychosocial evaluation and counseling. Couples should be encouraged to discuss the decision to attempt a pregnancy and how this decision will affect their lives and relationship. The couple's social, financial, and psychological readiness for pregnancy and commitment to parenthood should be assessed. In some communities, preconception classes are available through adult education programs. Preconception education has the potential to improve parenting skills and pregnancy outcomes. Providing information about fetal growth and development promotes intrauterine bonding between parent and child, as well as health-promotion behavior. Preconception counseling gives prospective parents the opportunity to make informed decisions and lifestyle adjustments in order to promote a successful pregnancy outcome.

Pregnancy

Psychological issues during pregnancy can include depression, emotional liability, low self-esteem, and body image disturbances. Changes in hormone levels during pregnancy can lead to fluctuations in feelings of anxiety, depression, sadness, elation, and confusion. Many women are unable to discuss their negative emotions and feelings for fear of being perceived as not wanting the pregnancy. Most women have self-esteem and body image issues as they go through a period of emotional adjustment to the changes occurring in their body.

The main health-promotion strategy is to help women understand that these feelings, emotions, and changes are normal and will resolve after the pregnancy. Health care providers must be able to recognize the spectrum of normal emotions, as well as to recognize the mental health problems during pregnancy and that have the potential of becoming serious and adversely affecting pregnancy outcomes. Mental health problems that can occur during pregnancy include anxiety and depression.

All pregnant women experience stress; however, high-level physical or emotional stress can be harmful for pregnant women, causing fatigue, sleeplessness, anxiety, poor appetite or overeating, headaches, and backaches. Pregnancy-related discomforts (nausea, fatigue, frequent urination, swelling, and backache) are temporary sources of stress that can be reduced with a healthy diet, regular exercise, and adequate rest and sleep. Pregnant women should not expect to do everything they did before pregnancy. Seeking support and assistance from the partner, family members, relatives, friends, and health care provider is important. The quality of social support for a woman during pregnancy is associated with positive pregnancy outcomes. The lack of social support has been identified as a risk factor for depression during pregnancy (Blanchard et al., 2009). In addition, the partner relationship is the most important aspect of social support during pregnancy (Blanchard et al., 2009). Health care providers may be able to discuss stress reduction/relaxation techniques, as well as find resources in the community to help in coping with the stress and emotional changes of pregnancy. The majority of women are able to adjust to the physical and psychological changes of pregnancy; however, some women need additional assistance and support.

The reported prevalence of depression during pregnancy is approximately 14–23% of pregnant women (Yonkers et al., 2009). Depression during pregnancy can affect the mother's ability to obtain prenatal care and avoid negative behaviors.

BOX 9-3

SYMPTOMS OF DEPRESSION

A depressed mood lasting for 2 weeks or longer with five or more of the following:

- Sleep disturbances or excessive sleeping
- Lack of interest or pleasure in activities that were once enjoyable
- Feelings of guilt, worthlessness, or helplessness
- Feelings of hopelessness or pessimism
- Persistent sad, anxious, or empty mood
- Decreased energy and fatigue
- Difficulty concentrating and difficulty with memory
- Difficulty making decisions
- Changes in appetite and/or weight
- Restlessness or slowed movement and irritability
- Suicidal thoughts, thoughts of death, or suicide attempts
- Persistent somatic complaints

Source: National Institute of Mental Health, National Institutes of Health (n.d.). http://www.nimh.nih.gov/health/publications/depression-in-women/index.shtml

---

These women are also more likely to smoke cigarettes, drink alcohol, or use illegal drugs (Yonkers et al., 2009). The negative behaviors that can result from depression during pregnancy can lead to adverse effects that result in poor maternal and fetal pregnancy outcomes. Box 9-3 lists the symptoms associated with depression.

Given the prevalence of depression during pregnancy, an important health-promotion strategy is to screen all pregnant women for depression and to arrange for the appropriate treatment and monitoring. Adding to the importance of screening is that depression during pregnancy is one of the greatest predictors of postpartum depression (Bansil et al., 2010). Risk factors associated with the incidence of depression during pregnancy are a personal and/or family history of mood disorder, marital conflict and domestic violence, limited social support, a history of significant stress, and substance abuse (Gossler, 2010).

Nurses can play a valuable role in identifying women experiencing depression during pregnancy; therefore, they must be able to understand the prevalence, signs and symptoms, and risk factors associated with depression during pregnancy. Nurses should also provide education about depression to pregnant women, their partners, and their family. In addition, nurses must support pregnant women experiencing depression in their treatment decisions. Treatment for depression during pregnancy can be very effective using both pharmacological and/or nonpharmacological methods (Goodman & Tyer-Viola, 2010). An example of a nonpharmacological, first-line treatment modality is behavioral therapy in the form of support groups, counseling, or psychotherapy. The pharmacologic treatment choice depends on weighing the benefits of a medication versus the possible adverse effects on the fetus from the medication (Yonkers et al., 2009).

The screening of all pregnant women should also include assessment for domestic violence. Domestic violence occurs across all social, economic, educational, and professional settings. Domestic violence encompasses domestic abuse, intimate partner violence, or battery. The term *intimate partner violence* (IPV) is the one of choice in this section. Violence during pregnancy poses a significant threat to maternal and fetal health and a significant risk of death for both. The prevalence of IPV is approximately 4.8–5.3 million annually among women over 18 years of age in the United States (CDC, 2011; Kramer, 2007). The prevalence of IPV among pregnant women is reported to be approximately 5–22% of all women (Antoniou, Vivilake, & Daglas, 2008). Unintended pregnancy is a risk factor associated with IPV. The prevalence of IPV is reported to increase by 25% during the postnatal period (Antoniou, Vivilake, & Daglas, 2008). Intimate partner violence may include coercion, threatening or harassing behavior, intimidation, and isolation, in addition to emotional, sexual, and physical abuse.

The nurse and the health care team usually have multiple opportunities to perform risk and physical assessment for IPV. Screening questions can be found in Box 9-4. IPV in pregnancy is a serious health care issue and is associated with an increased risk of miscarriage, infection, preterm labor, placental

---

BOX 9-4

SCREENING FOR DOMESTIC VIOLENCE (INTIMATE PARTNER VIOLENCE)

Preliminary questions:

- Are you in immediate danger?
- Are you afraid your life may be in danger?
- Do you ever feel unsafe at home?
- Has your partner ever threatened to kill you, himself/herself, or your children?
- Has your partner ever held you or your children against your will?
- Do you want to or feel like you have to go home with your partner?
- Has your partner physically hurt or threatened you?
- Are you afraid your partner will harm you or someone close to you?
- Do you have somewhere safe to go?

Additional questions for positive responses:

- Have you ever felt afraid of your partner or expartner?
- Has your partner or expartner:
  - Ever hit, grabbed, slapped, choked, or kicked you?
  - Forced you to have sexual activities you did not want to do?
  - Threatened to hurt you, your children, or someone close to you?
  - Stalked, followed, or monitored you?
- Has your partner emotionally abused you?

abruption, and low–birth-weight babies. Intimate partner violence during pregnancy has a significant impact on the maternal outcomes associated with depression, anxiety, delay or inadequate attendance of prenatal care, and drug and alcohol use (Shoffner, 2008). IPV has been found to be one of the strongest predictors of depression during pregnancy (Shoffner, 2008).

The prevalence of IPV and the associated maternal and fetal outcome indicates a crucial need to assess for IPV. The American College of Obstetricians and Gynecologists (ACOG) recommends screening all women for abuse during every trimester of pregnancy and postpartum (Kramer, 2007). Clinical studies have proven the effectiveness of the abuse assessment screen (AAS), which is a very brief screening tool designed to detect abuse in pregnant women (Rabin et al., 2009). Nurses are in a key position to help identify pregnant women experiencing IPV through the use of a screening tool along with establishing a caring and trusting therapeutic and patient-centered relationship with abused women. Nursing has long practiced active patient-nurse partnerships within a caring and therapeutic relationship (Swanson, 1993). The focus on patient-centered care for abused pregnant women, provided in a sensitive, honest, and respectful manner, is very helpful because it may be different from how they are treated by others and can help to establish a trusting relationship between the abused woman and the nurse. Nurses should honor the woman's right and capacity for self-direction and autonomy (Kramer, 2007). The nurse can facilitate the abused women in a healthier and safer direction by listening and learning about her experiences and perceptions of the abuse (Kramer, 2007). Nurses can offer guidance based on the woman's goals, needs, and values rather than impose their advice about what the women "should do." Nurses and other health care providers can significantly help abused pregnant women by showing empathy, genuine concern, and respect.

Cultural and psychological factors and possibly hormone changes may cause the expectant father to experience pregnancylike symptoms. The symptoms experienced by the expectant father are grouped as a syndrome that has a medical term known as **couvade**, which means sympathetic pregnancy experienced by the father. This term was first used to describe the practice in which the expectant father simulates labor and childbirth; the term now includes the sharing of pregnancylike symptoms. Couvade is thought to be a universal phenomenon that occurs across cultures.

It is estimated that 11–65% of expectant fathers experience pregnancylike symptoms that vary widely and typically occur during the first and third trimesters. The physical symptoms may include nausea and other gastrointestinal complaints, weight gain, fatigue, and difficulty sleeping; all of these symptoms are very similar to those of their pregnant partner. In addition, they may experience psychological symptoms such as anxiety, depression, restlessness, appear detached, and reduced libido (Melrose, 2010).

Nurses can help expectant fathers identify concerns and prepare for the reality of a new baby by asking questions about what the father expects the new baby to look like, what he thinks the experience of being a father will be like, and what thoughts he has about holding a crying baby, changing diapers, and being awakened at night (Melrose, 2010). The nurse should encourage the expectant father to ask questions especially as the birthday approaches. The nurse should also tell the father about the unborn baby's ability to respond to sound and encourage him to touch the mother's pregnant abdomen and

to talk to the fetus. Doing so helps to establish paternal-fetal bonding. One very helpful activity is attending prenatal classes. The nurse has a key role in promoting a positive pregnancy and birth experience for the father as well as for the mother.

Postpartum

Rapid hormonal changes, the lack of sleep, and meeting the demands of new infant care frequently cause the new mother to experience mood swings, depression, difficulty concentrating, and lack of appetite. These so-called baby blues usually start about 3–4 days after delivery and may last for several days. The baby blues are considered a normal part of early motherhood and usually goes away within about 10 days after delivery. Health-promotion strategies for dealing with these normal feelings are found in Box 9-5. Health care providers should note that baby blues are normal and that this condition is not the same as postpartum depression. Postpartum depression is a serious psychological disorder that requires immediate medical attention.

Women who have more severe symptoms than those of the baby blues or whose symptoms last longer may have postpartum depression (PPD) and requires immediate attention. This type of depression has significant negative effects on the new mother and is especially detrimental to the infant. Risk factors for the development of this more serious severe form of depression include previously having postpartum depression; a previous diagnosis of depression not related to pregnancy; relationship problems with the significant other; a lack of social support; and the presence of stressful life events (Baker & Oswalt, 2008). The single greatest predictor of postpartum depression has been found to be depression during pregnancy (Knudson-Martin & Silverstein, 2009). Postpartum depression is reported to occur in 10–20% of women in the first 6 months after delivery.

The harmful effects to the infant and family associated with postpartum depression are a lack of maternal-infant bonding, cognitive and social developmental delays, psychological issues later in life, and inadequate family functioning (Leahy-Warren & McCarthy, 2007). Postpartum depression is considered a medical emergency and, if left untreated, can lead to suicide and infanticide (Spinelli, 2003).

BOX 9-5

HEALTH-PROMOTION STRATEGIES FOR THE COMMON AND NORMAL BABY BLUES

Talk to someone such as a friend, relative, or health care provider.

Find someone to help you with child care, household chores, and errands.

Take 15 minutes a day for yourself: Read, exercise, take a bath, or meditate.

Keep a diary, and write down your emotions as a way of letting them out.

Don't be upset if you can't get everything done. Don't try to be a super mom.

Recognize that it's OK to feel overwhelmed with the changes and challenges.

RESEARCH NOTE

Detection, Treatment, and Referral of Perinatal Depression and Anxiety by Obstetrical Providers

STUDY PROBLEM/PURPOSE

Depression can occur in pregnant women and can affect birth outcomes. The purpose of the study was to assess the rates of detection, treatment, and referral of maternal depression by obstetrical providers during pregnancy and at 6 weeks postpartum.

METHODS

Four hundred ninety-one women receiving obstetrical care at a large urban teaching hospital were recruited from two hospital-affiliated obstetrical clinics that serve an ethnically and socioeconomically diverse population of pregnant and postpartum women. The women were assessed for symptoms of depression and anxiety using a questionnaire; electronic medical records were also reviewed 2 months after delivery for the documentation of psychiatric symptoms, psychiatric diagnosis, psychiatric treatments, and referrals to psychiatric services. Sixty-one percent of the participants completed the 6-week postpartum questionnaire. Participant race/ethnicity included 279 White, 129 Latina, and 81 who reported Other as race/ethnicity. All participants were in the third trimester of pregnancy, able to read or speak English or Spanish, and 18 years of age or older. Household income ranged from $19,999 to $100,000.

FINDINGS

One hundred thirteen women (23%) screened positive for symptoms of depression or anxiety during the third trimester; only 46 (41%) had any documentation of psychiatric symptoms or diagnosis in medical record; of these, only 17 (37%) had documented mental health treatment. Nine women who had documented psychiatric symptoms or diagnosis in the medical record had no documentation of treatment or referral. At 6 weeks postpartum, 51 (17%) women screened positive for symptoms of depression or anxiety; only 15 (29.4%) of these had any documentation of psychiatric symptoms or diagnosis in the medical record; and only 13 (25.5%) had documented postpartum mental health treatment.

IMPLICATIONS

Determining the optimal time for screening is important. Almost half of the women who screened positive for postpartum depression had screened positive prenatally. Screening women for symptoms of depression and anxiety during pregnancy can identify women at high risk for postpartum depression. The early identification and effective management of prenatal depression and anxiety would have the greatest overall impact and minimize negative maternal and newborn outcomes.

Source: Goodman, J. H., & Tyer-Viola, L. (2010). Detection, treatment, and referral of perinatal depression and anxiety by obstetrical providers. *Journal of Women's Health, 19*(3): 477–486.

Postpartum depression affects the entire family. New fathers often experience symptoms of postpartum depression. The prevalence of depression in new fathers is approximately 4–25% with 1 in every 4 men being affected. The prevalence of paternal postpartum depression is higher when maternal postpartum depression is present. In addition, maternal postpartum depression is the strongest predictor of depression in new fathers (Melrose, 2010). Paternal symptoms of depression include some that are similar to maternal symptoms of depression. The hallmark symptoms of PPD in the new father are withdrawal from social situations, indecisiveness, cynicism, and an irritable mood (Melrose, 2010). Another typical manifestation of paternal depression is an affect that presents more as anxious or angry instead of sad. New fathers experiencing depression are at higher risk of engaging in avoidance behavior, drinking, drug use, extramarital affairs, and intimate partner violence (Melrose, 2010).

Risk factors for paternal depression include a personal history of depression, maternal depression, and changes in the couple's relationship and functioning. In new fathers, financial concerns associated with a new baby lead to a great deal of stress, which can become chronic and lead to paternal depression. The children of depressed parents are more likely to develop social, behavioral, physical, and psychological impairments (Melrose, 2010). Untreated paternal depression may limit the father's capacity to provide emotional support to his partner and child. Paternal depression can also significantly limit the father's ability to function at work, compounding the problem by creating financial problems. Untreated depression in new fathers can persist for up to a year, if not longer (Melrose, 2010).

A health-promotion strategy is to identify new fathers for paternal depression. The nurse should remain aware of the potential predisposition to depression in new fathers and should take advantage of any contact with the new father, asking candidly if he feels depressed, anxious, or angry. This type of encounter can open communication for further exploration and may help the new father feel that he has support and understanding. Nurses can significantly help new fathers by telling them that this disorder is real and that it occurs in many new fathers. The nurse should emphasize that they are not alone and that treatment is available. In addition, nurses should provide new fathers with verbal and written information about paternal depression. The nurse should also be familiar with Internet Websites regarding paternal depression and share these with new fathers. Nurses should advocate for the inclusion of information about paternal depression in existing maternal postpartum depression programs and increase public awareness about this disorder in new fathers.

The most important health-promotion strategy is screening for postpartum depression in order to identify and treat women as early as possible because of the potential serious adverse effects to the mother and the infant. The best opportunity for the identification of maternal postpartum depression is at the mother's postpartum visit or the infant's checkup. New fathers may accompany the mother to these visits. The nurse should take advantage of any opportunity for contact with new fathers to identify depression. Maternal and paternal postpartum depression is treated much like any other depression with support, counseling, and medication.

Some women feel better within a few weeks, but others feel depressed for several months. Some postpartum women may experience psychosis. This situation is critical and a medical emergency requiring immediate intervention to prevent possible harm to the infant. The nurse should counsel the new mother by telling her that postpartum depression occurs in many new mothers, offering support by telling her that help is available and that she can get better. The nurse should reassess women with postpartum depression at every contact to monitor for worsening symptoms and the risk of developing psychosis. Box 9-5 describes health-promotion strategies for dealing with the baby blues.

Another psychosocial issue that may occur during the postpartum period is sibling rivalry. Parents can encourage older children to verbalize their emotions, role-play the safe handling of a newborn with a doll, tolerate some regression, and give the older children individual attention each day. Encouraging grandparents and other visitors to pay attention to the older children first is also helpful.

POLITICAL DOMAIN

The political domain in health-promotion encompasses governmental efforts in legislating environmental and behavioral changes that promote health. Laws affecting the mother's mental and physical health during the preconception, pregnancy, and postpartum periods are discussed in the following sections.

Preconception

Women should have the right to make informed reproductive decisions without interference from social and political entities. This right should include access to infertility care, contraception, abortion services, and adequate information about these reproductive options. There has not been any social or political assault on access to infertility care, but contraception and abortion continue to generate controversy in the political and social arenas. Not until 1965 did the use of contraception became legal, but only by married individuals, as the result of the 1965 Supreme Court ruling in *Griswold v. Connecticut,* which overturned a Connecticut law that prohibited contraception use by anybody. This law was ruled as unconstitutional by violating marital privacy. In 1972, the Supreme Court declared the ban on the use of contraceptives by unmarried individuals as unconstitutional in the case of *Eisenstadt v. Baird.* The result of this case was that the Supreme Court extended the right to use contraceptives to all people, married or single. Although contraceptive use is now legal in the United States, a significant barrier exists to the access of contraceptives. Health insurance does not cover prescription contraceptives, and a lack of access to contraceptives can result in increased unintended pregnancies. Primarily due to the cost of unintended pregnancy, the expense to an employer/insurer is 15–17% more than providing contraceptive health insurance coverage. Contraceptive equity legislation requiring health insurance coverage of prescription contraceptives can significantly impact women's health by

making contraceptives affordable. And it will increase the use of contraceptives and lower the numbers of unintended pregnancies. In addition, the drop in unintended pregnancies can lessen the adverse effects to the mother and fetus that are associated with unintended pregnancies, in addition to reducing the costs associated with poor pregnancy outcomes.

Access to safe and effective prescription contraception is an essential component of women's health care, yet many health insurance plans exclude coverage for such prescriptions. In addition, self-insured employers are exempt from state contraceptive equity law. As of 2011, 34 states mandate some form of contraceptive equity laws that impose requirements on insurers to provide coverage of FDA-approved prescription contraceptive drugs and devices on terms comparable to those of other prescription drugs (Lee, 2011). Twenty-eight states out of the 34 states with contraceptive impose exemptions and partial mandates for certain employer groups and insurers (Lee, 2011). The state contraception equity laws contain a loophole, or so-called refusal clause, which is imposed on the basis of religious objection to contraception. Some states use this to escape the imposed requirements of contraceptive equity laws. Eighteen states permit religious employers to refuse to provide contraceptive coverage, and three states permit religious insurers to refuse coverage (Lee, 2011). Seven states do not offer exemption provisions for insurers to refuse contraceptive coverage on religious grounds (Lee, 2011). Currently, 18 states out of the 26 that have contraceptive equity laws impose the refusal clause due to religious objection to contraception.

The availability and use of safe and effective emergency contraception (EC) has also been a subject of political and legal controversy. Emergency contraception is used to reduce the risk of pregnancy after unprotected sexual intercourse or contraception failure. It is not a method of terminating pregnancy. Emergency contraception in the United States originated in the 1960s only as a treatment for rape victims, required a physician's prescription, and had to be administered in a health care setting. In 1999, the FDA approved a form of EC known as Plan B. This was the first progestin-only EC in the United States and available only with a prescription (Sanap, Laddha, & Singh, 2011). The dosing of Plan B involved taking two pills. The first pill was taken as soon as possible after unprotected sexual intercourse or contraceptive failure. The second pill was 12 hours after the first pill. The FDA decision to allow Plan B to be available without a prescription for women 18 years and older was delayed due to political opposition and pressure. In 2006, the FDA approved Plan B for women 18 years and older without a prescription (Sanap, Laddha, & Singh, 2011). Plan B was approved for women younger than 18 years of age only with a prescription. In March of 2009, a U.S. District Court ordered the FDA to lower the age for the use of Plan B to women 17 years and older without a prescription (Sanap, Laddha, & Singh, 2011).

A few months later, in September 2009, the FDA approved a new EC known as Plan B One Step, which was intended to replace the old Plan B. Plan B One Step was the first safe and effective single-pill dose of EC in the United States and is currently available for women 17 years and older without a prescription, although a prescription is required if younger than 17 years of age (Sanap, Laddha, & Singh, 2011). The Plan B One Step pill, as directed by the FDA, should be taken as soon as possible following unprotected sexual intercourse or contraception failure. Plan B One Step is frequently taken after the recommended 72-hour period and has still been effective in some women. However, if the Plan B One Step pill is taken after the first 24 hours, the efficacy fades slightly; when taken after 72 hours, the efficacy drops significantly.

A generic equivalent of the old Plan B, known as Next Choice (single-pill dose), was available in the United States shortly after the FDA approval of Plan B One Step in 2009 (Sanap, Laddha, & Singh, 2011). The generic Next Choice is 10–20% less expensive than Plan B One Step and is equally safe and effective (Sanap, Laddha, & Singh, 2011). The current cost of Plan B One Step is approximately $35–45 on average in the United States.

In 2010, the FDA approved a new safe and effective form of prescription-only EC known as Ella. The significant distinction of Ella is that it can be taken up to 5 days (120 hours) after unprotected sex or contraceptive failure. Ella should not be taken if pregnancy is known or suspected.

The use of EC is best known for use by women who have been raped. EC, when used correctly, can help many rape victims avoid the additional trauma of facing an unwanted pregnancy. Emergency contraception is also appropriate for women who have experienced contraceptive failure such as condom breaks, who failed to use contraception because they were not planning on having sex, or who had unprotected intercourse for any other reason. Emergency contraception is underused in the United States with 1 in 3 women of reproductive age being unaware of emergency contraception. Although the American College of Obstetricians and Gynecologists recommends that physicians routinely discuss emergency contraception with women of reproductive age during their annual visit, only 1 in 4 obstetricians/gynecologists actually discuss emergency contraception with their patients. This strongly suggests the need for greater health care provider patient education. Health-promotion demands strategies to educate women of reproductive age about emergency contraception. This education can impact women's health by potentially preventing as many as 1 million unwanted/unintended pregnancies annually in the United States. This educational opportunity is most often at a women's annual exam or a well child visit. The nurse must encourage questions about the information provided. Nurses, especially community health nurses, can be very helpful in promoting public awareness campaigns targeting women and health care providers about emergency contraception. This can help to widely disseminate knowledge about emergency contraception as an important means of pregnancy prevention to women in the United States. A toll-free hotline and a Website with information about emergency contraception are listed at the end of this chapter.

Throughout the centuries, unwanted and unplanned pregnancies worldwide have resulted in abortion, whether legal or illegal. In 1973, the right to privacy was extended to abortion in the *Roe v. Wade* Supreme Court decision, which legalized abortion. Since the 1973 legalization of abortion, many states have proposed bills and enacted laws that restrict women's reproductive rights and create obstacles for women obtaining abortion services. In 1976, a state statute mandated that a husband must provide consent for married women to have an abortion procedure. The same year, 1979, the Supreme Court ruled in *Planned Parenthood v. Danforth* to invalidate the requirement of a husband's consent for married women to obtain an abortion. In the 1992 case *Planned Parenthood v. Casey*, some of the requirements in the Supreme Court ruling included a detailed informed consent with abortion-specific medical information and a waiting period between the abortion and the informed consent.

Currently, at least 23 states include information that is not in keeping with the fundamental tenets of informed consent. Some of these states use graphic, inflammatory language to describe the abortion procedure especially in a late abortion (Gold & Nash, 2007). All states now include objective information about the size and weight of the fetus at various stages. According to Gold & Nash (2007), information required to be provided by some states includes that "the fetus now has a distinct human appearance, the eyelids are formed, and the fetus sleeps and awakens" (p. 10). In 2005, South Dakota law required the physician performing the abortion to make the statement to the woman that the embryo/fetus is a "unique human being" (Siegel, 2007). Some states include in their abortion-specific informed consent material a statement, dictated by the state, that "the unborn child has the physical structures necessary to experience pain" (Richardson & Nash, 2006). Mandatory-delay state laws, which require women to wait at least 24 hours after receiving required information about abortion, can be an obstacle for women seeking abortion services. In some cases, delay period laws that require a second trip to the abortion provider can potentially place women at increased risk for intimate partner violence if the partner becomes aware of the woman's plans.

Since 1996, several states began proceedings for legislation to make ultrasound part of abortion services. Sixteen states currently have enacted some form of ultrasound legislation, and similar bills have been introduced in 14 other states (Sanger, 2008). However, the requirement of an ultrasound creates an obstacle. Some of the states that require an ultrasound prior to an abortion are required to offer women the ultrasound image (Wiebe & Adams, 2009). In 2010, Nebraska was the first state to pass into law and enact the Unborn Child Pain Awareness and Prevention Act. This law requires the physician performing an abortion at 20 weeks of gestation or greater to inform the woman, through written material or verbally and at least 24 hours prior to the procedure, that the unborn child is capable of feeling pain and that she has the option of having pain-reducing medication administered to the fetus (Gold & Nash, 2007). Following Nebraska, seven other states passed into law the Unborn Child Pain Awareness and Prevention Act in 2010–2011.

Pregnancy

During pregnancy, women are provided protections under the law. Although working women are not guaranteed paid maternity leave or insurance reimbursement during pregnancy, pregnant women do have protection against discrimination and, in many cases, are allowed unpaid leave. They also have protection against the risk of exposure to hazards in the workplace that might injure the fetus.

The Pregnancy Discrimination Act of 1978 requires employers with 15 or more employees to treat pregnant workers as any other employees with medical or disability conditions. It prevents an employer from firing a pregnant woman based on her pregnancy or a pregnancy-related illness or from forcing her to take a mandatory pregnancy or maternity leave. Pregnant women have the right to modified work tasks, to work as long as they are able, and to have their jobs protected during maternity leave.

Postpartum

The Family and Medical Leave Act of 1993 requires companies with 50 or more employees to allow a pregnant mother or her partner to take up to 12 weeks of unpaid leave in the 12-month period following the birth of their baby. Pregnant women may take this leave intermittently or for the full 12 weeks at one time. Typically, an employee must have worked a minimum of one full year with the company to qualify for benefits under the Family Leave Act. Information about pregnancy rights and family leave can be obtained from the U.S. Department of Labor. Recent federal legislation has positively affected mothers that are breast-feeding through the Patient Protection and Affordable Care Act (2010). This Act requires employers to provide reasonable break time for nursing employees to express breast milk. This applies to nursing mothers for one year after the birth of their baby. In addition, the employer must provide a place to express breast milk, other than the bathroom, that is shielded from view and free from intrusion to allow for privacy. This legislation has the potential to significantly impact the health of women and infants by promoting a longer duration of breast-feeding because working is one of the barriers to continue breast-feeding.

Environmental Domain

The environmental domain is defined as **exogenous** (originating outside the body) and includes conditions and substances that impact the reproductive health of women. A woman of childbearing age and in pregnancy can be exposed to various chemicals in the work setting, her home, or other environments.

Preconception and Pregnancy

During the preconception period and pregnancy (primarily the first trimester when organogenesis occurs), exposure to

---

✳ NURSING **ALERT**

Seat Belt Use during Pregnancy

Motor vehicle crashes are the leading cause of accidental fetal mortality worldwide. In the United States each year, approximately 130,000 pregnant women are involved in a motor vehicle crash during the second half of pregnancy (Acar & van Lopik, 2009). Among these women, 30,000 sustain nonfatal injuries and approximately 160 die. The pregnant women who survive have between 300 and 3800 fetal deaths (Acar & van Lopik, 2009). When traveling in a car, all pregnant women should use shoulder and lap belts for three-point restraint. The lap portion should be placed below the abdomen and across the upper thighs. The shoulder portion should rest between the breasts. Both belts should be worn snugly. A driver-side airbag also provides protection for pregnant women. Acar & van Lopik (2009) found that the use of a three-point seat belt (shoulder and lap belt), together with a driver airbag, offers the greatest protection to the fetus (p. 891). Health care providers should urge the consistent, proper use of seat belts at every opportunity throughout the pregnancy.

---

chemicals should be avoided in the home. Areas in the home should be well ventilated household cleaning products are being used; these may contain chemicals that can produce toxic fumes. Also, while using cleaning products, pregnant women should wear protective equipment such as gloves. Chemical fumes, particularly from paint or turpentine, should be avoided, and any chemical spills on the skin should be immediately washed.

Lead exposure is considered a public health problem for women of childbearing age and pregnant women because lead is a confirmed toxic substance. Prenatal exposure to lead has long been known to readily cross the placenta; therefore, it is a significant mode of lead exposure to the fetus (Schnaas et al., 2006). The toxic fetal effects of lead are especially damaging to the developing central nervous system; however, lead can potentially damage all fetal organ systems. The damage to the fetal brain can result in mental retardation, central nervous system anomalies, and decreased intellectual development. This damage can be permanent and lead to lifelong deficits.

The Agency for Toxic Substances and Disease Registry (ATSDR), as well as the CDC, has established that there is no safe blood lead level for a fetus or the mother. Preconception and prenatal lead exposure results when lead is swallowed or inhaled and in some cases when the mother uses cosmetics or topical products containing lead. Lead poisoning (known as elevated blood lead levels) in pregnant women can occur over a period of months or years before pregnancy as lead accumulates in the body over time. Accumulated lead is deposited in bone, and it can be released or mobilized from lead stores in bone when bone turnover increases. This increase often occurs during pregnancy and lactation because both situations place significant demands on the availability of calcium from the diet (exogenous) and from physiological stores (endogenous). Physiological maternal calcium comes from bone demineralization, also known as bone turnover, which releases lead and results in increased maternal blood lead levels. This ultimately results in fetal lead exposure.

Environment sources of lead include drinking water from lead plumbing, unwashed fruits and vegetables, lead solder on canned imported foods, cigarette smoke, imported herbal remedies, and leaded crystal glass. Other sources of lead exposure are imported products, such as cosmetics or glazed pottery for food preparation or storage. Hobbies such as pottery making and lead-soldered stained glass may also expose pregnant women to lead. Major risk factors for lead exposure in pregnant women are women practicing pica, poor nutritional status, and renovation of a home built before 1978, which may have lead-based paint on the walls. Houses should be inspected for lead before home improvements are done. Health-promotion community education programs are the primary prevention strategy, which can significantly lessen lead exposure for pregnant women and women planning to become pregnant.

There are environmental safeguards for the working pregnant woman. The Occupational Safety and Health Administration (OSHA) requires that employers provide either a workplace free of hazards that are likely to cause fetal death or serious harm and a written Material Safety Data Sheet (MSDS), listing hazardous substances or ionizing radiation that might be encountered in the workplace. In 2011, the American College of Occupational and Environmental Medicine (ACOEM) Task Force on Reproductive Toxicology developed a document known as "Reproductive and Developmental Hazard

Management Guidance" to assist occupational health professionals and agencies in managing reproductive and developmental risks and uncertainties in the workplace (RDHMG, 2011). This guide describes measures to assess the magnitude of potential risks and provides options to manage the uncertainty associated with these risks.

Postpartum

A breast-feeding mother must remember that any toxic environmental exposure that affects her may also affect her infant. Chemicals, medications, radiopharmaceuticals, and illegal drugs have all been shown to be transmitted in breast milk, often in highly increased concentrations.

SEXUAL DOMAIN

The sexual domain encompasses all the characteristics that differentiate the male and the female as well as the individual's expression of those differences. **Sexuality** is a broad term that includes not only the dimensions of sexual desire and response but also the individual's view and presentation of self. The expression of an individual's identity and reflection of the basic need for emotional and physical closeness with another is a uniquely human quality.

Preconception

Women of childbearing age have health care needs related to sexuality. Health-promotion strategies prior to conception involve assessing the individual's knowledge and practices regarding sexuality. Health care providers should also assess their own personal attitudes and values about sex and sexuality, which helps them discuss sexuality-related issues. When health care providers are comfortable discussing sexuality and intimacy they can help women also feel comfortable in disclosing information and asking questions about sexuality. Health care providers should furnish information about health problems and diseases that may have an effect on sexuality and sexual functioning, as well as the prevention and treatment for sexually transmitted infections. Provided in an open and nonjudgmental manner, education about sexual functioning, safe sex practices, and the dynamics of a sexual relationship can enhance the positive aspects of sexuality. The nurse can help identify individuals with sexual dysfunction by establishing good rapport and a trusting relationship with them. Individuals then feel safe in discussing or revealing sexuality issues and are more likely to ask questions. Individuals with sexual dysfunction should be referred to experts in this area.

Pregnancy

Sexual desire and response during pregnancy are affected by physical, hormonal, and psychosocial factors. Sexuality is an important part of a woman's self-concept, which may change as a result of pregnancy (Foux, 2008). Health care providers should counsel and provide information as these women experience sexual activity. Some pregnant women and their male partners have increased sexual desire, whereas others may have less. Sexual desire in the woman commonly increases during the second and third trimester. Sexual activity during pregnancy is perfectly safe for women experiencing a normal pregnancy. Only women with a history of miscarriage or a high-risk pregnancy may need to abstain from intercourse. Many couples continue to have sex up to the time of delivery. However, as the couple approaches the delivery date, different positions may be necessary due to the enlarging uterus (e.g., side-lying, woman on top). Often couples are concerned or fearful about what can happen to the fetus if they have sex. Health care providers should reassure pregnant women and the partner that sex during pregnancy does not hurt the fetus if pregnancy has no complications. Pregnant women may experience strong contractions during orgasm, but these should not be painful and are safe unless the woman is at risk for preterm labor. Toward the end of the third trimester, these contractions may help stimulate or strengthen labor, and the deposited semen contains chemicals that can help the cervix prepare for labor. Health-promotion strategies include education for the couple about the nature of sexual response, the need for communication, and alternative forms of sexual expression during pregnancy.

Postpartum

A couple is usually advised that they may resume sexual intercourse approximately 6 weeks following delivery. However, it is safe to begin having intercourse as soon as lochia stops and there are no other complications. When the lochia stops, the vagina, cervix, and uterus have healed. Often a return to prepregnant sexual response patterns may be delayed for up to 12 weeks postpartum because of decreased genital vasocongestion, vaginal lubrication, and orgasmic intensity. Interest in sexual activity varies considerably during the early postpartum period. Most women report low or absent sexual desire due to fatigue, weakness, painful intercourse, vaginal irritation, and fear of injury; however, the majority of women resume sexual relations 6–8 weeks postpartum. A well rested, emotionally supported new mother may feel more interest in resuming sexual activity. Sharing family tasks and responsibilities, sharing child and infant care, alone time for parents, and loving communication all facilitate readjustment to the marital relationship. Other health-promotion strategies include advising postpartum women to use water-soluble gels for vaginal lubrication, lubricated condoms, and positions that reduce the depth of penetration. Breast-feeding mothers can nurse the baby prior to sexual intimacy if milk ejection during sex is a concern. Before the new mother leaves the hospital, she should be counseled about the fluctuations of sexual interest, strategies to reduce discomfort, the importance of sleep and rest, the value of emotional support and sharing of tasks, and contraceptive methods. Discussing contraception in the postpartum period prior to discharge is especially important because the absence of menstrual periods does not mean that ovulation has not occurred.

SPIRITUAL DOMAIN

For some women, spirituality may be heightened and a source of personal support during pregnancy. Spirituality affects behavior. Religious beliefs, as part of spirituality, may become more important and can affect decision making, such as the selection of the type of birthing experience, circumcision, or naming of the newborn. For couples with different religious faiths, unresolved conflicts may surface or become heightened. Referral to professional counseling may be needed to help the couple accommodate each other and accept their differing religious beliefs or spiritual orientation in order to enhance the experience of pregnancy and parenthood.

Table 9-4 summarizes health-promotion in pregnancy according to pertinent domains.

TABLE 9-4 Health Promotion in Pregnancy

RELATED DOMAIN	RISK ASSESSMENT	HEALTH-PROMOTION ACTION
Biological	Nutrition	Well-balanced diet with increased calories, calcium, vitamin C, and a 400 mcg/day folic acid supplement
	Exercise	Daily exercise
	Chemical substance and medication use	Avoidance of tobacco, alcohol, illegal drugs, herbal supplements, over-the-counter or prescribed medications that are considered teratogens
	Genetic abnormalities	Screening for neural tube defects and chromosomal abnormalities
	Infection	Screening for asymptomatic bacteriuria, syphilis, rubella, hepatitis B, HIV, and group B streptococcal infection
	Isoimmunization	Assessment of blood type, Rh status, and atypical antibody titer
	Pregnancy complications	Assessment for gestational diabetes, pregnancy-induced hypertension, and fetal growth abnormalities
Psychological and Sociological	Psychological and physical well-being	Screening for depression and intimate partner violence
Political	Legal protection	Education about the pregnancy Discrimination Act, the Family and Medical Leave Act, breast-feeding at work law
Environmental	Environmental hazards	Avoidance of exposure to toxic chemicals, fumes, lead, and ionizing radiation
Sexual	Sexual response	Education about the nature of sexual response and alternative forms of sexual expression

© Cengage Learning 2013

THE INFANT AND TODDLER

Infant mortality is an important indicator of the health of a nation (MacDorman & Mathews, 2009). Infant mortality is defined as the death of an infant before 1 year of age. The infant mortality rate is the number of infant deaths per 1000 live births. The National Center for Health Statistics reports the U.S. infant mortality rate in 2008 as reported to be 6.59 infant deaths per 1000 live births (Minino, Xu, & Kochanek, 2010). This rate has remained the same to date. Statistics on infant mortality in the United States reinforces the need for providing parents with health-promotion and disease and accident prevention strategies in the infant, toddler, and maternal populations.

The top five leading causes of infant mortality in the United States are, in leading order (1) congenital malformations and chromosomal abnormalities, (2) disorders related to prematurity, (3) sudden infant death syndrome (SIDS), (4) death related to maternal complications, and, (5) complications with placenta, umbilical cord, and membranes (Minino, Xu, & Kochanek, 2010). Statistics also indicate that infant mortality rates continue to be higher among Black and Hispanic infants than among White non-Hispanic infants in the United States (Minino, Xu, & Kochanek, 2010). This can be a result of health disparities among racial and ethnic groups. The increasing emphasis in the health care system on reducing disparities with

health-promotion and disease prevention strategies can lead to potential decreases in infant mortality in the future.

There are numerous health-promotion needs between infancy (0–1 years of age) and toddlerhood (1–3 years of age). Meeting these needs offers a significant opportunity to make an impact on the lifetime health of an individual. Parents or other caregivers carry out health-promotion strategies for the infant because infants are completely dependent on caregivers. The term *caregiver*, here, is used interchangeably with parent.

BIOLOGICAL DOMAIN

The biological domain encompasses the biologic factors and physiologic processes involved in the functioning of the body. The areas of nutrition, elimination, sleep and activity, immunization, and screening are addressed for the infant and toddler.

Nutrition

The most important nutrition health-promotion strategy is to encourage the mother to breast-feed her infant (see Figure 9-1). The American Academy of Pediatrics (AAP) currently upholds the breast-feeding recommendation in the 2005 Policy Statement on Breastfeeding. This policy statement is supported by the CDC, and in January of 2011 the Surgeon General released *A Call to Action to Support Breastfeeding* (Breastfeeding Report Card—United States, 2010; Surgeon General's Report,

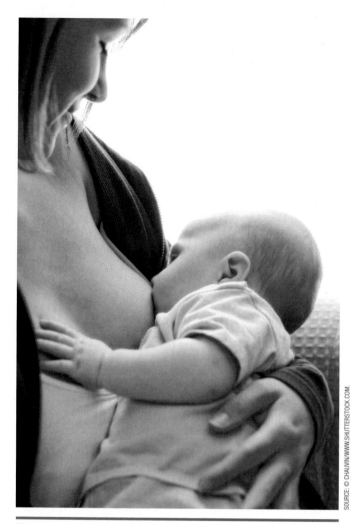

SOURCE: © CHAUVIN/WWW.SHUTTERSTOCK.COM.

FIGURE 9-1 Breast-feeding gives an infant the optimal start for growth and development. It is the preferred source of infant nutrition.

2011). Breast milk is considered the preferred source of nutrition for infants to promote adequate growth and development (American Academy of Pediatrics, 2011). Breast milk contains optimal sources of fat, protein, carbohydrates, and minerals. In addition, breast milk also contains certain immunoglobulins and antibodies to support the immature immune system of the infant by protecting against infections. Infants who are exclusively breast-fed have been found to have a decreased incidence of upper/lower respiratory tract infections, gastrointestinal infections, and otitis media (Duijts et al., 2010). In addition, breast-feeding decreases the risk of developing atopic dermatitis during infancy and childhood (Duncan & Sears, 2008). The American Academy of Pediatrics (AAP) recommends exclusive breast-feeding for at least the first 4 months but preferably for the first 6 months of age (AAP, 2011). This recommendation includes that breast-feeding should be continued, with the addition of complimentary foods, through the first 12 months of age and thereafter, as long as both the mother and the infant desire it (AAP, 2011).

The most recent CDC report on breast-feeding mothers indicate that 3 out of every 4 new mothers (75%) in the United States start out breast-feeding (Breastfeeding Report Card—United States, 2010). This report also indicates that rates of continued breastfeeding at 3, 6, and 12 months remain low. According to the CDC, fewer than 20% of mothers who

start out breast-feeding will continue to breast-feed 6 months later (Breastfeeding Report Card—United States, 2010). The high breast-feeding initiation rates indicate that most mothers want to breast-feed their babies and that they attempt to do so. The decline in breast-feeding rates at 3, 6, and 12 months after birth indicates that mothers in the United States continue to face barriers to breast-feeding. Health-promotion strategies to encourage the initiation and continuation of breast-feeding are found in Box 9-6.

The AAP recommends that all exclusively breast-fed infants should receive 200 IU of oral vitamin D daily, beginning the first 2 months of life and continuing until the daily consumption of vitamin D-fortified formula or milk is 500 ml (AAP, 2011). Breast milk does not contain fluoride, and the AAP recommends that exclusively breast-fed infants receive regular fluoride supplementation. The recommendation for fluoride supplementation is only for after 6 months of age and should be discussed with a health care provider (AAP, 2011).

Maternal contraindications to breast-feeding are uncommon. The AAP recommendation for a mother not to breast-feed extends to women infected with human immunodeficiency virus (HIV), infants diagnosed with galactosemia, women with herpetic lesions on the breasts, women who have active tuberculosis, and women ingesting illicit drugs or alcohol (AAP, 2011). Exposure to alcohol during infancy through breast milk has been found to cause delayed motor development and is detrimental to early learning (Mannella, n.d.). An important health-promotion strategy is to advise lactating women who ingest alcohol about the detrimental effects to

---

BOX 9-6

HOW TO PROMOTE BREAST-FEEDING

Provide structured breast-feeding education and behavioral counseling programs led by specially trained nurses or lactation specialists during the prenatal period; continued the strategy during the postpartum period, if necessary.

Discuss the importance of adequate rest, a healthy diet, and adequate fluid intake with the breast-feeding mother.

Provide resources on breast-feeding and information about support groups in the mother's locale.

Encourage early maternal contact with the newborn through rooming-in with the infant.

Teach the mother about infant hunger cues, and encourage her to feed on demand in response to these cues.

Encourage the mother to provide frequent, round-the-clock feedings in response to hunger cues.

Teach mothers who will be returning to work how to use a breast pump to maintain sufficient milk supply.

A breast-feeding mother should be encouraged to avoid formula supplementation while breast-feeding.

their infants, while urging the lactating women not to drink alcohol while breast-feeding.

Cow's milk is not an appropriate nutritional source for any infant under one year of age. Cow's milk-based formulas, with adjusted nutrient percentages and reduced mineral content, provide appropriate, relatively inexpensive nutrition when the mother is unable to breast-feed or chooses not to do so. Soy-based infant formula is another appropriate option for mothers who are not breast-feeding. Infants with an allergy or intolerance to cow's milk protein may also have an allergy to soy protein. A casein or whey hydrosylated formula is recommended instead of a soy-based formula. Table 9-5 compares the contents of breast milk, cow's milk, and prepared cow's milk-based formula.

Infants who are formula fed should always be given an iron-fortified infant formula (AAP, 2011). There is no scientific evidence that iron in infant formula increases diarrhea, constipation, or colic, so there is no contraindication for feeding iron-fortified formula. Breast-fed infants may need iron supplementation beginning at 6 months of age. The American Academy of Pediatrics recommends screening all infants for iron-deficiency anemia between 6 and 9 months of age. Infants fed premixed formula need fluoride supplementation, just as breast-fed infants do. If powdered or concentrated formula is mixed with fluoride-containing water, no supplementation is needed.

Infants are not physiologically or developmentally ready for solid foods until about 6 months of age when they have sufficient control of their head and neck and are able to sit up with only a little help. A diet of breast milk or iron-fortified infant formula is nutritionally adequate until this time. Solid foods should be introduced one at a time, with new foods spaced several days apart to assess for food intolerances. The sequence of food additions is largely a matter of preference; however, delaying the introduction of egg whites, wheat, corn, shellfish, and peanuts for at least the first year may reduce the development of lifelong allergies to these foods. Infants also do not need sugar or salt added to foods to enhance flavor. The caregiver should read the labels of all prepared foods before feeding them to the infant to avoid unnecessary food additives.

NURSING ALERT

Infant Botulism

Parents must be informed to completely avoid giving their infant honey, in any form, during the infant's first year. Often parents add honey to food or place it on pacifiers as a sweet enticement. Discourage this practice. Honey is an unpasteurized food and a source of bacterial spores that produce a toxin that causes the condition known as infant botulism. The infant immune system is immature and unable to fight off this bacterium. Symptoms of infant botulism are constipation, weak suck and cry, poor muscle tone with generalized weakness, and progression to flaccid paralysis, including apnea resulting from paralysis of the diaphragm.

TABLE 9-5 Nutritional Comparison: Breast Milk, Cow's Milk, and Cow's Milk-Based Formula

NUTRIENT	BREAST MILK (% OF TOTAL)	COW'S MILK (% OF TOTAL)	FORMULA (% OF TOTAL)
Protein:			
Calories	7	20	20
Casein	40	80	40–80
Whey	60	20	18–60
Fat:			
Calories	50	50	30–54
Linoleic acid	7	1	10
Carbohydrate:			
Calories	42	30	40–50
Minerals per 100 kcal:			
Calcium (mg)	50	186	75
Phosphorous (mg)	25	145	65
Sodium (mEq)	1	3.3	1.7
Chloride (mEq)	2.1	6	2.7
Potassium (mEq)	1.6	4.6	2.3
Iron:			
Content	0.3 to 0.5 mg/L	0.5 mg/L	0.5 mg/L
Absorption	50	10	4

Adapted from Pennington, J. A. T., & Douglass, J. S. (2004). *Bowe's and Church's food values of portions commonly used* (18th ed.) Philadelphia: Lippincott Williams & Wilkins.

The toddler age range is considered to be 1–3 years of age. During this period, toddlers typically consume so-called table food. An important nutrition health-promotion strategy for this age group is to provide a wide variety of foods, such as fruits, vegetables, whole grain breads and cereal, meats, and fats. This enables the toddler to experience different tastes and textures, as well as obtain an adequate balanced diet. Parents often complain that their toddler is a picky eater or that they have difficulty introducing new foods. Many parents are not aware that the toddler's acceptance of new foods is normally a lengthy course. Inform parents that it may require 10–15 attempts to introduce a new food before the toddler is willing to taste and swallow it. Parent education should also include that touching, smelling, and playing with new foods as well as spitting them out is normal exploratory behavior in toddlers.

Toddlers may be at risk for inadequate nutrition if the family does not eat a balanced diet with a wide variety of foods. A diet consistent with the Dietary Guidelines for Americans is nutritionally sound and can be recommended to parents (Dietary Guidelines, 2010). Chapter 15 has a detailed discussion of the role of nutrition in health promotion. Diets for infants and toddlers under 2 years of age should not have a fat limitation because calories in the form of fat are needed to fuel rapid growth and brain development during this time. The American Academy of Pediatrics does not recommend cow's milk for children under 1 year of age. When starting cow's milk, whole milk should not be substituted with reduced fat milk until at least 2 years of age. Toddlers who eat a balanced diet with a variety of foods do not need vitamin supplementation. Some toddlers may be poor eaters and should be evaluated by a health care provider for possibly needing vitamin supplementation. Fluoride supplements are needed if it is not supplied in the local water source.

A safety concern related to a toddler's eating table food is choking. The ability to control food in the mouth through the coordination of chewing and swallowing, as well as the skill of chewing food adequately, is not fully developed in the toddler. Educating parents about precautions to avoid the risk of choking is necessary. In addition, the nurse must reinforce that following these precautions consistently is crucial to the safety of their toddler. These precautions should include giving the toddler foods that gradually build self-feeding skills, always having the caregiver present during feeding, and placing the toddler in a high chair during mealtimes. Precautions also include avoiding certain foods. Teach parents to avoid hard foods and foods that may be difficult for toddlers to control in their mouths, such as nuts, raw carrots, popcorn, hot dogs, hard candy, and grapes.

Elimination

Renal development is not complete until the end of the first year of life; therefore, an infant's urine is usually a very pale yellow with little odor. An infant who voids 6–12 times a day indicates sufficient fluid intake. Urination should increase as fluid intake increases. The infant begins life with a relatively small bladder that gradually increases in size with the infant's age and increased growth, resulting in increasingly longer periods of dryness. Preventing dehydration is an important health-promotion strategy. Parent awareness of conditions that lead to dehydration is important: fever, vomiting, diarrhea, and elevated environmental temperatures. Caregivers should be informed of the need for increased fluids when these conditions

occur. Dehydration can also occur with reduced daily fluid intake, as well as prolonged periods without fluid intake.

Urinating and stooling are the body's modes of elimination. Infant stools vary in consistency, color, and frequency, depending on whether the infant is breast-fed or formula-fed. Breast-fed infants tend to have bright yellow, loose stools from 5–6 times a day to once every 3–4 days. Formula-fed infants tend to have lighter yellow, firmer stools from 2–3 times a day to once every 3–4 days.

A health-promotion strategy for elimination is educating caregivers about normal stooling patterns, variations in stooling patterns, and the definitions of diarrhea and constipation. This information helps eliminate unnecessary concern and anxiety over whether the infant is having diarrhea or constipation. **Diarrhea** is the frequent passage of watery, unformed fecal material. Infants have long intestines in proportion to their size. This characteristic provides greater surface area for the absorption of nutrients by a growing infant; however, this places the infant at greater risk than older age groups for dehydration resulting from diarrhea. **Constipation** is the difficult or infrequent passage of hard, dry fecal material.

Most infant and toddler constipation is functional. This results from the interaction between the child's development, gastrointestinal physiology, nutritional intake, and parental expectations. Organic or anatomic problems cause only 5% of constipation in infants and toddlers. Difficulty with expulsion and drying of the fecal mass in the rectum are the most common causes of functional constipation (Zheng-Hong, Dong. & Wang, 2008). Infant constipation frequently begins when the baby transitions from breast milk to formula or begins eating solid foods. Trying simple interventions, such as increasing the baby's water consumption, can reduce constipation. If the water does not help, offering the baby fruit juices might help. If the baby is eating solid foods, offer pureed pears or prunes. Offering barley cereal instead of rice cereal might also help. To ease the passage of hard stools, apply a lubricant to the baby's anal area. If the baby seems to be struggling with the constipation, glycerin suppositories are available without a prescription and can help alleviate the occasional constipation (Hoecker, 2011).

Toddlers may also experience functional constipation. Health-promotion strategies to prevent and treat functional constipation in toddlers before it becomes chronic include parental dietary education and behavioral training. Dietary education includes a diet with adequate fiber intake (high-fiber breakfast cereals, breads, and crackers, as well as fresh fruits and vegetables) and adequate intake of water. Adequate water intake is 2 oz of water for each gram of fiber intake (Zheng-Hong, Dong. & Wang, 2008). Behavioral training involves instituting a regular toilet-sitting schedule following meals, if the toddler is already potty trained, and at bedtime for approximately 5 minutes each time; minimizing distractions during toilet sitting times; and demonstrating proper toilet sitting position with upper body slightly flexed forward and having foot support. Behavioral training also includes providing praise for cooperative behavior, positive reinforcement for stooling, exhibiting a neutral attitude for undesirable results, and avoiding punitive approaches or embarrassment regarding any aspect of stooling.

Toilet training is a developmental task of toddlerhood. Brain and spinal cord maturation takes approximately 2 years, affecting readiness for bowel and bladder control. The toddler is relatively unaware of body functions until about 18–24 months of age; therefore, attempting to initiate toilet training prior to readiness will meet with less than satisfactory results

RESEARCH NOTE

The Association of Maternal Food Intake and Infants' or Toddlers' Food Intake

STUDY PROBLEM/PURPOSE

Studies with older children and adolescents suggest that parental food intake is associated with children's food intake. The purpose of this study is to determine whether the association of maternal food intake starts as early as infancy and toddlerhood.

METHODS

A convenience sample of 98 primarily African American mothers of infants and toddler of 6–18 months of age completed questionnaires on their own and child's food intake. Participants were recruited from an ambulatory care clinic in a Midwestern teaching hospital in the United States. Mothers were predominately African American (94%), and most received food and nutrition services through the Special Supplemental Nutrition Program for Women, Infants and Children (WIC) (89%). The mean age of mothers was 24.3 years; the mean age of infants was 11.1 months. Infants were predominately male (61%) and African American (93%). Mothers completed questionnaires that assessed demographic information, mothers' and children's food intake, and mother's perceptions of how healthy foods are.

FINDINGS

By maternal report, their children consumed fruit 1.79 times a day, vegetables 1.51 times, and snack foods 2.22 times. Mothers reported consuming fruit 1.91 times a day, vegetables 1.54 times, and snack foods 3.37 times. Mothers reported that vegetables were the healthiest foods and that snacks were "good" for their children. Findings suggested that the maternal intake of fruits, vegetables, and snack foods is significantly correlated to infant and toddler intake of the same foods. Findings from this study regarding eating patterns parallel those found in previous studies with diverse populations.

IMPLICATIONS

Study findings have important clinical implications for effective interventions to improve infants' and toddlers' eating habits and to prevent obesity in young children that may persist into childhood. Findings suggest that prevention and intervention programs for the adoption of healthy eating behaviors should start very early, perhaps just prior to the introduction of complementary foods. Interventions directed toward changing eating habits can be more beneficial. Effective behavior change strategies targeted at mothers' eating behaviors are important in influencing positive changes in young children's eating behavior. Interventions in this young age group should focus not only on the promotion of healthy eating behaviors, but on the prevention of unhealthy eating habits, including snack food and high-sugar-content beverages.

Source: Hart, C. N., Raynor, H. A., Jelalian, E., and Drotar, D. (2009). The association of maternal food intake and infants' and toddlers' food intake. *Child: Care, Health and Development, 36*(3); 396–403. DOI: 10.1111/j.1365-2214.2010.01072.x.

(Felt et al., 2004). As a rule, boys are not ready to toilet train as soon as girls, and they tend to take longer to toilet train than girls. Educating caregivers to be aware of the physiological and developmental signs of readiness (or lack of it) for toilet training is a health-promotion strategy for this age group. Signs of toilet training readiness are longer periods of dryness and being free of bowel movement overnight, being aware of having a "dirty" or "wet" diaper, voluntary participation and interest in toilet training, and following parents into the bathroom (Felt et al., 2008). Successful toilet training may positively influence an individual's elimination practices and concerns throughout the life span.

Sleep and Activity

Sleep patterns of the infant are related to the growth and development of the nervous system. As the nervous system matures and the rate of growth slows, the infant has decreased periods of sleep and increased periods of wakefulness. The infant sleeps up to 80% of a 24-hour period at birth and up to 50% of a 24-hour period by one year of age and into toddlerhood.

The major health-promotion strategy for infants is educating caregivers regarding sleep position to reduce the risk of sudden infant death syndrome (SIDS). SIDS is the sudden, unexplained death of an infant up to the age of 1 year. It is the leading cause of death among infants 1–12 months of age and is the third leading cause overall of death among infants in the United States (AAP, 2011) Studies examining SIDS found that sleeping in the prone (stomach down) position increased the incidence of SIDS (AAP, 2011). Infants sleeping on their sides also have an increased incidence of SIDS; therefore, the most recent AAP recommendation is that infants should be placed in a fully supine (on-the-back) sleeping position (AAP, 2011). In addition, AAP recommends that infants sleep in the same room as adults (but not in the same bed) and that a pacifier be offered at naptime and bedtime for at least the first year (AAP, 2011). The AAP further recommends that soft bedding and soft objects in the infant's sleeping environment, such as pillows or stuffed toys, should be avoided. The benefit of the supine sleeping position has been significant. Since the Back to Sleep campaign began in 1994, which promoted the supine position for sleep in infants, the overall SIDS rates have declined by more than 50%. This campaign was developed as a way to educate parents, caregivers, and health care providers about ways to reduce the risk of SIDS based on the AAP recommendations (AAP, 2011) The so-called back-to-sleep, or supine, position recommendation applies only to infants during sleep.

Awake and supervised infants should be allowed and encouraged to spend some time on their stomachs (prone position) for muscular and neurological development and to prevent flat spots on the occiput. As the infant matures and is able to turn from the supine to the prone position, the recommendation is that caregivers continue to place the infant in the supine position at bedtime but allow the infant to adopt whatever position is preferred.

The toddler usually sleeps about 12 hours at night and takes one daytime nap. As the toddler matures, the daytime nap is gradually no longer needed. The toddler's increasing independence may be exerted in resisting bedtime. The nurse should recommend a consistent bedtime routine that is quiet with reduced physical and emotional stimuli. Reading a favorite story and taking a favorite blanket or soft toy to bed should help establish the structure and security needed by the toddler. A nightlight may also promote feelings of security at bedtime.

Infants receive their activity during play by themselves, with their caregivers, and with toys or other objects. Caregivers may need to be educated as to the importance of frequent stimulation through play for physical and neurological development; however, structured exercise programs have not been shown to be therapeutically beneficial for healthy infants. The infant's bones are susceptible to trauma, and the infant lacks the strength and reflexes for protection from external forces. Opportunities for touching, holding, face-to-face contact, and the use of safe toys provide sufficient activity and motivation for infant physical development.

Obtaining sufficient activity and exercise is rarely a problem for the toddler. The ability to walk independently is only the first of many motor skill accomplishments. Toddlers, such as the ones pictured in Figure 9-2, seem to be constantly in motion as they learn, practice, and refine their motor skills. The health-promotion strategy during this time is encouraging and reinforcing cognitive and motor skill development by providing opportunities for safe new learning. Part of this health-promotion strategy is to educate parents that toddler's can often experience frustration with new learning experiences. Understanding that frustration in learning new things is common for this age group can help reduce parent concern and anxiety when encountering this behavior.

IMMUNIZATION

The first disease for which an immunization was discovered was smallpox. This disease was responsible for approximately 20% of deaths, and those who survived suffered from disfigurement and sometimes blindness. Edward Jenner successfully tested an immunization against smallpox in 1796. The discovery that certain infectious diseases could be prevented was a significant disease prevention strategy. Until this time, human beings were subject to sudden, devastating epidemics of infectious diseases.

The advent of immunizations changed the major cause of death from infectious diseases, such as diphtheria, smallpox, and yellow fever, to chronic diseases associated with aging. Vaccines, antibiotics, and improved sanitation are responsible for making infectious diseases a relatively minor cause of death in the United States. In fact, the global eradication of smallpox was certified by the World Health Organization in 1980, following a worldwide program of immunization and case hunting.

Immunization decreased the incidence of childhood diseases, such as measles, diphtheria, rubella, and pertussis, to such an extent that the general public became complacent about following immunization schedules. These common childhood diseases, which were almost eradicated during the 1970s, are reoccurring. Many individuals consider the common childhood diseases to be relatively mild and a part of growing up; however, serious complications, as well as mortality, are associated with these diseases. Encouraging caregivers to follow the recommended immunization schedule as closely as possible is a significant health-promotion and disease-prevention strategy. This strategy can have a significant impact on preventing the spread of communicable and vaccine preventable illnesses, as well as potential life-threatening complications of the diseases. The recommended immunization schedule for children 0–6 years of age can be found at the CDC Website (http://www.cdc.gov).

The yearly influenza (flu) vaccination is especially important for children who are at high risk for complications from

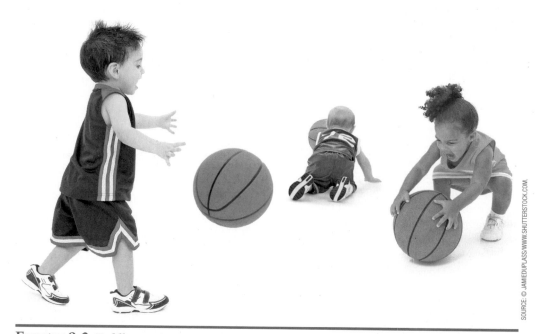

FIGURE 9-2 **Toddlers are in constant motion and need an appropriate place to expend their energy.**

contracting influenza (CDC, 2011a). This high risk group includes children that are less than two years of age; children with neurological disorders; those with chronic lung disease; and children with congenital heart disease (CDC, 2011a). In addition, all children with conditions that may result in breathing or swallowing difficulties should be vaccinated. According to the CDC the flu vaccine should be administered to infants starting at six months of age (CDC, 2011a). Immunization recommendation for hepatitis A currently includes all children beginning at one year of age. A vaccination for respiratory syncytial virus (RSV) is not currently available; this virus is the most common cause of bronchiolitis and pneumonia in infants younger than one year. Respiratory syncytial virus remains a significant cause of hospitalization among young infants, and research for the development of a vaccine remains a high priority in the United States.

Immunization practices and recommendations change frequently. Staying up-to-date on childhood vaccinations, including schedule and administration, is a priority nursing responsibility. Immunization information can be obtained through the Centers for Disease Control and Prevention and the American Academy of Pediatrics' Advisory Committee on Immunization Practices.

NURSING **ALERT**

Illness and Immunizations

Children with mild illnesses, such as the common cold, flu, and ear infections (with or without fever), should still get their immunizations on schedule. There is no decrease in the effectiveness of the vaccines, and the vaccination do not make the child sicker.

SCREENING

Screening is the use of a diagnostic procedure, such as a laboratory test or an evaluation tool, to determine the presence of a disease or risk factors associated with a health problem. Screening is a secondary intervention strategy that has the potential to provide early intervention and cost-effective preventive care. Screening is done for conditions that can have devastating effects on the quality and quantity of life. When these conditions are diagnosed before symptoms begin, treatment can reduce morbidity and mortality. In addition, during infancy, screening for abnormal growth patterns and developmental delays is important. Significant for the infant and toddler is newborn screening for inborn errors of metabolism, genetic defects, hemoglobinopathies, and hearing deficits. Newborn screening is mandatory in all states, the District of Columbia, and the U.S. territories of Puerto Rico and the U.S. Virgin Islands. The exceptions to this mandate are the states of Wyoming and Maryland, both of which require consent for newborn screening and permit the refusal of screening.

Which diseases to include in the newborn screening program is determined by the state, thus explaining the lack of screening uniformity throughout the United States. Each state analyzes the cost-to-benefit ratio of performing the newborn screening testing versus not performing it. Substantial costs are associated with newborn screening, including the actual cost of the test and confirmatory testing. In addition to cost, other problems are false negatives and false positives, along with parental anxiety associated with false positives. The ethical and financial dilemma that arises with newborn screening relates to the availability and assumption of treatment costs and follow-up services for the treatable disorders identified in the screening. Although the financial cost of screening for a selected group of treatable devastating disorders is certainly less than the financial cost of long-term care of individuals not identified and treated, the actual human costs have not been fully analyzed.

The American College of Medical Genetics identified 29 core conditions and 25 secondary conditions for newborn screening in the United States. All 29 core conditions are screened for in 24 states and the District of Columbia. The states of New Jersey and Minnesota screen for all 54 conditions. The state of Oklahoma is the only state that does not screen for biotinidase, and the District of Columbia is the only area in the United States that screens for glucose 6-phosphate dehydrogenase deficiency. All 50 states, the District of Columbia, and the U.S. territories of Puerto Rico and the U.S. Virgin Islands screen for the minimum following conditions: congenital adrenal hyperplasia, congenital hypothyroidism, galactosemia, phenylketonuria, and sickle cell disease/anemia.

An additional concern associated with newborn screening is timing. Tests to identify the congenital conditions of phenylketonuria, hypothyroidism, homocystinuria, and galactosemia measure the concentrations of analytes in the blood that increase over time; therefore, timing of the test is crucial. With the current trends of early hospital discharge, specimens are sometimes collected before the newborn is 24 hours old, which can result in false-negative results. The primary health-promotion strategy is to avoid false-negative test results in the newborn screening. A second specimen should be collected within two weeks after birth if the first specimen was collected before the newborn was 24 hours old.

Defects of Metabolism

The primary purpose of newborn screening for defects of metabolism is to identify infants with treatable metabolic disorders that can have devastating life-long health affects if untreated. These disorders are rare genetic disorders in which the body cannot properly metabolize specific components of food into energy that can be used by the body (Raghuveer, Garg, & Graf, 2006). The components of food that are not metabolized build up in the body, causing damage and resulting in a wide array of symptoms. Most defects of metabolism cause severe

SPOTLIGHT **ON**

Who Pays?

If mandatory newborn screening detects a defect in metabolism in a newborn, who is responsible for the cost of treatment and follow-up? What if the family has no insurance or income?

mental retardation and developmental delay if undetected and if not treated early. Some of the metabolic disorders that are screened for in all 50 states plus the District of Columbia and the U.S. territories of Puerto Rico and the U.S. Virgin Islands are galactosemia, phenylketonuria, congenital adrenal hyperplasia, and maple syrup urine disease.

Anemia

Iron deficiency is the most common cause of anemia in infants and toddlers. Any infant with a history of low birth weight, consumption of cow's milk starting before 6 months of age, or consumption of a non-iron-fortified formula should have a measurement of the hemoglobin or hematocrit level at 6–9 months of age. The prevention of untreated anemia is an important health-promotion strategy to enhance normal growth and development and resistance to infection.

Hearing Deficits

The ability to hear is essential to the infant and toddler for the development of speech and language, as well as psychosocial and intellectual development. Hearing loss is one of the most common **congenital** (present at birth) anomalies and is estimated to affect approximately 2–3 per 1,000 infants in the United States each year (Stevens-Wrightom, 2007). The early identification and intervention of hearing deficits in infants can prevent potential lifelong psychosocial, intellectual, and speech and language deficits. Infants with hearing deficits who are not identified before 6 months of age have been found to exhibit delays in speech and language (Stevens-Wrightom, 2007). Newborn hearing screening programs are currently established, but not necessarily required, in all 50 states and the District of Columbia, as well as the U.S. territories. Newborn infant hearing screening programs are designed to identify hearing loss in infants before one month of age. In the United States, 95% of newborn hearing tests are done prior to discharge from the hospital or birthing clinic. The identification of all newborns with hearing loss before 6 months of age has now become an attainable and realistic goal in the United States. In addition to assessing infants who did not receive newborn hearing screening, the startle or turning response to a noise produced outside the infant's field of vision should be conducted at every well child visit to identify delayed onset hearing loss. Although the observation of the startle or turning response is at best subjective and imprecise, the absence of babbling at six months, coupled with any parental reports of lack of response to noise, warrants evaluation by an audiologist. The health-promotion strategy for sensory development is to conduct hearing screening at every well child visit and to increase the number of visits of infants who fail the hearing screen for follow-up examinations. Nurses can play a crucial role in increasing the number of follow-up evaluations by communicating test results and the importance of follow-up evaluation accurately, clearly, and in a culturally sensitive manner. A very important part of this explanation is how hearing loss can hamper a child's speech and language development and have lifelong effects. A child whose hearing impairment is not discovered within the first three years of life may suffer permanently impeding communication ability.

Growth Retardation

The measurement of height, weight, as well as head and chest circumferences, is a health-promotion strategy to assess growth patterns in the infant and toddler. Each child has an individual pattern; however, comparison to known average patterns and to the infant's or toddler's pattern of growth history enables the identification of any deviations or dramatic changes. Growth pattern changes may be the result of one or all of the following factors—genetic, nutritional, emotional, or disease-related.

Developmental Delays

The early screening and identification of developmental disabilities in children enable an early intervention with effective therapy for treatable problems and accessing resources for non-reversible problems. Although early detection and intervention for developmental delays have substantial benefits, a large portion of healthy children are not routinely screened. The use of direct screening tools for developmental delays can be costly primarily because a trained professional is required for their administration and interpretation. Periodic screening for delays or deviations from expected milestones should be conducted at every well child visit; however, at a minimum, screening should occur when parents express concern about their infant's or toddler's development. Additionally, children at high risk for developmental delays should be routinely screened. High-risk infants are those who were premature, had a low birth weight, or had other abnormalities at birth.

The most widely used screening tool for developmental delays is the Denver Developmental Screening Test (DDST) II, which was revised and standardized in 1990. The DDST II is a brief, validated test with a high rate of sensitivity. It screens for a variety of mental, language, and social items, as well as for sensory and motor achievements. It can be used from birth to 6 years of age to provide mean ages and normal ranges of variation in the accomplishment of fine and gross motor tasks. The predictive value in culturally and economically diverse populations has been improved with the addition of norms for subgroups based on place of residence, ethnicity, and mother's education.

PSYCHOLOGICAL DOMAIN

The psychological domain involves application of theories of individual behavior and changes of behavior. For the infant and toddler, Jean Piaget's stages of cognitive development and Erik Erikson's stages of emotional development are the most applicable.

Cognitive Development

Jean Piaget's interest in intellectual development led to his belief that each child had a biological blueprint for cognitive development. He believed that the brain does not just mature on its own but that it is stimulated by experiences the child has in the environment. He postulated a framework to describe the evolution of learning and adaptation that demonstrates the processing of interactions (or experiences) between the child and the environment (Brainerd, 1978). This cognitive development theory (see Table 9-6) provides an explanation of how the child learns.

Children pass through definite stages of cognitive growth demonstrated by changes in behavior or thought. In the sensorimotor period. the infant is attempting to coordinate simple motor activities to adapt to and interact with the environment. Health-promotion strategies during this period involve teaching the caregivers to stimulate the infant's cognitive development through use of patterns on toys or crib attachments that encourage gazing. Observing moving objects helps develop the infant's ability for visual pursuit. Having safe, brightly colored toys within reach encourages reaching, grasping, and cause-effect development ("If I can reach it, I can bring it closer").

TABLE 9-6 Stages of Cognitive Development According to Jean Piaget

AGE	COGNITIVE STAGE	CHARACTERISTICS
Birth to 2 years	Sensorimotor	Moves from pure reflex adaptations to having a beginning grasp of cause and effect
		Able to complete small goal-directed tasks
		Realizes objects only if in sight
2–7 years	Preoperational	Has representational thoughts of past, present, and future
		Able to use and understand symbols such as language
		Makes simple classifications
		Has difficulty differentiating real from not real
		Believes he or she can influence reality through thought (magical thinking)
		Sees world only from egocentric point of view
7–11 years	Concrete operations	Able to perform concrete, action-oriented logical reasoning for familiar situations
		Increases use of symbols to represent reality
		Groups, sorts, and orders objects and concepts
		Analyzes relationships
		Able to reverse mental operations
		Understands concepts of reversibility, conservation, and transformation
11–15 years (and possibly up to 18–20)	Formal operations	Has true logical thinking
		Has capacity for abstract thought
		Able to predict and formulate hypotheses

Source: Brainerd, C. J. (1978). *Piaget's theory of intelligence*. Englewood Cliffs, NJ: Prentice Hall.

HEALTH PROMOTION
THEORY LINK

Barnard's Parent-Child Interaction Model and Infant Health Outcomes

The most immediate influence on the health outcomes of infants is the quality of parent-child interactions. Positive parent-child interactions throughout the first year of life promote neurophysiologic, physical, and psychological growth and development. The quality of parent-child interactions can also predict later cognitive and mental health in childhood. According to Barnard's Model, parent-child interaction is a process of mutual adaptation. The infant sends clear cues concerning his or her internal states, communicates needs, and is responsive to the parent. The parent must recognize and respond to the infant's cues, meet all needs, alleviate distress, and provide opportunities for growth and development. Parent responsiveness is defined as the ability to consistently recognize and act on infant cues. This fosters a sense of security in the infant and is key in development. Sensitive, warm parent interactions are just as important as consistent responsiveness to the infants needs, leading to the infant's feeling loved and cared for.

The World Health Organization recognizes the promotion of positive parent-child interactions as an important aspect in the health care of infants. Health care providers should be able to identify the adverse effects in the infant that are a result of inadequate parent-child interactions. Maternal behavior that can interfere with positive parent-child interactions should be identified: feeling overwhelmed, insecurity about parenting skills, difficulty with breast-feeding, anxiety, and depression. The early identification and intervention of new mothers at risk for conflict can promote breast-feeding. Health care providers in various settings are key in educating new mothers on recognizing their infants' behavioral cues.

Source: Barnard, K. E. (1994). Parent-child interaction model. In A. Marriner-Tomey (ed.). *Nursing theorists and their work*. St. Louis, MO: Mosby, pp. 406–422.

TABLE 9-7 Stages of Psychological Development According to Erik Erikson

LEVEL	CONFLICT	DEFINITION	BEHAVIORS
Infant	Trust	Optimism, warmth	Smiling, responsive to interactions
	Mistrust	Sense of deprivation	Feeding disorders, failure to thrive
Toddler	Autonomy	Self-control, adequacy	Curiosity, assertiveness, self-feeding
	Shame and doubt	Sense of inner failure	Extreme separation anxiety, sleep disturbances, toilet training disturbances
Preschool	Initiative	Ability to direct own actions	Independence
	Guilt	Anxiety about being bad	Temper tantrums, withdrawal
School age	Industry	Skill competence	Self-confident, cooperative Perseveres, completes tasks
	Inferiority	Sense of inadequacy	Passive, moody, depressed Incomplete tasks, isolated
Adolescent	Identity	Image of self as unique	Confident Develops loyal friendships
	Role confusion	Doubt about identity	Delinquent behavior Sense of futility Psychotic episodes
Young adult	Intimacy	Close relationships	Committed in relationships Self-abandonment
	Isolation	Distance from others	Loner in relationships Avoids social situations
Middle-aged adult	Generativity	Concern for future generations	Involved in family and community
	Stagnation	Self-concern	Self-absorbed, loner, depression
Old adult	Ego integrity	Satisfaction with life	Dignified, shows pride Sees death as part of life
	Despair	Nonacceptance of life	Fear of death, anger, depression

Source: Adapted from Erikson, E. (1950). *Childhood and society*. New York: Norton.

The toddler begins to depend less on physical manipulation and more on mental problem-solving. Exploratory behavior continues, with toddlers demonstrating curiosity about everything in their environment. The toddler touches, samples, and moves everything within reach: food, objects, and even people. The toddler can complete simple tasks, such as putting away one or two toys or obtaining a requested object. Toddlers are great mimics of observed behaviors, both in humans and nonhumans. Health-promotion strategies involve encouraging safe exploration and the verbal development that is the basis for representational thoughts and symbols.

EMOTIONAL DEVELOPMENT

Erik Erikson studied the psychological development of the child (see Table 9-7). He felt that psychological growth was the result of resolution of developmental crises from infancy through older adulthood. Without crisis resolution at each stage, the individual does not have a firm foundation for succeeding in the following stages (Erikson, 1950).

In the first stage of trust versus mistrust, resolution occurs when the infant learns that basic needs for food and comfort will be met. Infants should be fed whenever they show signs of hunger: alertness, activity, and mouthing. Crying is considered a late-stage indicator of hunger. Quick attention to the infant's needs develops the infant's belief that the world is a safe and predictable place. An infant who does not get sufficient food or comforting attention may always have a sense of deprivation and lack of trust in caregivers. Health-promotion strategies at this stage involve teaching the parents or caregivers about infant nutritional needs, infant hunger cues, feeding patterns and encouraging them to hold and comfort their infant as much as possible.

Resolution of the second stage, autonomy versus shame and doubt, occurs for toddlers as they learn that they can control their own behavior. Toddlers whose independent behavior is restricted will doubt their ability. If their efforts are greeted with a lack of acceptance, they develop shame. Health-promotion strategies at this stage involve encouraging appropriate independent behaviors so that toddlers can develop confidence in their abilities.

SOCIAL DOMAIN

Issues in the social domain for the infant and toddler are the use of day care facilities, child abuse and neglect, and cultural influences.

Family

For the infant, the social network consists of the family and caregivers. This social network creates the growth-promoting environment necessary for infant well-being, the basis for which is the development of attachment between the parent and infant. **Attachment** is a unique, specific, and enduring relationship involving mutual trust, responsiveness, and caring (Klaus & Kennel, 1985). It starts with development of a unilateral relationship (bonding), initiated by the parents, and then develops into attachment, which is a reciprocal relationship where the infant is able to respond to and elicit responses from the parents.

During attachment building, parents use eye contact, touching, and talking to get to know their infant. An important health-promotion strategy is to facilitate and encourage this acquaintance behavior as early and as frequently as possible. Extreme stress or illness may interfere with development of attachment. Nurses must observe for negative patterns of parenting behaviors, such as verbal expressions of dissatisfaction with the baby, a failure to respond to the infant's crying, and reduced touching or holding of the infant. Parental support, education, role modeling, and encouragement may enable the parent-infant relationship to progress positively.

By the time the infant becomes a toddler, a reciprocal relationship with the parents and older siblings has developed; however, the addition of a new infant to the family may cause jealousy and regression in interactive social skills if parents do not prepare for the event. Including the toddler (as much as is appropriate) in preparatory activities, reading books on anticipating a new baby, and spending special time alone with the toddler following the arrival of the new baby may assist the toddler in adjusting to the new social position.

Day Care

In many families, all available caregivers are working outside the home and must place their children in day care settings. There are two types of day-care facilities. One is the center-based facility (private, church, or community center–related), which is staffed by professional child care workers and aides and usually has a large number of children. The second is the family day care center, which is licensed to care for a limited number of children in a private home.

The health-promotion strategy for children of working parents is to educate the parents about how to evaluate the safety and quality of a day care facility. The nurse should inform working parents to assure that the day care center of choice is licensed for child care by the state. The primary purpose of licensing a child day care center is to protect the well-being of the children served. A day care center license is clear evidence that the building and grounds are safe, that staff are appropriately trained, and that the program reflects an understanding of the healthy growth and development of children. Further, the license is an assurance that children are being cared for in a safe, healthy environment where appropriate activities, time

schedules, food, equipment, and staff are consistently available, encouraging and supporting the children's physical, social, emotional, and intellectual growth. In addition, a licensed day care center requires the staff to have criminal background checks, further assuring parents of their child's safe care. The nurse should encourage parents to visit day care centers when children are in the facility and observe, in addition to the cleanliness and safety of the facility, the interaction between the children and the staff. Parents need to be aware of the staff-to-child ratio. Frequent unannounced parental visits should be conducted both before and after enrolling the infant or toddler.

Child Abuse and Neglect

Child abuse and neglect occur in all races, ethnicities, and socioeconomic classes throughout the world. In 2008, the U.S. state and local child protective services (CPS) received 3.3 million reports of children being abused or neglected (Centers for Disease Control and Prevention, 2008). Child protective services estimated that 772,000 (10.3 per 1000) children were victims of abuse or neglect. Unfortunately, many cases are unknown because they are not reported. More children suffer neglect than any other form of maltreatment. The investigations conducted by child protective services in 2008 on reported cases of child abuse and neglect revealed that approximately 71% of children were victims of neglect, 16% were victims of physical abuse, 9% were victims of sexual abuse, and 7% were victims of emotional abuse. Statistics reported by the CDC indicate that there are gender and race disparities among children who are victims of child abuse and neglect. In 2008, the rates of child abuse indicate higher incidence among certain races: African American, 16.6 per 1000 children; American Indian and Alaska Native, 13.6 per 1000 children; and multiracial children, 13.8 per 1000 children. The overall rates of victimization were slightly higher for girls at 10.8 per 1000, compared to the rate among boys at 9.7 per 1000. The World Health Organization reports that global estimates of child abuse, including fatal cases, are highest for the 0–4-year-old age group. In 2008, an estimated 1740 U.S. children died as a result of child abuse or neglect—a rate of 2.3 per 100,000 children. Among this estimate, 80% of deaths occurred among children younger than 4 years of age.

Any child is vulnerable to abuse or neglect. Child abuse occurs in both genders, across all socioeconomic classes, and among all races. Sadly, most children are abused by their parents rather than by other relatives or caregivers. Factors that tend to increase a child's risk of abuse include being 0–4 years of age; prematurity or low birth weight; being perceived as looking "unusual"

✿ NURSING **ALERT**

Everyone's Responsibility

All 50 states, the District of Columbia, and the U.S. territories have mandatory child abuse and neglect reporting laws. The report must be made to the local or state agency designated to receive and investigate suspected child abuse and neglect cases. Hotline numbers to report abuse and neglect are usually listed with community services in the front section of the telephone directory. Reporting agency numbers are also readily available at all child health care agencies.

GLOBAL HIGHLIGHTS IN HEALTH PROMOTION

Intimate Partner Violence during Pregnancy: A Global View

Women of reproductive age (15–49 years old) are more vulnerable to abuse by intimate partners than by any other perpetrator. Prevalence of intimate partner violence (IPV) during pregnancy differs across populations globally and has a significant impact on maternal and newborn outcomes. The documented worldwide prevalence of IPV is thought to be higher due to possible underreporting. Approximately as many as 300,000 pregnant women in the United States are affected by IPV every year. A World Health Organization study reported prevalence estimates of IPV during pregnancy from 10 participating countries, with the highest rate occurring in Africa. In addition, IPV was reported to be among the severest in Africa compared to other continents. A recent systematic review of African studies on IPV during pregnancy revealed prevalence as high as 57% of pregnant women suffering abuse from an intimate partner. Information from this review can be used for the development of policies for prevention and screening, advocacy programs, and screening of IPV and can ultimately lead to healthy maternal and newborn outcomes.

Shamu, S., Abrahams, N., Temmerman, M., Musekiwa, A., & Zarowsky, C. (2011). A systematic review of African studies on intimate partner violence against pregnant women: Prevalence and risk factors. *PloS ONE, 6*(3): e17591. DOI: 10.1371/journal.pone.001759.

or "different"; having a disease or congenital abnormality; being physically, emotionally, or developmentally disabled or delayed; having a high level of motor activity or being fussy and irritable; living in poverty; and living in an environment where substance abuse, high crime rates, and violence are present.

An important health-promotion strategy to prevent and identify child abuse or neglect is for health care professionals to be well enough educated to detect and report the early signs and symptoms. The early identification of victims of child abuse and neglect is vital for the interventions necessary to treat the child and prevent further victimization. Nurses have a key role in identifying and reporting suspected child abuse and neglect.

Nurses must know what to look for and be very vigilant in identifying any signs or symptoms of abuse or neglect in the child, as well as suspicious parent behavior and parent-supplied information. **Bruising** (the leakage of blood into skin tissue damaged by a direct blow or a crushing injury) is often the earliest and most visible sign in a child. Bruises observed in infants, especially on the face and buttocks, should always raise suspicion. Other signs the nurse should be alert for are bruises at different stages of healing, abrasions, hematomas, poor skin care, burns on the lower extremities, malnutrition, bite marks, retinal hemorrhage, and discrepancies between the reported cause of the injury and the observed injuries. In toddlers, injuries to the upper arms, trunk, front of the thighs, sides of the face, ears, neck, genitalia, stomach, and buttocks are likely associated with

intentional, nonaccidental injuries. Bruising on the shins, hips, lower arms, forehead, hands, or bony prominences are more consistent with accidental injuries among toddlers.

Parental behaviors may also alert the nurse. Typically, when a child has an accident, the parents seek help quickly, offer consistent details about the accident, are concerned about the child's status, have difficulty leaving the child, and may express guilt over not preventing the accident. Abusive parents, however, seem evasive about the injury, offer fewer or even conflicting details about the accident, appear inconvenienced or angry, and are not as concerned about the child's condition and progress as would be expected.

CULTURAL INFLUENCES

The infant is profoundly influenced by the culture/ethnicity of the parents or caregivers. The family's perceptions of illness, the cause of illness, childrearing practices, nutrition, and child behavior reflect cultural heritage. Because the infant depends totally on caregivers for nutrition, health care, affection, and safety, nurses must plan health-promotion strategies with adequate knowledge of and sensitivity to the family's culture/ethnicity. Also, nurses have to communicate health-promotion information in a culturally sensitive manner. They must be aware of their own cultural influences and be able to avoid allowing these influences to dictate health-promotion strategies and communication in any way. Knowledge of previous encounters with the health care community and any problems that might have occurred due to language barriers, religious values, and family lines of authority, family roles, or use of traditional (folk) medicine form the basis for collaboration with the family in planning health-promotion strategies for the infant or toddler. Cultural sensitivity on the part of the nurse is crucial when asking probing questions. Family cultural beliefs, values, and practices continue to mold the toddler, who is now able to participate in some of the family's cultural activities, such as celebrations and religious observances. Culturally sensitive collaboration continues to be key in developing health-promotion strategies for the infant and toddler.

POLITICAL DOMAIN

Three U.S. initiatives have an impact on health promotion for the infant and toddler: (1) the Supplemental Food Program for Women, Infants, and Children (WIC); (2) the second concerns safety legislature on requiring car safety seats; (3) legislation affecting lactating mothers in the workplace.

WIC Program

The Supplemental Food Program for Women, Infants, and Children is a grant program administered by the Food and Nutrition Service of the U.S. Department of Agriculture. It provides nutrition assessment and education, breast-feeding guidance and support, food supplements, and referral for health and social services to low-income pregnant, breast-feeding, and postpartum women, as well as to infants, and children under the age 5 who are at nutritional risk. Eligibility is based on income and nutritional need.

Safety Legislation

The key safety legislation that affects the health of the infant and toddler is the mandate for the use of car safety seats. All 50 states require infants traveling in any motor vehicle (car) to be restrained in a car safety seat. According to the National Highway Traffic Safety Administration, a properly used car safety

INFANT AND TODDLER CAR SAFETY

- Always place the infant/toddler in the car safety seat, even for short trips.
- Ensure that the car's seat belt holds the safety seat firmly without sliding.
- Use rear-facing safety seats for infants/toddlers less than 20 lb.
- Place the car safety seat in the center of the back seat.
- Never place an infant or toddler in a front seat with an operational airbag.
- Never use an infant carrier in place of a car safety seat.
- Ensure that straps lie flat and are held on the shoulders with a harness retainer clip.
- Watch for product recalls of car safety seats.
- Always leave a purse, cell phone, or important papers in the back seat with the infant/toddler so that the infant/toddler will not be forgotten in the back seat when the parent or caregiver arrives at a destination.

seat reduces the risk of infant mortality in a crash by 71% and the risk for a toddler by 54%. This is a significant impact on infant and toddler survival in a motor vehicle crash. The health-promotion strategy for infant and toddler safety related to car safety seat usage is parental education about the proper size, placement, and use of the seats. The safest place for a car seat is in the middle of the rear seat. Tips for infant and toddler car safety are listed in Box 9-7.

Although airbags save hundreds of lives each year, the deployment force and velocity of passenger-side airbags has resulted in the deaths of children placed in the front seat of cars, even if they are in car safety seats. Infants in rear-facing front safety seats are too close to the airbag housing and have been injured or killed by the force of the deployment. Toddlers, restrained or not, have also been injured or killed by passenger airbags.

Legislation Supporting Breast-Feeding

The most recent legislation to have a significant impact on health promotion for the infant and toddler is the Affordable Care Act, which was signed into law in 2010. This act requires employers, for 1 year after the child is born, to provide reasonable break time and a private, nonbathroom place for lactating mothers to express breast milk during the workday. One of the occasions for the discontinuation of breast-feeding is the mother's return to work. This legislation will have a significant impact on the continuation of breast-feeding through the first year of life and as a result will promote infant optimum health.

ENVIRONMENTAL DOMAIN

Accidents are responsible for the deaths of thousands of infants and toddlers annually, and more than 90% of these deaths are preventable. Specific environmental safety precautions for infants and toddlers are listed in Table 9-8.

Educating parents and caregivers on how to prevent accidents is the primary health-promotion strategy. Reminding parents that toddlers mimic adult behavior as part of their normal development at this age is very important. Toddlers often learn dangerous and harmful behavior from watching their parents and caregivers. Therefore, parents should refrain from doing anything in front of the toddler that they do not want the toddler to imitate: taking medication; not washing hands; holding pins or nails in the mouth; smoking, drinking alcohol, or taking illegal drugs; not wearing seat belts; using lighters or matches; and handling a firearm.

Parents should be instructed to keep all important numbers by every phone or even affixed to every phone in the house and the cell phone contact list. Some important numbers are emergency response for ambulance, police, and fire department; the poison control center; the family doctor; and a parent's or relative's work phone number.

Parents also need appropriate medical supplies kept in a first aid kit, with one kit kept in the house and one kit kept in each car. The first aid kit should contain items such as sterile gauze pads, adhesive tape/bandages, elastic bandage, antibiotic ointment, antiseptic wipes/soap, tweezers, scissors, calamine lotion, and a thermometer. Syrup of ipecac (used to induce vomiting) is no longer recommended for home management of poisoning in children.

Parents should be urged to learn cardiopulmonary resuscitation (CPR) for infants and children. Knowing CPR is vital when the infant or toddler is choking or not breathing. Reinforce the critical importance of knowing CPR if the house has a pool. Parents should be cautioned to be especially vigilant away from home. The toddler's natural curiosity in an unfamiliar place may lead to tragedy.

SEXUAL DOMAIN

Although the full expression of sexuality is an adult phenomenon, its development begins in infancy. An infant's sex (or gender) is determined at conception, and intrauterine development occurs in response to hormones. After birth, the infant's sexuality continues developing through the influence of hormones and by parental (or caregiver) interactions and role model influences. The infant develops gender-specific responses influenced by the caregiver's responses. If the caregiver, either consciously or unconsciously, believes that boys should be treated differently from girls, then a sex role differentiation is being taught and learned.

An important health-promotion strategy is to educate caregivers about an infant's natural exploration of the body. By 5–6 months of age, infants locate their genital area through the exploration and discovery of their body during bathing or diaper change. Just as these infants explored and manipulated their hands and feet, they manipulate their genitals. Males often experience an erection, and females may have some lubrication.

Assuring caregivers of this natural sequence of events may prevent undue concern and anxiety about this activity and set the stage to promote the healthy development of the infant's self-image and sexuality. The differences caused by gender-specific caregiving practices become apparent in the toddler. Toddlers can identify themselves as boys or girls and usually display the behaviors expected of their gender. They observe and imitate their same-sex parent. Children of both genders should be allowed to play with dolls, trucks, and other toys formerly considered gender-specific without parents being concerned that such play is "sissy" or "tomboyish." By toddlerhood, the self-concept as a girl or boy is completed.

TABLE 9-8 Environmental Safety for Infants and Toddlers

ACCIDENT	PREVENTION STRATEGIES
Falls	Place infant in crib for sleeping. Never place infant on a couch for sleeping. Never leave toddler unattended in high chair or shopping cart. Use safety gates to block stairways. Lock closed windows and use window guards when open. Anchor top-heavy furniture to wall: bookcases, TVs, fish tanks. Be sure floor rugs don't slip. Always light a room when entering. Hold toddler's hand while climbing stairs.
Suffocation/ choking	Place infant on back (supine) to sleep. Avoid soft bedding, pillows, or stuffed toys in the crib; avoid sheepskins under infants. Avoid bed sharing or cosleeping with adults or siblings. Place window blind or curtain cords out of reach. Avoid bibs with ties, and always remove a bib before bedtime. Crib slats should not be more than 2⅜ in. apart (the size of a soda can) and have no broken or missing rails. Keep small objects out of reach. Check floors and countertops for small objects daily. Cut table food into small pieces, no larger than ½ in. Supervise all eating, and never allow toddler to play while eating. Avoid giving toddler hard food or candy. Avoid giving toddlers food that can obstruct the airway, such as hot dogs, sliced carrots, grapes. Avoid uninflated or broken balloons or plastic bags. Provide toys no smaller than 1¾ in., with no removable small parts, and with no strings or cords. Do not allow toddlers to wear necklaces, purses, scarves, or clothing with drawstring.
Electrocution	Plug unused electrical outlets with clear covers (no cartoon characters or bright colors). Fill all empty light sockets with bulbs. Unplug any unused extension cords. Keep all electrical appliances unplugged, out of reach, and away from water.
Poisoning	Lock up household cleaning products. Keep all medication and vitamins out of reach. All medication and vitamin containers should have child-proof caps. Avoid taking any medication or vitamins in front of toddlers. Keep liquor cabinets locked. Keep poison control number by phone. Do not use syrup of ipecac for home treatment of poisoning.
Gun safety	Keep guns in locked case and keys out of reach. All guns should be unloaded and ammunition kept separately
Drowning	Never leave infant/toddler alone in the bathtub or near any water (pool, mop bucket, washing machine). Close toilet lids. CPR course is necessary for all adults if house has as pool.
Burns	Hand-test temperature before placing infant/toddler in bath water. Water temperature limit throughout the house should not exceed 120° F. Use back burners on stove as often as possible. Turn pot handles toward back of stove. Never leave an iron unattended. Install smoke detectors and check/replace batteries regularly Never leave a cigarette burning. Keep lighters and matches out of reach. Never leave a burning candle in the presence of an infant or toddler.
Cuts	Prevent toddlers from using glass drinking cups. Use easily identifiable decals on glass doors at toddler's eye level. Place breakable objects out of reach. Keep scissors and knives out of reach.

TABLE 9-9 Health Promotion for Infants and Toddlers

RELATED DOMAIN	RISK ASSESSMENT	HEALTH-PROMOTION ACTION
Biological	Nutrition	Breast-feeding for the first year of life
	Elimination	Education about identification and management of diarrhea and constipation
		Education about toilet training in the toddler
	Sleep	Back sleeping only until infant can turn without help
		Establishment of consistent bedtime routine for toddlers
	Play	Frequent stimulation for infants
		Provision of a safe learning environment and new learning opportunities for toddlers
	Immunization	Maintenance of recommended immunization schedule
Psychological	Screening for abnormalities	Assessment for defects of metabolism, anemia, hearing deficits, growth retardation, and developmental delays
Social	Development	Assessment for appropriate cognitive and emotional development
Political	Abuse and neglect	Assessment and mandatory reporting of child abuse and neglect
	Lactating mothers in the workplace	Law mandates that lactating mothers are provided with appropriate time and place to express breast milk at work.
	Care safety seats	Mandatory to use a care safety seat.
Environmental	Protection	Education about availability of supplemental food program and about car safety seats
	Safety	Anticipatory guidance about potential for accidents such as falls, suffocation/choking, electrocution, poisoning, drowning, burns, cuts, and gun safety

© Cengage Learning 2013

Toddlers have increasing control over their own bodies (running, jumping, toileting, self-feeding) and may increase their genital stimulation. Caregivers who are comfortable with their own sexuality can view this exploration as a natural extension of the toddler's curiosity. Parents should never react to this behavior by embarrassing or shaming the child. A neutral attitude is the most appropriate reaction.

SPIRITUAL DOMAIN

The spiritual domain relates to the essence of life, encompassing religious values and practices. The outward expression of spirituality is often through an organized church or religious institution. An individual's daily interactions with others, goals, and feelings of self-worth come from spiritual beliefs. These beliefs affect the individual's definition of health, life, quality of life, and health care practices. Spiritual and religious values are instilled in infants and toddlers by helping them develop a sense of trust and a belief in the security of their environment, which includes their caregiver. The foundation of values and a sense of trust and safety in these early years mske up the initial step in developing self-esteem and self-love. The health-promotion strategy for this domain is to encourage parents to show love and comfort to their infants and toddlers. Table 9-9 summarizes health promotion for infants and toddlers according to pertinent domains.

SUMMARY

Promoting the health of mothers, infants, and toddlers begins prior to conception with the education of the prospective parents, ideally beginning in high school. Educational programs focusing on personal health and wellness, conception, fetal development, and infant care can reduce infant mortality and morbidity.

There are many health-promotion and preventive-care interventions for the mother. This chapter grouped health-promotion strategies into three opportunities for intervention:

preconception, pregnancy, and postpartum. Each period of intervention was viewed through the biological, psychological and sociological, environmental, political, sexual, and spiritual domains.

Health-promotion strategies for the infant and toddler were viewed through the biological, psychological and sociological, environmental, political, sexual, and spiritual domains. These provided a comprehensive look at health-promotion in the infant and toddler age groups.

Individual: Nicole Lee Chang

TOPIC: Teenage pregnancy and intimate partner violence

OBJECTIVES/GOALS: Through discussion of this case study, participants will have the opportunity to:

1. Discuss how it is possible to deny being pregnant as an adolescent.
2. What techniques can be used to probe for information about intimate partner violence.
3. Discuss the risk factors associated with Nicole's sexual activity.

HEALTH PROMOTION CONCERN, HISTORY AND PHYSICAL, PRESENT HEALTH STATUS, PAST HEALTH STATUS, FAMILY HISTORY, AND SOCIAL HISTORY

Nicole Lee Chang is a 16-year-old, sexually active Asian American female who has been brought to the Women's Care Clinic by her mother. Her mother expresses concern that Nicole might be pregnant because she has not had a menstrual period in 2 months. Her mother shares that her daughter has had a previous pregnancy that resulted in abortion. Nicole denies that she is pregnant at this time. Her mother states that she does not think that Nicole is sexually active at present because she does not have a boyfriend.

During the physical exam, the nurse notes that the inner aspects of Nicole's arms are bruised, and there is an unusual mark on her breast that could be a bite mark as well and bruises on her thighs and her back. Some suspicious bruises appear to be in the healing stages on her legs and back. When Nicole is questioned about the bruises, she states, "Oh, that's nothing. My boyfriend gets a little carried away sometimes."

REVIEW OF PERTINENT DOMAINS

Biological Domain

Physical examination reveals height of 5 ft, 5 in,, and weight is 103 lb. Her BMI is 17, which places her in the below-normal category. Blood pressure is 98/64. Oral temperature is 98.7° F. Breasts are firm, without masses and nontender. Abdomen is soft, nontender, no hernias, or organomegaly. Signs of secondary sexual characteristics are present, which include hair pattern growth in the genital area, breast development, and development of a maturing body shape. External genitalia is normal, vagina is pink, with a moist, yellowish discharge noted; cervix shows no abnormalities. All other systems are unremarkable. Because she is underweight, eating disorders need to be explored.

GENITOURINARY: Last menstrual period was approximately 2 months ago.

Psychological Domain

Nicole does not want her mother present in the room during examination and health history interview. She appears anxious that her mother might find out something about the exam and interview.

Social Domain

Nicole is a sophomore in high school. She lives with her parents and two younger brothers. She states that she has a boyfriend but that no one in her family knows him; she spends most of her time with him because they are in love. Nicole is adamant that she is not pregnant but acknowledges that she was pregnant 6 months ago but chose to have an abortion. She admits that she engages in oral sex and some heavy petting but that she does not consider that having sex.

EDUCATIONAL ISSUES

Nicole needs education about the risks of sexually transmitted disease that can occur with oral sex as well as petting and intercourse. She also needs education about birth control because she may be having intercourse although she does not admit this.

QUESTIONS FOR DISCUSSION

1. Since Nicole is underage and requires her mother's consent to have medical care, is it necessary for her mother to be present in the room during the history and physical exam?
2. Does Nicole need testing for sexually transmitted diseases, and what evidence would suggest this?
3. What questions should specifically be intended to explore intimate partner violence?
4. What should be shared with Nicole and her mother regarding the possibility of Nicole's being pregnant?
5. What can the nurse do if she suspects that Nicole is the victim of intimate partner violence?

KEY CONCEPTS

1. Health promotion for mothers-to-be begins prior to conception. Women need education about the physiological and psychological changes related to pregnancy as well as fetal development. Healthy behaviors should be initiated prior to conception. These behaviors include an exercise program, a healthy and well-balanced diet, folic acid supplementation, and avoidance of substances known to be harmful to the fetus. Potential parents should have genetic history screening for inheritable abnormalities, and mothers should have screening for chronic diseases that might adversely affect the fetus.

2. During pregnancy, the mother-to-be should continue with a healthy lifestyle. Screening during this time is for gestational diabetes, Rh factor isoimmunization, fetal congenital anomalies, and prenatal depression because this is a risk factor for postpartum depression. Health promotion involves helping the mother reduce common discomforts that occur during pregnancy and to begin discussing and supporting the mother's choice to breast-feed.

3. Following delivery, the mother undergoes as many physiological and psychological changes as she did during pregnancy. Health promotion involves encouraging the mother to get adequate rest and nutrition, providing breast-feeding teaching and support, and helping the mother to access social and emotional support. The mother should be immunized during the immediate postpartum period for rubella, varicella, and pertussis if nonimmune, and she should be informed that she must avoid becoming pregnant for one month after vaccination and that contraception must be used. The new mother should also be screened for postpartum depression.

4. Health promotion for infants and toddlers in the biological domain includes strategies related to nutrition, elimination, sleep and activity, and immunizations.

5. Screening for actual or potential health problems in infants and toddlers is vital for promoting the quality and quantity of life. Nurses assist in screening for metabolic defects, anemia, hearing problems, and growth and developmental delays.

6. Promoting health in the psychological domain for infants and toddlers requires an understanding of normal cognitive and emotional development. Theoretical frameworks developed by Jean Piaget and Erik Erikson provide a foundation for evaluating the development of infants and toddlers.

7. Health promotion in the social domain for infants and toddlers evolves from the need for the family to include day care in their networks.

8. Child abuse and neglect affect more than 3.3 million children annually. Nurses need to be able to identify signs of child abuse and neglect. Some physical signs to look for are bruising, hematomas, poor skin care, malnutrition, bite marks, and retinal hemorrhage. Parental behavior and discrepancies between the reported cause of injury and the injury seen can also be important keys to identifying abuse. By law, any suspicion of abuse or neglect must be reported to the appropriate authorities.

9. In addition to legislation mandating the reporting of suspected child abuse, the political domain encompasses other social actions for health promotion: the Supplemental Food Program for Women, Infants, and Children (WIC), car safety seat requirement laws, and legislation that requires employers to provide adequate time and an appropriate location for a lactating mother to express breast milk uninterruptedly while in the workplace.

10. Nurses and parents share the responsibility for promoting the safety of infants and toddlers. Safety strategies, including immunizations, foods appropriate for age and providing toys that are not choking hazards, car seats, and hazard proofing the home are all important measures. Preventing physical and psychological trauma is vital to ensure healthy development throughout the life span.

11. Important in the sexual domain is the education of parents and caregivers about the normal sexual development of infants and toddlers.

12. Spiritual beliefs and practices of the parents and caregivers influence health promotion in the spiritual domain.

CHAPTER REVIEW

Learning Activities

1. Observe an infant's behavior, and compare it to Erikson's stages of psychological development.
2. Use local or Internet sources or both to find the infant mortality rate for your area.
3. With classmates, discuss approaches to reduce infant mortality.
4. List the immunization schedule for an infant through childhood.
5. Develop a pamphlet for a new mother that addresses the symptoms of depression.

Multiple Choice

1. The nurse is providing parent teaching regarding scheduled child immunizations. Which statement made by the parent indicates that further teaching is necessary?
   a. "Children with a mild illness such as a cold or flu should not receive their scheduled immunizations."
   b. "Children should be kept up-to-date on all scheduled immunizations, and catch immunizations should be administered if the schedule is missed."
   c. "Children with mild illness such as a cold or flu should not avoid their scheduled immunization."
   d. "Children should have their immunization records kept up-to-date for required school documentation of immunizations."

2. A two-day-old newborn girl will be discharged with her mother tomorrow. The mother asks the nurse when her baby will receive her first hepatitis B immunization. What should be the nurse's response?
   a. Only if you are positive for hepatitis B positive.
   b. She will receive her first hepatitis B vaccine prior to discharge.
   c. She should receive her first hepatitis B vaccine when she is one year old.
   d. She should receive her first hepatitis B vaccine when she is six months old.

3. A three-day postpartum woman, who is not immune to rubella, will receive the rubella vaccine prior to discharge. What should the nurse include in the discharge teaching regarding this vaccine?
   a. The mother should not become pregnant for at least 4 weeks.
   b. The mother should pump and discard her breast milk for one week.
   c. The mother should wear a surgical mask when caring for her baby for at least two weeks.
   d. Passive antibodies transported across the placenta will protect her baby.

4. The parents of a nine-month-old infant are attending a class on child safety. Following the class, what should the parents understand as one of the common causes of injury and death for a nine-month-old infant?
   a. Poisoning when with babysitter
   b. Dog bite while playing with pet
   c. Foreign object aspiration
   d. Child abuse by a parent

5. A woman is being seen in the gynecology clinic. The nurse notes that the woman has a swollen eye and a bruise on her neck. Which is an appropriate statement for the nurse to make?
   a. "I am required by law to notify the police department of your injuries."
   b. "Women who are physically abused often have injuries like yours."
   c. "You must leave your partner before you are injured again."
   d. "It is important that you refrain from doing things that anger your partner."

6. A nurse is counseling a new mother about postpartum blues. What statement should the nurse include in the discussion?
   a. Breast-feeding might make this condition worse.
   b. Postpartum blues last about a week or two.
   c. Medications are available and should be taken as soon as possible.
   d. Very few women experience postpartum blues, and this is a problem.

7. In the gynecologic clinic, the nurse is counseling a woman who is of childbearing age, is capable of getting pregnant, and who is sexually active. What supplement should the nurse recommend the woman to take because of the risk of becoming unknowingly pregnant?
   a. Extra calcium
   b. Folate
   c. Iron supplements
   d. Vitamin A

8. The nurse is advising the parents of a newborn being discharged from the hospital regarding car seat safety. What should be included in the teaching plan?
   a. Put the car seat facing forward only after the baby reaches 20 lb.
   b. The car seat should be placed facing the rear in the front seat of the car.
   c. A fist should fit between the straps of the car seat and the baby's body.
   d. Place the car seat in the center of the back seat facing forward.

ORGANIZATIONS AND WEBSITES

Administration for Children and Families (a division of the U.S. Department of Health and Human Services): Provides information about services, policies, and programs affecting children; includes information on child abuse and neglect, early child development, and child care: **http://www.acf.hhs.gov**

Advisory Committee on Immunization Practices (ACIP): Provides immunization recommendations and updated schedules; includes information on vaccine administration: **http://www.cdc.gov/vaccines/recs/acip**

American Academy of Pediatrics—Children's Health Topics: Breastfeeding: Provides breast-feeding education and includes family/community resources: **http://www.aap.org/ healthtopics/breastfeeding.cfm**

Centers for Disease Control and Prevention: Provides infant and child growth charts: **http://www.cdc.gov/growthcharts**

Coalition to End Childhood Lead Poisoning: Provides information on lead and has links to other websites (hotline 1-800-370-LEAD): **http://www.leadsafe.org**

National Domestic Violence Hotline: Provides crisis intervention and referrals (in English and Spanish) to in-state and out-of-state resources, such as women's shelters and crisis centers (1-800-799-SAFE or 1-800-799-7233.): **http:// www.thehotline.org** or **http://www.thehotline.org/ get-help/help-in-your-area/**

National Women's Health Information Center: Federal government source for women's health information; topics on healthy pregnancy and includes information on before getting pregnancy, preconception health, contraception, and unplanned pregnancy: **http://www.womenshealth.gov/pregnancy**

Not-2-Late: Provides information (in English and Spanish) about emergency contraception and resources; includes frequently asked questions: **http://www.not-2-late.com**

Office for Victims of Crime (Office of Justice Programs): Provides information and resources such as crime victims' rights, help for crime victims, sexual assault, date rape, child abuse, and teens: **http://www.ojp.usdoj.gov/ovc/**

Vaccine safety and effectiveness: Includes information on disease prevention and infectious diseases; provides childhood immunization schedule and where to get vaccinated in your local area: **http://www.vaccines.gov**

REFERENCES

Acar, B. S., & van Lopik, D. (2009). Computational pregnant occupant model, "expecting" for crash simulations. Proceedings of the Institution of Mechanical Engineers, Part D. *Journal of Automobile Engineering, 223,* 891–902. DOI: 10.1243/0954407JAUTO7072.

American Academy of Pediatrics. (2011). Policy statement SIDS and other sleep-related infant deaths: Expansion of recommendations for a safe infant sleeping environment task force on sudden infant death syndrome, Retrieved from http://aappolicy.aappublications.org/cgi/content/full/pediatrics;128/5/1030

American Academy of Pediatrics. (2011). Policy Statement on Breast-feeding and the use of human milk released in 2005. Retrieved from http://www.aap.org/breastfeeding

Antoniou, R. M., Vivilake, R. M., & Daglas, M. (2008). Correlation of domestic violence during pregnancy with postnatal depression: Systematic review of bibliography. *Health Science Journal, 2*(1), 15–19.

Asary, A., Palacios, C., De-Regil, L. M., & Pena-Rosas, J. P. (2010). Vitamin D supplementation for women during pregnancy. *Cochran Database of Systematic Reviews, 12,* CD008873. DOI: 10.1002/14651858.cd008873.

Ayoola, A. B., Nettleman, M. D., Stommel, M., & Canady, R. B. (2010). Time of pregnancy recognition and prenatal care use: A population-based study in the United States. *Birth, 37*(1), 37–43.

Badell, M. I., Ramin, S. M., & Smith, J. A. (2006). Treatment options for nausea and vomiting during pregnancy. *Journal of Maternal Child Nursing, 34*(2), 98–105.

Baker, L., & Oswalt, K. (2008). Screening of postpartum depression in a rural community. *Community Mental Health Journal, 44,* 171–180.

Bansil, P., Kuklina, E., Meikle, S., Posner, S., Kourtis, A., Ellington, S. & Jamieson, D. (2010). Maternal and fetal outcomes among women with depression. *Journal of Women's Health, 19*(2), 329–334. DOI: 10.1089/jwh.2009.1387

Barnard, K. E. (1994). Parent-child interaction model. In A. Marriner-Tomey (ed.). *Nursing theorists and their work.* St. Louis, MO: Mosby, pp. 406–422.

Blanchard, A., Hodgson, J., Gunn, W., Jesse, E., & White, M. (2009). Understanding social support and the couple's relationship among women with depression symptoms in pregnancy. *Issues in Mental Health Nursing, 30*(12), 764–776. DOI: 10.3109/01612840903725594.

Boyles, S. (2010). High doses of vitamin D may cut pregnancy risks. *WebMD Health News.* Retrieved from http://www.webmd.com/baby/news

Brainerd, C. J. (1978). *Piaget's theory of intelligence.* Englewood Cliffs, NJ: Prentice Hall.

Breastfeeding Report Card—United States (2010). Center for Disease Control and Prevention, Section on Breastfeeding. Retrieved from http://www.cdc.gov/breastfeeding/data/reportcard.htm

Bruhn, K., & Tillet, J. (2009). Administration of vaccinations in pregnancy and postpartum. *The American Journal of Maternal Child Nursing, 34*(2), 98–105.

Centers for Disease Control and Prevention (CDC). (2008a). Prevention and control of influenza: Recommendations of the advisory committee on immunization practices. *Morbidity and Mortality Weekly Report, 57*(RR-4), 2–3.

Centers for Disease Control and Prevention (CDC). (2008b). Violence prevention data sheet. Retreived from http://www.cdc.gov/ViolencePrevention/pdf/SV-DataSheet-a.pdf

Centers for Disease Control and Prevention. (CDC). (2010). Pertussis prevention: vaccination. Retrieved from http://www.cdc.gov/pertussis/about/prevention.html

Centers for Disease Control and Prevention (CDC). (2011a). Recommendation of the Advisory Committee on Immunization Practices. *Morbidity and Mortality Weekly Report, 57*(RR-4), 2–3. Retrieved from http://www.cdc.gov/mmwr/PDF/rr/rr5704.pdf

Centers for Disease Control and Prevention (CDC). (2011b). Understanding intimate partner violence. Retrieved from http://www.cdc.gov/ViolencePrevention/intimatepartnerviolence/

Chang, J. J., Pien, G. W., Duntley, S. P., & Macones, G. A. (2010). Sleep deprivation during pregnancy and maternal and fetal outcomes: Is there a relationship? *Sleep Medicine Reviews, 14*(2), 107–114. DOI: 10.1016/i.smrv.2009.05.001

Child Health USA. (2011). Maternal mortality. Retrieved from http://mchb.hrsa.gov/chusa11/hstat/hsi/pages/208mm.html

Cleveland Clinic (2011). Good nutrition during pregnancy for you and your baby. Health Information, Retrieved from http://my.clevelandclinic.org/healthy_living/pregnancy/hic_good_nutrition_during_pregnancy_for_you_and_your_baby.aspx#

Coleman, T. (2007). Recommendation for the use of pharmacological smoking cessation strategies in pregnant women. *CNS Drugs, 21*(2), 983–993.

Corbiett, R., Ryan, C., & Weinrich, S. (2011). Pica in pregnancy: Does it affect pregnancy outcomes? *Journal of Maternal Child Nursing*, 36, 183–189.

Davidoff, F., & Trussell, J. (2006). Plan B and the politics of doubt. *The Journal of the American Medical Association, 296*(14), 1775–1778. DOI: 10.1001/jama.296.14.1775.

Dietary guidelines for Americans. (2010). The Center for Nutrition Policy and Promotion of the U.S. Department of Agriculture. Retrieved from http://www.cnpp.usda.gov/DietaryGuidelines.htm

Down syndrome facts. (2011). The National Center on Birth Defects and Developmental Disabilities of the Centers for Disease Control and Prevention. Retrieved from http://www.cdc.gov/ncbddd/birthdefects/DownSyndrome.html

Duijts, L., Jaddoe, V. W., Hofman, A., & Moll, H. A. (2010). Prolonged and exclusive breastfeeding reduces the risk of infectious diseases in infancy. *Pediatrics, 126*(1), e18.

Duncan, J. M., & Sears, M. R. (2008). Breastfeeding and allergies: Time for a change in paradigm? *Current Opinion in Allergy and Clinical Immunology, 8*, 388–405. DOI: 10.1097/ACI.0b013e32830d82ed.

Einarson, A., & Riordan, S. (2009). Smoking in pregnancy and lactation: A review of risks and cessation strategies. *European Journal of Clinical Pharmacology, 65*(4), 325–330. DOI: 10.1007/s00228-008-0609-0,

Emergency Contraception: Frequently asked questions (2009). The National Women's Health Information. Retrieved from http://www.womenshealth.gov/faq/emergency-contraception.cfm

Erikson, E. (1950). *Childhood and society.* New York, NY: Norton.

Facts About Down Syndrome (2011). The National Center on Birth Defects and Developmental Disabilities of the Centers for Disease Control and Prevention. Retrieved from http://www.cdc.gov/ncbddd/birthdefects/DownSyndrome.html

Felt, B. T., Brown, P., Coran, A. G., Kochhar, P., Opipari-Arrigan, & L. Van Harrison, R. (2004). Functional constipation and soiling in children. *Clinics in Family Practice, 6*(3), 709–730.

Foux, R. (2008). Sex education in pregnancy: Does it exist? A literature review. *Sexual and Relationship Therapy, 23*(2), 271–277.

Gold, R. B., & Nash, E. (2007). State abortion counseling policies and the fundamental principles of informed consent. *Guttmacher Policy Review, 10*, 6–13.

Goodman, J. H., & Tyer-Viola, L. (2010). Detection, treatment, and referral of perinatal depression and anxiety by obstetrical providers. *Journal of Women's Health, 19*(3), 477–489.

Gossler, S. M. (2010). Use of complementary and alternative therapies during pregnancy, postpartum, and lactation. *Journal of Psychosocial Nursing & Mental Health Series, 48*(11), 30–36. DOI: 10.3928/02793695-20100930-02.

Guidelines for vaccinating pregnant women. (2011). Centers for Disease Control and Prevention. Retrieved from http://www.cdc.gov/vaccines/pubs/pre-guide.htm

Hamilton, B. E., Martin, J. A., & Ventura, M. A. (2010). Births: Preliminary Data for 2009. *National Vital Statistics Reports, 59*(3). http://www.cdc.gov

Hart, C. N., Raynor, H. A., Jelalian, E., & Drotar, D. (2010). The association of maternal food intake and infants' and toddlers' food intake. *Child: Care, Health and Development, 36*(3), 396–403. DOI: 10.1111/j.1365-2214.2010.01072.x.

Hoecker, J. (2011). What are the signs of infant constipation? And what is the best way to treat it? *Infant and Toddler Health,* Mayo clinic. Retrieved from http://www.mayoclinic.com/health/infant-constipation/AN01089

Institute of Medicine (IOM) and the National Research Council. (2009). *Weight gain during pregnancy: Reexamining the guidelines.* Washington, DC: The National Academic Press. Retrieved from http://iom.edu/Reports/2009/Weight-Gain-During-Pregnancy-Reexamining-the-Guidelines.aspx

Khresheh, R. (2011). How woman manage nausea and vomiting during pregnancy: A Jordanian study. *Midwifery, 27*(1), 42–45. DOI: 10.1016/j.midw.2009.12.002.

Klaus, M. H., & Kennel, J. H. (1985). Parent-infant bonding. St. Louis, MO: Mosby Press.

Knudson-Martin, C., & Silverstein, R. (2009). Suffering in silence: A qualitative meta-data-analysis of postpartum depression. *Journal of Marital and Family Therapy, 35*(2), 145–158.

Kramer, A. (2007). Stages of change: Surviving intimate partner violence during and after pregnancy. *Journal of Perinatal and Neonatal Nursing, 21*(4), 285–295.

Leahy-Warren, P., & McCarthy, G. (2007). Postnatal depression: Prevalence, mothers' perspectives and treatments. *Archives of Psychiatric Nursing, 21*, 91–100.

Lee, K. A., & Caughey, A. B. (2006). Sleep disorders in women: A guide to practical management, Evaluating insomnia during pregnancy and postpartum. In H. P. Attarian (ed.), *Current clinical neurology.* Totowa, NJ: Human Press, pp. 185–198. DOI: 10.1007/978-1-59745-1154_15.

Lee, J. (2011). A quick fix solution for the morning after: An alternative approach to mandatory contraceptive coverage. *The Georgetown Journal of Law & Public Policy, 9*, 189–216. Retrieved from http://ijptp.iomcworld.com/files/Gajanan.pdf

Lindbald, F., & Hjern, A. (2010). ADHD after fetal exposure to maternal smoking. *Nicotine and Tobacco Research, 12*(4), 408–415.

MacDorman, M. F., & Mathew, T. J. (2009). *Behind international rankings of infant mortality: How the United States compares with Europe* (NCHS data brief No. 23). National Center for Health Statistics. Hyattsville, MD: National Center for Health Statistics.

Mannella, J. (n.d.). Alcohol's effects an lactation. National Institute on Alcohol Abuse and Alcoholism (NIAAA) of the National Institutes of Health. Retrieved from http://pubs.niaaa.nih.gov/publications/arh25-3/230-234.htm

Melrose, S. (2010). Paternal postpartum depression: How can nurses begin to help? *Contemporary Nurse. Journal for the Australian Nursing Profession, 34*(2), 199–210. DOI: 10.5172/conu.2010.34.2.199.

Minino, A. M., Xu, J., Kochanek, K. D. (2010). *Infant mortality: Final data for 2008.* National Vital Statistics Reports 59(2). Retrieved from National Center for Health Statistics website: http://www.cdc.gov/nchs/data/nvsr/nvsr58/nvsr58_19.pdf

Mosher, W. D., & Jones, J. (2010). Use of contraception in the United States: 1982–2008. *National Center for Health Statistics. Vital Health Statistics, 23*(29).

Murray, R. B., Zentner, J. P., & Yakimo, R. (2009). Prenatal and other developmental issues. In M. Connor (ed.). Health promotion strategies through the life span (8th ed.). Upper Saddler River, NJ: Prentice Hall, p. 220.

Oken, E., Osterdal, M. L., Gillman, M. W., Knudsen, V. K., Halldorsson, T. I., Strom, M., Bellinger, D. C., Hadders-Algra, M., Michaelsen, K. F., & Olsen, S. F. (2008). Associations of maternal fish intake during pregnancy and breastfeeding with attainment of developmental milestones in early childhood: A study from the Danish National Birth Cohort. *American Journal of Clinical Nutrition, 88*(3), 789–796.

Oncken, C. A., & Kranzler, H. R. (2009). What do we know about the role of pharmacotherapy for smoking cessation before or during pregnancy? *Nicotine and Tobacco Research, 11*(11), 1273–1278. DOI: 10.1093/ntr/ntp136.

Ozgoli, G., Marjan, G., & Masoumen, S. (2009). Effects of ginger capsules on pregnancy, nausea, and vomiting. *The Journal of Alternative and Complementary Medicine, 15*(3), 243–246. DOI: 10.1039/acm.2008.0406.

Perry, S. E., Hockenberry, M. J., Lowdermilk, D. L., & Wilson, D. (2010). Pregnancy at risk: Preexisting conditions. In P. F. Barrera (ed.), *Maternal child nursing care* (4th ed.). Maryland, MO: Mosby Elsevier, pp. 298–309.

Pregnancy statistics (2011). American Pregnancy Association. Retrieved from http://www.americanpregnancy.org/main/statistics.html

Rabin, R. F., Jenning, J. M., Campbell, J. C., & Bair-Merritt, M. H. (2009). Intimate partner violence during screening tools: A systemic review. *American Journal of Preventive Medicine, 36*(5), 439–445.

Raghuveer, T., Garg, U., & Graf, W. D. (2006). Inborn errors of metabolism in infancy and early childhood: An update. *American Family Physician, 73*(11), 1981–1990.

Reproductive and Developmental Hazard Management Guidance (RDHMG) (2011). The American College of Occupational and Environmental Medicine (ACOEM) Task Force on Reproductive Toxicology. Retrieved from http://www.acoem.org/Reproductive_Developmental_Hazard_Management.aspx

Richardson, C. T., & Nash, E. (2006). Misinformed consent: The medical accuracy of stat-developed abortion counseling materials. *Guttmacher Policy Review, 9*(4), 6–11.

Rifampin: Special precautions with contraception. (2011). U.S. National Library of Medicine of the National Institutes of Health. Retrieved from http://www.nlm.nih.gov/medlineplus/druginfo/meds/a682403.html

Robyn, L. M., Ponsonby, A. L., Pasco, J. A., & Morley, R. (2008). Future health implications of prenatal and early-life vitamin D status. *Nutrition Reviews, 66*(12), 710.

Ross, A. C., Russell, R. M., Miller, S. A., Munro, T. C., Rodricks, J. V., Yetley, E. A., & Julien, E. (2009). Application of a key event dose-response analysis to nutrients: A case study with vitamin A (retinol). *Critical Reviews in Food Science and Nutrition, 49*, 708–717. DOI: 10.1080/10408390903898749.

Sanap, G. S., Laddha, S. S., & Singh, A. (2011). Emergency contraceptive pills—A review. *International Journal of Pharmacy Teaching Practices, 2*(1), 27–33. Retrieved from http://ijptp.iomcworld.com/files/Gajanan.pdf

Sanger, C. (2008). Seeing and believing: Mandatory ultrasound and the path to a protected choice. *UCLA Law Review, 56*(2), 351–408. Retrieved from http://uclalawreview.org/pdf/56-2-2.pdf

Sayal, K., Heron, J., Golding, J., Alti, R., Smith, G. D., Gray, R., & Emond, A. (2009). Binge pattern of alcohol consumption during pregnancy and childhood mental health outcomes: Longitudinal population based study. *Pediatrics, 123*(2), e289-296. DOI: 10.1542/peds.2008-1961.

Schnaas, L., Rothenberg, S., Flores, M., Martinez, S., Hernandez, C., Osorio, E., Velasco, S. R., & Perroni, E. (2006). Reduced intellectual development in children with prenatal lead exposure. *Environmental Health Perspectives, 114*(5), 791–787.

Shamu, S., Abrahams, N., Temmerman, M., Musekiwa, A., & Zarowsky, C. (2011). A systematic review of African studies on intimate partner violence against pregnant women: Prevalence and risk factors. *PloS ONE, 6*(3): e17591. DOI: 10.1371/journal.pone.0017591.

Shoffner, D. H. (2007). We don't like to think about it: Intimate partner violence during pregnancy and postpartum. *Journal of Perinatal and Neonatal Nursing, 22*(1), 39–48.

Siegel, R. B. (2007). The new politics of abortion: An equality analysis of women-protective abortion restrictions. Braun Lecture, Yale Law School, Public Working Paper (No. 9). University of Illinois Law Review, Champaign, IL.

Shoffner, D. H. (2008). We don't like to think about it: Intimate partner violence during pregnancy. *Journal of Perinatal and Neonatal Nursing, 21*(4), 285–295.

Spinelli, M. (2003). *Infanticide: Psychosocial and legal perspectives on mothers who kill.* Washington, DC: American Psychiatric Association.

Stevens-Wrightom, A. (2007). Universal newborn hearing screening. *American Family Physician, 75*(9), 1349–1352.

The Surgeon General's Call to Action to Support Breastfeeding (2011). Office of the Surgeon General of the U.S. Department of Health and Human Services. Retrieved from http://www.surgeongeneral.gov/topics/breastfeeding/index.html

Swanson, K. M. (1993). Nursing as caring for the well being of others. *Journal of Nursing Scholarship, 23*(4), 452–457.

Teen births: A fact sheet reporting national, state, and city trends in teen childbearing for 2009. Publication 2011. Retrieved from http://www.childtrends.org/Files/Child_Trends-2011_04_14_FG_2011.pdf

Tremellen, K. (2008). Oxidative stress and male fertility, a clinical perspective. *Human Reproductive Update, 14*(3), 243–258.

U.S. Preventive Services Task Force. (2009). Folic acid to prevent neural tube defects. Retrieved from http://www.uspreventiveservicestaskforce.org/uspstf/uspsnrfol.htm

Van de Brock, N., Dou, L., Othman, M., Neilson, J. P., Gates, S., & Gulmezoglu, A. M. (2010). Vitamin A supplementation during pregnancy for maternal and newborn outcomes. *Cochran Database of Systematic Reviews, 11*, No: CD008999. DOI: 10.1002/13651858.CD008666.pub2.

Weber, S. E. (2009). An attempt to legislate morality: Forced ultrasound as the newest tactic in antiabortion legislation. *The University of Tulsa Law Review, 45*(359).

Whitehouse, C. R., Boullata, J., & McCauley, L. A. (2008). The potential toxicity of artificial sweeteners. *The American Association of Occupation Health Nurses Journal, 56*(6), 329–334.

Wiebe, E. R., & Adams, L. (2009). Women's perceptions about seeing the ultrasound picture before an abortion. *European Journal of Contraception & Reproduction Health Care, 14*(2), 97–102. DOI: 10.1080/13625180902745730.

Wiwanitkit, V. (2009). Rabies vaccination in pregnancy and lactation. *Anatolian Journal of Obstetrics & Gynecology, 4*(2), 1–3.

Wolff, T., Witkop, C. T., Miller, T., & Shamsuzoha, B. S. (2009). Folic acid supplementation for the prevention of neural tube defects: An update of the evidence for the U.S. Preventive Services Task Force. *Annals of Internal Medicine, 150*, 632–639.

World Health Organization (WHO). (2011). Child and adolescent health: Adolescent health and development. Retrieved from http://www.searo.who.int/en/Section13/Section1245_4980.htm

Yonkers, K. A., Wisner, K. L., Stewart, D. E., Oberlander, T. F., Dell, D. L., Stotland, N., Ramin, S., Chandron, L., & Lockwood, C. (2009). The management of depression during pregnancy: A report from the American Psychiatric Association and the American College of Obstetricians and Gynecologists. *General Hospital Psychiatry, 4*, 1–11. DOI: 10.1016/j.genhosppsych.2009.04.003.

Young, S. L. (2010). Pica in pregnancy: New ideas about an old condition. *Annual Review of Nutrition, 30*, 403–422. DOI: 10.1146/annurev.nutr.012809.10473.

Zheng-Hong, L., Dong, M., & Wang, Z. F. (2008). Functional constipation in children: Investigation and management of anorectal motility. *World Journal of Pediatrics, 4*(1), 41–53.

CHAPTER 10
The Child

BEATRIZ G. BAUTISTA, DNP, APRN, FNP-BC, CCD

KEY TERMS

acanthosis nigricans (AN)
attention-deficit/hyperactivity
   disorder (ADHD)
body mass index (BMI)
egocentric
encopresis

enuresis
incontinence
nightmares
night terror
obesity
overweight

peers
rickets
scoliosis
underweight

OBJECTIVES

Upon completion of this chapter, the reader should be able to:

- Examine health-promotion strategies in the biological domain for children.
- Identify nursing responsibilities for screening to promote the health of children.
- Relate theories of cognitive and emotional development to health-promotion strategies in children.
- Identify social networks and their importance in child health.
- Describe the occurrence, signs and symptoms, and nursing responsibilities relating to child abuse and neglect.
- Identify legislative actions designed to improve the health of children.
- Describe parental and nursing responsibilities for promoting child safety.
- Relate normal sexual development to strategies designed to promote sexual health in children.
- Describe spiritual influences on health promotion in children.

INTRODUCTION

Childhood is typically divided into two periods: the preschool years and the school-age years. The preschool years include ages 3–6. Physical growth has slowed, but significant social, emotional, and cognitive growth is occurring. Preschool children are learning how to get along with others and understand another's feelings and needs. They enjoy playing games, reading books, and being with other children, and they can be away from parents and caregivers for longer periods. Preschoolers are beginning to gain mastery over their bodies as they learn to toilet, feed, and dress themselves. They are gaining mastery over language and can often be great conversationalists, talking about all sorts of subjects, asking innumerable questions, and expressing their own ideas about things. All these developments help prepare the preschooler for entrance into formal education.

The school-age years include ages 6–12, where development is focused on mental abilities, competence, and self-esteem. Although growth in height and weight is slower, growth in learning and motor skills is impressive. School-age children learn to read, write, do mathematics, and understand a wide variety of other subjects, such as geography, history, and music. Their world is no longer focused on themselves and the family unit, expanding to include peers and the school environment. The major developmental tasks are achievement in school and acceptance by peers. The school-age years are often the so-called calm before the storm of adolescence.

THE PRESCHOOL AND SCHOOL-AGE CHILD

The enormous physical and psychological development of the preschool and school-age years makes health promotion critical. Health-promotion strategies can begin to involve the child in a more active role.

BIOLOGICAL DOMAIN

The biological areas of nutrition, elimination, sleep and activity, immunization, and screening are discussed in this section as they relate to health promotion for the preschool and the school-age child. The health-promotion strategies recommended are largely the responsibility of the parents/caregivers and the nurse.

Nutrition

Both the preschool and the school-age child need a balanced diet that includes a wide variety of choices from the five major food groups. MyPlate (see Chapter 15), recommended by the American Academy of Pediatrics, serves as a guide to food planning. In contrast to infants, who require up to 50% of their calories from fat (because the brain in particular needs dietary fat for proper growth and development), both preschool and school-age children benefit from a diet lower in total fat (30–35 percent and 25–35% of their total calories, respectively). The permanent switch from whole milk to skim or 2% milk at this time is imperative and should comply with the recommendations made for the rest of the family. Saturated fat, cholesterol, sugar, and salt should also be monitored. Sweetened beverages, such as sodas and fruit drinks, should be avoided because they have no nutritional value and can quickly lead to weight gain. To prevent obesity and tooth decay, the American Academy of Pediatrics (AAP) recommends no more than 4–6 oz/day of 100% fruit juice. Fruit juices offer no nutritional benefits over whole fruits, which can also provide fiber and other nutrients (AAP, 2011a). The nurse needs to encourage a diet of poultry, fish, lean meat, low-fat and skim milk products, dried peas and beans, whole grain breads and cereals, vegetables, and fruits.

The nurse needs to remind the parents of the differences in food portions. The child usually eats one-fourth to one-third of the adult portion or roughly one tablespoon of each food for each year of the child's age. Parents should allow children to ask for more food if they are still hungry instead of overfilling the child's plate (AAP, 2011a).

The first step in assessing a child's weight and nutrition is to determine the **body mass index (BMI)** for age and gender. The BMI is a number that shows body weight adjusted for height and can be calculated using inches and pounds or meters and kilograms. The CDC provides a calculator at http://www.cdc.gov; from that page, search for "BMIcalculator." In children, BMI is used to assess for underweight, normal or healthy weight, overweight, and obesity. Because body fat changes in children as they grow older and differences exist between boys and girls, BMI should be plotted on a gender-specific growth chart that uses percentiles to show how the child's BMI compares to that of children of the same gender and age. Nurses use the established percentile cutoff point in Table 10-1 to identify underweight, overweight, and obesity in children. BMI is a useful tool for assessment because it provides a reference for adolescents that can be used beyond puberty, it compares well to laboratory measures of body fat, and it can be used to track body size throughout life.

Assessing a child's weight should also include a review of the child's growth pattern: weight for height before the age of 2 and BMI after the age of 2. A weight problem can be detected if the child moves either up or down across percentile lines. Asking about the child's eating habits and activity levels is also important.

Parents of preschoolers often become concerned with their child's food preferences and lack of interest in eating. Preschoolers' emerging ability to control their environment is frequently demonstrated by adamant food preferences and rejections. Many reject cooked vegetables, mixed foods, and new foods. Experts tell us that it often takes about a dozen times for a child to develop a taste or flavor for an unfamiliar food item. The nurse can help frustrated parents review the overall nutritional adequacy of the diet, evaluate for the presence of pressure and stress during mealtimes, and learn a variety of ways to introduce adequate nutrition to the diet. Suggestions for managing the picky eater are presented in Box 10-1.

Parents have a major influence over the nutritional adequacy of the child's diet that goes beyond purchasing and preparing the food. Providing the child with role models who eat and enjoy a wide variety of nutritious foods is essential because

TABLE 10-1 Weight Classification by Body Mass Index (BMI)	
Underweight	BMI-for-age/sex < 5th percentile
Normal or healthy weight	BMI-for-age/sex 5th to < 85th percentile
Overweight	BMI-for-age/sex 85th to < 95th percentile
Obese	BMI-for-age/sex ≥ 95th percentile

© Cengage Learning 2013

BOX 10-1
MANAGING THE PICKY EATER

1. Serve vegetables raw and cut into finger-sized pieces. Use them for snacks.
2. Use cookie cutters to cut sandwiches into fun shapes.
3. Use special dishware, such as their favorite theme or character.
4. "Tea-time" can be the occasions to introduce items for snacks.
5. Provide a sauce for dipping vegetables such as melted cheese, salad dressing, or yogurt.
6. Serve foods plain and separated, rather than in casseroles, in stews, or creamed.
7. Serve small portions, arranged attractively and separately on the plate.
8. Cut easily chewable meat into bite-sized pieces.
9. Continue to introduce new foods even if they are met with rejection at first.
10. Serve one food on the child's like-list at each meal.
11. Incorporate pureed vegetables (carrots, squash, and spinach) into sauces for pizza or spaghetti.
12. Avoid allowing excessive eating between meals.
13. Encourage participation with meal planning and preparation (selecting a nutritious menu, setting the table, stirring an instant pudding).

the child's food preferences generally reflect those of the parents. Healthy habits are established in the first five years of life. Parents should seek to make mealtime a comfortable, social experience without coaxing, threatening, or bribing. Making food an issue is certain to make the child more adamant about not eating. Parents should be reassured that the appetite and the acceptance of new foods usually increase as the child gets older.

Vitamins may be a good supplement to the preschooler's diet, especially during periods of increased food fussiness. Fluoride supplements are needed if the local water supply does not contain it. Calcium and vitamin D intake needs to be assessed. National data show that many children do not get enough calcium or [MP2] vitamin D, increasing their risk of developing **rickets** (a preventable condition resulting in poor bone mineralization, leading to soft bones and skeletal deformities) and, later, osteoporosis. Children need calcium and vitamin D for bone formation and weight-bearing exercise to strengthen bones. The American Academy of Pediatrics (2008) has doubled the recommended intake of vitamin D to 400 IU/day for infants, children, and adolescents. The best source of vitamin D comes from sunlight exposure, but the risk of skin cancer concerns have added to this deficiency. Substituting soft drinks for milk or calcium-fortified juice and increased time in sedentary activities also place bones at risk. Screening for calcium intake and bone health should occur at age 2–3 after weaning from breast milk or formula, at age 8–9 before the adolescent growth spurt, and again during puberty when the peak rate of bone mass growth occurs.

The school-age child may continue to display some food preferences, occasionally eating only one specific food.

Health-promotion strategies are similar to those for the preschool child but should include an assessment of meals eaten at school. Although the majority of schools use the USDA school lunch guideline of less than 30% of calories from fat, some schools also sell or have vending machines with high-fat, high-calorie, and high-sugar items. Most school-age children drink at least one high-sugar soft drink daily, with some consuming three or more. In a recent research study exploring the relationship between childhood obesity and school type, statistically significant effects on BMI were found. The children attending public schools (eating the National School Lunch Program and School Breakfast Program) had a much higher BMI then did the children attending private schools. This finding highlights the need for more parent involvement at the local and state level (Li & Hooker, 2010).

Although the majority of parents of preschoolers are concerned about children who will not eat, an increasing minority are concerned about overweight children. Obesity has become epidemic in the United States, now reaching down from adults to children and even to infancy. Studies have reported that almost 10% of our infants and toddlers are now considered obese (weight at or above the 95th percentile sex-specific). Childhood overweight rates (weight at or above the 85th percentile of BMI for age) in the United States have nearly doubled among 2- to 5-year-olds and more than tripled among 6- to 19-year-olds in the past three decades (Ogden et al., 2010). This childhood obesity epidemic is a significant health-promotion problem in the United States that should prompt us to take time to educate

SPOTLIGHT **ON**

Let's Take a Second Look at the Sunshine Vitamin

Recent studies show that millions of children in the United States may not be getting enough vitamin D, which is known as the sunshine vitamin, for proper growth and development. Vitamin D is produced by the body in response to sunlight exposure. It can also be found in foods such as fish, egg yolks, and fortified dairy products. We have always known that vitamin D helps the body use the calcium derived from the diet to keep bones healthy. Numerous research studies have also uncovered the relationship between vitamin D deficiency and conditions such as Type 1 and Type 2 diabetes, epilepsy, cardiovascular disease, glucose intolerance, and multiple sclerosis.

Experts recommend 5–10 minute/day of sun exposure to the arms and legs. Children with darker skin may need more exposure than fair-skinned children to get an adequate amount of vitamin D. The health care provider should determine whether a child's level of vitamin D is sufficient.

Source: Kumar, J., Muntner, P., Kaskel, F. J., Hailpern, S. M., Melamed, M. L. (2009). Prevalence and associations of 25-Hydroxyvitamin D deficiency in the US children: NHANES 2001–2004. *Pediatrics, 124* (3), 362–370.

the parents. To assess for overweight and obesity in children, plot the BMI on age- and gender-specific growth charts. Plotting weight for age and weight for height percentiles instead may result in the failure to recognize almost 73% of overweight children (Looney, Spence, & Raynor, 2011). In children, **underweight** is defined as being under the 5th percentile; **overweight** is being between the 85th and 94th percentile; and **obesity** is being at or above the 95th percentile for age-/sex-specific BMI. A red flag for a weight problem is moving up across percentiles. Family history, eating habits, activity levels, and social relationships are also important. Laboratory studies include fasting serum glucose, lipoprotein panel, and insulin levels, as well as a serum alanine transaminase (ALT).

The increase in preschool obesity has serious implications for future child health because it affects physiologic measures, such as blood pressure and cholesterol, and jeopardizes mental health. Childhood obesity affects self-esteem, peer relationships, inclusion in social events, and participation in sports. Influenced by the media and societal attitudes, children as young as 6 years of age have been found to develop negative attitudes toward obesity, associating or labeling obesity with ugliness and laziness (Camden, 2009). Nationwide, over 33% of children and adolescents are considered overweight. Among 2–5-year-olds, the prevalence of overweight is close to 25%. Statistics show that children who are overweight become obese adults, making this issue a public health concern. Adults who were overweight as children have increased morbidity and mortality rates associated with high blood pressure, diabetes, and certain cancers (Ogden et al., 2010)

Childhood obesity is associated with increased risk of dyslipidemia, hypertension, insulin resistance, and Type 2 diabetes mellitus, which can contribute to heart disease later in life. Recognizing and reducing childhood obesity is important not only because of its relationship with adult obesity and the associated medical complications but also because these same complications are now being demonstrated by children. Overweight children are developing Type 2 diabetes mellitus and hypertension, diseases formerly found almost exclusively in adults. Asthma and obstructive sleep apnea have also increased. Overweight children have orthopedic problems, especially in weight-bearing joints, and psychosocial problems related to poor self-esteem. In addition, overweight girls may have an early menarche.

Interventions to prevent childhood obesity should be initiated in the early years because we know that during this period healthy behaviors and the basic building blocks for learning are being formed (Shonkoff & Phillips, 2000). Nursery schools, Head Start centers, and day care centers could initiate comprehensive health education programs that can be continued into the school years. In addition, schools can promote physical activity. Unfortunately, many schools are reducing or cutting physical education from the curriculum, just as the obesity epidemic is being documented.

Prevention and treatment requires the whole family to make healthful lifestyle changes. Parental education is essential. Parents are in control: They buy the food, cook the food, and decide where food is eaten. Box 10-2 lists ways parents can help their overweight children. Primary prevention, health-promotion strategies include altering food preferences by introducing children to a wide variety of fruits and vegetables, reducing the time for exposure to television (and food advertising) and to computers (limiting snacking and making time for more active behaviors).

Obesity treatment programs for children do not have weight loss as a goal. The aim is to halt weight gain so that

---

BOX 10-2

PARENTS' GUIDE TO PROMOTING NORMAL WEIGHT IN CHILDREN

- Be a good role model. Be more active and improve your own diet.
- When grocery shopping, choose fruits and vegetables over convenience foods high in sugar and fat.
- Have healthy snacks available (fresh fruit, low-fat popcorn, low-fat frozen yogurt), and eliminate high-fat, high-sugar foods from the home (chips, pizza, cookies, ice cream, etc.).
- Limit sweetened beverages, including those containing fruit juices.
- Select recipes and methods of cooking that are low in fat (baking or broiling instead of frying).
- Put colorful foods on the table: green and yellow vegetables, fruits of various colors, brown whole grain breads. Limit white carbohydrates: rice, pasta, white bread, sugar (desserts).
- Sit down together for family meals.
- Limit television and computer time to fewer than 2 hours daily.
- Encourage physical activity such as riding a bike 20 minutes a day, scheduling regular family walks, using the stairs rather than the elevator, parking far back in the mall lot.

---

children grow into their body weight over a period of months to years. Programs for the school-age child should have three components: physical activity, healthy eating, and behavior modification.

Adopting a formal exercise program or simply becoming more active is valuable to burn fat, increase energy expenditure, and keep off lost weight. Even if body weight and body fat percentage do not change, 50 minutes of aerobic exercise three times per week results in improvements in blood lipid profiles and blood pressure. Diet management must be combined with physical activity to be effective.

ASK YOURSELF

Preventing Childhood Obesity

Prevention of childhood obesity should begin as early in life as possible. Nurses are in a position to teach parents so that they can guide their children. Health-promotion strategies involve the parents, the children, and the schools. How can the nurse be involved personally, professionally, politically, or in all three ways to promote the prevention of childhood obesity?

Fasting or extreme caloric restriction is not advisable for children. This approach not is only psychologically stressful but may adversely affect growth and the child's perception of normal eating. Changes in metabolism from severe calorie restriction, followed by binge eating, may cause children to gain rather than lose weight (AAP, 2003). Helping children to adopt good eating habits without severe calorie restriction is a better health-promotion choice. Balanced diets with moderate caloric restriction, especially reduced dietary fat, have been successful in treating obesity. Nutritional education is also beneficial.

Behavioral modification has been successful: self-monitoring and recording food intake and physical activity, slowing the rate of eating, limiting the time and place of eating, and using nonfood rewards and incentives for desirable behaviors. Including parents in behaviorally based treatments is particularly effective. Parents should be taught to avoid using food as a reward and to allow children to leave food on their plates when their appetites are satisfied.

Elimination

The majority of preschool children have attained independent toileting with only occasional accidents, which are usually due to not wanting to interrupt play activities. The school-age child usually has an elimination pattern similar to that of an adult, urinating every 3–4 hours with a bowel movement every 1–2 days. Some children, however, may have a problem with elimination.

Enuresis is involuntary urinary incontinence in a child 5 years of age or older who has no physical abnormality causing the incontinence. **Incontinence** is defined as the inability to retain urine or feces. Enuresis refers to urine. Over 90% of children with enuresis have primary nocturnal enuresis (bedwetting). These children wet only at night during sleep, and they have never had a sustained period of nocturnal dryness. The occurrence of primary nocturnal enuresis is common and decreases with age: 15–20% in 5-year-olds, 5% in 10-year-olds, and 2–3% in 12- to 14-year-olds (Makari & Rushton, 2006). Boys are more likely than girls to be enuretic, and there is frequently a family history of enuresis, especially in the father.

Less common is secondary enuresis, which develops after a child has a sustained period of bladder control. This development is frequently associated with a stressful event in the child's life: birth of a sibling, loss of a significant person, or extreme family disharmony.

The major health-promotion strategy for families with an enuretic child is to help prevent low self-esteem and decreased self-confidence in the child. The nurse should be sure that the child has been evaluated for a possible organic problem, such as bladder infection, neurologic abnormality, seizure disorder, diabetes mellitus, and urinary tract abnormality, because these conditions may cause enuresis. Once an organic cause is ruled out, the nurse may recommend a bladder exercise program or a wet alarm system. The nurse can provide support through sharing information about the condition, the treatment modalities, and the emotional distress that enuresis causes.

Encopresis is fecal incontinence in a child 4 years of age or older who has no physical abnormality causing the incontinence. *Incontinence* in this case refers to the inability to retain feces. Functional encopresis affects 1–1.5% of school-age children, with males affected four times more commonly

RESEARCH NOTE

Is There a Link between Obesity, Asthma, and Inactivity?

STUDY PROBLEM/PURPOSE

Obesity and asthma are two major public health problems in children that are associated with multifactorial morbidity and mortality rates. The overlap between the two have been reported in numerous research studies. The purpose of this integrative review of literature is to investigate the relationship between obesity and asthma as it relates to clinical application.

METHOD

A review of literature that included statistics on the prevalence of childhood obesity and asthma and their relationship. Data bases used in this review were MEDLINE, PubMed, OVID, and CINAHL.

FINDINGS

Both asthma and obesity are considered inflammatory diseases. Inactivity is compounded by the physiological changes that occur with excessive body fat and by the restrictive pathology found in asthma. Studies have concluded that obesity can very well lead to increased asthma symptoms, which, in turn, results in less physical activity. Decreased activity, in turn, predisposes the child to obesity and long-term respiratory complications, thereby prolonging the vicious cycle of inactivity, obesity, and worsening asthma.

IMPLICATIONS

The nurse can be a key role in making sure that the parents of asthmatic children are aware of the *Guidelines for the Diagnosis and Management of Asthma* (National Heart, Lung and Blood Institute: National Asthma Education and Prevention Program Expert Panel-3) and that the child is properly evaluated by a health care provider. A child with properly controlled asthma can participate in physical activity in order to prevent obesity.

Source: Rance, K., & O'Laughlen, M. (2011). Obesity and asthma: A dangerous link in children: An integrative review of the literature. *The Journal for Nurse Practitioners,* 7 (4), 287–292.

than females. Many are also enuretic. The health-promotion strategy for this condition involves support by the nurse for the family and child as they undergo a bowel training program and professional counseling.

Sleep and Activity

The preschool child typically sleeps 8–12 hours at night. The need for napping varies among children. Many preschoolers may benefit from a quiet time in the afternoon. Others do

BOX 10-3
HELPING THE PRESCHOOLER AT BEDTIME

1. Develop a bedtime ritual of 30–45 minutes (stories, prayers, music, sitting quietly).
2. Adhere to the ritual as much as possible.
3. Be firm about bedtime.
4. Allow the child to take a special soft toy or blanket to bed.
5. Try putting a night-light in the child's room, if one is not already there.
6. If the child awakens during the night, reassure the child but keep the child in bed.
7. Avoid vigorous activity, sweet treats, and frightening stories or television before bedtime.

better with approximately 0.5–1 hour of sleep to supplement their nighttime sleep.

Bedtime becomes a time of ritual, which preschoolers may resist in an attempt to prolong going to bed. Box 10-3 lists ways to facilitate preschooler bedtime.

Getting the child to stay in bed is not always easy. One innovative method is to give preschool and school-age children a free pass to get out of bed once each night. A card embossed with the child's name can be turned in for one brief visit out of the bedroom for a specific purpose: a drink of water, a hug, or a bathroom visit. If the child cries or leaves the room after the pass has been used, parents should ignore the crying and return the child to bed without eye contact and without a word. Many children save the pass for later and then fall asleep, secure in the knowledge that they have it. Also, knowing that leaving the bedroom is no longer forbidden removes some of its allure.

Preschoolers commonly waken during the night. Providing reassurance without restarting the bedtime ritual is usually sufficient. If awakening is due to a **night terror** (where the child screams out, cries, and does not respond to parents), the parent should understand that the child is not fully awake and that the terror will abate in 10–15 minutes. The child will fall back asleep without remembering the dream. **Nightmares** (or anxiety dreams) are more common than night terrors. The child fully awakens and can describe the dream to the parents. Calm reassurance is helpful at this time.

The school-age child usually sleeps between 8–12 hours at night. Most do not take naps during the day. Bedtime is not usually a source of struggle between the school-age child and the parents. Parents who establish an agreed-upon bedtime with the child and allow flexibility when appropriate usually receive cooperation from the child. Nightmares and night terrors may still occur, but sleepwalking and sleeptalking are more common. The health-promotion strategy is to reassure parents that these sleep disturbances tend to be outgrown. Parents should protect the sleepwalking child from injury and gently guide the child back to bed.

As for activity, the preschool child receives exercise through play. The preschooler's natural tendency to explore the environment should provide enough motor activity to achieve an adequate level of physical fitness. As shown in Figure 10-1, motor skill development occurs best in an unstructured,

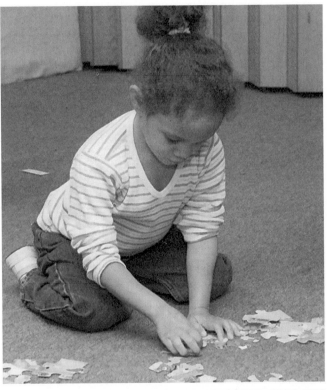

FIGURE 10-1 The preschooler develops motor skills through repetition and trial and error.

noncompetitive environment, allowing the preschooler to experiment and learn by trial and error. The primary health-promotion strategy is to provide a safe environment for this play and exploration. The majority of children are not ready to participate in organized sports before 6 years of age.

The American Academy of Pediatrics recommends that school-age children get 20–30 minutes of vigorous physical activity at least 6 times a week as a minimum (AAP, 2011a). The nurse should assess the activity level of the child by means of questions about interest and participation in active and sedentary hobbies, time spent watching television, participation in organized physical activity programs, and family exercise habits. The primary health-promotion strategy for this age group is to encourage the physical activity habits that form the lifelong behaviors important to improving general well-being and preventing illness.

IMMUNIZATION

Immunizations for the preschool or school-age children include a booster for diphtheria-pertussis-tetanus, measles-mumps-rubella, varicella, and polio. The inactive poliovirus (IPV) vaccine is normally used. Table 10-2 provides the recommended immunization schedule for children under age 7 who were not immunized in infancy. It also outlines a catch-up vaccination schedule for children ages 7–18.

Since the advent of the varicella vaccine in 1995, severe cases of chickenpox are rare; however, mild to moderate cases are being found in children who received the vaccine more than 3 years earlier. A second dose of varicella is now recommended between the ages of 4–6 years for children who have received only one dose (Centers for Disease Control and Prevention [CDC], 2011).

© CENGAGE LEARNING 2013

TABLE 10-2 Recommended Immunization Schedule for Children

Recommended Immunization Schedule for Persons Aged 0 Through 6 Years—United States • 2011
For those who fall behind or start late, see the catch-up schedule

Vaccine ▼ Age ►	Birth	1 month	2 months	4 months	6 months	12 months	15 months	18 months	19–23 months	2–3 years	4–6 years	
Hepatitis B[1]	HepB	HepB				HepB						Range of recommended ages for all children
Rotavirus[2]			RV	RV	RV[2]							
Diphtheria, Tetanus, Pertussis[3]			DTaP	DTaP	DTaP	see footnote[3]	DTaP				DTaP	
Haemophilus influenzae type b[4]			Hib	Hib	Hib[4]	Hib						
Pneumococcal[5]			PCV	PCV	PCV	PCV				PPSV		
Inactivated Poliovirus[6]			IPV	IPV		IPV					IPV	
Influenza[7]						Influenza (Yearly)						Range of recommended ages for certain high-risk groups
Measles, Mumps, Rubella[8]						MMR		see footnote[8]			MMR	
Varicella[9]						Varicella		see footnote[9]			Varicella	
Hepatitis A[10]						HepA (2 doses)				HepA Series		
Meningococcal[11]										MCV4		

This schedule includes recommendations in effect as of December 21, 2010. Any dose not administered at the recommended age should be administered at a subsequent visit, when indicated and feasible. The use of a combination vaccine generally is preferred over separate injections of its equivalent component vaccines. Considerations should include provider assessment, patient preference, and the potential for adverse events. Providers should consult the relevant Advisory Committee on Immunization Practices statement for detailed recommendations: **http://www.cdc.gov/vaccines/pubs-list.htm**. Clinically significant adverse events that follow immunization should be reported to the Vaccine Adverse Event Reporting System (VAERS) at **http://www.vaers.hhs.gov** or by telephone, **800-822-7967**. Use of trade names and commercial sources is for identification only and does not imply endorsement by the U.S. Department of Health and Human Services.

1. **Hepatitis B vaccine (HepB).** (Minimum age: birth)
   At birth:
   • Administer monovalent HepB to all newborns before hospital discharge.
   • If mother is hepatitis B surface antigen (HBsAg)-positive, administer HepB and 0.5 mL of hepatitis B immune globulin (HBIG) within 12 hours of birth.
   • If mother's HBsAg status is unknown, administer HepB within 12 hours of birth. Determine mother's HBsAg status as soon as possible and, if HBsAg-positive, administer HBIG (no later than age 1 week).
   Doses following the birth dose:
   • The second dose should be administered at age 1 or 2 months. Monovalent HepB should be used for doses administered before age 6 weeks.
   • Infants born to HBsAg-positive mothers should be tested for HBsAg and antibody to HBsAg 1 to 2 months after completion of at least 3 doses of the HepB series, at age 9 through 18 months (generally at the next well-child visit).
   • Administration of 4 doses of HepB to infants is permissible when a combination vaccine containing HepB is administered after the birth dose.
   • Infants who did not receive a birth dose should receive 3 doses of HepB on a schedule of 0, 1, and 6 months.
   • The final (3rd or 4th) dose in the HepB series should be administered no earlier than age 24 weeks.
2. **Rotavirus vaccine (RV).** (Minimum age: 6 weeks)
   • Administer the first dose at age 6 through 14 weeks (maximum age: 14 weeks 6 days). Vaccination should not be initiated for infants aged 15 weeks 0 days or older.
   • The maximum age for the final dose in the series is 8 months 0 days.
   • If Rotarix is administered at ages 2 and 4 months, a dose at 6 months is not indicated.
3. **Diphtheria and tetanus toxoids and acellular pertussis vaccine (DTaP).** (Minimum age: 6 weeks)
   • The fourth dose may be administered as early as age 12 months, provided at least 6 months have elapsed since the third dose.
4. *Haemophilus influenzae* **type b conjugate vaccine (Hib).** (Minimum age: 6 weeks)
   • If PRP-OMP (PedvaxHIB or Comvax [HepB-Hib]) is administered at ages 2 and 4 months, a dose at age 6 months is not indicated.
   • Hiberix should not be used for doses at ages 2, 4, or 6 months for the primary series but can be used as the final dose in children aged 12 months through 4 years.
5. **Pneumococcal vaccine.** (Minimum age: 6 weeks for pneumococcal conjugate vaccine [PCV]; 2 years for pneumococcal polysaccharide vaccine [PPSV])
   • PCV is recommended for all children aged younger than 5 years. Administer 1 dose of PCV to all healthy children aged 24 through 59 months who are not completely vaccinated for their age.
   • A PCV series begun with 7-valent PCV (PCV7) should be completed with 13-valent PCV (PCV13).
   • A single supplemental dose of PCV13 is recommended for all children aged 14 through 59 months who have received an age-appropriate series of PCV7.
   • A single supplemental dose of PCV13 is recommended for all children aged 60 through 71 months with underlying medical conditions who have received an age-appropriate series of PCV7.

   • The supplemental dose of PCV13 should be administered at least 8 weeks after the previous dose of PCV7. See *MMWR* 2010:59(No. RR-11).
   • Administer PPSV at least 8 weeks after last dose of PCV to children aged 2 years or older with certain underlying medical conditions, including a cochlear implant.
6. **Inactivated poliovirus vaccine (IPV).** (Minimum age: 6 weeks)
   • If 4 or more doses are administered prior to age 4 years an additional dose should be administered at age 4 through 6 years.
   • The final dose in the series should be administered on or after the fourth birthday and at least 6 months following the previous dose.
7. **Influenza vaccine (seasonal).** (Minimum age: 6 months for trivalent inactivated influenza vaccine [TIV]; 2 years for live, attenuated influenza vaccine [LAIV])
   • For healthy children aged 2 years and older (i.e., those who do not have underlying medical conditions that predispose them to influenza complications), either LAIV or TIV may be used, except LAIV should not be given to children aged 2 through 4 years who have had wheezing in the past 12 months.
   • Administer 2 doses (separated by at least 4 weeks) to children aged 6 months through 8 years who are receiving seasonal influenza vaccine for the first time or who were vaccinated for the first time during the previous influenza season but only received 1 dose.
   • Children aged 6 months through 8 years who received no doses of monovalent 2009 H1N1 vaccine should receive 2 doses of 2010–2011 seasonal influenza vaccine. See *MMWR* 2010;59(No. RR-8):33–34.
8. **Measles, mumps, and rubella vaccine (MMR).** (Minimum age: 12 months)
   • The second dose may be administered before age 4 years, provided at least 4 weeks have elapsed since the first dose.
9. **Varicella vaccine.** (Minimum age: 12 months)
   • The second dose may be administered before age 4 years, provided at least 3 months have elapsed since the first dose.
   • For children aged 12 months through 12 years the recommended minimum interval between doses is 3 months. However, if the second dose was administered at least 4 weeks after the first dose, it can be accepted as valid.
10. **Hepatitis A vaccine (HepA).** (Minimum age: 12 months)
    • Administer 2 doses at least 6 months apart.
    • HepA is recommended for children aged older than 23 months who live in areas where vaccination programs target older children, who are at increased risk for infection, or for whom immunity against hepatitis A is desired.
11. **Meningococcal conjugate vaccine, quadrivalent (MCV4).** (Minimum age: 2 years)
    • Administer 2 doses of MCV4 at least 8 weeks apart to children aged 2 through 10 years with persistent complement component deficiency and anatomic or functional asplenia, and 1 dose every 5 years thereafter.
    • Persons with human immunodeficiency virus (HIV) infection who are vaccinated with MCV4 should receive 2 doses at least 8 weeks apart.
    • Administer 1 dose of MCV4 to children aged 2 through 10 years who travel to countries with highly endemic or epidemic disease and during outbreaks caused by a vaccine serogroup.
    • Administer MCV4 to children at continued risk for meningococcal disease who were previously vaccinated with MCV4 or meningococcal polysaccharide vaccine after 3 years if the first dose was administered at age 2 through 6 years.

The Recommended Immunization Schedules for Persons Aged 0 Through 18 Years are approved by the Advisory Committee on Immunization Practices (**http://www.cdc.gov/vaccines/recs/acip**), the American Academy of Pediatrics (**http://www.aap.org**), and the American Academy of Family Physicians (**http://www.aafp.org**).

Department of Health and Human Services • Centers for Disease Control and Prevention

TABLE 10-2 *(Continued)*

Recommended Immunization Schedule for Persons Aged 7 Through 18 Years—United States • 2011
For those who fall behind or start late, see the schedule below and the catch-up schedule

Vaccine ▼ Age ▶	7–10 years	11–12 years	13–18 years	
Tetanus, Diphtheria, Pertussis[1]		Tdap	Tdap	Range of recommended ages for all children
Human Papillomavirus[2]	see footnote[2]	HPV (3 doses)(females)	HPV Series	
Meningococcal[3]	MCV4	MCV4	MCV4	
Influenza[4]	Influenza (Yearly)			
Pneumococcal[5]	Pneumococcal			Range of recommended ages for catch-up immunization
Hepatitis A[6]	HepA Series			
Hepatitis B[7]	Hep B Series			
Inactivated Poliovirus[8]	IPV Series			
Measles, Mumps, Rubella[9]	MMR Series			Range of recommended ages for certain high-risk groups
Varicella[10]	Varicella Series			

This schedule includes recommendations in effect as of December 21, 2010. Any dose not administered at the recommended age should be administered at a subsequent visit, when indicated and feasible. The use of a combination vaccine generally is preferred over separate injections of its equivalent component vaccines. Considerations should include provider assessment, patient preference, and the potential for adverse events. Providers should consult the relevant Advisory Committee on Immunization Practices statement for detailed recommendations: **http://www.cdc.gov/vaccines/pubs/acip-list.htm**. Clinically significant adverse events that follow immunization should be reported to the Vaccine Adverse Event Reporting System (VAERS) at **http://www.vaers.hhs.gov** or by telephone, **800-822-7967**.

1. **Tetanus and diphtheria toxoids and acellular pertussis vaccine (Tdap).** (Minimum age: 10 years for Boostrix and 11 years for Adacel)
   - Persons aged 11 through 18 years who have not received Tdap should receive a dose followed by Td booster doses every 10 years thereafter.
   - Persons aged 7 through 10 years who are not fully immunized against pertussis (including those never vaccinated or with unknown pertussis vaccination status) should receive a single dose of Tdap. Refer to the catch-up schedule if additional doses of tetanus and diphtheria toxoid–containing vaccine are needed.
   - Tdap can be administered regardless of the interval since the last tetanus and diphtheria toxoid–containing vaccine.
2. **Human papillomavirus (HPV).** (Minimum age: 9 years)
   - Quadrivalent HPV vaccine (HPV4) or bivalent HPV vaccine (HPV2) is recommended for the prevention of cervical precancers and cancers in females.
   - HPV4 is recommended for prevention of cervical precancers, cancers, and genital warts in females.
   - HPV4 may be administered in a 3-dose series to males aged 9 through 18 years to reduce their likelihood of genital warts.
   - Administer the second dose 1 to 2 months after the first dose and the third dose 6 months after the first dose (at least 24 weeks after the first dose).
3. **Meningococcal conjugate vaccine, quadrivalent (MCV4).** (Minimum age: 2 years)
   - Administer MCV4 at age 11 through 12 years with a booster dose at age 16 years.
   - Administer 1 dose at age 13 through 18 years if not previously vaccinated.
   - Persons who received their first dose at age 13 through 15 years should receive a booster dose at age 16 through 18 years.
   - Administer 1 dose to previously unvaccinated college freshmen living in a dormitory.
   - Administer 2 doses at least 8 weeks apart to children aged 2 through 10 years with persistent complement component deficiency and anatomic or functional asplenia, and 1 dose every 5 years thereafter.
   - Persons with HIV infection who are vaccinated with MCV4 should receive 2 doses at least 8 weeks apart.
   - Administer 1 dose of MCV4 to children aged 2 through 10 years who travel to countries with highly endemic or epidemic disease and during outbreaks caused by a vaccine serogroup.
   - Administer MCV4 to children at continued risk for meningococcal disease who were previously vaccinated with MCV4 or meningococcal polysaccharide vaccine after 3 years (if first dose administered at age 2 through 6 years) or after 5 years (if first dose administered at age 7 years or older).
4. **Influenza vaccine (seasonal).**
   - For healthy nonpregnant persons aged 7 through 18 years (i.e., those who do not have underlying medical conditions that predispose them to influenza complications), either LAIV or TIV may be used.
   - Administer 2 doses (separated by at least 4 weeks) to children aged 6 months through 8 years who are receiving seasonal influenza vaccine for the first

time or who were vaccinated for the first time during the previous influenza season but only received 1 dose.
   - Children 6 months through 8 years of age who received no doses of monovalent 2009 H1N1 vaccine should receive 2 doses of 2010-2011 seasonal influenza vaccine. See *MMWR* 2010;59(No. RR-8):33–34.
5. **Pneumococcal vaccines.**
   - A single dose of 13-valent pneumococcal conjugate vaccine (PCV13) may be administered to children aged 6 through 18 years who have functional or anatomic asplenia, HIV infection or other immunocompromising condition, cochlear implant or CSF leak. See *MMWR* 2010;59(No. RR-11).
   - The dose of PCV13 should be administered at least 8 weeks after the previous dose of PCV7.
   - Administer pneumococcal polysaccharide vaccine at least 8 weeks after the last dose of PCV to children aged 2 years or older with certain underlying medical conditions, including a cochlear implant. A single revaccination should be administered after 5 years to children with functional or anatomic asplenia or an immunocompromising condition.
6. **Hepatitis A vaccine (HepA).**
   - Administer 2 doses at least 6 months apart.
   - HepA is recommended for children aged older than 23 months who live in areas where vaccination programs target older children, or who are at increased risk for infection, or for whom immunity against hepatitis A is desired.
7. **Hepatitis B vaccine (HepB).**
   - Administer the 3-dose series to those not previously vaccinated. For those with incomplete vaccination, follow the catch-up schedule.
   - A 2-dose series (separated by at least 4 months) of adult formulation Recombivax HB is licensed for children aged 11 through 15 years.
8. **Inactivated poliovirus vaccine (IPV).**
   - The final dose in the series should be administered on or after the fourth birthday and at least 6 months following the previous dose.
   - If both OPV and IPV were administered as part of a series, a total of 4 doses should be administered, regardless of the child's current age.
9. **Measles, mumps, and rubella vaccine (MMR).**
   - The minimum interval between the 2 doses of MMR is 4 weeks.
10. **Varicella vaccine.**
   - For persons aged 7 through 18 years without evidence of immunity (see *MMWR* 2007;56[No. RR-4]), administer 2 doses if not previously vaccinated or the second dose if only 1 dose has been administered.
   - For persons aged 7 through 12 years, the recommended minimum interval between doses is 3 months. However, if the second dose was administered at least 4 weeks after the first dose, it can be accepted as valid.
   - For persons aged 13 years and older, the minimum interval between doses is 4 weeks.

The Recommended Immunization Schedules for Persons Aged 0 Through 18 Years are approved by the Advisory Committee on Immunization Practices (**http://www.cdc.gov/vaccines/recs/acip**), the American Academy of Pediatrics (**http://www.aap.org**), and the American Academy of Family Physicians (**http://www.aafp.org**).
Department of Health and Human Services • Centers for Disease Control and Prevention

SPOTLIGHT **ON**

Illness and Immunizations

Children with mild illnesses such as colds, flu, and ear infections (either with or without fever) should still get their immunizations on schedule. There is no decrease in the effectiveness of the vaccines, and they do not cause the child to be more ill.

Additional immunizations should be considered for at-risk preschool or school-age children. Hepatitis A is an acute, self-limiting virus that is transmitted from person to person, usually by the fecal-oral route. Children living in communities with high infection rates of hepatitis A or who are traveling to areas with known hepatitis A infections should be immunized with the two-dose series. Children with chronic pulmonary or cardiovascular disease should be immunized for pneumococcal diseases such as pneumonia and meningitis, as well as annually for influenza. Children with immune system deficiencies need immunization against bacterial meningitis. The prevention of contagious diseases for which immunization is available is a key health-promotion strategy.

Screening

Annual health maintenance visits are opportunities to screen for disease as well as to provide health teaching and anticipatory guidance. The preschooler is mature enough to cooperate with objective vision and hearing screening using standardized pictures and pure-tone audiometry. A tumbling E chart (Figure 10-2) should be used if the child is not familiar with the letters of the alphabet. This chart has the capital letter E facing in different directions, and the child is asked to point either up, down, left, or right. A normally farsighted (hyperopia) preschool child has 20/20 vision by age eight. Screening for anemia and blood abnormalities, such as sickle cell anemia and thalassemia when indicated, should be accompanied by screening for lead. Explaining these tests gives the nurse the opportunity to discuss ways to prevent lead ingestion.

Screening blood cholesterol levels is recommended only when there is a family history of hyperlipidemia or early myocardial infarction. Blood pressure screening begins during the preschool years; hypertension in children younger than 10 years of age usually has an organic cause.

The preschooler should be screened for tuberculosis (TB) around four years of age, and children at high risk for TB should be screened annually. High-risk groups include medically underserved low-income populations, foreign-born children from high-prevalence countries, children in close contact with a prison resident, someone with infectious TB or HIV cases, and children with compromised immune systems. Some schools require TB screening prior to enrollment. As shown in Table 10-3. the American Academy of Pediatrics (APA, 2011a) has provided recommendations for preventive pediatric health care from infancy through adolescence.

The preschooler should have the first visit to the dentist by age three. Follow-up discussions about proper dental care and toothbrushing can be done at each health maintenance visit, along with encouraging regular visits to the dentist.

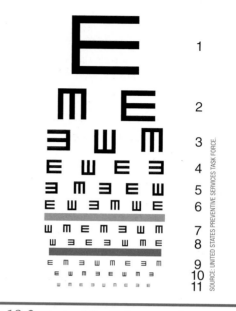

FIGURE 10-2 The tumbling E chart is used to assess visual acuity in the child who is not familiar with the letters of the English alphabet.

The school-age child should have vision screening prior to entering school and yearly during the school years. Vision problems, such as accommodation problems, strabismus, and astigmatism, are common during the school-age years. Vision screening should also include testing for color blindness. Warning signs for vision problems in children are listed in Box 10-4.

Recurrent or chronic ear infections are common in school-age children, making periodic hearing tests an important screen for hearing loss. Blood pressure screening is important for all school-age children and especially those in identified groups at high risk: obese, premature or low birth weight, and those with hypertensive parents.

NURSING **ALERT**

Accurate Anemia Screening

Screening for anemia is not accurate if the child has had a fever or infection within the 2–3 weeks prior to testing. The hemoglobin testing during this time results in a false-positive test—an inaccurate diagnosis of anemia in an otherwise healthy child.

BOX 10-4

WARNING SIGNS FOR VISION PROBLEMS IN CHILDREN

- Squinting
- Tilting the head to look at something
- Reluctance to do close work
- Poor school performance by a child with a prior history of good performance
- Complaining of frequent headaches

TABLE 10-3 American Academy of Pediatrics Recommendations for Preventive Pediatric Health Care, Infancy through Adolescence

Catch-up Immunization Schedule for Persons Aged 4 Months Through 18 Years Who Start Late or Who Are More Than 1 Month Behind—United States • 2011

The table below provides catch-up schedules and minimum intervals between doses for children whose vaccinations have been delayed. A vaccine series does not need to be restarted, regardless of the time that has elapsed between doses. Use the section appropriate for the child's age

Vaccine	Minimum Age for Dose 1	Minimum Interval Between Doses			
		Dose 1 to Dose 2	Dose 2 to Dose 3	Dose 3 to Dose 4	Dose 4 to Dose 5
PERSONS AGED 4 MONTHS THROUGH 6 YEARS					
Hepatitis B[1]	Birth	4 weeks	8 weeks (and at least 16 weeks after first dose)		
Rotavirus[2]	6 wks	4 weeks	4 weeks[2]		
Diphtheria, Tetanus, Pertussis[3]	6 wks	4 weeks	4 weeks	6 months	6 months[3]
Haemophilus influenzae type b[4]	6 wks	4 weeks if first dose administered at younger than age 12 months; 8 weeks (as final dose) if first dose administered at age 12–14 months; No further doses needed if first dose administered at age 15 months or older	4 weeks[4] if current age is younger than 12 months; 8 weeks (as final dose)[4] if current age is 12 months or older and first dose administered at younger than age 12 months and second dose administered at younger than 15 months; No further doses needed if previous dose administered at age 15 months or older	8 weeks (as final dose) This dose only necessary for children aged 12 months through 59 months who received 3 doses before age 12 months	
Pneumococcal[5]	6 wks	4 weeks if first dose administered at younger than age 12 months; 8 weeks (as final dose for healthy children) if first dose administered at age 12 months or older or current age 24 through 59 months; No further doses needed for healthy children if first dose administered at age 24 months or older	4 weeks if current age is younger than 12 months; 8 weeks (as final dose for healthy children) if current age is 12 months or older; No further doses needed for healthy children if previous dose administered at age 24 months or older	8 weeks (as final dose) This dose only necessary for children aged 12 months through 59 months who received 3 doses before age 12 months or for children at high risk who received 3 doses at any age	
Inactivated Poliovirus[6]	6 wks	4 weeks	4 weeks	6 months[6]	
Measles, Mumps, Rubella[7]	12 mos	4 weeks			
Varicella[8]	12 mos	3 months			
Hepatitis A[9]	12 mos	6 months			
PERSONS AGED 7 THROUGH 18 YEARS					
Tetanus, Diphtheria/ Tetanus, Diphtheria, Pertussis[10]	7 yrs[10]	4 weeks	4 weeks if first dose administered at younger than age 12 months; 6 months if first dose administered at 12 months or older	6 months if first dose administered at younger than age 12 months	
Human Papillomavirus[11]	9 yrs	Routine dosing intervals are recommended (females)[11]			
Hepatitis A[9]	12 mos	6 months			
Hepatitis B[1]	Birth	4 weeks	8 weeks (and at least 16 weeks after first dose)		
Inactivated Poliovirus[6]	6 wks	4 weeks	4 weeks[6]	6 months[6]	
Measles, Mumps, Rubella[7]	12 mos	4 weeks			
Varicella[8]	12 mos	3 months if person is younger than age 13 years; 4 weeks if person is aged 13 years or older			

1. **Hepatitis B vaccine (HepB).**
   - Administer the 3-dose series to those not previously vaccinated.
   - The minimum age for the third dose of HepB is 24 weeks.
   - A 2-dose series (separated by at least 4 months) of adult formulation Recombivax HB is licensed for children aged 11 through 15 years.
2. **Rotavirus vaccine (RV).**
   - The maximum age for the first dose is 14 weeks 6 days. Vaccination should not be initiated for infants aged 15 weeks 0 days or older.
   - The maximum age for the final dose in the series is 8 months 0 days.
   - If Rotarix was administered for the first and second doses, a third dose is not indicated.
3. **Diphtheria and tetanus toxoids and acellular pertussis vaccine (DTaP).**
   - The fifth dose is not necessary if the fourth dose was administered at age 4 years or older.
4. ***Haemophilus influenzae* type b conjugate vaccine (Hib).**
   - 1 dose of Hib vaccine should be considered for unvaccinated persons aged 5 years or older who have sickle cell disease, leukemia, or HIV infection, or who have had a splenectomy.
   - If the first 2 doses were PRP-OMP (PedvaxHIB or Comvax), and administered at age 11 months or younger, the third (and final) dose should be administered at age 12 through 15 months and at least 8 weeks after the second dose.
   - If the first dose was administered at age 7 through 11 months, administer the second dose at least 4 weeks later and a final dose at age 12 through 15 months.
5. **Pneumococcal vaccine.**
   - Administer 1 dose of 13-valent pneumococcal conjugate vaccine (PCV13) to all healthy children aged 24 through 59 months with any incomplete PCV schedule (PCV7 or PCV13).
   - For children aged 24 through 71 months with underlying medical conditions, administer 1 dose of PCV13 if 3 doses of PCV were received previously or administer 2 doses of PCV13 at least 8 weeks apart if fewer than 3 doses of PCV were received previously.
   - A single dose of PCV13 is recommended for certain children with underlying medical conditions through 18 years of age. See age-specific schedules for details.
   - Administer pneumococcal polysaccharide vaccine (PPSV) to children aged 2 years or older with certain underlying medical conditions, including a cochlear implant, at least 8 weeks after the last dose of PCV. A single revaccination should be administered after 5 years to children with functional or anatomic asplenia or an immunocompromising condition. See *MMWR* 2010;59(No. RR-11).

6. **Inactivated poliovirus vaccine (IPV).**
   - The final dose in the series should be administered on or after the fourth birthday and at least 6 months following the previous dose.
   - A fourth dose is not necessary if the third dose was administered at age 4 years or older and at least 6 months following the previous dose.
   - In the first 6 months of life, minimum age and minimum intervals are only recommended if the person is at risk for imminent exposure to circulating poliovirus (i.e., travel to a polio-endemic region or during an outbreak).
7. **Measles, mumps, and rubella vaccine (MMR).**
   - Administer the second dose routinely at age 4 through 6 years. The minimum interval between the 2 doses of MMR is 4 weeks.
8. **Varicella vaccine.**
   - Administer the second dose routinely at age 4 through 6 years.
   - If the second dose was administered at least 4 weeks after the first dose, it can be accepted as valid.
9. **Hepatitis A (HepA).**
   - HepA is recommended for children aged older than age 23 months who live in areas where vaccination programs target older children, or who are at increased risk for infection, or for whom immunity against hepatitis A is desired.
10. **Tetanus and diphtheria toxoids (Td) and tetanus and diphtheria toxoids and acellular pertussis vaccine (Tdap).**
    - Doses of DTaP are counted as part of the Td/Tdap series.
    - Tdap should be substituted for a single dose of Td in the catch-up series for children aged 7 through 10 years or as a booster for children aged 11 through 18 years; use Td for other doses.
11. **Human papillomavirus vaccine (HPV).**
    - Administer the series to females at age 13 through 18 years if not previously vaccinated or have not completed the vaccine series.
    - Quadrivalent HPV vaccine (HPV4) may be administered in a 3-dose series to males aged 9 through 18 years to reduce their likelihood of genital warts.
    - Use recommended routine dosing intervals for series catch-up (i.e., the second and third doses should be administered at 1 to 2 and 6 months after the first dose). The minimum interval between the first and second doses is 4 weeks. The minimum interval between the second and third doses is 12 weeks, and the third dose should be administered at least 24 weeks after the first dose.

Information about reporting reactions after immunization is available online at **http://www.vaers.hhs.gov** or by telephone, **800-822-7967**. Suspected cases of vaccine-preventable diseases should be reported to the state or local health department. Additional information, including precautions and contraindications for immunization, is available from the National Center for Immunization and Respiratory Diseases at **http://www.cdc.gov/vaccines** or telephone, **800-CDC-INFO** (800-232-4636).
Department of Health and Human Services • Centers for Disease Control and Prevention

(Continues)

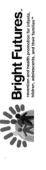

TABLE 10-3 American Academy of Pediatrics Recommendations for Preventive Pediatric Health Care, Infancy Through Adolescence (*Continued*)

American Academy of Pediatrics
DEDICATED TO THE HEALTH OF ALL CHILDREN™

Bright Futures.
prevention and health promotion for infants, children, adolescents, and their families™

Recommendations for Preventive Pediatric Health Care

Bright Futures/American Academy of Pediatrics

Each child and family is unique; therefore, these **Recommendations for Preventive Pediatric Health Care** are designed for the care of children who are receiving competent parenting, have no manifestations of any important health problems, and are growing and developing in satisfactory fashion. **Additional visits may become necessary** if circumstances suggest variations from normal.

Developmental, psychosocial, and chronic disease issues for children and adolescents may require frequent counseling and treatment visits separate from preventive care visits.

These guidelines represent a consensus by the American Academy of Pediatrics (AAP) and Bright Futures. The AAP continues to emphasize the great importance of **continuity of care** in comprehensive health supervision and the need to avoid **fragmentation of care**.

The recommendations in this statement do not indicate an exclusive course of treatment or standard of medical care. Variations, taking into account individual circumstances, may be appropriate.

Copyright © 2008 by the American Academy of Pediatrics.

No part of this statement may be reproduced in any form or by any means without prior written permission from the American Academy of Pediatrics except for one copy for personal use.

AGE[1]	INFANCY									EARLY CHILDHOOD								MIDDLE CHILDHOOD							ADOLESCENCE												
	PRENATAL[2]	NEWBORN[3]	3–5 d[4]	By 1 mo	2 mo	4 mo	6 mo	9 mo	12 m	15 mo	18 mo	24 mo	30 mo	3 y	4 y	5 y	6 y	7 y	8 y	9 y	10 y	11 y	12 y	13 y	14 y	15 y	16 y	17 y	18 y	19 y	20 y	21 y
HISTORY Initial/Interval	•	•	•	•	•	•	•	•	•	•	•	•	•	•	•	•	•	•	•	•	•	•	•	•	•	•	•	•	•	•	•	•
MEASUREMENTS																																
Length/Height and Weight		•	•	•	•	•	•	•	•	•	•	•	•	•	•	•	•	•	•	•	•	•	•	•	•	•	•	•	•	•	•	•
Head Circumference		•	•	•	•	•	•	•	•	•	•	•																				
Weight for Length		•	•	•	•	•	•	•	•	•	•																					
Body Mass Index												•	•	•	•	•	•	•	•	•	•	•	•	•	•	•	•	•	•	•	•	•
Blood Pressure[5]		★	★	★	★	★	★	★	★	★	★	★	★	•	•	•	•	•	•	•	•	•	•	•	•	•	•	•	•	•	•	•
SENSORY SCREENING																																
Vision		★*	★	★	★	★	★	★	★	★	★	★	★	•	•	•	•	★	•	★	•	•	★	★	•	★	•	★	•	★	•	★
Hearing		★	★	★	★	★	★	★	★	★	★	★	★	★	•	•	•	★	•	★	•	★	•	★	★	★	★	★	★	★	★	★
DEVELOPMENTAL/BEHAVIORAL ASSESSMENT																																
Developmental Screening[8]								•			•		•																			
Autism Screening[9]											•																					
Developmental Surveillance[8]		•	•	•	•	•	•		•	•		•	•	•	•	•	•	•	•	•	•	•	•	•	•	•	•	•	•	•	•	•
Psychosocial/Behavioral Assessment		•	•	•	•	•	•	•	•	•	•	•	•	•	•	•	•	•	•	•	•	•	•	•	•	•	•	•	•	•	•	•
Alcohol and Drug Use Assessment																						★	★	★	★	★	★	★	★	★	★	★
PHYSICAL EXAMINATION[10]		•	•	•	•	•	•	•	•	•	•	•	•	•	•	•	•	•	•	•	•	•	•	•	•	•	•	•	•	•	•	•
PROCEDURES[11]																																
Newborn Metabolic/Hemoglobin Screening[12]		★	↕	↕																												
Immunization[13]		•	•	•	•	•	•	•	•	•	•	•	•	•	•	•	•	•	•	•	•	•	•	•	•	•	•	•	•	•	•	•
Hematocrit or Hemoglobin[14]				★		★		★	★or★[16]		★	★	★	★	★	★	★	★	★	★	★	★	★	★	★	★	★	★	★	★	★	★
Lead Screening[15]							★	★	★or★[16]		★or★[16]	★or★[16]		★																		
Tuberculin Test[17]					★				★					★																		
Dyslipidemia Screening[18]												★		★		★		★		★		★		★		★	★or•[20]					
STI Screening[19]																						★	★	★	★	★	★	★	★	★	★	★
Cervical Dysplasia Screening[20]																													★	★	★	★
ORAL HEALTH[21]						★		★	★or★[22]		★or★[22]	★or★[22]	★	★			•															
ANTICIPATORY GUIDANCE[23]	•	•	•	•	•	•	•	•	•	•	•	•	•	•	•	•	•	•	•	•	•	•	•	•	•	•	•	•	•	•	•	•

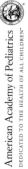

1. If a child comes under care for the first time at any point on the schedule, or if any items are not accomplished at the suggested age, the schedule should be brought up to date at the earliest possible time.
2. A prenatal visit is recommended for parents who are at high risk, for first-time parents, and for those who request a conference. The prenatal visit should include anticipatory guidance, pertinent medical history, and a discussion of benefits of breastfeeding and planned method of feeding per AAP statement "The Prenatal Visit" (2001) [URL: http://aappolicy.aappublications.org/cgi/content/full/pediatrics;107/6/1456].
3. Every infant should have a newborn evaluation after birth, breastfeeding encouraged, and instruction and support offered.
4. Every infant should have an evaluation within 3 to 5 days of birth and within 48 to 72 hours after discharge from the hospital to include evaluation for feeding and jaundice. Breastfeeding infants should receive formal breastfeeding evaluation, encouragement, and instruction as recommended in AAP statement "Breastfeeding and the Use of Human Milk" (2005) [URL: http://aappolicy.aappublications.org/cgi/content/full/pediatrics;115/2/496]. For newborns discharged in less than 48 hours after delivery, the infant must be examined within 48 hours of discharge per AAP statement "Hospital Stay for Healthy Term Newborns" (2004) [URL: http://aappolicy.aappublications.org/cgi/content/full/pediatrics;113/5/1434].
5. Blood pressure measurement in infants and children with specific risk conditions should be performed at visits before age 3 years.
6. If the patient is uncooperative, rescreen within 6 months per the AAP statement "Eye Examination in Infants, Children, and Young Adults by Pediatricians" (2007) [URL: http://aappolicy.aappublications.org/cgi/content/full/pediatrics;111/4/902].
7. All newborns should be screened per AAP statement "Year 2000 Position Statement: Principles and Guidelines for Early Hearing Detection and Intervention Programs" (2000) [URL: http://aappolicy.aappublications.org/cgi/content/full/

pediatrics;106/4/798]. Joint Committee on Infant Hearing. Year 2007 position statement: principles and guidelines for early hearing detection and intervention programs. *Pediatrics*. 2007;120:898–921.
8. AAP Council on Children With Disabilities, AAP Section on Developmental Behavioral Pediatrics, AAP Bright Futures Steering Committee, AAP Medical Home Initiatives for Children With Special Needs Project Advisory Committee. Identifying infants and young children with developmental disorders in the medical home: an algorithm for developmental surveillance and screening. *Pediatrics*. 2006;118:405–420 [URL: http://aappolicy.aappublications.org/cgi/content/full/pediatrics;118/1/405].
9. Gupta VB, Hyman SL, Johnson CP, et al. Identifying children with autism early? *Pediatrics*. 2007;119:152–153 [URL: http://pediatrics.aappublications.org/cgi/content/full/119/1/152].
10. At each visit, age-appropriate physical examination is essential, with infant totally unclothed, older child undressed and suitably draped.
11. These may be modified, depending on entry point into schedule and individual need.
12. Newborn metabolic and hemoglobinopathy screening should be done according to state law. Results should be reviewed at visits and appropriate retesting or referral done as needed.
13. Schedules per the Committee on Infectious Diseases, published annually in the January issue of *Pediatrics*. Every visit should be an opportunity to update and complete a child's immunizations.
14. See AAP *Pediatric Nutrition Handbook*, 5th Edition (2003) for a discussion of universal and selective screening options. See also Recommendations to prevent and control iron deficiency in the United States. *MMWR*. 1998;47(RR-3):1–36.
15. Mutilation at risk of lead exposure; consult the AAP statement "Lead Exposure in Children: Prevention, Detection, and Management" (2005) [URL: http://aappolicy.aappublications.org/cgi/content/full/pediatrics;116/4/1036]. Additionally, screening should be done in accordance with state law where applicable.
16. Perform risk assessments or screens as appropriate, based on universal screening requirements for patients with Medicaid or high prevalence areas.
17. Tuberculosis testing per recommendations of the Committee on Infectious Diseases, published in the current edition of *Red Book: Report of the Committee on Infectious Diseases*. Testing should be done on recognition of high-risk factors.
18. "Third Report of the National Cholesterol Education Program (NCEP) Expert Panel on Detection, Evaluation, and Treatment of High Blood Cholesterol in Adults (Adult Treatment Panel III) Final Report" (2002) [URL: http://circ.ahajournals.org/cgi/content/full/106/25/3143] and "The Expert Committee Recommendations on the Assessment, Prevention, and Treatment of Child and Adolescent Overweight and Obesity," Supplement to *Pediatrics*. In press.
19. All sexually active patients should be screened for sexually transmitted infections (STIs).
20. All sexually active girls should have screening for cervical dysplasia as part of a pelvic examination beginning within 3 years of onset of sexual activity or age 21 (whichever comes first).
21. Referral to dental home, if available. Otherwise, administer oral health risk assessment. If the primary water source is deficient in fluoride, consider oral fluoride supplementation.
22. At the visits for 3 years and 6 years of age, it should be determined whether the patient has a dental home. If the patient does not have a dental home, a referral should be made to one. If the primary water source is deficient in fluoride, consider oral fluoride supplementation.
23. Refer to the specific guidance by age as listed in Bright Futures Guidelines. (Hagan JF, Shaw JS, Duncan PM, eds. *Bright Futures: Guidelines for Health Supervision of Infants, Children, and Adolescents*; 3rd ed. Elk Grove Village, IL: American Academy of Pediatrics; 2008).

KEY
• = to be performed   ★ = risk assessment to be performed, with appropriate action to follow, if positive   ↔ • = range during which a service may be provided, with the symbol indicating the preferred age

The spine should be assessed for **scoliosis**, a lateral curvature of the spine that begins during the school-age years and is aggravated by the adolescent growth spurt. The early identification of scoliosis is extremely important in order to prevent long-term consequences of the problem. Extreme curvature can impinge on lung expansion and cardiac action and can lead to the need for corrective surgery.

The skin should be assessed for **acanthosis nigricans (AN)**, a skin condition associated with insulin resistance and Type 2 diabetes mellitus. AN is characterized by symmetrical, velvety, light brown to black, poorly marginated plaques of hyperpigmentation. AN usually develops in flexural areas, especially the axillae, nape of the neck, the groin, and the anogenital areas. Obesity is the most common abnormality associated with AN between the ages of 10–30. Individuals with AN usually exhibit fasting plasma insulin levels markedly higher than those in obese individuals without these cutaneous changes. Obese children with insulin resistance are at a high risk of developing Type 2 diabetes. Screening for AN can lead to health-promotion strategies that reduce obesity in children with AN. Weight loss and daily exercise can reverse the pathophysiological process responsible for AN by reducing both insulin resistance and compensatory hyperinsulinemia, thereby reducing the risk of Type 2 diabetes mellitus.

PSYCHOLOGICAL DOMAIN

Preschool children are in Piaget's preoperational stage of cognitive development, in which they are able to perform symbolic functioning: making and verbalizing mental images (Brainerd, 1978). Symbolic functioning is especially noted during play when children use symbolic games to represent reality. They use play objects in their environment to represent real objects, such as using a popsicle stick to represent a spoon to eat a make-believe lunch or a rock to represent a cookie. The social rules and interactions of society are imitated during play, sometimes with an imaginary friend or pet. Thought processes are very concrete and **egocentric**; that is, they concentrate on themselves with little or no regard to others or the external world. The preschoolers have difficulty concentrating on more than one aspect of a situation and cannot fathom a point of view other than their own. Through play, preschoolers experience and learn about their environment, learn social roles, and develop both fine and gross motor skills. The primary health-promotion strategy for this cognitive development is having a loving caretaker for the child to imitate; this is someone who encourages safe exploration of the real world and the development of imagination, logical thinking skills, and creative activities.

The emotional assessment of the preschooler finds children in Erikson's third stage of development, wrestling with resolution of the initiative-versus-guilt conflict. In resolving this developmental crisis, children become more assertive and exuberantly initiate new tasks using their developing physical and mental mastery. This quest for power may bring with it feelings of guilt for being too forceful. Health-promotion strategies seek to promote the development of physical and mental mastery in situations that the child can control. Achieving mastery of new actions and situations encourages the preschooler to continue exploration and experimentation. Criticism or ridicule promotes feelings of guilt and inadequacy, inhibiting further initiative.

The school-age child moves into Piaget's concrete operational stage of cognitive development (Brainerd, 1978). In this stage, the child demonstrates cooperative rather than egocentric interactions, the ability to classify and order objects, and an understanding of the concepts of reversibility, transformation, and conservation. A school-age child begins to be able to see another's point of view, even requesting another's advice or including another person in conversation. The ability to classify and order objects forms the basis for learning mathematics and understanding relationships. Realizing that objects and activities can be reversed or changed, or that they remain the same despite a slight change in form, is an important development in the child's ability to understand the world. The concept of time also develops during this period.

Although the preschool child may participate in a formal type of educational experience, the school-age child faces the prospect of the next 12 years in the school establishment. The changes in personal and social relationships encountered with entry into school often present a developmental challenge for both the child and the family. The school-age child is under constant pressure to learn new skills. The developmental task according to Erikson is industry versus inferiority (Erikson, 1950). The mastery of both personal and social tasks gives children a sense of industry: the beliefs that they can learn, solve problems, and be a part of the real world.

Health-promotion strategies involve giving the child an opportunity to learn competence without an excessive fear of the consequences of failure. The child who is given no cushion for the experience of learning becomes fearful and withdrawn, resisting trying new skills or activities. Occasionally, these children seek attention in an inappropriate manner by acting-out behaviors: bossiness, lying, and destructive activities.

Attention-Deficit/ Hyperactivity Disorder

Attention-deficit/hyperactivity disorder (ADHD) is a neurobehavioral disorder found in approximately 3–17% of children and adolescents (McDonnell & Moffett, 2010). Increased impulsivity, the inability to concentrate, hyperactivity, and difficulties in school and family relationships are the most common symptoms. The majority of children with this disorder do not have a learning disability, but they usually have difficulty with schoolwork. Children with ADHD should be evaluated by a multidisciplinary team to determine the need for assistance. Sometimes medications are needed to allow the students to more fully participate in their education, improve their academic and social skills, and decrease their impulsivity. Numerous studies have demonstrated the benefit of appropriate therapy in improving the educational and psychosocial outcomes in these children (Biederman et al., 2009). Parent education classes, advocacy group conferences, support groups, social skill classes, and counseling for both the child and the family may also help with behavioral management. In the classroom, numerous strategies can help the child with ADHD (see Box 10-5).

Children diagnosed with ADHD are entitled to a free and appropriate public education, as well as special education programs as needed (see the Political Domain section later in this chapter). The health-promotion strategy is to educate parents and teachers about the symptoms of ADHD, so that the condition can be recognized earlier in the child's educational career and methods and strategies can be implemented to prevent academic and psychosocial delays.

BOX 10-5

CLASSROOM STRATEGIES FOR A CHILD WITH ADHD

- Seat the child in the front of the room, away from sources of distraction like doors or windows.
- Seat the child near a task-focused child.
- Teach the child to make a list and to cross off completed tasks.
- Provide frequent bathroom breaks, and allow the child to move around the classroom as needed.
- Allow the child to leave the room for a few minutes if frustrated.
- Develop consistent routines.
- Help the child keep the work space neat and uncluttered.
- Communicate regularly with the parents about the child's behavior and progress.

SOCIAL DOMAIN

The social domain for the preschool and school-age child is focused on relationships with the family, peers, and the community. Other significant social influences are television and culture.

Relationships

Exploring their own roles, as well as trying out others, helps preschoolers understand who they are in relation to their families and the world. The ability to imagine how others feel and behave moves the child from total egocentrism toward cooperation in the world. Most preschoolers have one or more siblings—older, younger, or both. The health-promotion strategy recommended consists of observing and guiding the social relationship between the siblings.

Preschoolers with older siblings may find themselves envious of all the attention the older siblings receive and frustrated at being unable to do similar things. Praising preschoolers for their own accomplishments helps them have positive feelings about themselves, thus building self-esteem.

Preschoolers who have been presented with a younger sibling may display jealousy and regressive demanding behaviors. If parents inform preschoolers about the upcoming addition to the family involve them in preparations and encourage them to express their personal opinions, the experience of the transition will be less difficult. Once the new arrival is in the home, spending special time alone with preschoolers, encouraging them to help the parents in caring for the baby, and giving them a doll to promote role-play as caregivers may also assist in the transition.

People outside the immediate family may begin to influence the child if they are in contact frequently enough. Grandparents, aunts and uncles, and peers provide the child with insights into different social situations, preparing the child to interact in group situations, to cooperate with others, and to increase personal independence. All these social accomplishments prepare the child for school. Again, praise for the child's accomplishments and positive reinforcement for cooperative behaviors are the needed strategies to promote the child's social health.

The broadening of social contacts outside the home continues for the school-age child. **Peers** (individuals of the same age) play a central role in the development of the child's identity, often competing with that of the parents. During the first half of the school-age years (6–9), same-gender peers are preferred. This preference changes as the child moves toward adolescence. Interactions with peers often lead to the testing of rules and values learned from the parents. Peer acceptance helps build the child's self-esteem and feelings of self-worth, but the lessening of parental influence may cause anxiety in some parents. Parents with high self-esteem who have demonstrated an affectionate, supportive relationship with the child will continue to be the primary role models and support for the developing child. Health-promotion strategies for the child are the approval and reinforcement of appropriate behaviors and accomplishments. For the parents of the school-age child, strategies involve exploring parental concerns and guiding or validating supportive parental behaviors.

TELEVISION

Outside the family, the most significant social influence on the preschool and school-age child is television. In the United States, children's TV- and other media-related activities average close to 40 hours per week (August et. al., 2008). A report from the U.S. Department of Health and Human Services found that children who watched more than three hours/day of television had a 54% higher odds of being overweight than those who watched less than one hour/day (Singh & Kogan, 2010). By the time they graduate from high school, children will have spent less time in the classroom than watching television. Children who watch 3–4 hours of television daily tend to perform more poorly in school, read and exercise less, be obese, play less well with friends, have fewer hobbies, and view the world as a dangerous and scary place. In addition, these children tend to have an increased potential for aggression, alcohol and drug use, and early involvement in sexual activity (Gidwani et al., 2002; Strasburger, 2006).

Watching television advertisements may be as harmful as watching television programs, such as soap operas, adult sitcoms, adult talk shows, and violent shows. Although preschoolers do not understand that the purpose of advertising is to sell a product, school-age children who watch a lot of television are more likely to believe the advertising claims. A review of advertisements during typical Saturday morning children's programming finds that 90% are selling sugary cereals, candy, salty snacks, fatty foods, junk food, and toys. Children also see tens of thousands of alcohol commercials before they reach the legal age to consume such beverages. There is approximately 1 hour of commercials for every five hours of programming.

Not all television watching is detrimental. With guided program selection, the preschooler can develop imagination and learn letters, numbers, colors, and shapes. The school-age child, with appropriate guidance in program selection, can learn historical information, geography, and positive behaviors such as cooperation and friendship.

An added concern is the effect of interactive home video games on children. Psychologists and neuroscientists have recognized the deleterious effects that video games have on the brain, and, because the effects are subtle, they are considered harmless. Noting that research on the effects of home video games have identified both positive effects (increased dexterity, peripheral vision, sense of mastery, etc.) and negative effects (decreased exercise, obesity, aggression, isolation, etc.), researchers have recommended focusing on five attributes in investigations: amount of use, content, structure, mechanics,

GLOBAL HIGHLIGHTS IN HEALTH PROMOTION

The Relationship between Violent Video Games and Aggression

A review of numerous studies demonstrated an association between violent video games and aggressive behavior in children. Video games allow the player to interact with the game physically, emotionally, and psychologically in such a way that can increase frustration and anger. Compared to earlier studies that linked violent TV watching with an increased antisocial and aggressive behavior in children, the effects are greater with violent video games. Because these studies are less than 25 years old, the effects of long-term exposure to violent video games is not yet known. Reports by reputable professional health associations (e.g., American Academy of Pediatrics, Australian College of Paediatrics, Canadian Paediatric Society and the American Psychological Association) and health agencies suggest reducing the exposure of youth to these violent video games. Nurses can educate parents, teachers, and community leaders to help promote age-related activities that can be easily accessible.

Source: Anderson, C. A., Ihori, N., Bushman, B. J., Rothstein, H. R. Shibuya, A., Swing, E. L., & Saleem, M. (2010). Violent video game effects on aggression, empathy, and prosocial behavior in eastern and western countries: A meta-analytic review. Psychological Bulletin, 136 (2), 151–173.

and social context (Gentile, 2009). Box 10-6 describes the health-promotion strategies that can be recommended to parents and to caregivers who want to use television watching in a healthy and positive way.

Cultural Influences

As preschoolers take a more active role in family practices, rituals, and holidays, they may begin to notice differences between their cultural heritage and that of their playmates or neighbors. The natural curiosity about the world demonstrated by this age group provides an excellent opportunity to begin education about diversity in cultures, races, and individuals. Health-promotion strategies involve imparting an appreciation for the contribution that diversity brings to the world. Preschoolers rapidly adopt the prejudices demonstrated by their parents, caregivers, or playmates.

School-age children have increased opportunities to interact with individuals from different cultures. Parents and teachers can promote respect and appreciation for cultural differences through reading assignments, classroom interactions, and participation in cultural events. Knowledge of the beliefs, values, and practices of diverse cultures reduces the development of ethnocentrism and prejudice.

Political Domain

Political initiatives that have had a direct impact on the preschool and school-age child are Medicaid, the State Children's Health Insurance Program, and the National School Lunch Program. Each of these federal initiatives addresses child health through health promotion. In addition, the Individuals with Disabilities Education Act (IDEA) and Section 504 of the Rehabilitation Act have had a strong impact on the education provided for preschool and school-age children.

Medicaid and the State Children's Health Insurance Program

Medicaid and the State Children's Health Insurance Program (SCHIP) provide health care coverage for about 34 million poor and near-poor children in the United States; yet nearly nine million children are uninsured. These two types of public health care coverage provide age-related preventive health (well child visits, immunizations, screening) and acute care

BOX 10-6
GUIDE TO THE HEALTHY USE OF TELEVISION, HOME VIDEO GAMES, AND MOVIES

PRESCHOOL CHILDREN	SCHOOL-AGE CHILDREN
1. Limit time in front of a screen to 2 hours daily.	1. Limit time in front of a screen to 2 hours daily, and limit handheld game time.
2. Choose shows and videos developed especially for preschoolers.	2. Select developmentally appropriate shows.
3. Make a weekly plan for appropriate shows.	3. Discuss unrealistic role models and values when viewed on a program.
4. Discuss fantasy and what is real in TV programs, games, or movies.	4. Encourage activities other than television watching: sports, hobbies, play.
5. Prohibit watching violence.	5. Prohibit watching violence.
6. Turn off TV during family mealtime.	6. Turn off TV while completing homework.
7. Set an example for responsible TV watching.	7. Do not allow children to have a TV in their bedrooms.
8. Join them in watching their favorite program, a movie, or playing an appropriate game or video activity such as Wii.	8. Join them in watching their favorite program, a movie, or playing an appropriate game or video activity such as Wii.

visits (Kenney & Dorn, 2009). Reaching the millions of children who are eligible but who remain uninsured continues to be an important health-promotion challenge and strategy.

National School Lunch Program

Another federal benefit with a significant impact on the health of school-age children is the National School Lunch Program. Enacted in 1946 to provide the opportunity for children to receive at least one healthy meal every school day, the program reimburses schools for providing eligible children with a meal that meets the Federal nutrition requirements. Over 31 million children participated in the lunch program in 2010 through 101,000 public and nonprofit private participating schools.

Individuals with Disabilities Education Act

Two federal laws entitle children with disabilities to get assistance with their educational needs. The Individuals with Disabilities Education Act (IDEA) (replacing the Education of the Handicapped Act) provides funding to guarantee 3- to 21-year-olds a free and appropriate education, based on the assessment of individual needs, in the least restrictive environment that is racially and culturally unbiased, as well as an individualized education program (IEP) prepared by a team of professionals. The language was changed to focus more on the child with disabilities than on the so-called handicapped child (U.S. Department of Education, 2011). The act requires school systems to pay for related services such as transportation, audiology, recreation, psychological services, and social work services. It requires a written IEP for each child with parental input in educational planning and decision making.

Section 504 of the Rehabilitation Act was passed to end discrimination against any person with a handicap. When a child has emotional or behavioral problems in school, Section 504 protects the child from discrimination and provides interventions in the classroom. If a child with a disability has been identified and confirmed by school testing, accommodations must be made to assist the child in succeeding in the classroom. Children who do not qualify for special education (IDEA) can be evaluated for a Section 504 accommodation, so that behavior and curriculum modification can be implemented.

ENVIRONMENTAL DOMAIN

The accident rate for preschoolers is less than for toddlers; however, preschoolers are still impulsive and lack sufficient maturity to recognize all potential dangers. Table 10-4 lists common sources of injury for preschool children, along with health-promotion strategies to prevent accidental injury. Two areas of health promotion should be emphasized: street safety and firearm safety.

The preschool child is not mature enough to play close to streets or cross streets without adult supervision. The use of riding toys should be confined to sidewalks and other protected areas, with particular care if there are driveway intersections.

Firearm safety has been receiving needed attention, especially with the passage of state laws allowing an individual to carry handguns. Many of these states have also passed laws holding the owners responsible for accidents or injuries caused by their guns. There is no truly safe place for a loaded gun in any household, especially where a child might be living or visiting. The only safe gun is unloaded, with the gun and the ammunition stored separately, both under lock and key.

An environmental hazard that affects both the preschool and the school-age child is exposure to tobacco smoke. According to a CDC (2010) report, approximately 54% of children from 3 to 11 years of age are exposed to secondhand smoke. Epidemiologic studies have associated increased rates of sudden infant death syndrome and low birth weight, acute respiratory illness, asthma, and increased rates of middle ear infections with exposure of children to environmental smoke. Childhood exposure may also increase rates of cancer development in adulthood. Promoting a smoke-free environment is a health-promotion strategy that benefits individuals across the life span.

Bicycling is a fun and healthy activity during childhood, with over 70% of children ages 5–14 years of age riding bicycles in 2009. Bicycle riding is, however, responsible for over 300,000 injuries (Castleet al., 2010). The use of helmets has been shown to reduce the risk of head injury and fatalities related to head injury related (Castle et al., 2010). Helmets must be properly fitted and meet the standards developed by the Snell Memorial Foundation and the American National Standards Institutes. The American Pediatrics Association has recommended that retail stores sell inexpensive approved helmets as a package deal to individuals buying bicycles. Positive factors that influence a child's compliance with wearing a bicycle helmet are parental ownership and use of a helmet while cycling, parental rules enforcing helmet use, and peers and siblings who use a helmet. Children were 100 times more likely to own and use a helmet if their parents used one (Clements, 2005). Negative factors include cost, appearance, comfort, inconvenience, and not seeing a need for a helmet when riding close to home.

The potential for injuries from contact sports and playground equipment for this age group makes adult supervision during these activities imperative.

In the United States, over 3 million cases of child abuse and neglect are reported each year, and, as a result, three children die each day (AAP, 2011b). There are four types of abuse including physical abuse, sexual abuse, emotional abuse, and child neglect. Nurses need to look for physical signs of abuse, including bruising, hematoma, bite marks, and retinal hemorrhage; and signs of neglect including malnutrition, poor skin care, cleanliness, and medical and dental care. Parental behavior and discrepancies between the reported cause of injury and the injury seen can be an important in identifying abuse or neglect. Emotional abuse takes many forms and may not be overtly apparent. It includes more than the suffering of verbal abuse from constantly being yelled at, humiliated, or belittled. Coldness, harassment, being ignored, or forced into corruptive behavior from parents, other caregivers, or family members are a few of the forms that emotional abuse can take. Depending on the level of resiliency or hardiness, children of abuse are prone to developing poor or maladaptive social behavior even to the extent of depression and acts of self-destruction. All states have a law that requires reporting any suspicion of abuse or neglect to the appropriate authorities.

SEXUAL DOMAIN

The preschool child recognizes gender differences and has a developing sexual curiosity. Negative reactions from caregivers toward this curiosity make the child repress these feelings and may be detrimental to the child's developing body and self-image. The preschool age is the age of "1000 questions," and some of those questions are about sex. Parents need accurate information in order to give factual responses. The ability to supply age-appropriate information with honesty is essential to helping the child develop. Choosing the right time and

TABLE 10-4 Environmental Safety for Preschool and School-Age Children

SOURCE OF INJURY	PREVENTION STRATEGIES
Automobiles	Supervise children younger than 10 when crossing streets.
	Teach street-crossing techniques.
	Use a booster seat if child is under 70 lb.
	Always use both lap and shoulder restraints.
	If a shoulder restraint crosses child's face, place it behind the child.
	Encourage riding in the back seat.
	Keep car doors locked when moving.
	Do not allow child to ride in the cargo area of a pickup, van, or station wagon.
	Be a good role model.
Sports/play	Participate in a bicycle training course.
	Use bicycle helmets for rider and passenger.
	Use bike lanes if available.
	Watch traffic, and encourage off-peak riding times.
	Use safety helmet and pads when skating.
	Use safety lenses for indicated sports and hobbies.
	Provide adequate adult supervision for playground and team sports activities.
	Watch for exhaustion and heat exposure.
	Restrict play around stairs and windows or on furniture.
Poison	Keep medicines and dangerous chemicals in a locked cabinet.
	Keep the Poison Control number readily available.
	Buy vitamins and other over-the-counter medications in small quantities.
Water	Teach children to swim.
	Never let children swim alone.
	Use a personal flotation device in boats and around lakes and rivers.
Fire/burns	Always supervise children cooking.
	Keep hot water heater set at 120–130° F.
	Install smoke and carbon monoxide detectors, and test regularly.
	Use flame-retardant clothing around stoves, fires, and adults who smoke.
	Have a fire escape plan.
	Review the fire escape plan by means of role-playing.
	Teach children the use of emergency phone numbers, such as 911, or key-family members, etc.
Firearms	Keep all firearms unloaded and locked up.

© Cengage Learning 2013

place and taking advantage of teachable moments may help parents deal with the barrage of questions more comfortably. The questions that naturally arise when the child notices that the mother has breasts or that the father has a penis or sees a sexually oriented program or advertisement on television may create a teachable moment. Parents can also use books, pamphlets, or situations to stimulate teachable moments.

Sexuality education (factual information about anatomy, physiology, birth control, and sexually transmitted diseases) should occur during the school-age years. Although school-age children are at the height of their sexual curiosity, their sexual urges are dormant, making this the ideal time to prepare them for the upcoming changes of puberty. Age-appropriate information about puberty and reproduction can be presented before children become self-conscious about their emerging sexuality. The understanding of the information should be evaluated because the child can misinterpret, pick up on limited parts, or be influenced by misinformation from peers. A vital health-promotion strategy for the nurse is to encourage parents and schools to collaborate in providing factual, complete sexuality information for the school-age child.

SPIRITUAL DOMAIN

The preschool child begins more active participation in the spiritual and religious life of the family. Reading books, saying simple prayers, and participating in the celebration of religious holidays and family rituals are appropriate methods for developing the spiritual health of young children. Both the preschool and the school-age child should be taught the value of kindness, goodness, patience, faithfulness, gentleness, and self-control.

The school-age child is mature enough for reading, study, and discussion about the family's religious and spiritual beliefs. In addition to participating in celebrations and rituals, the school-age child can observe and understand the application of religious principles to everyday life.

HEALTH PROMOTION
THEORY LINK

Orem's Self-Care Deficit Theory Applied to Children

Nurse theorist Dorothea Orem viewed patients as individuals with health-related limitations that make them incapable of continuous self-care and dependent on others for care. Children are maturing persons who, due to their lack of knowledge, skills, motivation, experience, or orientation, require the assistance of others for promoting and maintaining health across all domains. Guidance and intervention from parents, caregivers, and health care providers are necessary to meet the eight self-care requisites identified by Orem:

1. Maintenance of sufficient air
2. Maintenance of sufficient intake of food
3. Maintenance of sufficient intake of water
4. Provision of care associated with elimination processes and excrements
5. Maintenance of balance between activity and rest

6. Maintenance of balance between solitude and isolation
7. Prevention of hazards to human life, human functioning, and human well-being
8. Promotion of human functioning and development within social groups in accordance with human potential, known human limitations, and the human desire to be normal (with consideration of genetic and other characteristics and talents of individuals).

These requisites are part of the daily life of children as they mature and take greater responsibilities for themselves. This theory is applicable to all children considering that the guidance and direction from others influence their development of increased independence and responsibility for self-care.

Source: Adapted from Berbiglia, V. A., & Banfield, B. (2010). Self-care deficit theory of nursing. In M. R. Alligood & A. M. Tomey (eds.). *Nursing theorists and their work*. Maryland Heights, MO: Mosby-Elsevier, pp. 265–285.

TABLE 10-5 Health Promotion in Children

RELATED DOMAIN	RISK ASSESSMENT	HEALTH-PROMOTION ACTION
Biological	Nutrition	Well-balanced diet consisting of a variety of low-fat foods. Foods with so-called empty calories, such as soda, should be used sparingly. Identify underweight, overweight, and obese children through the body mass index.
	Elimination	Assess for enuresis, encopresis, or both with appropriate follow-up.
	Sleep and activity	Bedtime routines and rituals.
		Regular physical activity (20–30 minutes at least six times weekly).
	Immunization	Adhere to immunization schedule and catch-up if needed.
Psychological	Cognitive and emotional development	Assess for appropriate cognitive and emotional development according to age and stage.
Social	Relationships	Approve of and reinforce appropriate behaviors with family and peers.
		Supervise and guide television watching.
Environmental	Accidents	Anticipatory guidance to prevent accidental injury.
Sexual	Knowledge	Encourage factual, age-appropriate information from parents and schools.
Spiritual	Values	Encourage application of religious principles to everyday life.
	Beliefs	

SUMMARY

Promoting the health of the preschool and school-age child recognizes the significant social, emotional, and cognitive growth that is occurring. Providing adequate nutrition without causing overweight or obesity requires education about wholesome diets and the need for regular physical activity. Screening for immunization status, vision and hearing problems, delayed development, and learning and behavior problems as well as physical problems is essential. Keeping preschool and school-age children safe and preventing accidents play a crucial role in helping them grow up healthy.

This chapter grouped health-promotion strategies into sections for the preschool and the school-age child. Each age group was viewed through biological, psychological, social, political, environmental, sexual, and spiritual domains for a comprehensive look at health promotion in the early years of life. Table 10-5 provides suggested health-promotion actions related to areas of risk assessment for the domains that specifically apply to children.

CASE STUDY

Shauney Williams: Overweight and at Risk for Type 2 Diabetes Mellitus

OBJECTIVES/GOALS: Through participation in discussion of this case study, participants will have the opportunity to:

1. Discuss the assessment of a child for weight and nutrition.
2. Investigate the relationship between overweight and development of Type 2 diabetes.
3. Discuss dietary and activity changes to prevent childhood obesity.

HEALTH PROMOTION CONCERN, HISTORY AND PHYSICAL, PRESENT HEALTH STATUS, PAST HEALTH STATUS, FAMILY HISTORY, AND SOCIAL HISTORY

Shauney Williams is a 10-year-old Black female who was referred for evaluation of acanthosis nigricans on the nape of her neck. She reports noticing darker skin markings to her neck and underarms about 1 year ago and denies any problems, including GI or GU. She is in the fourth grade in a local elementary school and is making As and Bs in her schoolwork. She is the youngest of three children in the family. Her birth was a spontaneous vaginal delivery, and she weighed 8 lb, 12 oz. Her mother is 5 ft, 4 in., weighs approximately 180 lb, and had gestational diabetes with her last two pregnancies. She weighed about the same before Shauney's birth. Shauney has always been between the 85th–90th percentile for her age-/sex-specific body mass index (BMI) according to the CDC chart. She is up-to-date with her immunizations.

REVIEW OF PERTINENT DOMAINS

Biological Domain

PHYSICAL EXAM: Reveals a 4 ft, 10 in. female weighing 106 lb (90th percentile for BMI). Thyroid is without enlargement or nodules.

INTEGUMENTARY: She has a velvety, hyperpigmented brown plaque with accentuated skin markings on the nape of her neck. The hyperpigmentation is a lighter brown in her axillae.

CARDIOVASCULAR/RESPIRATORY: Her blood pressure is normal for her age. Her heart rate and rhythm are within normal limits, and her lungs are clear to auscultation.

GASTROINTESTINAL: Soft, round, and mildly protruded abdomen with normal bowel sounds

24-HOUR DIET RECALL: 10 oz of Sugar Frosted Flakes and whole milk for breakfast. The school lunch consisted of a hamburger with cheese and mayonnaise, two servings of French fries (her friends give her some of their food), two servings of orange juice, plus an ice cream bar for dessert. After-school snack was 10 Oreo cookies and 12-oz cola drink. She had three pieces of fried chicken, green beans, corn, and mashed potatoes with gravy for dinner. At bedtime she had a small piece of cake and whole milk.

(Continues)

CASE STUDY

(Continued)

ACTIVITY RECALL: Played softball in physical education for 20 minutes at school. She watched TV and played video games on the computer after school; then she watched more TV after dinner with the family, making a total of five hours of viewing time.

DIAGNOSTIC TESTING: Shauney's hematocrit, urinalysis, TSH, ALT, and fasting serum glucose and lipid panel are within normal limits. Her fasting serum insulin level is slightly elevated.

Psychological Domain

Shauney's grades are above average, and she has no trouble completing assignments on time. Shauney's and the family's readiness to make lifestyle changes needs to be assessed.

Social Domain

Shauney is a bright, sociable child who makes friends easily.

Environmental Domain

Shauney's family is upper middle-class and surrounds her with love, but, as the youngest in the family, she is always rewarded with lots of candies and rich foods, which she likes to eat in abundance. No limits are placed on Shauney's eating habits, and, as a consequence, she is considered big for her age. Shauney and her family need education about the presence of acanthosis nigricans as a marker for insulin resistance, the relationship between overweight and development of Type 2 diabetes, and the need for a wholesome, low-fat diet, daily exercise, including limiting her TV/video game time.

QUESTIONS FOR DISCUSSION

1. What risk factors does Shauney have for being overweight?
2. Why should Shauney's mother be concerned about her daughter having acanthosis nigricans?
3. What changes in lifestyle should be recommended for Shauney and her family?

KEY CONCEPTS

1. Health promotion for infants and children in the biological domain includes strategies related to nutrition, elimination, sleep and activity, and immunization.

2. Screening for actual or potential health problems in children is vital for promoting the quality and quantity of life. Nurses assist in screening for hypertension, TB, vision and hearing problems, scoliosis, and acanthosis nigricans for school-age children.

3. Promoting health in the psychological domain requires an understanding of normal cognitive and emotional development. Theoretical frameworks developed by Jean Piaget and Erik Erikson provide a foundation for evaluating the development of children.

4. Health promotion in the social domain for children evolves from the family to include day care networks, school, and the community. The influence of television should be consistently evaluated and regulated.

5. Child abuse and neglect occur in more than 3 million children annually. Nurses need to look for physical signs including bruising, hematomas, poor skin care, malnutrition, bite marks, and retinal hemorrhage. Parental behavior and discrepancies between the reported cause of injury and the injury seen can also be important keys to identifying abuse. Any suspicion of abuse or neglect must, by law, be reported to the appropriate authorities.

6. In addition to legislation mandating the reporting of suspected child abuse, there are other social actions for health promotion in the political domain: the Supplemental Food Program for Women, Infants, and Children (WIC), car occupant safety requirement laws, Medicaid, SCHIP and IDEA programs, and the National School Lunch Program.

7. Nurses and parents share responsibility for promoting the safety of children. Safety strategies include providing age-appropriate foods; giving immunizations; using seat belts, car seats, and protective helmets; and teaching behaviors for healthy lifestyles. Preventing physical and psychological trauma is vital to ensure healthy development throughout the life span.

8. Important in the sexual domain is the education of parents and caregivers about the normal sexual development of children. The provision of complete, accurate sexuality education is critical for the development of sexual health.

9. Spiritual beliefs and practices of the parents and caregivers influence health promotion in the spiritual domain.

CHAPTER REVIEW

Learning Activities

1. Plan an educational program designed to assist parents with the management of the preschooler or school-age child who is a picky eater.

2. Develop a brochure for parents related to the prevention of overweight in children.

3. List positive findings for acanthosis nigricans. Participate in a screening for acanthosis nigricans.

Multiple Choice

1. You are performing a preschool assessment of a 5-year-old male child. Which of the following would be your first step in assessing his nutritional status?
   a. Assessment of the child's food preferences
   b. Assessment of the child's visual acuity
   c. Determination of the child's body mass index (BMI)
   d. Recording the child's vital signs

2. A mother reports that her 9-year-old daughter and 11-year-old son are spending at least three hours daily watching TV and playing home video games. Your response to her is based on the American Academy of Pediatrics recommended screen-time for a school-aged child, which is:
   a. between 2–4 hours/day.
   b. between 4–6 hours/day.
   c. maximum of 1 hour/day.
   d. no more than 2 hours/day.

3. Your supervising nurse assigns you to develop a teaching module titled "Taking Baby Home" for parents of newborns who have siblings. The aim of the module is to provide helpful information and guidance for parents to use in facilitating successful adjustment of preschool children to the addition of a new baby in the family. Which of the following strategies would you include?
   a. Assure the preschooler that she or he will love the new baby.
   b. Avoid discussion about the new baby until 1–2 weeks before its arrival because of the short attention span of most preschoolers.
   c. Give the preschooler a doll to promote role-play as a caregiver.
   d. Wait until the new baby arrives to move the preschooler to a new room.

4. Which of the following is a significant influence on whether a child wears a bicycle helmet?
   a. The bicycle will be ridden over one mile from home.
   b. The child has had a previous accident with a head injury.
   c. The helmet fits properly.
   d. The parents wear helmets while cycling.

5. To evaluate for a healthy sleep pattern in an 8-year-old child, you know that school-aged children will usually sleep:
   a. 7–8 hours at night.
   b. 8–12 hours at night.
   c. 10–14 hours at night.
   d. 7–14 hours depending on what time they get to bed.

6. Advice to parents regarding the best way to respond to the numerous questions preschoolers might have regarding sexuality is to:
   a. explain that all those questions will be answered in school.
   b. ignore the questions because it is too early to talk about sex.
   c. supply age-appropriate information with honesty.
   d. try to avoid these situations until the child is school-aged.

7. You are a school nurse, and parents have questioned you about who sets the guidelines for lunch programs in your state. Your response is based on the knowledge that the National School Lunch Program follows which nutritional guidelines?
   a. Individual guidelines set forth by the local registered dietician
   b. The federal nutritional requirements
   c. The nutritional guidelines mandated by their board of directors
   d The nutritional guidelines mandated by their state

8. The incidences of child abuse and neglect have continued to escalate all over the world. In the United States alone, how many cases of child abuse and neglect are reported each year?
   a. 1–2 million cases
   b. less than 1 million cases
   c. unknown
   d. over 3 million cases

9. Child abuse encompasses many aspects. What are the three major categories, or types, of child abuse?
   a. Physical, sexual, and emotional/psychological
   b. Poor nutrition, poor hygiene, and neglect
   c. Poor hygiene, tobacco exposure, and neglect
   d. Tobacco exposure, sexual abuse, and neglect

10. Which of the following is an environmental hazard that affects both preschool and school-aged children and increases their susceptibility to numerous respiratory infections?
    a. Air pollution
    b. Allergens
    c. Household carpets
    d. Tobacco smoke

ORGANIZATIONS AND WEBSITES

American Academy of Pediatrics: An excellent resource for topics related to children and adolescents: **http://www.aap.org**

American Diabetes Association: Offers a wealth of information on diabetes for all ages: **http://www.diabetes.org**

American Dietetic Association: Offers a current search engine to help locate useful nutrition-related content accurately and quickly: **http://www.eatright.org/**

Center for Nutrition Policy and Promotion: Dietary Guidelines for Americans 2010: **http://www.dietaryguidelines.gov**

Centers for Disease Control and Prevention: Has a link to explain and calculate body mass index: **http://www.cdc.gov**

Children's Safety Network (CNS) National Injury and Violence Prevention Resource Center: A National center for the prevention of childhood injuries and violence: **http://www.childrenssafetynetwork.org**

Department of Child and Adolescent Health and Development (CAH): Provides resources for child and adolescent health and development throughout the world: **http://www.who.int**

Partnership for Children's Health and the Environment: Provides information on ways to protect children from harmful environmental exposures. **http://partnersforchildren.org**

U.S. Department of Health and Human Services: Childhood obesity intervention tool kit that provide resources for community leaders: **http://www.hhs.gov/intergovernmental/letsmove**

REFERENCES

American Academy of Pediatrics. (AAP). (2003). Prevention of pediatric overweight and obesity. *Pediatrics, 112*(2), 424–430.

American Academy of Pediatrics. (AAP). (2008). *New guidelines double the amount of recommended vitamin D*. Retrieved from http://www.aap.org/pressroom/nce/nce08vitamind.htm

American Academy of Pediatrics. (AAP). (2011a). *Healthy children*. Retrieved from http://www.healthchildren.org/English/healthy-living/nutrition/pages

American Academy of Pediatrics. (AAP). (2011b). *Child abuse and neglect*. Retrieved from http://www.aap.org/healthtopics/childabuse.cfm

American Academy of Pediatrics. (AAP). (2011c). *Recommendations for preventive pediatric health care (Periodicity schedule)*. Retrieved from http://practice.aap.org/content.aspx?aid=1599

August, G. P., Caprio, S., Fennoy, I., Freemark, M., Kaufman, F. R., Lustig, R. H., & Montori, V. M. (2008). Prevention and treatment of pediatric obesity: An endocrine society clinical practice guideline based on expert opinion. *Journal Clinical Endocrine and Metabolic, 93*(12), 4576–4599. DOI: 10.1210/jc.2007–2458

Barroso, C. S., Kelder, S. H., Springer, A. E., Smith, C. L., Ranitt, N., Ledingham, C., & Hoelscher, D. M. (2009). Senate bill 42: Implementation and impact on physical activity in middle schools. *Journal of Adolescent Health, 45*, S82–S90.

Biederman, J., Monuteaux, M. C., Spencer, T., Wilens, T. E., & Faraone, S. V. (2009). Do stimulants protect against psychiatric disorders in youth with ADHD? A 10-year follow-up study. *Pediatrics, 124*(1), 71–78. DOI: 10.1542/peds.2008–3347

Brainerd, C. J. (1978). *Piaget's theory of intelligence*. Englewood Cliffs, NJ: Prentice Hall.

Camden, S. G. (2009). Obesity: An emerging concern for patients and nurses. *The Online Journal of Issues in Nursing, 14*(1). Retrieved from http://www.nursingworld.org/MainMenuCategories/ANAMarketplace/ANAPeriodicals/OJIN

Castle, S. L., Burle, R. V., Arbogast, H., & Upperman, J. S. (2010). Bicycle helmet legislation and injury patterns in trauma patients when under age 18. *Journal of Surgical Research*, 1–5. DOI:10.1016/j.jss.2010.10.031.

Centers for Disease Control and Prevention. (CDC). (2010). Press Release: *Half of children still exposed to secondhand smoke*. Retrieved from http://practice.aap.org/content.aspx?aid=1599

Centers for Disease Control and Prevention. (CDC), (2011). *The recommended immunization schedules*. Retrieved from http://www.cdc.gov/vaccines/recs/acip

Clements, J. (2005). Promoting the use of bicycle helmets during primary care visits. *Journal of the American Academy of Nurse Practitioners, 17*(9), 350–354.

Erikson, E. (1950). Childhood and society. New York, NY: Norton.

Gentile, D. A. (2009, July). Video Games Affect the Brain—for Better and Worse. *Cerebrum, The DANA Foundation*. Retrieved from http://www.dana.org/news/cerebrum/detail.aspx?id=22800

Gidwani, P., Sobol, A., DeJong, W., Perrin, J., & Gortmaker, S. (2002). Television viewing and initiation of smoking among youth. *Pediatrics, 110*(3), 505–508.

Kenney, G. M., & Dorn, S. (2009). Health care reform for children with public coverage: How can policymakers maximize gains and prevent harm? *Robert Wood Johnson Foundation*. Retrieved from http://www.rwjf.org/healthpolicy/product.jsp?id=44068

Koshy, G., Delpisheh, A., & Brabin, B. J. (2011). Childhood obesity and parental smoking as risk factors for childhood ADHD in Liverpool children. *Attention Deficit Hyperactivity Disorder, 3*, 21–28.

Kumar, J., Muntner, P., Kaskel, F. J., Hailpern, S. M., & Melamed, M. L. (2009). Prevalence and associations of 25-Hydroxyvitamin D deficiency in the US children: NHANES 2001–2004. *Pediatrics, 124*(3), 362–370.

Li, J., & Hooker, N. H. (2010). Childhood obesity and schools: Evidence from the national survey of children's health. *Journal of School Health, 80*(2),

Looney, S. M., Spence, M. L., & Raynor, H. A. (2011). Use of body mass index and body mass index growth charts for assessment of childhood weight status in the United States: A systematic review. *Clinical Pediatrics, 50*(2), 91–99. DOI: 10.1177/0009922810379911

Makari, J., & Rushton, H. G. (2006). Nocturnal enuresis. *American Family Physician, 73*(9), 1611–1614.

McDonnell, M. A., & Moffett, C. (2010). Pharmacology treatment for ADHD. *Advance for NPs & PAs, 1*(4). Retrieved from http://nurse-practitioners-and-physician-assistants.advanceweb.com/Archives/Article-Archives/Coming-into-Focus.aspx

Ogden, C. L., Carroll, M. D., Curtin, L. R., & Lamb, M. M. (2010). Prevalence of high body mass index in US children and adolescents, 2007–2008. *Journal of the American Medical Association, 303*(3), 242–249.

Rance, K., & O'Laughlen, M. (2011). Obesity and asthma: A dangerous link in children; An integrative review of the literature. *The Journal for Nurse Practitioners, 7*(4), 287–292.

Salmeron, P. A. (2009). Childhood and adolescent attention-deficit hyperactivity disorder: Diagnosis, clinical practice guidelines, and social implications. *Journal of the American Academy of Nurse Practitioners, 21*, 488–497.

Seal, N. (2011). Introduction to genetics and childhood obesity: Relevance to nursing practice. *Biologic Research for Nursing, 13*(1), 61–69. DOI: 10.1177/1099800410381424

Shonkoff, J. P., & Phillips, D. A. (2000). *From neurons to neighborhoods: The science of early childhood development*. Washington, DC: The National Academies Press.

Singh, G. K., Siahpush, M., & Kogan, M. D. (2010). Rising social inequalities in US childhood obesity, 2003–2007. *Annuals of Epidemiology, 20*(1), 40–52. DOI: 10.1016/j.annepidem.2009.09.008.

Strasburger, V. (2006). "Clueless": Why do pediatricians underestimate the media's influence on children and adolescents? *Pediatrics 117*(4), 1427–1431. DOI:10.1542/peds.2005–2336.

U.S. Department of Education. (2011). Special education & rehabilitative services. Retrieved from http://www2.ed.gov/policy/speced/guid/idea/monitor/index.html

CHAPTER 11
The Adolescent and Young Adult

JOYCE ENGEL, PhD

KEY TERMS

abuse	gonads	meditation
acne	gynecomastia	melanoma
alpha brain waves	homosexuality	menarche
anorexia nervosa	hypothalamus	Papanicolaou (Pap) test
bulimia nervosa	incest	premenstrual syndrome (PMS)
cohabitation	intimate partner violence	puberty
dental caries	masturbation	substance abuse

OBJECTIVES

Upon completion of this chapter, the reader should be able to:

- Examine health-promotion strategies in the biological domain for adolescents and young adults.
- Identify nursing responsibilities for screening to promote the health of adolescents and young adults.
- Relate theories of cognitive and emotional development to health-promotion strategies in adolescents and young adults.
- Describe the occurrence of, signs and symptoms of, nursing responsibilities for, and strategies to reduce or prevent abuse and domestic violence.
- Identify political influences on the adolescent and young adult.
- Describe strategies to reduce accidental deaths in adolescents and young adults.
- Relate normal emotional and sexual development to strategies designed to promote sexual health in adolescents and young adults.
- Describe spiritual development in adolescents and young adults.

INTRODUCTION

Individuals in the adolescent and young adult period of their lives are generally the healthiest they have ever been or will be. Their mortality rates are among the lowest of all age groups, and they have the lowest morbidity rates for chronic medical conditions of the entire population. This healthy condition may lessen the adolescent's or young adult's perceived need for health promotion. However, the major causes of death for older adults have their roots in the behaviors adopted during the adolescent and young adult stages. Unhealthy eating patterns and low levels of physical activity are important factors in the later development of cardiovascular disease. An equal threat to health are the social morbidities of unintended pregnancy, sexually transmitted infections, homicide, suicide, injuries related to violence, and substance abuse. The prevention of health risk behaviors and the development of health-promoting behaviors during the adolescent and young adult periods has a lifelong positive effect on health status.

This chapter is divided into two sections: the adolescent and the young adult. To provide a guiding framework for organization, health-promotion strategies are viewed through the biological, psychological, social, political, environmental, sexual, and spiritual domains.

THE ADOLESCENT

The period between childhood and adulthood is called adolescence. This period is characterized by physical, sexual, and psychological maturation. Maturation signals the transference of health-promotion responsibilities from the caregivers, or parents, to the individual.

BIOLOGICAL DOMAIN

In chronological terms, adolescence is generally a period of 10–12 years beginning with the onset of puberty. By definition, **puberty** is the period in life during which members of both genders become capable of reproduction. This period of change usually occurs between the ages of 11 and 15 in boys and between 9 and 16 in girls, ending in the attainment of sexual maturity (Kaplan and Love-Osborne, 2007). In addition, physical growth to adult stature is also completed.

PUBERTY

Puberty is a dynamic biological process that is determined by highly organized mechanisms intrinsic to each individual. It depends on a complex interaction between the hypothalamus, anterior pituitary, the **gonads** (ovaries and testes), and the body's muscles and skeleton.

Control over these events is primarily in the **hypothalamus**, the gland in the brain responsible for controlling metabolic activities, the regulation of body temperature, the integration of sympathetic and parasympathetic activities, and the secretion of releasing (stimulating) and inhibiting hormones (Guyton & Hall, 2011). The hypothalamus secretes two releasing hormones to stimulate the anterior pituitary gland. One stimulates the pituitary gland to release sex steroids, and the other stimulates the pituitary to release growth hormones. The sex steroids (follicle-stimulating hormone and luteinizing hormone) stimulate the maturation of the gonads. The hormones produced by the gonads are responsible for the development of the secondary sex characteristics. The estrogenic activity of the ovaries causes growth and development of the vagina, uterus, Fallopian tubes, and breasts. The androgenic activity of the testes causes growth and development of the penis, scrotum, prostate, and larynx. Figure 11-1 illustrates hormone stimulation in puberty.

The hypothalamus also plays a part in stimulating the maturation of the adrenal glands. This adrenal and gonadal maturation provides the hormones that are responsible for developing pubic hair.

Musculoskeletal growth is controlled by the hypothalamus, with each individual having his or her own maturation and growth schedule. Adolescents grow at varying rates, and the rate of growth is not related to ultimate size. Unless there is a pathologic condition, the boy who gets his height early will fall into the same average adult height range as the boy who gets his height later (Kaplan and Love-Osborne, 2007).

The primary health-promotion strategy is educating adolescents and their parents about the normal variation among individuals. Applying the standardized growth charts used for younger age groups is not appropriate for normal individual adolescents in puberty. Early developers may jump from the 75th percentile to the 95th percentile and then plateau, while late developers may fall from the 25th percentile to the 10th percentile and have a late spurt. In general, tall children tend to be tall adults, and short children tend to be short adults. Key factors in eventual height are genetics and nutrition, not growth tempo.

The disturbance in the androgen-estrogen balance found in puberty is one of the causes of acne, the bane of existence in 85% of adolescents. **Acne** is an inflammatory process of the sebaceous follicles of the skin, characterized by papules, comedones, and pustules (Kyle, 2008). The increased secretion of androgen in both males and females increases the size and activity of the sebaceous glands, primarily on the face, chest, and upper back. The presence of sebum and keratin in the follicles creates an excellent medium for the growth of the bacteria, *Poprionibacterium acnes* (Kyle, 2008).

Acne can be treated both topically and systemically, depending on its severity. The nurse needs to encourage the parents of adolescents with severe acne in which there are pustules, cysts, and nodules to seek treatment to prevent scarring. Severe acne may require systemic antibiotics, oral retinoids, or both to decrease sebum production and inflammation (Thiboutet et al. 2009). Moderate acne responds to topical antibiotics and topical keratolytic agents to relieve follicular obstruction. Adolescents on antibiotic therapy need to be carefully monitored for evidence of effectiveness and cautioned to use medications as ordered to avoid the development of antibiotic resistance. Adolescents with mild acne can reduce its effects by following the guidelines found in Box 11-1. Restricting dietary intake of certain substances, such as chocolate, has not proven to affect acne formation; however, the link between diet and acne can no longer be completely ignored. Recent evidence suggests that there may be a link between high glycemic loads and acne and that vitamin D may be helpful in the treatment of acne (Bowe, Smith, & Shalita, 2010). A hereditary tendency toward the development of acne has also been noted. Providing emotional support and understanding is a key health-promotion strategy for adolescents with acne.

Early or late physical maturation can put adolescents at risk. Early maturing girls may be unprepared for the emotional and social demands placed on them. They may not have the social maturity to handle advances from older males, putting them at risk for unwanted pregnancies and sexually transmitted diseases. They are also at risk for depression and substance

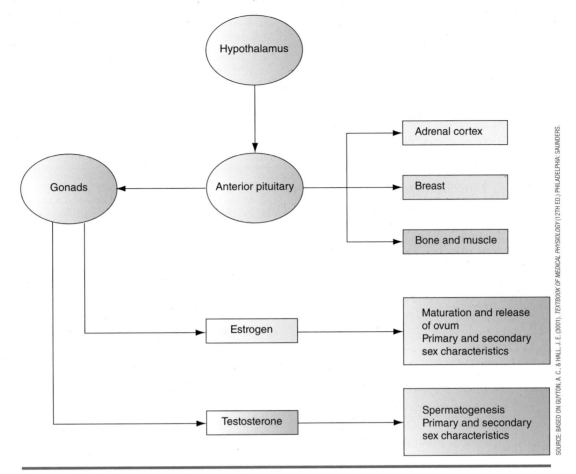

SOURCE: BASED ON GUYTON, A. C., & HALL, J. E. (3001). *TEXTBOOK OF MEDICAL PHYSIOLOGY* (12TH ED.) PHILADELPHIA: SAUNDERS.

FIGURE 11-1 Hormone stimulation in puberty.

abuse. Late maturing boys, whose development is out of sync with their peers, are at increased risk for depression and being bullied. To prove their maturity, they may be tempted to participate in high-risk behaviors such as sexual activity, smoking, or delinquency. Helping parents understand that adolescent autonomy should be determined by the teen's chronological age and by social and emotional development and not by the level of physical maturation is an important health-promotion strategy.

Female Puberty

Breast development in girls is one of the earliest observable signs of female puberty. The average age for beginning breast development is 9–11 years (Kyle, 2008). Late developers may gain reassurance from the knowledge that there is no relationship between the timing of breast development and eventual breast size (Kaplan & Love-Osborne, 2007). One breast may even be noticeably larger than the other during early development. The nurse should make it a point to discuss this potential asymmetry with the adolescent in order to reassure her of its normalcy. Boys may also have some breast development, called **gynecomastia**, during early puberty. They need reassurance that it is a transient condition that regresses within a year or two.

Menarche (the initiation of menstruation) usually occurs about 2.5 years after breast development begins (Kaplan & Love-Osborne, 2007). Ninety-five percent of females begin menstruation between 11 and 15 years of age. This wide variation in mean age appears to be influenced by ethnic, socioeconomic, and athletic factors, as well as by other considerations such as family structure, relative weight, stress, and maternal

Global trends in menarche present significant concerns for the well-being of adolescents and women. Early menarche is associated with a heightened risk for breast cancer and has been associated with metabolic syndrome and obesity. Early menarche may present a number of other health concerns in adolescent girls, including early sexual activity, depression, eating disorders, and poor school performance. The age of menarche in the United States has continued to decrease and was estimated to be 12.34 years in the period 1999–2002. The average age for Canadian adolescents is 12.72 years, which is lower than for Australia (13 years), Russia (13 years), and Norway (13.2 years).

Source: Al-Sahab, B., Ardern, C. I., Hamadeh, M. J., & Tamin, H. (2010). Age at menarche in Canada: Results from the National Longitudinal Study of Children and Youth. *BMC Public Health, 10,* 736.

age at menarche (Al-Sahab, Ardern, Hamadeh, & Tamim, 2010). The time between cycles is frequently irregular in the first year or two and should not be a cause for alarm if there is no other evidence of organic pathology. The primary health-promotion strategy is to prepare the adolescent and her parents for menarche through education. This anticipatory guidance can help the participants view the experience in a significantly healthier and more positive manner.

Male Puberty

In male puberty, testicular growth and development begin prior to penile growth. The mean age for the initiation of testicular growth is 11 years with about 4 years needed to attain full development (Kaplan & Love-Osborne, 2007). The left testicle hangs lower than the right once puberty begins. Penile growth begins around 12 years of age and takes about 3 years to complete. The release of sperm generally begins between 12 and 14 years of age. Erections occur more frequently and are common upon awakening. Preparing and reassuring the adolescent male of the normalcy of frequent erections and release of sperm during sleep (nocturnal emissions, or wet dreams) is an important health-promotion strategy.

NUTRITION

It is well recognized that an adolescent in the midst of a growth spurt needs adequate nutrition; however, adolescence tends to be the time when nutrition receives less than optimal attention. Skipping meals and snacking, as well as dining at fast-food restaurants, result in high intakes of calories and fat (Van Groningen, Barksdale, & McCarthy, 2010). Young adolescent boys and older adolescents in particular are more likely to eat fast foods and to drink nondiet sodas (Cutler, Flood, Hannan, & Neumark-Sztainer, 2009). Adolescents on average get 34% of their calories from fat and 53% from carbohydrates (Mandleco, 2004). Calcium, iron, and protein intake are frequently less than adequate to support growth in males

and females. National data shows that the highest prevalence rates of iron deficiency anemia are found in adolescent girls 12–19 years of age (Mandleco, 2004).

The home environment can be a positive influence on healthy eating behavior; however, the prevalence of eating out suggests that the influences of the family may be weakened. The school environment attempts to offer nutritionally adequate foods, but a large portion of adolescents choose nutritionally empty, high-calorie, high-fat foods from vending machines or fast-food sources. A primary prevention strategy is dietary modification for youths at risk of chronic diseases, such as coronary artery disease, before atherosclerotic lesions can cause irreparable damage. The need to promote the benefits of a low-fat eating pattern in youth has been supported by the finding of atherosclerotic occlusions on the aorta and right coronary arteries when adolescents who died in accidents were autopsied The most important health-promotion strategy for achieving adequate adolescent nutrition is educating adolescents and their families about the immediate effect of eating behaviors on health and their long-term effect on adult eating patterns. Lifestyle changes may be easier to make before life-long habits are established.

Both malnutrition and obesity are found in the adolescent age group. Malnutrition (an inadequate intake of calories) may be a result of lack of access to food due to poverty, a result of poor eating habits, or an effect of anorexia nervosa or bulimia nervosa or both (Dwyer, Stuart, & Hendricks, 2008)). **Anorexia nervosa** is an eating disorder in which the individual voluntarily refuses to eat because of an excessive concern over body shape or weight. **Bulimia nervosa** is related to anorexia and is characterized by binge eating followed by purging through self-induced vomiting, laxatives, diuretics, or excessive exercise. Both conditions result in inadequate nutritional support for the rapid physiological development of adolescence. The most prominent signs and symptoms of anorexia nervosa and bulimia nervosa are listed in Table 11-1. Disordered eating can be seen in both genders, across socioeconomic levels, and in most ethnic groups. There is an increasing incidence of very young girls with obsessive concern over dieting, fitness, weight

TABLE 11-1 Signs and Symptoms of Anorexia Nervosa and Bulimia Nervosa	
ANOREXIA NERVOSA	**BULIMIA NERVOSA**
1. Refusal to eat	1. Binge eating followed by purging
2. Plays with food and eats only very small amounts	2. Loss of tooth enamel, especially on posterior front teeth
3. Perceives body or body part as being fat even though thin	3. Calluses on dorsum of fingers or scars on dorsum of hand
4. Dry skin, fine downy body hair	4. Reddened knuckles
5. Absent menses	5. Enlarged parotid gland
6. Hypothermia, hypotension, bradycardia	6. Increased peristalsis, rectal bleeding, or constipation

© Cengage Learning 2013

BOX 11-2
MAJOR RISK FACTORS FOR EATING DISORDERS

Biological

- History of excessive dieting, skipped meals, compulsive exercise
- Obesity
- Depression
- History of obstetrical complications (maternal stress, prematurity, anoxia)
- Genetic family traits or characteristics
- Puberty
- Female gender

Psychological

- Body image distortion or dissatisfaction
- High level of concern with weight
- Low self-esteem
- Increased sensitivity to stress

- Personality traits such as perfectionism
- Physical or sexual abuse

Family

- Maternal history of eating disorder or obesity (younger adolescents)
- Parental attitudes, behaviors, or comments regarding appearance
- Affective illness or alcoholism in first-degree relatives

Sociocultural

- Participation in "visual sports" such as ballet, gymnastics, modeling
- Peer pressure
- Media influence: TV, magazines

Source: Based on White, J. H. (2001.) The prevention of eating disorders: A review of the research on risk factors with implications for practice. *Journal of Child and Adolescent Psychiatric Nursing, 13*(2), 76–88; Martinez-Gonzalez, M. A., et al. (2003). Parental factors, mass media influences, and the onset of eating disorders in a prospective population-based cohort. *Pediatrics, 111*(2), 315–321; Laird Birmingham, C., & Treasure, J. (2010). *Medical management of eating disorders*. New York: Cambridge University Press.

---

loss, and body image. A partial listing of risk factors for the development of eating disorders can be found in Box 11-2.

Even though the symptoms of eating disorders are physical, the cause is psychiatric, and treatment needs to be sought from a mental health practitioner. The longer the duration of the eating disorder, the harder it is to achieve recovery; therefore, patients need to be diagnosed early in the disease process (Rome & Blazar, 2008). Parents, educators, and coaches can help with early recognition of the first signs of disordered eating, such as a preference for eating alone, severe limitation in food choices, ritualized eating habits, excessive fluid intake, excessive chewing of ice or gum, or recent vegetarianism. Health care practitioners should screen for body image, changes in diet or dietary habits, and alterations of growth patterns (Rome & Blazar, 2008). A lack of treatment may result in numerous complications throughout the body, including death.

The incidence of obesity in adolescence has increased from 5% in the period 1976–1980 to 18.1% in the period 2007–2008 (Ogden & Carroll, 2010). This increase has been related to a decrease in physical activity coupled with the typical high-fat, high-carbohydrate diet consumed by youths. Eight out of ten obese adolescents continue to be obese in adulthood. The medical risks of adolescent obesity include hypertension, atherosclerosis, cerebrovascular accidents, gallbladder disease, degenerative arthritis, and adult onset diabetes, which has assumed dramatic increases in adolescents. Of equal importance are the psychosocial hazards. Obese adolescents may experience social discrimination, poor self-esteem, and depression (Cochran, 2008). Recommendations out of ProjectEAT, a large, population-based survey of eating and weight-related behaviors, include five strategies to prevent obesity and eating disorders in adolescents:

- Encouraging healthy eating and physical activity and discouraging unhealthy eating

- Encouraging families to focus on "doing" healthy eating and physical activity, rather than talking about weight
- Encouraging enjoyable healthy meals
- Promoting a healthy body image
- Assuming that adolescents have experienced mistreatment because of weight and addressing this possibility, both with adolescents and their families (Neumark-Sztainer, 2009)

ACTIVITY

The physical condition of adolescents is steadily declining. Today's children and adolescents are less fit and have a higher body fat percentage than their parents had, as determined through the measurement of body mass index (BMI) (American Heart Association, 2011). This may be the first generation whose life expectancy will be less than that of their parents. Obesity and physical activity are closely related. The rate of obesity is higher in rural areas, and the rate of participation in physical activity is substantially lower than in urban areas (Cochran, 2008).

The majority of actual physical activity for the adolescent centers around organized sports. Teenage boys and girls should be encouraged to participate in team-centered or individual physical activities or both to promote bone and muscle development as well as to enhance psychosocial development, self-esteem, and academic performance. Adolescent physical activity has many positive long-term effects, such as helping control weight, promoting psychological well-being, reducing depression and anxiety, decreasing the likelihood of using drugs or alcohol, and reducing the risk of smoking (Hales & Lauzon, 2010). In addition, regular physical activity reduces the risk of dying from cardiovascular disease and developing diabetes, hypertension, colon cancer, and osteoporosis. Health-promotion strategies should focus on improving opportunities for recreation and play and on promoting fitness through appropriate role models. It takes only moderate physical activity on a daily basis to produce the desired benefits and to establish a pattern for lifelong fitness.

SCREENING

Although screening is classified as secondary prevention, it is an important health-promotion strategy. Screening for the presence of disease or risk factors during adolescence may include assessment for signs and symptoms of hypertension, dental caries and periodontal disease, substance use, and sexually transmitted infections.

Blood Pressure

As blood pressure determination has become more routine in children, systemic hypertension has become more widely recognized in this age group. Blood pressure should be routinely measured at any office visit because hypertension is a known risk factor for heart disease. To obtain an accurate blood pressure reading, use the widest cuff that will fit between the axilla and the antecubital fossa. Using too large a cuff may decrease the readings by 5 mm Hg, while too small a cuff will increase readings by 10–50 mm Hg. Health-promotion for adolescents with hypertension starts with losing weight if obese, avoiding excessive salt intake, starting a regular exercise program, and avoiding cigarette smoking and oral contraceptives.

Dental Caries and Gum Disease

Although the addition of fluoride to municipal water supplies and the emphasis on daily toothbrushing have reduced the prevalence of **dental caries** (progressive decalcification of the enamel of a tooth), the majority of adolescents have at least one cavity in their permanent teeth by the age of 17. In addition, up to one-third have gum disease. Dietary habits may increase the incidence of cavities. Snacking, unbalanced diets with low levels of calcium, and high intake of carbonated beverages place the adolescent at risk for tooth decay. Carbonated beverages reduce the pH of the mouth to 2.5, a level conducive to tooth decay. In addition, hormones, orthodontic appliances, and the natural rebellion and desire for independence may contribute to poor adolescent oral hygiene. Oral screening should also include observation for malalignment, crowding of teeth, and mismatching upper and lower dental arches. Adolescents with any of these problems need a dental referral.

The oral health status of adults depends on their preventive care as adolescents. Daily flossing, brushing after meals, and maintaining a regular schedule for dental cleaning and

screening are all part of health-promotion activities for oral health. Peer pressure and the developmental focus of adolescents on appearance often provide the motivation for good oral hygiene. The minimum goal should be one thorough cleaning with brushing and flossing teeth before bedtime.

Substance Use

Screening for dental caries provides the nurse with an excellent opportunity to provide health-promotion counseling about the hazards of tobacco use. The average age at which smokers first try a cigarette is 15.08 years (National Cancer Institute, 2010). Eighty percent of all adult smokers started habitual tobacco use by age 18 [Centers for Disease Control and Prevention (CDC), 2010a]. Although the use of tobacco is declining, the 2009 Youth Risk Behavior Surveillance System (YRBSS) surveys of high school students conducted by the Centers for Disease Control and Prevention (CDC) found that 22.5% of White non-Hispanic students, 9.5% of Black students, and 18% of White Hispanic students report having smoked at least one out of the last 30 days (CDC, 2010b). The addictiveness of nicotine is considered comparable to that of heroin and alcohol (CDC, 2010a). Once an adolescent is a regular smoker, the effectiveness of recruitment and retention in a smoking cessation program is extremely low. Risk factors related to the initiation of tobacco use are found in Box 11-3.

Adolescents are knowledgeable about the long-term health problems of cardiovascular disease and lung cancer associated with tobacco use; however, this knowledge is not a sufficient deterrent to keep them from smoking. The most effective health-promotion strategy is to concentrate on broad strategies that target advertising and policy at the system level and the short-term effects of tobacco at the individual level. Emphasizing the detrimental cosmetic effects of yellowed teeth and bad

---

NURSING ALERT

The Effects of Nicotine and Caffeine on Blood Pressure

Adolescents should be questioned about tobacco use (including smokeless) or caffeine ingestion (coffee or cola products) prior to blood pressure measurement because these raise blood pressure. The blood pressure should be taken no sooner than 30 minutes after use or ingestion to obtain an accurate reading.

BOX 11-3
TOBACCO USE RISK FACTORS

Sociodemographic Factors
- Low socioeconomic status
- Early adolescence (11–15 years)
- Single-parent family

Environmental Factors
- Accessibility of tobacco
- Promotion of tobacco products
- Parental, sibling, and teacher use
- Peer use

Behavioral Factors
- Poor academic achievement
- Rebelliousness and impulsivity
- Use of other tobacco products
- Alcohol use

Personal Factors
- Perceived acceptability
- Perceived benefits
- Low self-esteem

RESEARCH NOTE

Contextual Factors and Smoking Behaviors in Adolescents

STUDY PROBLEM/PURPOSE

To measure the onset of the symptoms of nicotine symptoms in relation to cigarette smoking and to investigate a range of psychosocial, sociodemographic, contextual, and lifestyle-related influences on the initiation of smoking and the occurrence of nicotine dependence in adolescents.

METHOD

The sample included 877 students who were 12–13 years of age and who had never smoked at the time of initiation of the study. Baseline data included anthropometric measurements (height and weight) and a self-reported questionnaire that the students completed. The questionnaires were repeated every 3 months for a total of 5 years and 20 cycles. Follow-up anthropometric measures were completed in cycles 12 and 19. Students and school administrators in the 10 schools were asked to identify commercial outlets where students "hung out" within a 1-mile radius of the schools, and these were observed directly for access to tobacco products, tobacco promotions, and no smoking signs. School administrators completed self-report questionnaires regarding school policies and smoking.

FINDINGS

A number of factors were found to be significant in the initiation and maintenance of smoking behavior in adolescents in the study: younger age, poor academic performance, single-parent family, smoking by significant others (parents, siblings, peers, teachers), stress, impulsivity, susceptibility to tobacco advertisements (which were influenced by impulsivity and stress), use of alcohol and of other tobacco products, and lenient school policies related to smoking. Essentially, the study suggested that the determinants of smoking are multiple and diverse. The study also suggested that nicotine dependence led to increased smoking, rather than the reverse.

IMPLICATIONS

Prevention programs need to be directed toward social environments in the home and the school and are likely to be less successful if single factors in the initiation and maintenance of smoking are targeted. Broad strategies, such as public policy that bans advertisement of smoking, need to have priority.

Source: O'Loughlin, J., Karp, I., Koulis, T., Paradis, G., & DiFranz, J. (2009). Determinants of first puff and daily cigarette smoking in adolescents. *American Journal of Epidemiology, 170*, 585–597.

breath as well as the health effects of decreased stamina and athletic performance is an important health-promotion strategy to discourage tobacco use. Personal appearance is highly important in adolescence, and knowledge about long-term detrimental effects of smoking, such as facial wrinkles and nicotine-stained fingers, can also be a deterrent to smoking. In addition, adolescents with low self-image, poor social skills, or other risk-taking behaviors need skills to identify and resist the social influences to smoke.

The adolescent also should be asked about the use of smokeless tobacco products such as dip and chewing tobacco. Although the use of smokeless tobacco products has remained stable overall among adolescents during the 5-year period 2002–2007, the levels of current use among 12- to 17-year-old males has increased significantly from 3.4% to 4.4% (Substance Abuse and Mental Health Services Administration, 2009). Smokeless tobacco can be more addicting than cigarettes because nicotine is easily absorbed by the oral mucosa. The intensity of the withdrawal symptoms makes quitting difficult. Again, an emphasis on the cosmetic effects of bad breath, discoloration of teeth, dental caries, and gum recession is more effective than emphasis on the potential danger for the development of oral cancer.

There is an association between tobacco use and the use of alcohol and other drugs (O'Loughlin et al., 2009); therefore, screening for the use of other substances is essential. The pressure produced by the tremendous physical and emotional growth and development experienced by adolescents may cause them to experiment with substances that make them feel less insecure, more confident, or simply different. Substances may also be used to reduce the stress of transitioning through the developmental tasks of adolescence. Drinking is viewed as normal experimental behavior by society, but adolescents are at increased risk because of their limited experience with alcohol, their smaller body size, and the more rapid progression toward dependence. Experimentation may lead to **substance abuse**, frequently defined as the habitual use of alcohol or illegal substances such as marijuana, cocaine, methamphetamine, and numerous other substances. The 2009 added the use of prescription drugs to the survey for the first time, in recognition of the growing concern with the nonprescription use of drugs such as Oxycontin and Percocet by adolescents (CDC, 2010c). Box 11-4 illustrates the percentage of high school students who reported drug-related behaviors.

The pressures generated by the tremendous changes occurring during adolescence do not account for all adolescent substance abuse; therefore, to prevent substance abuse, the risk factors for it must be examined. The nurse who is aware of the influence of all these factors on the adolescent's potential for alcohol and substance abuse can assist the individual and the family in developing health-promotion strategies to reduce the potential. An individual adolescent's potential for alcohol or drug abuse is most likely influenced by genetic, familial, environmental, and/or developmental factors. Twin and sibling studies on alcoholism have revealed a genetic vulnerability in some individuals. The children of alcoholics have a 25% chance of becoming alcoholics themselves (American Academy of Child & Adolescent Psychiatry, 2002). There is also an increased vulnerability in individuals from dysfunctional families, especially if the parents are substance abusers themselves. These adolescents may have low self-esteem, decreased feelings of belonging, high levels of frustration and anger, and a reduced ability to negotiate the social environment. The school and peer environments form an important social environment for adolescents. Belonging to a

BOX 11-4

SUBSTANCE USE BY HIGH SCHOOL STUDENTS

SUBSTANCE USED	PERCENTAGE (%)
Tobacco	46.3 had ever smoked.
Alcohol	72.5 had ever used alcohol/24.5 had five or more drinks in a row within last 30 days.
Marijuana	36.8 had ever used marijuana.
Cocaine	2.8 had ever used any form.
Solvent use	11.7 had ever used solvents to get high.
Methamphetamine	4.1 had ever used methamphetamine.
Steroids	3.3 had taken steroids without a doctor's prescription.
Ecstasy	6.7 had ever used ecstasy.
Prescription abuse	20 had ever used Oxycontin, Percocet, Vicodin, Adderall, Ritalin, Xanax without a doctor's prescription.

Source: *2009 YRBSS* (Centers for Disease Control and Prevention, 2010c; 2010d).

substance-using peer group is one of the strongest predictors of substance use. The excessive use of alcohol usually starts in the home but may be reinforced by the peer group.

The use of alcohol, as well as other substance abuse, is widely advertised and frequently seen on television and in movies by adolescents. Advertising portrays alcohol use as sophisticated and a natural part of life, essential to social acceptance, and a reward after work, at a sporting event, or for relaxing. The risks of alcohol are minimized or totally omitted. The home is the primary source of alcohol for adolescents; however, parental attitudes and behaviors may vary drastically. Families who do not use alcohol or who do not drink excessively usually reinforce appropriate alcohol use. Families who accept and encourage excessive drinking or who have a history of antisocial behavior and poor parenting skills increase the risk of having children who use alcohol and other substances inappropriately. An assessment of the adolescent's genetic heritage, level of family support, educational environment, and freedom to experiment with new role development forms the basis for developing health-promotion strategies to prevent alcohol and substance abuse. Table 11-2 describes risk factors and prevention strategies for adolescent alcohol use.

Adolescents who do not abuse alcohol or other substances have been found to have social competence, problem-solving skills, autonomy, and a sense of purpose and future. Adolescents who are depressed or who have been physically or sexually abused may use alcohol or other substances to help cope with their psychological distress.

There is a relationship between substance abuse and sexual activity. Drugs and alcohol can lower an adolescent's inhibition against sexual activity, or sex can be a means to obtain drugs or alcohol. During 2009, 22% of adolescents reported having sexual intercourse in the past 3 months after drinking [Centers for Disease Control and Prevention (CDC), 2010e].

TABLE 11-2   Risk Factors and Prevention Strategies for Adolescent Alcohol Use

SOURCE	RISK FACTOR	PREVENTION STRATEGIES
Society/community	Acceptability of alcohol use behavior as portrayed through media. Availability of alcohol.	Reduce alcohol advertising and media portrayal of unacceptable alcohol use. Enforce minimum legal drinking age.
School	Decreased commitment and involvement in school. Presence of behavioral or attention problems or both.	Promote academic involvement and achievement. Refer students with problem behavior.
Family	Family role models; use of alcohol inappropriately. Poor family nurturing, communication, or both. Decreased familial interaction.	Family role models avoid inappropriate alcohol use. Parent communication and parenting training. Parent involvement in school and home activities.
Peers	Peers are alcohol users. Rejection by peers.	Monitor alcohol use by peers. Supervise recreational outlets.
Individual	Genetic susceptibility. Decreased social or problem-solving skills.	Teach about hereditary potential for susceptibility to alcoholism. Foster self-esteem and use of life skills.

BOX 11-5
GUIDELINES FOR EFFECTIVE CONDOM USE

- Handle condoms carefully to avoid damaging them with fingernails or sharp objects.
- Use a new condom in good condition for each act of intercourse.
- Check the expiration date on the package. Do not use condoms beyond the date of expiration.
- Place the condom on an erect penis before any intimate contact, and unroll it completely to the base.
- Leave a space at the tip of the condom and remove air pockets in the space.
- Ensure adequate lubrication during intercourse. Water-based lubricants (e.g., K-Y jelly, spermicidal foam or gel) should be used. Petroleum jelly, mineral oil, hand lotion, baby oil, cold cream, massage oil, and other oil-based lubricants should not be used because they may damage latex condoms.
- Hold the condom firmly against the base of penis during withdrawal, and withdraw while the penis is still erect so that the condom remains in place.

Sexually Transmitted Infections

The adolescent period is characterized by sexual curiosity, experimentation, and risk-taking behavior, increasing the adolescent's risk of exposure to sexually transmitted infections. Approximately 46% of high school students have engaged in sexual intercourse, with 14% reporting more than four sex partners (CDC, 2010e). Screening for sexually transmitted infections is a health-promotion strategy for all sexually active adolescents, especially those with a history of substance abuse.

Each year, there are approximately 19 million new sexually transmitted infections, and over half of these occur among 15- to 24-year-olds. Despite these statistics, 34% of adolescents in 2009 reported not using a condom during their last sexual intercourse (CDC, 2010e). In 2006, 1 million adolescents were reported as having chlamydia, gonorrhea, or syphillis, and 20,000 were living with HIV/AIDS (CDC, 2010e). Screening for sexually transmitted diseases is critical to prevent transmission and later problems with infertility and cancer.

Sexually active adolescents should receive complete information on their risk for acquiring sexually transmitted infections. Counseling about the effective measures to reduce risk includes abstaining from sexual activity, maintaining a mutually faithful monogamous relationship with an uninfected partner, using condoms regularly, and avoiding casual sexual contact with high-risk individuals. Guidelines for effective condom use are found in Box 11-5.

PSYCHOLOGICAL DOMAIN

The psychological domain for the adolescent includes both cognitive and emotional development. In addition to cognitive development, the concepts of invulnerability, body image, and moral development are discussed. Depression and suicide are discussed with emotional development.

Cognitive Development

According to Jean Piaget, as adolescents mature, they move beyond using concrete, actual experience as the only basis for their thought processes to using abstract, logical, and hypothetical processes (Brainerd, 1978). Cognitively mature adolescents are able to think in abstraction and demonstrate logical analyses. They are able to think about thinking, which enables them to become more introspective. This permits reflections on self, prior relationships, and future interactions. Adolescents spend a great deal of time contemplating the limitless variety of roles, situations, or both that might arise in their lives. Their world has numerous partly developed theories about themselves and life. Thoughts go beyond immediate situations and current interpersonal relationships to personally relevant future possibilities. Increased cognitive maturity enables the adolescent to think hypothetically and to anticipate the possible consequences of actions on such things as the selection of an occupation, a marriage partner, and future lifestyle. Health-promotion strategies promote this introspection, reflection, and projection.

Invulnerability

It has been hypothesized that younger adolescents exhibit a cognitive egocentrism characterized by an exaggerated sense of uniqueness (Elkind, 1967). This egocentrism is demonstrated by a belief in their invulnerability and lack of susceptibility to the natural laws that pertain to others. Elkind felt that this belief was one of the causes of adolescent risk-taking behaviors; however, studies have demonstrated that adolescents do not underestimate their vulnerability any more than adults (Millstein & Igra, 1995). The expectation that adolescents move toward adult decision making and self-determination may push the adolescent toward experimentation and risk taking as a means to accomplish autonomy and mastery. Other proposed reasons for adolescent risk-taking behaviors are curiosity, resentment of authority, anxiety, low self-esteem, and feelings of inadequacy or isolation. A health-promotion strategy is to determine the most likely etiology of a particular risk-taking behavior and the developmental processes that may be contributing factors before proposing solutions or behavior changes.

Body Image

The rapid changes in physical appearance occurring during the adolescent period cause adolescents to constantly evaluate and reevaluate their own bodies. They compare and contrast their bodies with those of their peers as well as some imaginary ideal. Judgments are influenced by reactions from others, their own level of self-esteem, and prevailing standards of attractiveness. Young adolescents are often self-critical. They believe that others are constantly evaluating them and are as critical of them as they are of themselves. The belief in an "imaginary audience" helps explain the adolescent self-consciousness, need for privacy, and fear of scrutiny. This egocentrism also helps explain the development of tight peer groups, which seek to diminish individual differences among themselves by promoting extreme conformity. Cognitive egocentrism is less evident as the adolescent undergoes advanced cognitive development.

Moral Development

The development of a sense of values and ethical behavior is a cognitive process that develops through maturation and changing social relationships. Lawrence Kohlberg, a psychologist, presented various ethical dilemmas to males of school age through young adulthood and then compiled their responses and the reasons for their choices. He found three distinct levels of moral development, each having two types of motivation, represented as stages. The levels were sequential and depended significantly on cognitive development; however, only a small percentage of individuals progress to the most mature stages (Kohlberg, 1981).

Working with Kohlberg was Carol Gilligan, whose research focused on moral development in females. She found a difference in responses provided by women, indicating that women approach moral dilemmas from a different perspective than men (Gilligan, 1982). Women define a moral problem in terms of relationships with others, emphasizing caring and concern, whereas men have a justice perspective, emphasizing the preservation of rules, rights, and principles.

Understanding the different levels of development as well as individual perspectives helps the nurse in planning health-promotion strategies reflective of individual differences. Parents can facilitate moral development by modeling altruistic and caring behavior toward others. Certain behaviors can help adolescents take the perspective of others, express themselves, ask questions, clarify their values, and evaluate their reasoning. Parents can identify issues involving fairness and morality and initiate conversations about concepts such as racism, sexism, homophobia, ageism, and biases against persons with disabilities Encouraging adolescents to volunteer in the community promotes a sense of purpose and meaning, and it enhances moral development.

Emotional Development

According to Erik Erikson (1950), the central developmental task of adolescence is to develop a sense of identity. Adolescent attempt to discover who they are. Adolescents must leave behind childhood beliefs and fantasies and assume the responsibilities and decision making of adulthood. To do so, they explore various roles and beliefs in an attempt to develop individual identities separate from the family. Adolescents have the task of integrating themselves into society by confronting the potential for role confusion in order to establish an equilibrium in which a firm identity is developed (Erikson, 1950).

Helping adolescents raise their self-esteem is a significant health-promotion strategy for parents and health professionals. Identifying specific areas that are important to adolescents and finding resources to enable them to succeed in those areas help improve self-concept, contributing to self-esteem. Providing support and encouragement to help an adolescent face a problem instead of avoiding it also enhances self-esteem.

Promoting emotional health must be considered a significant strategy in reducing morbidity and mortality in adolescents. Recent findings of the Mental Health Commission of Canada (2009) suggest that 70% of all mental illness in adults begins in childhood and adolescence. Problems range from behavioral disorders such as depression, eating disorders, and substance abuse to severe depression, suicide, and schizophrenia.

Depression

There is a relationship between adolescent depression and alcohol or substance abuse. The risk for substance abuse and

---

> **BOX 11-6**
> ### WARNING SIGNS FOR ADOLESCENT DEPRESSION
>
> - Noticeable sadness, hostility, or irritability
> - Decreased interest in or withdrawal from usual family, school, or peer activities
> - Changes in eating, sleeping, personal hygiene, or activity patterns
> - Decline in school performance or refusal to attend school
> - Drug and alcohol use

subsequent mental health problems increases with a family history of substance abuse, early initiation of substance use, and association with peer group users.

Fourteen percent of 13- to 18-year-olds have experienced a mood disorder in their lifetime, and 4.7% have been diagnosed with a severe disorder (Merikangas et al., 2010). Stress in relationships at school or home, decreased social support due to divorce or moving, and the presence of learning, conduct, or attention disorders place adolescents at risk for depression. Warning signs for adolescent depression and suicide are found in Box 11-6. The depressed adolescent may progress to thoughts or actions relating to suicide. Feelings of hopelessness and anger, social isolation, overt family conflict, and poor communication have also been associated with adolescent suicide.

Suicide

In 2007, suicide was the third leading cause of death for 15- to 24-year-olds, and adolescent males are five times more likely than adolescent females to commit suicide. Firearms, suffocation, and poisoning are the preferred methods for suicide in adolescents. The number of suicides for young adults (20- to 24-year-olds) is 12.7 per 100,000, which is higher than in the population overall [National Institute of Mental Health (NIMH), 2010]. Nonfatal attempts are often unreported. Risk factors for suicidal behaviors are found in Box 11-7. Depressed adolescents who are planning to commit suicide may write about suicide, talk about suicide or not being around much

---

> **BOX 11-7**
> ### RISK FACTORS FOR SUICIDAL BEHAVIOR
>
> - Gender: Males > females
> - Ethnicity: Whites > minorities
> - Exposure to suicidal behavior
> - Substance abuse
> - Depression
> - Disruptive behavior
> - Prior suicide attempt
> - Feelings of hopelessness
> - Sexual/physical abuse
> - Homosexual orientation

Source: Strof, B. S., & Velsor, F. B. (2006). Health promotion in adolescents: A review of Pender's Health Promotion Model. *Nursing Science Quarterly, 26,* 366–373.

HEALTH PROMOTION THEORY LINK

Pender's Health Promotion Model and Interpersonal Influences in Adolescence

Adolescents have unique needs in relation to health promotion that may not be fully addressed by existing theoretical models such as Pender's Health Promotion Model (HPM). The belief in being able to control events in one's life, or self-efficacy, is foundational to HPM and one of the strongest predictors of health-promoting behavior in adolescents in studies to date. Environmental influences such as peers and families may be a source of self-efficacy, particularly in adolescents, but they are not reflected in the HPM. Further research and development is needed to explore links between self-efficacy, commitment to action, and the influence of factors such as interpersonal relationships in the application of HPM to adolescent health.

longer, clean out their rooms or school lockers, give or throw away important possessions, become suddenly cheerful, or all of these. Families of depressed adolescents should be made aware of these warning signs.

Prevention strategies focus on programs to develop social skills, self-esteem, communication, problem solving, crisis/stress management, and anger control. This support should come from the family, the school, and the community. Positive communication and social support from the family encourages interaction between the parents and the adolescent. Parental involvement in the school provides a bridge of support between the two places adolescents spend the majority of their time. Communities that have useful roles for adolescents in providing community service reinforce the support provided by parents and schools, thus increasing adolescent self-efficacy.

SOCIAL DOMAIN

The adolescent is seen by much of society as a source of concern because of their rising rates of adolescent substance abuse, pregnancy, suicide, and violence. Many have blamed changes in the structure of families for the unhealthy and maladaptive functioning in troubled adolescents, and cite the lack of character development in adolescents who are deprived of the stabilizing influence of familial experiences.

Family

The major social role of the family of an adolescent is to provide support for the adolescent's search for identity and independence. As the adolescent begins to spend more time away from home with peers, the family may overreact by either imposing strict rules on the adolescent's behavior or by discarding

all rules. Neither of these options provides the support needed by adolescents as they strive to develop their own identity and independence. The health-promotion strategy to be recommended to the family is emotional support of the adolescent, accompanied by encouragement of the adolescent's movement toward autonomy. Regardless of the family form—single parent, shared custody, adoptive, traditional—adolescents need warm, involved adults who provide firm guidelines and limits, have appropriate developmental expectations, and encourage the development of individual beliefs. Using reasoning and persuasion, explaining rules, discussing issues, and listening respectfully are hallmarks of effective parenting practices.

Peers

The expanded peer life and increased social activities of adolescents enable their movement toward personal identity formation and autonomy. The intense relationships in peer groups facilitate this movement. By identifying with peers, adolescents are able to individuate from parents and family. Peers provide the bridge of support between being a child in the family and being an autonomous adult in society. Although the intense pressure to conform and suppress individual personality may result in risk-taking behavior, the maturing cognitive development allows adolescents to consider the consequences of possible actions. Peer influence tends to be strongest in issues such as dress, music, language, and sexual behavior, while parental influence is more notable in issues of underlying moral and social values. The types of peers with whom an adolescent affiliates is a stronger predictor of behavior than family, school, or community characteristics. Affiliating with deviant peers is associated with a growth in delinquent behavior such as drug use, high-risk sexual behavior, antisocial actions, and violent offenses (Urberg, Luo, Pilgrim, & Degirmencioglu, 2003).

The health-promotion strategy during this time is to assure parents that peer influence tends to concern external issues and be short-lived, while parental influence affects long-range goals, values, and attitudes. Parents should be cautioned that it is important to monitor and control with whom their adolescents affiliate. Parents can be reassured that peer influence is strongest during early adolescence. Not all peer influence is negative. Peers can influence positive, health-promoting behaviors through the peer education and counseling programs available in many communities. The relationship with peers offers an opportunity for acceptance and a feeling of belonging, for trying different roles and behaviors within the safety of the group, for observing role models and developing a sense of identity, and for integrating a new body image and self-concept.

Abuse

Infants and toddlers are the most common victims of abuse, with adolescents ranking second. **Abuse** is defined as physical, emotional, or sexual maltreatment. Although the exact numbers of adolescents who have been abused or neglected cannot be known, almost a million cases of abuse are substantiated or indicated annually.

The dynamics of families with adolescents may make the adolescents more vulnerable to maltreatment and make the parents more likely to abuse. A disequilibrium is created by the interaction of the adolescent's emerging physical, cognitive, emotional, and sexual potential with the midlife readjustments that parents face. Parents may feel threatened by the adolescent's ability to find flaws in the parents' reasoning, to retaliate or leave home, and to make autonomous relationships outside the family. Adolescent abuse also has been linked to multiple problems within the family, such as divorce and separation, financial stress, and overt conflict. Adolescents with developmental problems and decreased social competency are at increased risk for maltreatment.

Abuse may also take the form of **incest**, defined as sexual contact with the adolescent by any member of the family or household. Girls are at highest risk, but boys are also victimized. In addition to creating psychological difficulties for the adolescent in the area of sexuality, incest puts the adolescent at risk for pregnancy, sexually transmitted infections contracted during the relationship, or both. The prevalence of incest is underestimated due to underreporting. Adolescents may be in a state of denial or may have been threatened with severe consequences for reporting the abuse.

When there is abuse, intense family conflict, or identity problems, adolescents may decide to leave home. Runaway youths are adolescents under 18 years of age who leave home without permission and whose whereabouts are unknown. Walkaway youths leave home but their whereabouts are known. Thrownaway youths have been told to leave, have been abandoned, or have been runaways not allowed to return home. Homeless youths have no place for shelter and are in need of care, services, and supervision. Many runaway or homeless youths in shelters report being physically or sexually abused. Runaway or homeless adolescents have little or no economic support and are at high risk for further abuse, illness, unintended pregnancy, sexually transmitted diseases, substance abuse, and violence.

Health promotion for these adolescents includes both prevention strategies and identification of maltreatment. Mandatory child abuse and neglect reporting laws have been in effect since 1968. Teens should be encouraged to report abuse or incest. Health care providers need to be educated about the signs of abuse. Box 11-8 lists both the physical and the behavioral signs of abuse. Intervention and prevention strategies must focus on providing age-appropriate and culturally sensitive counseling for adolescents, providing family education and training programs, and promoting positive sociocultural

---

BOX 11-8
SIGNS OF ABUSE

Physical Signs

- Bruising
- Muscle or bone injury
- Recurrent abdominal pain
- Frequent urinary tract infections
- Sexually transmitted infection
- Pregnancy

Behavioral Signs

- Withdrawal, guilt, or depression
- Sleep disturbances
- Appetite disturbances
- School problems
- Substance abuse
- Promiscuity

---

values that make family violence unacceptable. In addition, programs providing street outreach, shelter, food, education and job training, substance abuse rehabilitation, and health care services need to be made available.

Culture

The primary cultural influence in adolescence is the culture of peers. Childhood ethnic and cultural influences are less obvious as the adolescent attempts to conform to the predominant adolescent culture. Conflicts may arise as adolescents try to look or act like the model being promoted in the latest media advertising campaign. When minority adolescents attempt to emulate the majority adolescent culture, the family may feel that the adolescents are rejecting their cultural heritage or values. The primary health-promotion strategy is to help parents recognize the limited influence that peer culture has on long-term adolescent values. Supporting adolescent efforts at conformity in external issues while recognizing personal identities enables the adolescent to move through this developmental stage more easily.

Political Domain

Legislation affecting adolescents primarily deals with minimum age requirements for assuming adult responsibilities such as driving, using alcohol and cigarettes, marrying, and purchasing firearms. This legislation reflects society's belief that adolescents lack experience, adequate perspective, and the judgment needed to recognize and avoid danger. Knowledge of the significant diversity in maturational level diversity among 16-year-old adolescents illustrates the need to deal with adolescents individually, especially in matters of health care.

Encouraged by the National Highway Traffic Safety Administration, licensing systems that prolong the learning process for young, novice drivers now exist in 38 states. Graduated driver's licensing eases younger drivers into driving through a phased approach. It sets a minimum age for a learner's permit, requires a licensed adult in the vehicle and certification of practice hours, restricts teenage passenger numbers, and restricts nighttime driving hours. Despite the initiation of these measures, the risk of motor vehicle accidents among 16- to 19-year-olds remains higher than for any other age group (CDC, 2010f).

The establishment of school-based clinics has brought health care to children and adolescents who did not typically have access to care. Approximately one in eight children under the age of 18 has no health insurance. Although school-based clinics were initially developed to prevent adolescent pregnancies, most have expanded their roles to include primary health care, referral, health and nutrition education, preventive care, and substance-abuse counseling. Parental consent for treatment is generally required; however, some clinics provide services to mature adolescents without parental consent. Some adolescents are economically and emotionally independent from their families and are recognized as so-called emancipated minors, fully authorized to take responsibility for many aspects of their lives.

Adolescents are more likely to seek services where they can be guaranteed confidentiality, especially for contraception and sexually transmitted disease treatment. Conservative groups fear that confidential services usurp parental authority and are currently seeking to require parental consent for all services. Although ideally all adolescents should have the type of relationship with their parents that promoted communication on all issues, the reality is that many would risk emotional or physical harm in seeking permission for contraceptive care, pregnancy determination or termination, and sexually transmitted disease treatment. So the primary health-promotion strategy is to encourage appropriate communication between parents and adolescents while keeping confidential health care services available.

ENVIRONMENTAL DOMAIN

Accidents and violence are two important environmental factors influencing the health of adolescents. An accident is an unforeseen or unplanned event or happening, leading to an unintentional injury. Violence, however, is intentional. Violence can be defined as behaviors that threaten to or attempt to inflict physical harm on others.

Accidents

Traumatic injury is a serious health concern for adolescents, with motor vehicle accidents being the leading cause of death in 16- to 20-year-olds. The risk for accidents is high due to the enormous changes adolescents are undergoing physically, cognitively, emotionally, and socially. The characteristics of adolescent development, such as challenging adult authority, desiring autonomy, experimenting in risky situations, seeking peer approval, and seeking to enhance self-esteem, all contribute to the numbers of adolescent injuries. In 2009, 3,000 adolescents were killed, and 350,000 were treated for injuries from motor vehicle accidents (CDC, 2010f). Driving habits and the tendency to take risks may be influenced by emotions, peer group pressure, and other stresses. Adolescents are more likely than adult drivers to report that they speed, run red lights, make illegal turns, and do not wear seat belts. In addition, they are less likely to recognize or to respond to hazards because of inexperience. When compared on a per-mile-driven basis with the general population, 16-year-old drivers are four times more likely to have an accident. Although nighttime driving is challenging for all age groups, adolescents have a disproportionately greater rate of nighttime accidents and fatalities. In 2008, half of the deaths among adolescents from motor vehicle accidents occurred in the evening and on Fridays, Saturdays, and Sundays (CDC, 2010f).

ASK YOURSELF

Morals, Ethics, and Legalities: A Nurse's Dilemma

What would you do if a 14-year-old girl came to you stating that she thinks she is pregnant and that the father is her mother's new husband?

The availability of alcohol and the legal ability to drive a car interact with the adolescent's developmental characteristics to produce one of the greatest hazards to adolescent health: motor vehicle–related injuries. Three out of 10 adolescents report having ridden in the past month with a driver who had been drinking, and one in 10 report drinking before driving (CDC, 2010f).

Approximately 2.3 million adolescents worked in 2008. Many adolescents seek part-time jobs to earn money and to gain experience. Approximately 139,000 of these young workers suffered work-related injuries in 2008, and 436 died of work-related injuries (U.S. Department of Labor, 2010). The reasons for these injuries include insufficient training; inexperience; dangerous and/or inappropriate jobs in high-risk areas such as restaurants, fast food, and construction; and lack of supervision. The primary health-promotion strategy is assuring appropriate education, training, and supervision for young workers. Education should include body mechanics, hazardous chemicals, and the proper use of equipment. Other leading causes of unintentional injury are drowning, firearms, poisoning, and burns. Table 11-3 discusses injury risks and strategies for prevention.

Violence

Violence is a major contributor to the deaths, disabilities, and injuries of adolescents. The 2009 National Youth Risk Behavior Survey (NYRBS) reports that 17.5% of grade-9 to grade-12 students had carried a gun at least once in the 30 days prior to the survey and that 5.6% had carried a gun on school property. Nearly 8% reported being threatened or injured with a weapon in the 12 months prior to the survey, and 31.5% had been involved in a physical fight within the previous 12 months (CDC, 2010d). In a large, cross-sectional study that involved the 2007 Minnesota Student Survey, results from the survey of 6th-, 9th-, and 12th-grade students suggested that 11.6% of the adolescents had witnessed physical violence, approximately 13.6% had been victims of physical violence in their homes, and 2.6% had experienced sexual abuse by a family member. Those who had experienced an adverse event were more likely to engage in delinquent behavior themselves, such as bullying, dating violence, physical fighting, and self-directed violence. The occurrence of more than one adverse event at home dramatically increased the likelihood that adolescents would themselves engage in abusive behavior (Duke, Pettingill, McMorris, & Borowsky, 2010). Other factors associated with the rising incidence of adolescent violence are media influence, drug and alcohol use, peer influence from gangs, the availability of firearms, family violence, and poverty.

Violence has moved into the schools. Incidents involving fights, guns, alcohol, vandalism, and sexual assaults are commonly reported. Minority rates of homicide, especially for Black males, are an important problem. Firearms are involved in the majority of homicidal deaths, which are characteristically intraracial and among acquaintances. Gun control has been proposed as a health-promotion strategy to prevent injury to adolescents; however, no specific data is available to support this strategy. Programs to deal with conflict may have a more immediate and far-reaching impact on adolescent health. Violence prevention must include cooperative programs involving schools, law enforcement, health care providers, parents, and adolescents themselves. Issues that should be considered include poverty, health care access, abuse, racial/ethnic inequities, gun availability, alcohol and other substance use, and the influence of the media.

SEXUAL DOMAIN

Although humans are sexual beings from birth, during the adolescent period, the individual develops a personal sexual identity. The accomplishment of a stable sexual role and self-image is a significant developmental task of adolescence.

TABLE 11-3 Environmental Safety for Adolescents and Young Adults

ACCIDENT	PREVENTION STRATEGIES
Motor vehicle injury	Never drive after drinking.
	Never ride with anyone who has been drinking.
	Always use seat belts, both in front and in back.
	Encourage loss of driving privileges for driving rule infractions.
	Avoid night driving for adolescents when possible.
Firearm injury	Never keep a loaded gun unsecured in the house.
	Require gun safety courses before gun use.
	Wear bright clothing when hunting.
	Avoid alcohol use when using firearms.
Poisoning	Identify problems with alcohol and substance abuse.
	Discard all prescription drugs not used during the illness.
	Check labels of over-the-counter medications for expiration dates.
Sports injury	Wear proper safety equipment: bike helmets, knee and elbow protectors, football helmets, and pads.
	Observe proper safety practices during training as well as during competition.
	Confine bike riding to approved bike lanes and trails.
	Warm up before vigorous exercise.
	Do not combine alcohol and sports activities.
Drowning	Avoid swimming alone.
	Use a personal flotation device while sailing.
	Require supervised experience and training for boat driving.
	Do not combine alcohol and water sports.
	Dive only where water has sufficient depth.
Burns	Install smoke detectors, and check them regularly.
	Never leave an iron unattended.
	Never leave a cigarette burning.
	Never smoke in bed or when sleepy.
	Check bathwater or shower temperature before entering.

© Cengage Learning 2013

During early adolescence, males, more than females, express their sexuality through masturbation. **Masturbation** is the self-manipulation of the genitals for the purpose of sexual pleasure. This activity in either gender is considered normal sexual behavior unless it becomes so time-consuming that it interferes with activities of daily living or is conducted publicly.

Sexual curiosity and experimentation characterize the adolescent period. Males are more sexually active than females, possibly due to the prominence of their sexual organs, which are more easily manipulated, the increased levels of sexual aggressiveness caused by testosterone levels, and the female focus on love and affection rather than on sexual gratification (Sahler & Kreipe, 1991). Information gathered about adolescent sexuality shows that slightly less than half of adolescents begin having sex in their mid- to late-teens. Forty-six percent of adolescents report ever having sex. Of those who are currently sexually active (34.2%), 61.1% report using a condom, and 22.9% reported that either they or their partners used the birth control pill to prevent pregnancy (CDC, 2010d).

Predictive factors for early sexual intercourse are early puberty, sexual abuse, poverty, poor parental support, the lack of school or career goals, and poor school performance [American Academy of Pediatrics (AAP), 2005]. The delayed initiation of sexual intercourse is associated with living in a stable two-parent home, religious involvement, and increased family income.

Sexual exploration among same-gender adolescents is common, perhaps because it is less threatening than heterosexual relationships. The health-promotion strategy is to acknowledge that this behavior is a common form of experimentation and not a definite homosexual orientation; however, sensitive and thorough discussion with the adolescent can help the adolescent analyze this behavior. Adolescents struggling with their sexual identity needs confirmation of personal worth and acceptance.

Many homosexuals first become aware of their sexual orientation during adolescence. **Homosexuality** is the sexual orientation of a person who is sexually attracted to persons of the same sex. Both males and females can be homosexual. Male homosexuals are sometimes designated as gay, whereas female homosexuals are designated as lesbian. Although the cause is unknown, homosexuality may be a result of a combination of genetic, physiological, and environmental factors. Gay and lesbian adolescents, like their heterosexual counterparts, have the same developmental tasks of establishing a sexual identity and deciding on sexual behaviors. Health promotion for homosexual adolescents includes care that is confidential, nonjudgmental, and without heterosexual bias. Regardless of sexual orientation, all adolescents need encouragement to practice abstinence, as well as information and anticipatory guidance about the seriousness of sexually transmitted infections.

Adolescent Pregnancy

The U.S. society has changed from agricultural and manufacturing occupations to occupations dependent on technology and education. This has extended the time required for the educational process and delayed the time when individuals become independent with adult responsibilities. Adolescents become sexually mature long before they are ready or able to assume the responsibilities of adulthood, leading to a significant increase in the percentage of sexually active adolescents. Despite the increased use of contraceptives, many adolescents have been sexually active for a year or more before seeking information or prescriptions for contraception. Fifty percent of adolescent pregnancies occur within the first 6 months of sexual intercourse (AAP, 2005). Early onset of sexual activity with subsequent pregnancies, abortions, childrearing, and parenting responsibilities, presents a significant and complex societal problem.

Pregnant adolescents have a higher incidence of medical complications for both mother and child than do adult women (AAP, 2005). In the adolescent population, the risk is greater for low infant birth weight, premature birth, increased infant and maternal death rates, pregnancy-induced hypertension, anemia, and sexually transmitted infections. Psychosocial complications include not completing school, increased levels of poverty, limited vocational opportunities, and repeat pregnancies.

Health-promotion strategies need to directly address the prevention of adolescent pregnancy. Abstinence counseling to postpone early sexual activity lays the foundation for pregnancy prevention. Accurate and comprehensive education about sexuality starts in childhood and continues during adolescence. Assuring access to contraception for sexually active adolescents is imperative. When prevention has not been successful, confidential access to abortion services or comprehensive pregnancy programs can assure improved outcomes.

SPIRITUAL DOMAIN

Adolescent psychological development forms the basis for addressing the spiritual domain. As adolescents strive to discover who they are and what their role is, they question every aspect of themselves and their world. They attempt to reconcile the values, roles, and responsibilities learned from parents with the world they observe. Feelings and emotions are frequently labile and unexplainable. Parents need reassurance that this time of conflict and rebellion is a necessary activity by which the adolescent searches for a personal identity and purpose in life. Group contact and interaction with peers from a church or synagogue provide support, influence, and affirmation for the adolescent, strengthening commitment to religious belief. For many adolescents, churches serve as both a spiritual resource and a source of social support.

Health-promotion strategies include frankly and accurately discussing the relationship between sexuality and religious beliefs; encouraging involvement with youth groups and activities that provide spiritual, social, and peer support; involving the whole family in religious activities and recreation; and providing a mechanism for communication and sharing within the family. The spiritual health and well-being of the family provides the support needed for adolescents to feel that they are able to explore and discover who they are and what their role in life will be. Adolescents whose families place importance on church or synagogue attendance and prayer are less likely to participate in substance abuse and risky sexual behaviors (Hendricks, 2005).

THE YOUNG ADULT

Individuals are considered to be in the young adult stage from about age 18 through ages 35. Many of the physical and emotional changes initiated during the adolescent years continue through the early years of the young adult stage. Knowledge of these changes continues to focus health-promotion and disease-prevention strategies. The biological, psychological, social, political, environmental, sexual, and spiritual domains are the guiding framework for the organization of these strategies.

BIOLOGICAL DOMAIN

Generally, physical growth is complete by age 20–25; therefore, health-promotion strategies in the biological domain continue to focus on building and maintaining the body's health through appropriate nutrition, exercise, and rest. Intervention for common health problems such as obesity and stress may be needed. Secondary prevention activities include screening for substance abuse, sexually transmitted infections, and malignancies.

Nutrition

The health of an individual is based on a balanced and nutritious diet. Young adults understand this concept; however, knowledge alone is unlikely to influence their nutritional habits. Food choice is shaped by ethnic heritage, financial status, religious beliefs, and personal likes and dislikes. Food preferences and behaviors are developed from childhood through adolescence, and, by the time individuals are young adults, these habits and preferences have become an integral part of their perception of themselves as sociocultural beings. Chapter 15 discusses the components of a balanced and nutritious diet in depth.

Approximately 28% of males and 36% of females 20–39 years old in the 2007–2008 National Health and Nutrition Examination Survey (NHANES) were considered to be overweight or obese (Flegal et al., 2010). The relationship between being overweight and developing adult onset diabetes, hypertension, and cardiac disease has been well documented. In addition, obesity has been associated with an increased risk of certain cancers, gallbladder diseases, sleep disorders, venous blood clots, and osteoarthritis. Quality-of-life issues affected by obesity are mobility and physical endurance, as well as social, academic, and vocational functioning.

The health-promotion strategy to promote the intake of a balanced and nutritious diet is to appeal to the young adult's sense of social approval and self-esteem. Dietary modification

SPOTLIGHT **ON**

To Eat or Not to Eat, That Is the Question

Every few weeks, newspapers and magazines publish articles about the benefits or dangers of different foods. What is the nurse's responsibility in relation to this dietary information and related concerns discussed in the media?

BOX 11-9
MALIGNANT MELANOMA SKIN LESION CHARACTERISTICS

- *Asymmetry*—One half does not match the other half.
- *Border irregularity*—The edges are ragged, notched, or blurred.
- *Color*—The pigmentation is not uniform and may have shades of tan, brown, and black.
- *Diameter*—It is larger than 6 mm or has a sudden or continuing increase in size.
- *Evolving*—Any change in size, shape, color, elevation, or another trait, or any new symptom such as bleeding, itching or crusting.

is the most commonly used weight-loss strategy. Dietary information should be provided that is ethnically and religiously sensitive, as well as relevant to individual lifestyle and financial status. Recommending routine physical activity has been shown to increase the long-term effects of weight loss.

Dietary calcium intake by many young women is less than recommended and required for building and maintaining bones. Reduced calcium intake may be a risk factor in bone mineral loss and the weakening of bones in later life. The primary health-promotion strategy for adolescents and young women is to encourage eating foods with a high calcium content and taking calcium supplements to obtain 1,200 to 1,500 mg per day. Common foods high in calcium include broccoli, cheese, milk, sardines, soybeans, spinach, and yogurt. Physical activity, the avoidance of smoking, and the reduction of caffeine and alcohol use also benefit bone health.

Exercise

Incorporating regular physical activity into daily routines is recommended to help prevent coronary heart disease, hypertension, obesity, and diabetes. In addition, physical activity has been associated with improvements in self-esteem, as noted in self-efficacy, self-acceptance, self-concept, and physical competence. Recommended types (aerobic or anaerobic) and levels of exercise are those that are necessary to maintain physical fitness. Chapter 16 discusses exercise in depth.

In counseling the young adult, focusing on the long-term benefits of exercise is less effective than emphasizing the shorter-term effects of feeling good, improving appearance, and increasing self-esteem. The young adult also needs to be counseled about the potential risks of injury from overly vigorous exercise. Young adults have attained their maximum physical and motor functioning and can sustain an overuse injury from trying to push themselves to further limits. The type of activities usually engaged in for regular exercise are running, fast walking, cycling, and swimming, each of which lends itself to the potential for injury. Counseling moderation in distance, intensity, and speed is an appropriate health-promotion strategy.

Skin Cancer Prevention

The use of sunscreen should be recommended for any activities that take place outdoors. Sunscreen guards against the most common forms of skin cancer, wrinkling, and painful sunburns. Most people do not use enough sunscreen. For complete coverage, an adult needs to apply approximately 1 oz of

lotion initially and reapply as sunscreen is sweated, rubbed, or washed off. It should be reapplied hourly while swimming. Even though the day may be cloudy, up to 80% of ultraviolet radiation penetrates cloud cover. Other protective recommendations include avoiding being in the sun between 10 a.m. and 4 p.m, wearing tightly woven clothing with long sleeves and pants, wearing a broad-brimmed hat, and staying in the shade whenever possible. To protect the eyes from sun damage, the recommendations include wearing sunglasses with labels indicating that they meet ANSI UV requirements. The use of tanning beds is not recommended because tanning lights give out both UVA and UVB rays (American Cancer Society, 2010).

Sunscreen may not be effective in preventing **melanoma**, a malignant skin lesion that develops from repeated exposure to the sun. Melanoma is the leading cause of death from skin disease (FDA, 2011). Box 11-9 describes skin lesion characteristics of a potential melanoma.

Rest

Many young adults do not get enough sleep. Causative factors include work schedules, erratic hours, and stress. Young adults may be less senior in their work environments and subject to being placed on a schedule that includes evening or night shifts or both. Or they may be working more than one job in order to make ends meet or to obtain a higher education. In addition, young adults may stay up later socializing or be awakened

❊ NURSING **ALERT**

Sunscreen and UV Protection

For the greatest protection from ultraviolet-type sunrays, recommend a sunscreen with an SPF (sun protection factor) of 30 or higher that contains titanium dioxide, zinc oxide, ecamzule, or avobenzone as protection against UVB and most UVA rays (American Cancer Society, 2010). A bottle or tube of sunscreen is effective for up to 2 to 3 years, and so the expiration date needs to be checked carefully. Any sunscreen with a foul odor should be discarded.

during the night by small children in the family. Health promotion involves recognizing sleep deprivation and encouraging rest during the day.

In addition to contributing to sleep deprivation, stress and anxiety can affect the overall health of young adults. Stress stimulates the fight-or-flight response of the body. Cardiovascular responses are seen in preparation for the violent muscular activity for which the body is being prepared. The sympathetic stimulation of the adrenal glands releases epinephrine into the bloodstream to decrease digestive processes and to shunt blood from the internal organs to the skeletal muscle. Epinephrine also increases the clotting tendency of blood.

At the same time, there is a release of adrenocorticotropic hormone, which causes the release of fatty acids in the blood, interferes with the action of insulin to increase blood sugar, and suppresses the immune system. The combination of these factors explains the problems that accompany prolonged stress: hypertension, blood clots, and decreased immune system response.

One health-promotion strategy for stress reduction is meditation. **Meditation** is the intentional focusing of attention on a singular activity, thought, or object such as one's own breathing, a visual image, a religious symbol, or a phrase repeated silently to oneself. The physiologic changes that occur during meditation include reductions in heart rate and blood pressure, decreased breathing rates with lowered oxygen consumption, and an increase in alpha brain waves (Roth & Creaser, 1997). **Alpha brain waves** are rhythmical waves associated with a quiet, resting state in the brain and body (Guyton & Hall, 2011). These body responses are the opposite of those generated by the fight-or-flight response initiated by stress. Studies of individuals who practice meditation have shown that these individuals react differently to stress (Kang, Choi, & Ryu, 2009). They have a greater anticipatory mental alertness and recover from the psychological and physical effects of stress more rapidly.

Screening

Screening for risk factors or the presence of disease continues to be an important health-promotion strategy during young adulthood. The nurse's screening for this age group primarily focuses on substance use, sexually transmitted infections, and malignancies. When risk factors are present, screening for anemia, diabetes, hypercholesterolemia, tuberculosis, and cardiac disease may be needed.

The cost of screening young adults is an issue. More than 13 million young adults lacked health insurance in 2010, a number that has been steadily increasing since 1999 (Martinez & Cohen, 2011). Many of the jobs available to younger workers are low wage or temporary and lack health benefits. Young adults from low-income families are especially likely to lack coverage, which has helped to make this age group the most likely of all to be uninsured (Martinez & Cohen, 2011).

Tobacco, alcohol, marijuana, and cocaine continue to be the primary substances abused by young adults. The nurse should take every opportunity to discuss tobacco-related diseases and recommend cessation of tobacco use when it is encountered. Young adults may have to be told several times how tobacco use is a major threat to health before they attempt to stop. Box 11-10 illustrates the National Cancer Institute's recommendations for promoting smoking cessation.

Youthful experimentation with alcohol and other drugs may progress to misuse, abuse, and dependence. Although

---

BOX 11-10

HOW TO HELP CLIENTS STOP SMOKING

- *Ask*—Ask about smoking at every visit: "Do you smoke?" "Are you still smoking?"
- *Advise*—Make a clear statement of advice: "As your nurse, I must advise you to stop smoking now."
- *Assist*—Set a specific date and provide information about smoking cessation for those interested. For those not interested, refrain from nagging.
- *Arrange*—Make a follow-up visit within the first two weeks after cessation.

---

alcohol users may have occasional episodes of misuse, 15–20% of drinkers progress to the abuse category, and a smaller percentage become physiologically dependent. Health-promotion strategies should focus on helping individuals who do not have significant problems to take an active role in assessing their substance use and the consequences of continuing their risky behaviors. Changing these behaviors even moderately can have a significant impact on the health of these individuals and of their families.

Using a model similar to the National Cancer Institute's smoking cessation program is helpful. After elucidating a health risk from alcohol use or drug use or both, the nurse should share concerns about the effects of these substances. Educating the individual about the adverse consequences related to use and discussing options for behavioral change help to engage the individual in the process. Arranging for follow-up visits and supportive reinforcement of the individual's efforts can help make change more successful. Individuals with serious problems need referral to an addiction specialist.

One in six people out of the 16.2% of the United States population aged 14–49 years of age are infected with genital HSV-2,. and 1 million infected with HIV (CDC, 2010h), screening for sexually transmitted infections is a key health-promotion strategy. Increased personal freedom and the drive to establish meaningful intimate relationships may make young adults vulnerable to sexually transmitted infections. In addition, substance use can promote unsafe sexual behaviors. Information obtained from the sexual history provides direction for health-promotion strategies and interventions specifically geared to the individual's personal risk behaviors. The nurse should elicit information regarding:

- The individual's sexual orientation.
- Whether the individual is sexually active in a mutually monogamous relationship or active with multiple partners.
- Whether the individual has recently changed or added partners.
- Whether the individual has ever had a sexually transmitted infection.

If risks are identified, the nurse should provide health education and prevention counseling to help individuals avoid acquiring sexually transmitted infections or to prevent complications and the spread of those already acquired. Screening should always

---

BOX 11-11

BREAST SELF-EXAMINATION (BSE) TECHNIQUES

Inspection

- Examine the breasts in front of a mirror, looking for noticeable differences in contour, nipple placement, or dimpling.
- Reexamine with hands on hips, arms raised over the head, and leaning forward.

Palpation in bath or shower

- Using the hand opposite the breast, palpate the entire breast with the flat pads of the first three fingers, using a circular motion.
- Repeat with the other breast.

Palpation lying down

- Raise one arm, and tuck it behind the head.
- Using the same technique as in the bath or shower, palpate the breast with the fingers of the opposite hand.
- Repeat with the other breast.

BOX 11-12

RISK FACTORS FOR BREAST CANCER

- Being female
- Increasing age
- Never having children or having a first child after 30 years of age
- First-degree relative with breast cancer
- Inherited BRCA1 and BRCA2 genes
- Early menarche
- Late menopause
- Being overweight or obese
- Alcohol consumption
- Recent use of hormone therapy
- Breast biopsies
- Radiation exposure to chest in childhood for treatment of another cancer

---

be considered for sexually active individuals with multiple sex partners, with a history of sexually transmitted infections, or with a sex partner who has multiple partners or a known sexually transmitted infection.

Screening for malignancies such as breast cancer, cervical cancer, and testicular cancer are important health-promotion strategies. Breast self-examination has been a popular, noninvasive technique that was considered effective in the early detection of breast cancer tumors. Recent studies have called into question the use of BSE, although organizations such as the American Cancer Society continue to recommend teaching young women its use (see Box 11-11). When discussing the use of BSE, young women should be counseled as to its benefits (e.g., noninvasive, can be effective in detecting some cancer, and increased awareness of breast changes) and harms (e.g., increased number of benign biopsies and increased health care costs) (Allen, Van Groningen, Barksdale, & McCarthy, 2010). For young adult women who choose to do BSE, teaching should include the importance of doing BSE one week after the first day of the menstrual period when breasts are less sensitive. Teaching regarding breast cancer may also include lifestyle choices that can reduce the risk of breast cancer, including maintaining a healthy weight, limiting alcohol consumption to one drink or less per day, and engaging in physical activity for 45–60 minutes at least 5 days a week (American Cancer Society, 2011). Factors for breast cancer are listed in Box 11-12.

In the **Papanicolaou (Pap) test**, cells are collected from areas that shed cells and are microscopically examined for early changes that may be related to the development of cancer. Use of the Pap test to screen for cancer in the cervical portion of the uterus has decreased deaths from cervical cancer by 70% since the test was developed in the 1940s. Pap smears for cervical cancer should be conducted for all women who are or have been sexually active or who have reached age 20. The American Cancer Society recommends screening every 1–3 years, depending on the results of previous smears. The most important health-promotion strategy to prevent cervical cancer is to educate young adult women on risk reduction for sexually transmitted infections. Risk factors for cervical cancer are listed in Box 11-13.

Although testicular cancer has a low incidence rate in the overall population, it is the most commonly occurring cancer in males between ages 15 and 35 (National Cancer Institute, 2011). Young adult men can increase their chances of finding testicular cancer early by performing monthly testicular self-examination (TSE). The best time to perform the exam is after a warm bath or shower when the heat has caused the scrotal skin to relax, making it easier to feel anything unusual on the testicle. TSE techniques are described in Box 11-14 and should be performed monthly. Young men should be instructed to look for changes in the testicles. The earliest signs of testicular cancer are pain, swelling, or hardness of the testicle. A painless

---

BOX 11-13

RISK FACTORS FOR CERVICAL CANCER

- Cigarette smoking
- Family history of cervical cancer
- First intercourse at an early age
- High fasting glucose levels (above 140 mg/DL)
- Infection with human papillomavirus (HPV) (primary risk factor)
- Long-term use of birth control
- Low socioeconomic status
- Multiple sexual partners
- Multiple pregnancies
- Sexually transmitted infections
- Weakened immune system
- Young age (17 years or younger) with first full-term pregnancy

BOX 11-14
TESTICULAR SELF-EXAMINATION

- Place the index and middle fingers underneath the testicle and the thumb on top.
- Gently roll the testicle between the thumb and fingers.
- Feel for any changes or abnormal lumps.
- Repeat with second testicle.

lump, usually about the size of a pea, may also be cancerous. Risk factors for testicular cancer are listed in Box 11-15.

PSYCHOLOGICAL DOMAIN

The psychological domain for the young adult includes both cognitive and emotional development. Closely tied to Piaget's theory of cognitive development are both moral and ego development. Kohlberg's and Gilligan's theories of moral development were discussed in the adolescent section of this chapter. Loevinger's ego development theory is considered in this section. Several psychosocial theories describe the emotional development of young adults. Along with Erikson's young adult stage of development, observations described by Levinson and Sheehy are discussed.

Cognitive Development

According to Jean Piaget, the cognitive transformation of young adults has progressed to the formal operations reasoning stage with the ability to consider multiple hypothetical possibilities of the consequences of actions (Brainerd, 1978); however, it has been found that some persons may never reach this higher stage of development. Some may use their formal operational abilities in certain aspects of their lives but use concrete operational thinking in other aspects.

Closely tied to cognitive development are moral and ego development. Jean Piaget emphasized that moral judgment was a developing cognitive process that was stimulated by social relationships. The development of moral judgment was discussed earlier in this chapter.

Ego Development Cognitive and moral development support ego development. Jane Loevinger's ego development theory is based on the theoretical constructs of Piaget's cognitive developmental theory, Kohlberg's moral development theory,

BOX 11-15
RISK FACTORS FOR TESTICULAR CANCER

- Undescended testicle
- Gonadal defect
- Genetic abnormality
- First-degree relative with testicular cancer
- History of testicular cancer
- Age (9 out 10 cases of testicular cancer arise in the 20–54 age group)

RESEARCH
NOTE

College Men's Knowledge, Attitudes, and Beliefs about Testicular Cancer

STUDY PROBLEM/PURPOSE

To examine male college students' knowledge of testicular cancer.

METHOD

The study, which is part of a larger study, involved six focus groups of 4–7 young male students (aged 18–25 years) at one university. The focus group sessions were conducted by one moderator, who used a series of open-ended questions related to risk factors, diagnosis/screening, treatment, beliefs about cure, psychological effects, and health education related to testicular cancer.

FINDINGS

Participants reported recognition of concepts related to testicular cancer, its treatment, and prevention, but they had very little knowledge and even less understanding of the concepts. The participants thought that information about testicular cancer would have more impact if it were focused on how testicular cancer affects them rather than on facts. The impact of awareness campaigns by celebrities such as Lance Armstrong and Tom Green was seen as having a larger impact than traditional health education programs.

IMPLICATIONS

Awareness of the disease is important before preventative practices can occur. Health education approaches should include simple, short, clear statements about how testicular cancer impacts the lives of young adult males rather than emphasizing facts. Further study is required to determine whether these findings can be generalized to a larger population of young adult males.

Source: Daley, C. H. (2007). College men's knowledge, attitudes, and beliefs about testicular cancer. *American Journal of Men's Health, 1*, 173–182.

and Sullivan's development of the self system. Ego development refers to the individual's integrative processes and overall orientation to family, friends, and the larger society. Although these stages are defined independently of age, individuals can be characterized through descriptions specific to each stage. The ego development theory represents the individual's movement across the domains of personal relationships, impulse control, moral development, and cognitive style. Table 11-4 summarizes the distinctive features of each stage.

Emotional Development

According to Erik Erikson (1950), the central developmental task of young adulthood is to develop intimacy. Young adults

TABLE 11-4 Ego Development: Stages and Individual Behaviors

Impulsive
- Self-centered, concrete thinking
- Self-control viewed as undesirable
- No consideration for intent

Self-protective
- Obedience to rules motivated by self-interest
- Morality governed by pragmatism
- Manipulative relationships
- Developing independence

Ritual
- Increased conventionalist tendencies in responses

Conformist
- Beginning recognition of social norms and needs
- Increase in feelings of morality, interpersonal reciprocity
- Concern with material things, conventional behavior, reputation, and status

Self-aware transition
- Growing awareness of relativism in situations
- Able to be self-critical and to understand motivation
- Freedom from peer pressure

Conscientious
- Interest in differences in individuals, relationships, ideals, achievement, and obligations

Individualistic transition
- Toleration of paradoxical relationships
- Concern for interpersonal relationships
- Growing recognition of emotional interdependence

Autonomous
- Ability to cope with inner conflict and conflicts experienced by others
- Concerned with self-fulfillment and individuality of self and others

Integrated
- Ability to reconcile conflicting demands and let go of the unattainable

© Cengage Learning 2013

seek to develop intense, lasting relationships with other individuals, thereby increasing their feelings of competency and self-esteem. The developmental task of achieving intimacy is accomplished when an individual can develop an open, supportive relationship with another without fear of losing his or her own individual identity. The capacity to openly share feelings and thoughts, to be empathetic, and to develop mutually dependent emotional ties characterizes an intimate relationship (Sigelman & Rider, 2005). This intimacy may be expressed in a sexual relationship, either heterosexual or homosexual. Without intimate relationships, young adults remain isolated and self-absorbed, often engaging in promiscuous sexual behavior without commitment or psychological security.

Another psychosocial development theory applicable to the young adult stage was developed by Daniel Levinson, who made a biographical, longitudinal study of a group of young men (Levinson et al., 1976). Based on the biographies of the subjects, Levinson proposed a life cycle structure with five eras: Preadulthood, Early Adulthood, Middle Adulthood, Late Adulthood, and Late Late Adulthood. Early Adulthood is divided into four periods. Table 11-5 describes the ages and developmental occurrences Levinson observed. The sequences described male development and may not be descriptive of female development.

One writer who looked at the psychosocial development of adulthood with close attention to the perceptions of both

TABLE 11-5 Early Adulthood Periods

PERIOD	AGE	CHARACTERISTIC	EVENTS
Early adult transition	18–23 years	Modification of relationships with family, peers, and other groups	High school graduation
			College entry
		Initial exploration and choices in adult world	Moving out of family home
Getting into the adult world	Early to late 20s	Exploration and provisional commitment to adult roles and responsibilities	Marriage
			Occupation choice
Age 30 transition	28–33 years	Modification of provisional life structure	Divorce
Settling down	Early 30s to late 30s	Deeper commitments to occupation, family	Occupational change
			Long-range plans for specific goals

Source: Based on Levinson, D. J., Darrow, C. M., Klein, C. B., Levinson, M. H., & McKee, B. (1976). Periods in the adult development of men: Ages 18–45. *Counseling Psychologist, 6,* 21–25.

TABLE 11-6 Crises of Young Adulthood

PERIOD	AGE	CHARACTERISTIC	EVENTS
Pulling up roots	18–20	Separate individual worldview from family worldview Locate self in peer group role, sex role, and worldview	College Military service Travel
The trying twenties	Early to late 20s	Prepare for life work Form capacity for intimacy Construct safe structure for future	Marriage Occupation choice Life pattern choice
Catch 30	Late 20s to early 30s	Outgrow career and personal choices made in the 20s Desire to expand personal and professional life	Divorce/marriage Occupation change Job change Childbirth
Rooting and extending	Early 30s	Increase order, rationality Reduce social life outside family Focus on raising children	Buy home Seek career advancement

Source: Sheey. G. (1974). *Passages: Predictable crises of adult life.* New York: Dutton

men and women was Gail Sheehy (1974). Using a similar qualitative research approach of collecting individual biographies, she compared the developmental rhythms of men and women, finding them to be similar, but lacking synchrony. Both genders experience predictable crises in adulthood. Table 11-6 lists these crises for young adults.

SOCIAL DOMAIN

Individuals become adults through socialization. The individual learns and adopts the norms, values, expectations, and social roles required by the individual's social group. This ongoing process is initiated in infancy and continues throughout adulthood. Changes in role, occupation, family structure, or habitation may necessitate resocialization. For young adults, the major social change is establishing a separate residence from the family of origin and achieving emotional autonomy. (Sigelman & Rider, 2005). Social interaction continues to include the family of origin and may include financial and emotional support; however, there is a restructuring toward a more equal relationship of one adult to another. An individual's transition from adolescence to young adulthood is facilitated by a family that is accepting, empathetic, and supportive.

Heterosexual relationships during this young adult period may result in marriage or cohabitation. The median age at first marriage is increasing and currently 26.1 years for women and 28.2 years for men (U.S. Census Bureau, 2010). The 2009 provisional data shows a marriage rate of 6.8 marriages per 1,000 population, which reflects a decrease from earlier in the same decade. The steady decline in the divorce rate from 4.0 per 1,000 in 2000 to 3.5 in 2009 (CDC, 2010h) parallels the increase in age at first marriage, suggesting that increased age at marriage may be related to marriage stability. The most important health-promotion strategy to help young adults be successful at marriage is to promote communication between the partners. Many adjustments must be made in a marriage (emotional, sexual, personal, financial, and social).

The degree of marital satisfaction that couples can achieve depends on communication about these tasks during courtship and continued communication following marriage (Sigelman & Rider, 2005).

Marriage has the advantage of recognized social stability where partners share economic resources and property; however, some young adults may decide to live together without marrying. **Cohabitation**, as reported by the U.S. Bureau of the Census, refers to two unrelated adults of the opposite sex living together without a binding social or institutional contract. In 2010, data from the Current Population Survey indicated that the percentage of adults who were married had declined from 57.3% in 2000 to 54.1% in 2010 (U.S. Census Bureau, 2010). The number of couples who were cohabiting rose to 7.5 million, representing a continuing increase since 1990 and a dramatic increases in the last decade (Kreider, 2010). Many couples may decide to live together to see whether they are compatible for marriage and to cope with unemployment and income-related issues. However, research studies have shown increased levels of physical aggression, lower-quality marriages, and higher rates of divorce after marriage among cohabiting couples, perhaps due to a lack of a feeling of permanence. One health-promotion strategy for couples contemplating cohabitation is to review studies and statistics comparing marriage to cohabitation. Enhancing communication between the partners is also important.

The desire for intimacy may also be expressed in a homosexual relationship. There are no definitive statistics on the prevalence of homosexuality. According to the *2006–2008 National Survey of Family Growth*, approximately 5.2% of males and 13% of females have had same-sex contact in their lifetimes (Chandra et al., 2011). When asked, "Do you think of yourself as heterosexual, homosexual, bisexual, or something else?" 95.7% of men 18–44 years of age responded that they think of themselves as heterosexual, 1.7% answered homosexual, 1.1% bisexual, 0.2% "something else," and 1.3% did not answer the question (Chandra et al., 2011).

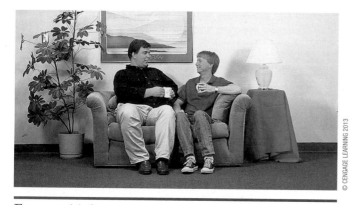

© CENGAGE LEARNING 2013

FIGURE 11-2 Families come in many shapes and configurations.

Societal attitudes of hostility, hatred, and isolation have created psychosocial difficulties for homosexual adolescents and young adults, leading to secrecy in relationships, a lack of opportunity for open socialization, and limited communication with healthy role models. Rejection or harassment by family, peers, or society has led to isolation, substance abuse, domestic violence, depression, and suicide.

Health-promotion strategies include finding ways to increase the comfort and confidence with which homosexual individuals can interact with health care providers. Essential to a healthy life for heterosexuals, as well as homosexuals, is the recognition of heterosexual bias (seeing the human experience in a strictly heterosexual context), homophobia (the irrational fear or hatred of homosexuality), stereotyping, stigmatizing, and social prejudice against homosexuals (see Figure 11-2.)

Intimate partner violence is a serious social problem affecting heterosexual and homosexual young adults. **Intimate partner violence** is a pattern of assault or coercion to force a partner to comply with the other partner's wishes. Abuse occurs across all cultures, all religions, and all socioeconomic groups; however, young women and those below the poverty line are disproportionately affected. Reliable reporting of abuse presents significant challenges because of the interpretation of terms and possible underreporting of incidents; in 2010, the National Intimate Sexual Violence Surveillance System began collecting data using standardized definitions and methodology (CDC, 2009). According to currently available data each year, nearly 5.3 million intimate partner victimizations occur among women age 18 and older, resulting in nearly 2 million injuries and 1,300 deaths (Rennison, 2003). Women experience over 10 times as many incidents of violence by an intimate partner as do men, accounting for 85–90% of partner abuse. Men are more likely to have been victimized by an acquaintance or a stranger rather than an intimate partner. Abusive relationships intensify during pregnancy, and violence escalates. Women assaulted during pregnancy are more likely to suffer miscarriage or deliver premature, low-birth-weight infants. Intimate partner violence occurs in both heterosexual and homosexual relationships. Violence within gay and lesbian relationships may go unreported for fear of harassment or ridicule.

For those who had experienced an incident, such as rape or physical assault, requiring treatment, most women reported that they were battered by their boyfriends or ex-boyfriends. Women reported being punched, kicked, and slapped; being hit with tools such as a hammer, nail gun, and crowbar; and being hit with household items such as pots, pans, dishes, a beer can, and a lamp. Jumping from a moving car, being choked, and

being burned with a cigarette caused other reported injuries. Knives and guns were also reported as weapons of injury.

Women with a history of intimate partner violence report higher rates of health problems such as sleeping disorders, arthritis, bowel problems, and mental health disorders than do women with no history of abuse (Wuest, 2010). Adolescents and young adult women who have been involved in intimate partner violence have been found to experience an increased incidence of eating disorders, substance abuse, suicidal ideation, and suicide attempts. Anxiety disorders are more commonly associated with young adult women who have been involved in these relationships than with adolescents. Intimate partner violence is particularly of concern among young adult women who are violent or who have recently given birth because a higher rate of partner violence is seen among these young women than among other groups involved in partner violence (Gee, 2006).

The most important health-promotion strategy to stop or prevent intimate partner violence is educating health care professionals to ask about and recognize signs of abusive relationships. Each encounter with an individual enables the health care provider to assess the type of relationship in which the individual is involved. Box 11-16 lists indications of chronic or acute abuse. Individuals tend to seek help several times before being able to leave an abusive situation. Support systems including health care providers, social services, law enforcement, and emergency shelters need to be in place. Intervening in a timely manner may prevent severe injury, even death. An abused individual returning to the same environment is only abused again.

POLITICAL DOMAIN

The young adult no longer is restricted by the minimum age requirements for adult activities. In fact, young adults, with the ability to vote in local, state, and national elections and to seek local, state, and national elected office, can be instrumental in determining which laws are passed and which are not. Young adults should be encouraged to be knowledgeable and to actively participate in the political system. They can seek

---

BOX 11-16

INDICATIONS OF INTIMATE PARTNER VIOLENCE

Physical indications

- Bruises on the face, head, breasts, abdomen, or genitals
- Bruises in various stages of healing
- Bite marks
- Repeatedly seeking medical attention for chronic, stress-related disorders

Subtle indications

- Delay seeking prenatal care
- Frequent missed appointments
- Unlikely explanations for bruising
- Overpossessive partner who does not allow the client to respond
- Belittling or oversolicitous partner

Source: Parker, V. F. (1995). Battered. *RN, 58*(1), 26–29.

RESEARCH
NOTE

Screening for Domestic Violence in Pregnant Women

STUDY PROBLEM/PURPOSE

To investigate relationships in perceived and self-reported parent aggression and the victimization and perpetuation of intimate partner violence among young adult children.

METHOD

A total of 200 undergraduate students from Midwestern University and 386 of their parents participated in a study. Students and their parents completed the Conflict Tactics Scale, which measures intimate violence violence victimization and parents' verbal aggression. Parents and students were cautioned not to discuss their individual responses with each other.

FINDINGS

Findings from the study supported relationships between parental aggression and victimization and perpetuation of intimate partner violence in young adult children. In particular, the behavior of the mother was found to be influential in sexual victimization and perpetuation among both sons and daughters.

IMPLICATION

Further study is recommended to differentiate the impact of parental violence on children, adolescents, and young adults. The results of this study suggest that the reports of young adult children correlate more strongly with parent reports than do those of adolescents and parents. The study suggests that interventions aimed at improving the communication efficacy of parents can reduce the risk of intimate partner violence among young adults and the resultant health problems.

Source: Palazzo, K. E., Roberto, A. J., & Babin, E. (2010). The relationship between parents' verbal aggression and young adult children's intimate partner violence victimization and perpetuation. *Health Communication, 25*, 357–364.

BOX 11-17
OCCUPATIONAL HAZARDS

Biological
- Bloodborne pathogens
- Infectious bacteria, mold, and fungi
- Contagious viruses
- Sanitation

Respiratory
- Indoor air quality
- Asbestos
- Tobacco smoke

Chemical
- Toxic substances
- Lead
- Machine fluids
- Pesticides

Physical
- Confined space
- Radiation
- Nonergonomic workstations
- Repetitive strain
- High noise levels

Safety
- Falls
- Machinery-related accidents
- Fire and explosions

Psychological
- Stress
- Harassment
- Workplace violence

Working conditions and environment are sources of hazards for both men and women; however, the safety and health standards and exposure limits are based on research with male populations and laboratory tests only. Some occupations, such as those in microelectronics, food production, teaching, office work, hospitals, banks, and domestic work, are predominantly female, exposing women to certain health disorders such as back injuries, repetitive strain injuries, reproductive hazards, and stress. Women are paid workers outside the home and unpaid workers at home, working an average of 1–3 hours per day longer than a man in the same society. Health problems arising from this situation include stress, chronic fatigue, and premature aging. Women also are more often victims of sexual harassment and discrimination in the workplace. To provide health-promotion strategies for young adults, the health care professional must be aware of occupational health hazards and potential gender differences.

SEXUAL DOMAIN

Young adults have accomplished the developmental task of establishing their sexual identity. They know whether they are heterosexual, homosexual, or somewhere along the continuum between the two. They may have selected life partners and be establishing their own homes and careers. The major health-promotion strategy in this domain is to help the young adult establish a healthy sexuality.

An assessment of sexuality should be included in the overall health assessment. Problems in sexual relationships for young adults frequently involve poor communication between partners. Facilitating communication between partners, teaching about sexuality, clarifying erroneous information, and providing frank, comprehensive information are health-promotion strategies to encourage sexual health.

Young adulthood is the time when many couples decide to raise a family. The tremendous economic, social, and emotional adjustments that accompany parenting responsibilities may affect a couple's sexual desire and responsiveness. Parents may have

out causes or political candidates that can make a difference in society and should be encouraged to devote time, energy, and effort to effect positive social change.

ENVIRONMENTAL DOMAIN

Accidents, especially motor vehicle accidents, are the primary cause of death among young adults. Firearms, poisoning, sports injury, drowning, and burns also contribute to accidental injuries in young adults. Table 11-3 presents accident prevention strategies applicable to the young adult population.

At least one-third of a young adult's time is spent on the job. Providing a thorough knowledge of the hazards associated with the individual's profession or occupation is the primary health-promotion strategy. Box 11-17 illustrates common occupational hazards.

less time and energy for promoting the marital relationship. Facilitating communication and encouraging couples to make time to be alone is an appropriate sexual health-promotion strategy.

A common health problem affecting sexuality as well as the overall quality of life is premenstrual syndrome. **Premenstrual syndrome (PMS)** is the cyclic recurrence of distressing physical, psychological, and/or behavioral changes related to the menstrual cycle. These changes may affect normal activities, relationships, or both. Eighty percent of women report some degree of PMS, with 10% having severe symptoms that significantly interfere with daily activities for 1–2 weeks each month (Dowd, 2005). Symptoms range from changes in mood, thinking, and eating behaviors to bloating, weight gain, headache, and breast tenderness. Researchers have investigated hormonal, nutritional, psychological, biochemical, and metabolic causes with no definitive answers found. Once diagnosis is made, PMS can be treated or controlled. Box 11-18 lists some of the treatments that have been successful.

SPIRITUAL DOMAIN

By the time adolescents reach young adulthood, they have established their own identity and are establishing an intimate relationship with another. They may also make a conscious commitment to their religious beliefs. They may struggle and question during the effort to test, learn, and make a decision about their commitment. As they continue to mature, they reexamine their purpose and focus in life, providing the opportunity to confirm their values, morals, and religious foundation. An appropriate health-promotion strategy is to encourage young adult participation in support, learning, fellowship, and

---

BOX 11-18

TREATMENT OF PREMENSTRUAL SYNDROME (PMS)

Changing diet
- Decreasing salt, caffeine, refined sugar, and fat
- Restricting alcohol and tobacco use

Changing activity
- Increasing anaerobic exercise such as walking, jogging, or swimming

Supplements
- Daily multivitamin tablet
- Evening primrose oil

Medication
- Oral contraceptives
- Diuretics

Counseling and support groups

---

spiritual-growth groups. Young adults also take on the responsibility for nurturing the spiritual development of their children. Providing a religious foundation that teaches the value of kindness, goodness, and faithfulness is a parental responsibility. Parents who do not have an active, faithful spiritual life will not be able to impart these values to their children.

SUMMARY

Health promotion in adolescents and young adults focuses on creating healthy lifestyle patterns. Individuals in the adolescent and young adult age groups are primarily healthy; therefore, the majority of health problems addressed in this chapter are potential problems.

Significant physical development, relational change, and emotional turmoil characterize the adolescent period. The potential hazards of adolescence transcend race, gender, and ethnicity; however, adolescents are pliable, adaptable, and responsive to challenge. Their ability to recover from periods of problem behaviors and emotional disorders enables them to mature into responsible and functional young adults. The opportunity to intervene and prevent lifelong health problems is greater and more effective in this age group than in any other. This chapter discussed a wide range of health-promotion and preventive care interventions for adolescents organized according to the biological, psychological, social, environmental, sexual, and spiritual domains.

Young adulthood is a period of stabilization in which individuals make career and relationship decisions that become the framework for the rest of their lives. Young adults develop a balance between autonomy and attachment, separateness and connectedness. Intimacy is expressed in sexual relationships and in the choice of a life partner. Health concerns are similar to those of the adolescent and middle-aged adult. Lifestyle decisions made during adolescence and young adulthood will determine the quality of life in later years. Health-promotion strategies were viewed through biological, psychological, social, political, environmental, sexual, and spiritual domains.

CASE STUDY

Lisa Flores: At Risk for Overweight and Constipation; Self-Concept Disturbance

OBJECTIVES/GOALS: Through participation in a discussion of this case study, participants will have the opportunity to:

1. Discuss the relationship between diet, exercise, and constipation.
2. Discuss the relationship between diet, exercise, and overweight.
3. Relate body image to maintenance of self-concept.

HEALTH-PROMOTION CONCERN, HISTORY AND PHYSICAL, PRESENT HEALTH STATUS, PAST HEALTH STATUS, FAMILY HISTORY, AND SOCIAL HISTORY

Lisa Flores is a 19-year-old Mexican American college student. She comes to the Student Health Center at the college complaining of abdominal pain. Her health in the past has been good with only minor illnesses such as colds and flu. She has no chronic illnesses, and her immunizations are all up-to-date. Her family history is positive for hypertension (maternal grandmother), coronary artery disease (paternal grandfather), and diabetes mellitus type 2 (paternal aunt). Lisa is single and is a freshman in college studying anthropology. She is currently living in a dormitory on campus and eats either in the cafeteria or at local fast-food vendors. She notes that she has gained 10 lb since coming to college.

She has one sister, 22 years old, and one brother, 15 years old. Both parents are living and well without chronic disease. She does not smoke, drink alcohol, or use street drugs. She uses no over-the-counter medications other than an occasional acetaminophen for headache.

REVIEW OF PERTINENT DOMAINS

Biological Domain

PHYSICAL EXAM: Reveals a well developed, well nourished young adult female, 64 in. tall, weighing 154 lb for a BMI of 26.4. No abnormal findings were found except for slight tenderness in the left lower quadrant of her abdomen and hard feces in the rectum on digital examination.

GASTROINTESTINAL: Reports that she used to have a soft, formed bowel movement daily but, since coming to college, has hard, dry bowel movements every 3–4 days. Her last bowel movement was 2 days ago. She does not use laxatives or enemas.

GENITOURINARY: No frequency, burning, urgency on urination. No vaginal itching, burning, or discharge. Her menstrual periods are approximately every 28 days, lasting 5–6 days, with no dysmenorrhea. Her last menstrual period was 2 weeks ago, and she is not sexually active.

24-HOUR DIET RECALL: Lisa skipped breakfast except for 4 oz of orange juice from the cafeteria. She had a 12-oz regular cola at midmorning, pepperoni pizza and a 10-oz glass of water for lunch, a 12-oz regular cola midafternoon, chicken-flavored ramen noodles for dinner, and a late-evening snack of potato chips and half a candy bar.

DIAGNOSTIC TESTING: Complete blood count (CBC) and urinalysis (UA) were in normal range.

Psychological Domain

COGNITIVE: Lisa has been making above-average grades in school. She appears to lack information about lifestyle changes that establish and promote consistent bowel habits. She also is unaware of the components of a balanced low-fat diet, daily exercise, and her body's daily calorie needs.

EMOTIONAL: Lisa is concerned about her body image since gaining extra weight. She says she feels stressed with studying and school activities.

Social Domain

Lisa has been declining invitations to go out socially because she feels unattractive. She stays in her dorm room most days.

Environmental Domain

Before starting college life, Lisa engaged in step aerobics three times weekly but says she does not have time anymore because she must study so much.

QUESTIONS FOR DISCUSSION

1. What is missing from Lisa's diet? How can daily bowel elimination be promoted? Are there any complications from chronic constipation?
2. What is the so-called Freshman Fifteen"? What should Lisa do to avoid becoming overweight?
3. What can be done to promote her self-concept?

KEY CONCEPTS

1. Education about the process and normal variations of attaining physical maturity is a key adolescent health-promotion strategy. Additional health promotion for adolescents and young adults in the biological domain includes strategies related to nutrition, activity/exercise, and rest.

2. Screening for actual or potential health problems in adolescents and young adults is vital for promoting the quality and quantity of life. Adolescent screening includes hypertension, dental disease, substance use, and sexually transmitted infections. Young adult screening focuses on substance use, sexually transmitted infections, and malignancies.

3. Promoting health in the psychological domain requires understanding normal cognitive and emotional development. Theoretical frameworks developed by Jean Piaget, Erik Erikson, Lawrence Kohlberg, Carol Gilligan, Daniel Levinson, Gail Sheehy, and Jane Loevinger provide a foundation for determining appropriate health-promotion strategies for adolescents and young adults. Depression and potential suicide are adolescent health problems that need careful attention and intervention. Developing the ability to make an intimate relationship during young adulthood is central to emotional security throughout life.

4. Health promotion in the social domain examines relationships with family and peers, as well as intimate relationships. Health problems related to abuse and intimate partner violence need significant attention.

5. Conservative political forces are attempting to prohibit adolescent access to confidential health care. Reduced access, especially for contraception and sexually transmitted infection treatment, has a far-reaching negative impact on adolescent health.

6. Accidents, especially motor vehicle accidents, are the leading cause of death for adolescents and young adults. Health promotion focuses on strategies that reduce or prevent accidents in these age groups.

7. The adolescent and young adult mature from a child to an individual capable of reproduction. Sexual health focuses on assisting individuals to develop a comprehensive, accurate knowledge of their own and others' sexuality, with relationships based on caring and responsibility between individuals.

8. Adolescents are capable of assuming responsibility for their own spiritual development. Young adults must assume responsibility for the spiritual development of their children.

CHAPTER REVIEW

Learning Activities

1. Describe environmental safety promotion strategies for adolescents and young adults.

2. Observe television news broadcasts for at least three evenings. List the types of crimes reportedly committed by adolescents or young adults or both, and compare these crimes with those committed by adults. Document your conclusions. With your classmates, discuss violence prevention measures for adolescents and young adults.

3. Design a presentation on skin cancer prevention for adolescents and young adults.

Multiple Choice

1. Environmental hazards for nurses in the workplace include:
   a. ergonomics.
   b. dementia.
   c. musculoskeletal injury.
   d. autonomy.

2. Breast development in male adolescents is called:
   a. gynecomastia.
   b. male puberty.
   c. menarche.
   d. asymmetry.

3. The most accurate blood pressure reading for an adolescent is obtained using a cuff that:
   a. is 4 in. wide or greater.
   b. fits the space between the axilla and the antecubital fossa.
   c. extends beyond the antecubital fossa.
   d. is no more than 2 in. wide.

4. The high rate of motor vehicle accidents in adolescence is related to adolescents':
   a. poor muscle development and motor coordination.
   b. short attention span and memory.
   c. risk taking and distractions.
   d. gender and socioeconomic status.

5. The type of rhythmic brain waves noted during a meditation session are:
   a. alpha waves.
   b. beta waves.
   c. gamma waves.
   d. delta waves.

6. Precancerous changes in the cells of the cervix are most likely to be caused by:
   a. early age onset of sexual intercourse.
   b. excessive douching.
   c. high-fat, high–caloric diet.
   d. sexually transmitted viral infection.

7. Which of the following groups would you target, in particular, for a health-promotion program related to fast food?
   a. Young adolescent girls
   b. Young adolescent boys
   c. Adolescents with a family history of eating disorders
   d. Urban adolescents

8. Which SPF would you recommend to an adolescent for adequate protection from the sun?
   a. 10
   b. 15
   c. 25
   d. 30

9. Current guidelines and opinions on breast self-examination (BSE) suggest that you would:
   a. recommend regular BSE to all adolescent girls from the age of 16 years and beyond.
   b. emphasize the need to show adolescent girls how to properly perform BSE.
   c. avoid discussing the use of BSE altogether with any age group.
   d. advise about the advantages and disadvantages of BSE during your teaching.

10. Meaghan, age 15, has numerous cysts, pustules, bumps, and scarring on her face and back. She washes her face faithfully twice a day and uses a commercial over-the-counter preparation with benoxyl perioxide. Despite her best efforts, her acne is getting worse. Your *best* approach would be to:
    a. reinforce the importance to Meaghan of maintaining her current routine.
    b. counsel Meaghan to avoid sunlight and chocolate.
    c. teach Meaghan which cosmetics cause breakouts and which do not.
    d. counsel Meaghan and her parents to seek treatment to prevent scarring.

ORGANIZATIONS AND WEBSITES

Centers for Disease Control and Prevention: Offers information related to physical activity and health from a report by the Surgeon General to the Centers for Disease Control and prevention, Division of the National Center for Chronic Disease Prevention and Health Promotion: **http://www.cdc.gov**

Division of Epidemiology and Community Health: Discusses the Center for Youth Health Promotion (CYHP) at the University of Minnesota that was designed to disseminate to schools and communities innovative youth health-promotion programs and materials created by the Division of Epidemiology of the School of Public Health: **http://www.epi.umn.edu**

Girls Health.gov Website: Developed by the Department of Health and Human Services' Office of Women's Health to respond to adolescent girls' health concerns; focuses on friends and family relationships, trust, sexuality, violence and abuse, peer pressure, and self-esteem; intended to motivate girls to choose healthy behaviors without the tediousness of a you-should-do-this message: **http://www.girlshealth.gov**

President's Council on Physical Fitness and Sports: Source for information on fitness and ways to motivate active lifestyles for better health through President's Challenge and program offerings: **http://www.fitness.gov**

Substance Abuse and Mental Health Services Administration with the United States Department of Health and Human Services: Focuses on cultural competence in serving children and adolescents with mental health problems in recognition that all cultures practice traditions that support and value their children and that prepare them for living in their society: **http://www.mentalhealth.samhsa.gov**

UCLA/RAND Center for Adolescent Health Promotion: A model for an academic-community partnership to improve adolescent health; funded by the Federal Centers for Disease Control and Prevention: **http://www.rand.org/health/centers/adolescent**

University of California Agriculture and Natural Resources: Has a nine-lesson educational intervention that uses computer technology to assist adolescents from low-income communities with diet assessment and "guided" goal setting for making healthy lifestyle choices; designed to be delivered by middle school teachers for skill building, social support, and goal attainment: **http://groups.ucanr.org**

World Health Organization: Provides information from the World Health Organization on the health, growth, and development of children from birth to 19 years of age throughout the world: **http://www.who.int**

REFERENCES

Allen, T. L., Van Groningen, B. J., Barksdale, D. J., & McCarthy, R. (2010). The breast self-examination controversy: What providers and partners should know. *Journal of Nurse Practitioners, 6,* 444–451.

Al-Sahab, B., Ardern, C. I., Hamadeh, M. J., & Tamim, H. (2010). Age at menarche in Canada: results from the National Longitudinal Study of Children and Youth. *BMC Public Health, 10,* 736.

American Academy of Child & Adolescent Psychiatry. (AACAP). (2002, November). Facts for families: Children of alcoholics. Retrieved from http://www.aacap.org/page.ww?name=Children+Of+Alcoholics&section=Facts+for+Families

American Academy of Pediatrics (AAP). (2005). Adolescent pregnancy—Current trends and issues: 2005. *Pediatrics, 116,* 281–286.

American Cancer Society. (2010). *Skin cancer: Prevention and early detection.* Retrieved from http://www.cancer.org/Cancer/CancerCauses/SunandUVExposure/SkinCancerPreventionandEarlyDetection/skin-cancer-prevention-and-early-detection-intro

American Cancer Society. (2011). Breast cancer: early detection. Retrieved from http://www.cancer.org/healthy/findcancerearly/cancerscreeningguidelines//american-cancer-society-guidelines-for-the-early-detection-of-cancer

American Heart Association. (2011). Overweight in children. Retrieved from http://www.heart.org/HEARTORG/GettingHealthy/overweight-in-children_UCM304054_Article.jsp.

Bowe, W., Smita, S. J., & Shalita, A. R. (2010). Diet and acne. *American Academy of Dermatology, 63,* 124–141.

Brainerd, C. (1978). *Piaget's theory of intelligence.* Englewood Cliffs, NJ: Prentice Hall.

Centers for Disease Control and Prevention (CDC). (2009). The National Intimate and Sexual Violence Surveillance System (NISVSS). Retrieved from http://www.cdc.gov/violenceprevention/nisvs/index.html

Centers for Disease Control and Prevention (CDC). (2010a). Vital signs: tobacco use: smoking. Retrieved from http://www.cdc.gov/vitalsigns/TobaccoUse/smoking/LatestFindings.html

Centers for Disease Control and Prevention (CDC). (2010b). Healthy youth! Tobacco use and the health of young people. Retrieved from http://www.cdc.gov/vitalsigns/TobaccoUse/smoking/LatestFindings.htm

Centers for Disease Control and Prevention (CDC). (2010c). CDC survey finds that 1 in 5 U.S. high school students have abused prescriptions. Retrieved from http://www.cdc.gov/HealthyYouth/yrbs/pdf/press_release_yrbs.pdf

Centers for Disease Control and Prevention. (CDC). (2010d). YRBSS 2009 National Youth Risk Behavior Survey overview. Retrieved from http://www.cdc.gov/HealthyYouth/yrbs/pdf/us_overview_yrbs.pdf

Centers for Disease Control and Prevention. (2010e). Healthy youth: sexual risk behaviours. Retrieved from http://www.cdc.gov/HealthyYouth/sexualbehaviors.

Centers for Disease Control and Prevention. (2010f). Teen drivers: fact sheet. Retrieved from http://www.cdc.gov/MotorVehicleSafety/Teen_Drivers/teendrivers_factsheet.html

Centers for Disease Control and Prevention (2010g). Genital herpes—CDC fact sheet. Retrieved from http://www.cdc.gov/MotorVehicleSafety/Teen_Drivers/teendrivers_factsheet.html

Centers for Disease Control and Prevention. (2010h). National marriage and divorce rates trends. Retrieved from http://www.cdc.gov/std/herpes/STDFact-herpes.htm

Chandra, A., Mosher, W. D., Copen, C., & Sionean, C. (2011). *National Health Statistics Reports: sexual behavior, sexual attraction, and sexual identity in the United States. Data from the 2006–2008 National Survey of Family Growth.* Retrieved from http://www.cdc.gov/nchs/data/nhsr/nhsr036.pdf

Cochran, J. (2008). Empowerment in childhood obesity and state of the science. *Online Journal of Rural Nursing and Health Care, 8*(1), 63–73.

Cutler, G. T., Flood, A., Hannan, P., & Neumark-Sztainer, D. (2009). Major patterns in dietary intake in adolescents and their stability over time. *The Journal of Nutrition, 139,* 323–328.

Daley, C. M. (2007). College men's knowledge, attitudes, and beliefs about testicular cancer. *American Journal of Men's Health, 1,* 173–182.

Dowd, S. (2005). Premenstrual dysphoric disorder: A clinical trial approach to assessment. *Advance for Nurse Practitioners, 13*(2), 57–59.

Duke, N. N., Pettingill, S. L., McMorris, B. J., & Borowski, I. (2010). Adolescent violence perpetuation: association with multiple types of diverse childhood experiences. *Pediatics, 125,* 778–786.

Dwyer, J., & Stuart, M. A., & Hendricks, K. M. (2008). Community nutrition and its impact on children: Industrialized countries. In C. Duggan, J. B. Watkins, & W. A. Walker (eds.), *Nutrition in Pediatrics: Basic Science, Clinical Applications.* Hamilton, ON: BC Decker, pp. 153–166.

Elkind, D. (1967). Egocentrism in adolescence. *Child Development, 38,* 1025–1034

Erikson, E. (1950). *Childhood and society.* New York, NY: Norton.

Flegal, K. M., Carroll, M. D., Ogden, C. L., & Curtin, L. R. (2010). Prevalence and trends in obesity among US adults 1999–2008. *Journal of the American Medical Association (JAMA), 303,* 235–241.

Food and Drug Administration (FDA). (2011). *FDA news release: FDA approves new treatment for a type of late-stage cancer.* Retrieved from http://www.fda.gov/newsevents/newsroom/pressannouncements/ucm1193237.htm

Gee, C. B. (2006). Abusive romantic relationships among adolescent and young adult mothers. Retrieved from http://crcw.princeton.edu/workingpapers/WP06-07-FF.pdf

Gilligan, C. (1982). *In a different voice: Psychological theory and women's development.* Cambridge: Harvard University Press.

Guyton, A., & Hall, J. (2011). *Textbook of medical physiology* (12th ed.). Philadelphia, PA: W. B. Saunder.

Hales, D., & Lauzon, L. (2010). *An invitation to health.* Toronto, ON: Nelson Education.

Hendricks, M. (2005). Risky business: Drug use, pregnancy, alcohol abuse, reckless driving. *Magazine of the Johns Hopkins Bloomberg School of Public Health Online Edition,* Spring.

Kang, Y. S., Choi, S. Y., & Ryu, E. (2009). The effectiveness of a stress coping program based on mindfulness meditation on the stress, anxiety, and depression experienced by nursing students in Korea. *Nursing Education Today, 29,* 538–543.

Kaplan, D. & Love-Osborne, K. (2007). Adolescence. In W. Hay, A. Hayward, M. Levin, & J. Sondheimer (eds.), *Current pediatric diagnosis and treatment* (18th ed.). New York, NY: Lange Medical Books/McGraw-Hill, pp. 102–143.

Kohlberg, L. (1981). *The philosophy of moral development* (Vol. 1). San Francisco, CA: Harper & Row.

Kreider, R. M. (2010). Increase in opposite sex cohabiting together in the annual social and economic supplement (ASEC) to the current population survey (CPS). Retrieved from http://www.census.gov/population/www/socdemo/Inc-Opp-sex-2009-to-2010.pdf

Kyle, T. (2008). *Essentials of pediatric nursing.* New York, NY: Wolters Kluwer/Lippincott Williams & Williams.

Laird Birmingham, C., & Treasure, J. (2010). *Medical management of eating disorders.* New York, NY: Cambridge University Press

Levinson, D. J., Darrow, C. M., Klein, C. B., Levinson, M. H., & McKee, B. (1976). Periods in the adult development of men: Ages 18–45. *The Counseling Psychologist, 6,* 21–25.

Mandleco, B. (2004). *Growth and development handbook: Newborn through adolescent.* Clifton Park, NY: Delmar Cengage Learning.

Martinez, M., & Cohen, R. (2011). Health insurance coverage: Early release of estimates from the national health interview survey January-eptember 2010. Retrieved from http://www.cdc.gov/nchs/data/nhis/earlyrelease/insur201106.htm

Martinez-Gonzalez, M., Gual, P., Lahortiga, F., Alonso, Y., de Irala-Estevez, J., & Cervera, S. (2003). Parental factors, mass media influences, and the onset of eating disorders in a prospective population-based cohort. *Pediatrics, 111*(2), 315–321.

Mental Health Commission of Canada. (2009). Toward recovery and well-being: a framework for a mental health strategy for Canada. Retrieved from http://www.mentalhealthcommission.ca

Merikangas, K. R., Burstein, M., Swanson, S. A., Avenevoli, S., Cui, L., Benjet, C., Georgiades, K., et al. (2010). Lifetime prevalence of mental disorders in U.S. adolescents: results from the National Comorbidity Study—Adolescent Supplement (NCS-A). *Journal of American Academy of Child and Adolescent Psychiatry, 49,* 980–989.

Millstein, S. G., & Igra, V. (1995). Theoretical models of adolescent risk-taking behavior. In J. L. Wallander & L. J. Siegel (eds.), *Adolescent health problems: Behavioral perspectives.* New York, NY: Guilford Press, pp. 52–71.

National Cancer Institute. (2011). Testicular cancer. Retrieved from http://www.cancer.gov/cancertopics/types/testicular

National Institute of Mental Health (NIMH). (2011). Suicide in the U.S.: statistics and prevention. Retrieved from www.nimh.nih.gov/health/publications/suicide-in-the-us-statistics-and-prevention/index.shtml

Neumark-Sztainer, D. (2009). Preventing obesity and eating disorders in adolescents: What can health providers do? *Journal of Adolescent Health, 44,* 206–213.

Ogden, C., & Carroll, M. (2010). NCHS health e-stat: prevalence of obesity among children and adolescents: United States trends 1963-1965 through 2007-2008. Retrieved from http://www.cdc.gov/nchs/data/hestat/obesity_child_07_08/obesity_child_07_08.htm

O'Loughlin, J., Karp, I, Paradis, G., & DiFranza, J. (2009). Determinants of first puff and daily cigarette smoking in adolescents. *American Journal of Epidemiology, 170,* 585–597.

Palazzo, K. E., Roberto, A. J., & Babin, E. (2010). The relationship between parents' verbal aggression and young adult children's intimate partner violence victimization and perpetuation. *Health Communication, 25,* 357–364.

Rennison, C. M. (2003). Intimate partner violence, 1993–2001. *Crime Date Brief.* Bureau of Justice Statistics. Retrieved from http://www.ojp.usdoj.gov/bjs/pub/pdf/ipv01.pdf

Rome, E. S., & Blazar, N. E. (2008). Adolescence: Healthy and disordered eating. In C, Duggan, J. B. Watkins, & W. A. Walker (eds.), *Nutrition in Pediatrics: Basic science, clinical applications.* Hamilton, ON: BC Decker, pp. 723–736

Roth, B., & Creaser, T. (1997). Mindfulness meditation-based stress reduction: Experience with a bilingual inner city program. *The Nurse Practitioner: The American Journal of Primary Health Care, 22,* 150–152.

Sahler, O. J., & Kreipe, R. E. (1991). Psychological development in normal adolescents. In W. R. Hendee (ed.). *The health of adolescents.* San Francisco: Jossey-Bass, pp. 55–88.

Sheehy, G. (1974). *Passages: Predictable crises of adult life.* New York, NY: Dutton.

Sigel, E. (2003). Eating disorders. In W. Hay, A. Hayward, M. Levin, & J. Sondheimer (eds.), *Current pediatric diagnosis and treatment* (16th ed.) New York, NY: Lange Medical Books/McGraw-Hill, 162–171.

Sigelman, C. K., & Rider, E. A. (2005). *Life-span human development* (5th ed.). Belmont, CA: Wadsworth Publishing Company.

Strof, B. S., & Velsor, F. B. (2006). Health promotion in adolescents: a review of Pender's Health Promotion Model. *Nursing Science Quarterly, 26,* 267–277.

Substance Abuse and Mental Health Services Administration. (SAMHSA). (2009). Levels of smokeless tobacco use increase among adolescent males. Retrieved from http://www.samhsa.gov/newsroom/advisories/0903041223.aspx

Thiboutet, D., Gollnick, H., Bettoli, V., Dreno, B., Kang, S., Leyden, J. J., et al. (2009). New insights into the management of acne: An update from the Global Alliance to improve outcomes in acne group. *Journal of the American Academy of Dermatologists, 60*(5), Supp11, S1–S50.

Urberg, L., Luo, Q, Pilgrim, C., & Degirmencioglu, S. (2003). A two-stage model of peer influence in adolescence substance use: Individual and relationship-specific differences in susceptibility to influence. *Addictive Behaviors, 28*(7), 1243–1256.

U.S. Census Bureau. (2010). Families and living arrangements. Retrieved from http://www.census.gov/population/www/socdemo/hh-fam.html

U.S. Department of Labor. (2010). Young workers. Retrieved from http://www.osha.gov/SLTC/teenworkers/index.html

Wuest, J. (2010). Health research: An exploratory study of the feasibility and efficacy of a primary health intervention for women in early years after leaving an abusive partner.

CHAPTER 12
The Middle-Aged Adult

Jeanette McNeill, DrPH, AOCNS, CNE, RN

KEY TERMS

andropause
chronic illnesses
climacteric
community-level interventions
genetics

genomics
menopause
outcomes
perimenopause
risk factors

sandwich generation
sensitivity of a
   screening test
specificity of a
   screening test

OBJECTIVES

Upon completion of this chapter, the reader should be able to:

- Describe the characteristics of middle adulthood that influence health-promotion activities.
- Discuss the function of health promotion for the middle adult in terms of improved physiological, psychological, sociological, spiritual, and sexual health.
- Identify genomic and environmental factors that influence health outcomes for the middle adult.
- Describe guidelines and prevention recommendations for healthy lifestyles for this age group.
- Examine nursing's role in the early detection (secondary prevention) activities based on recommended screening tests for middle adults based on age, gender, and risk status, including family history.
- Relate nursing theory to health promotion and health education activities of nurses.
- Explore health promotion for the middle adult as influenced by global health influences and practices.

INTRODUCTION

The middle adult years from 40 to 65 are usually characterized by relative stability in the job arena and increasing job-related responsibility. Middle adults reflect on their accomplishments, and consider the meaning of life. There is an increasing awareness of one's mortality, as many middle adults cope with the chronic illnesses and disabilities of their own or of parents, spouses or children.

Most in this age group demonstrate a heightened sense of caring, both for immediate family and for extended family and community. Members of this age group have been identified as the **sandwich generation**, the middle adult period in which individuals are sandwiched between their children who need nurturance and support and their aging parents, who also need care. As they are parenting teen and young adult children, they are also increasingly called on to care for their aging parents who are living longer. Health-promotion and health-maintenance activities are becoming increasingly critical for middle adults. This chapter addresses topics such as general wellness, exercise, the identification of personal risk factors including family history, and education regarding prevention and screening. The role of the nurse in promoting health in the middle-aged adult is presented. Primary prevention and screening (secondary prevention) recommendations specific for this age group are discussed. Primary prevention comprises activities taken to prevent illness or injury (e.g., immunizations), whereas secondary prevention refers to activities to detect illness at its earliest stages, when treatment can be most effectively begun and have the most beneficial effect.

IMPORTANCE OF HEALTH PROMOTION IN MIDDLE ADULTHOOD

The years between 40 and 65 are critical ones for health promotion. Actions taken during this life stage influence health in the older years when functional ability and quality of life are increasingly influenced by health status. Because of the developmental tasks of this age, the middle-aged adult is particularly receptive to the development of health-promotion lifestyles. Awareness of the aging process has begun, and middle adults are interested in keeping their health and maintaining functional status.

CURRENT PERSPECTIVE OF HEALTH PROMOTION IN MIDDLE-AGED ADULTS

Over the past few decades, great strides have been made in overall health for middle-aged adults. This age group formerly experienced a high rate of mortality and morbidity from heart disease and stroke, but rates continue to decrease due to early detection and treatment of cardiovascular disease. Changes in the ability to control high blood pressure, coupled with lower mean blood cholesterol levels and reduced rates of cigarette smoking, have largely been responsible for the 25% decrease in heart disease mortality rates (National Center for Health Statistics, 2011). Deaths from motor vehicle accidents, the highest death rate from nondisease causes, declined, a drop that is attributed predominantly to seat belt use and reduced rates of driving while intoxicated.

The shift in concern to preventing and reducing the impact of chronic illness is reflected in *Healthy People 2020*. Heart disease, stroke, cancer, and other **chronic illnesses** (a type of disease or disorder that limits activity for a prolonged period, such as chronic liver disease and cirrhosis) have emerged as leading causes of mortality. In fact, chronic diseases account for five of the six leading causes of death in the 45- to 64-year-old age group (National Center for Health Statistics, 2011). These trends are indicated in the objectives of *Healthy People 2020* that are focused on disease prevention by decreasing risk factors and increasing screening participation by those at high risk for development of chronic illness.

DEMOGRAPHICS OF MIDDLE ADULTHOOD

The 2010 Census report indicated that about 79 million people, or 26% of the population, were between the ages of 45 and 64. Projections are that this percentage will continue to increase because of the continued influx of baby boomers into middle adulthood (U.S. Census Bureau, 2009).

A corresponding increase in the numbers of persons living with chronic illness is also expected. The number of chronically ill persons, defined as noncommunicable illnesses of prolonged duration that are rarely cured, has been increasing each year and has affected 133 million Americans, nearly one in two adults (CDC, 2009). Over 75% of health care costs relate to chronic illness, and about one-fourth of those with chronic illness experience limitations in daily activities. The CDC launched an initiative specifically targeting heart disease, cancer, diabetes, arthritis, and obesity through the development of a National Center for Chronic Disease Prevention and Health-promotion. Three overarching goals are proposed: 1) to prevent, delay, detect, and control chronic diseases, 2) contribute to chronic disease research, and 3) achieve equity by eliminating racial and ethnic disparities (CDC, 2009). Costs of health care are influencing a shift in emphasis to prevention and early detection by some institutions, employers, and insurers in an attempt to maintain or reduce health care expenditures for the greater numbers of chronically ill middle and older adults.

MIDDLE ADULTHOOD: A TIME OF PLANNED CHANGE

Numerous changes in the physical, psychological, social, spiritual, environmental, political, and gender/sexual domains occur during middle adulthood. Some are common to most in this age group. Some are unique to the individual. Many are influenced by lifestyle and health-promotion efforts that have occurred during childhood, adolescence, and early adulthood. Many of the health outcomes of middle adulthood can be directly traced to health practices adopted in earlier developmental periods. However, health-promotion activities undertaken during this period can still reap benefits and are important to ensuring optimal functioning in late adulthood.

PHYSICAL DOMAIN

The middle adult enters the fourth decade usually in good health and in a highly efficient functional state (see Figure 12-1).

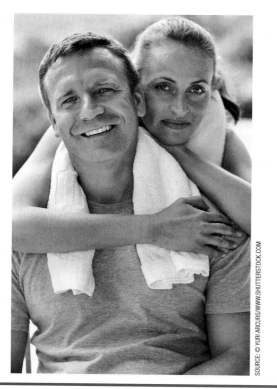

SOURCE: © YURI ARCURS/WWW.SHUTTERSTOCK.COM

FIGURE 12-1 Good health and the ability to enjoy physical activity accompany this couple into middle adulthood.

Although a number of physiological changes occur during this period, most are relatively gradual. General slowing of activity and metabolic rate results in the potential for weight gain and loss of muscle strength and elasticity. These factors predispose to muscle and joint stiffness and a tendency toward respiratory dysfunction. Reproductive changes are the most striking. This period is when perimenopause and menopause occur for women. For men, changes in sexual potency may occur, although reproductive potential for men continues into later years. The occurrence of chronic illnesses, of course, can influence this gradual pace of physical change and can profoundly affect psychosocial development, and affects an estimated 133 million Americans, nearly one in two adults (CDC, 2009). Table 12-1 depicts important physiological changes by body system.

FEMALE CLIMACTERIC

The female **climacteric**, or change of life, occurs gradually over years as ovarian function diminishes, resulting in permanent cessation of menses. Perimenopause and menopause are two stages leading to the female climacteric. **Perimenopause** is a time of transition that occurs gradually over 2–15 years as ovarian function gradually diminishes. During perimenopause, a woman may experience physical, psychological, and emotional changes related to decreasing levels of estrogen and progesterone.

The premenopausal stage, usually beginning around 40, is characterized by changes in the pattern of menstruation and heightened premenstrual syndrome symptoms. Between the ages of 45 and 55, 95% of women actually experience menopause.

The perimenopausal woman may experience hot flashes (flushes), palpitations, loss of muscle strength, increased facial hair, and various gynecological changes associated with decreased amounts of circulating estrogen. Emotional symptoms

such as nervousness, irritability, depression, or mood swings may also occur (Carroll, 2005). Although some women might experience adverse effects of perimenopause and menopause, others experience this passage with a sense of freedom, joy, confidence, and a greater wisdom of life and aging.

Menopause, or the cessation of menses, is considered complete after a year of amenorrhea. Menopause may be induced artificially from surgery such as oophorectomy (the surgical removal of the ovaries) or by other therapies causing sterility such as cancer chemotherapy. In some cases, hormone replacement therapy (HRT) can be helpful in alleviating symptoms. In other cases, such as some malignancies, this therapy may be contraindicated. Concern over the protective effects of estrogen for the skeletal system influences the decisions regarding HRT. Health care providers should discuss cardiovascular, osteoporosis, and cancer risks with women who are considering HRT, whether menopause occurred naturally or was surgically induced, so that an informed health-promotion decision can be made for each individual woman. In addition to HRT, other considerations for promoting a healthy life during perimenopause and menopause include healthy lifestyle changes, social support, and psychological support.

MALE CLIMACTERIC

This life change for men occurs at a much more gradual rate than for their female counterparts but begins in midlife. The time may be characterized by many of the same physical and emotional symptoms that women experience. Because many of the resulting symptoms parallel those of women during menopause, this time in a man's life has been termed the male climacteric, or **andropause**, reflective of the diminished levels of the androgen hormone, testosterone, in men. Loss of body hair, gradual weight gain, decreased strength, mood swings, irritability, decreased libido, and memory lapses may occur. By their mid-fifties, men begin to experience a decline in sexual function, but changes are gradual. For instance, the midlife male may notice he needs more stimulation to achieve an erection, needs more time between erections, and experiences a reduced force of ejaculation. Impotence during this period of life should always be completely assessed for physiological causes, such as diabetes, other chronic illness or treatment, and adverse effects of medications, particularly antihypertensives, as well as psychological causes. As with women, considerations for promoting a healthy life for men during this stage of life include healthy lifestyle changes along with social and psychological support.

PSYCHOLOGICAL DOMAIN

The dynamics of middle age are characterized by psychological changes as depicted in Table 12-2. According to Erikson's theory of human development, individuals in this stage of life are faced with the tasks of achieving generativity, or the passing on of their wisdom and experience to those in succeeding generations. The negative outcome of this stage is self-absorption. When middle life is a continued progression of increasing social influence and economic success, the task of generativity is more likely to be achieved, and the adult's self-concept and perception of fulfillment are enhanced. On the other hand, some may view this period as a time when opportunities become more limited or when the chance for achieving success or economic stability is reduced. Some may view midlife as a beginning of changes in health status and loss of earning power and influence in society.

TABLE 12-1 Body Changes in Middle Adulthood

BODY SYSTEM	PHYSIOLOGICAL CHANGE	IMPLICATIONS FOR HEALTH PROMOTION
Musculoskeletal	Decreasing bone mass in women Vertebral cartilage hardens Metatarsal spread Loss of muscle mass	Supplement calcium for women over 40. Take safety measures to prevent falls. Height decrease may be slowed by hormone replacement therapy. Wear properly fitting shoes. Maintain physical fitness.
Neurological	Presbyopia, a gradual decline in ability to focus on close objects Cataract development Presbycusis, progressive hearing loss caused by thickening of capillaries that supply inner ear	Have annual eye examinations. Avoid excessive noise. Have auditory examination if necessary.
Cardiovascular/ hematologic	Cholesterol and low-density lipoprotein (LDL) increases Blood pressure increases Varicosity development	Maintain physical fitness. Monitor cholesterol, LDL, triglycerides, BP for changes. Maintain regular exercise, use support stockings or socks, avoid dependent position of lower leg.
Respiratory	Less elasticity of lung tissue but no loss of functioning unless smoker, respiratory illness	Avoid tobacco use. Maintain physical fitness.
Integumentary	Loss of elasticity causing sagging and wrinkling Vitiligo and age spots May develop skin cancer Callus and corn formation Hair graying and hair loss	Maintain physical fitness and sound nutritional practices. Protect skin from sun with sunscreen and cover-ups. Participate in skin self-exam. Maintain positive body image.
Immunological	Slowed cellular repair and regeneration	Maintain physical and emotional well-being to avoid infection and injury.
Gastrointestinal	Periodontal disease, tartar build-up common Slowed GI motility and reduced hydrochloric acid and pepsin production Constipation, also hemorrhoid development Development of lactose intolerance	Have preventive and maintenance dental care. Balance diet and fluid needs; avoid troublesome foods. Exercise regularly.
Urinary	Gradual decline of glomerular filtration rate Decreased bladder tone Decreased sphincter tone, especially in females Prostate enlargement	Usually causes no dysfunction, may be important in chronic illness or diabetes. More frequent urination reduces problems. Monitor prostate size for problems with urinary retention; screen for malignancy.
Endocrine	Reduced thyroxine due to decreased metabolic rate Reduced pancreatic secretion of insulin	Monitor thyroid function, and note signs and symptoms of thyroid disease. Screen for non-insulin–dependent diabetes mellitus in high-risk persons or if symptoms occur.

(Continues)

TABLE 12-1 Body Changes in Middle Adulthood *(Continued)*

BODY SYSTEM	PHYSIOLOGICAL CHANGE	IMPLICATIONS FOR HEALTH PROMOTION
Reproductive	Diminished ovarian function leading to menopause	Maintain family planning mechanisms as desired by client.
	Increased risk of breast and other reproductive cancers increases	Participate in screening procedures and self-exams of breast and vulva.
	Diminished size and firmness of testes	Monitor perimenopausal symptoms, manage symptoms, do hormone replacement therapy for short-term symptom relief.
	Reduced testosterone production	
	Health states may affect erectile function and sex drive	Monitor symptoms; do physical and psychological workup for impotence to rule out treatable physical causes.

© Cengage Learning 2013

DEPRESSION

Depression has been associated with all age groups. Surveys conducted in the 1980s and 1990s showed the younger adult population to be at highest risk for depression, but an escalation of depression has recently been identified with middle-aged adults. In their lifetime, approximately half of Americans have a serious mental health condition; about 30% experience anxiety, and almost 20% experience a major depressive disorder (National Center for Health Statistics, 2010). Major depressive disorder (MDD), the most common type of major depression in adults, is characterized by one or more episodes that include the following symptoms: depressed mood, loss of interest or pleasure in activities, significant weight loss or gain, sleep disturbance, psychomotor agitation or retardation,

fatigue, feelings of worthlessness, loss of concentration, and recurrent thoughts of death or suicide (First, Frances, & Pincus, 2004). Minor depression, with fewer symptoms and less impairment, is not yet recognized as an official disorder, yet its occurrence can have negative consequences on health and well-being. The National Epidemiologic Survey of Alcoholism and Related Conditions (NESARC) (NIH, 2005), a longitudinal survey on the prevalence of psychiatric disorders among U.S. adults, reported the following findings:

1. Asian, Hispanic, and Black race/ethnicities have lower risk.
2. Women are twice as likely as men to experience MDD.
3. Women are somewhat more likely to receive treatment.

TABLE 12-2 Psychosocial Factors in Middle Adulthood

PSYCHOSOCIAL FACTORS	HEALTH-PROMOTION IMPLICATIONS
Family relationships	Social support can be a motivating factor for health promotion.
Spouses	Stress in family relationships can cause physical and emotional consequences; health-promotion activities, particularly exercise, can be an outlet for stress.
Children	
Aging parents	Demands of caregiving must be balanced with middle adults' own needs.
Extended family	
Career	Advise middle adults about the importance of balance in life between work and leisure activities.
Career changes	
Retraining/education	The perceived need to retrain to increase job security can be a real source of stress.
Responsibility for others	The perceived success as a mentor can be an important source of emotional satisfaction and contribute to self-esteem.
Hobbies and use of leisure time	Hobbies and recreational activities provide balance with work and career.
	Counsel regarding the safety implications of recreational activities is important.
	Include assessment for alcohol and recreational drug use by middle-aged clients.
Values clarification	Assist the middle adult in examining values, mortality issues, evidence of experiencing midlife crisis, and vulnerability to depression.
Facing one's mortality	
Midlife crisis	Assess for signs of depression, and counsel regarding resources available. Counsel regarding the importance of having a living will, advance directives, or both.
Planning for retirement	

© Cengage Learning 2013

4. There is a lag time of about 3 years between onset and treatment.

5. Of all persons who experienced MDD, age 18 and older, nearly one-half wanted to die, one-third considered suicide, and 9% reported a suicide attempt.

6. Among those with current MDD, 14% also have an alcohol use disorder, 5% have a drug use disorder, and 26% have nicotine dependence.

7. More than 37% have a personality disorder, and more than 36% have at least one anxiety disorder (Columbia University's Mailman School of Public Health, 2005).

Another study examined racial/ethnic differences in significant depressive symptoms among middle-aged women before and after adjustment for socioeconomic, health-related, and psychosocial characteristics (Bromberger, Harlow, & Avis, 2004). Using the Center for Epidemiologic Studies Depression [CES-D] Scale, it was found that, contrary to the NESARC report, Hispanic and African American women had the highest odds, and Chinese and Japanese women had the lowest odds for depression. It was noted that the variation was most likely due to health-related and psychosocial factors that are linked to socioeconomic status.

The effect of depression on function and health of 7,000 preretirement adults at peak earnings potential was the focus of another study (Crown, 2005). It was found that persons with depression were more likely to live alone; report chronic conditions (particularly cancer and lung disease), disabilities, or functional limitations; and have fewer economic resources in terms of income or wealth, or greater reliance on government health insurance such as Medicaid, compared with those who were not depressed. It was concluded that, compared to non-depressed peers, adults suffering from depression experience an increased burden of health needs caused by the effects from depression.

Undoubtedly, both major and minor depression are associated with significant disability in physical, social, and role functioning during middle adulthood.

SOCIOLOGICAL DOMAIN

Many of the changes of middle adulthood have to do with role transitions regarding family responsibilities. As children grow into adulthood, they establish independence from their parents, as the middle adult's aging parents become more dependent. Another prominent area of potential role alteration is that of job and career-related change. For many in this period, job security and feelings of accomplishment continue, with the middle adult moving into a mentorship role with younger colleagues. However, in times of economic constraints, downsizing, and technological progress, individuals in this age group may feel insecure in their career paths. They may pursue career change or cross-training opportunities to increase their options. As work is an extremely important part of life for most middle adults, threats to job security result in stress, the effects of which ripple into other aspects of life. Relationships with others are often affected.

A new trend that affects men and women in the middle adult years is the increasing number of grandparents raising grandchildren, due to death, disease, or inability of the parent. This shift in responsibility for child rearing may occur for the usual reasons but has been shown to be increasingly due to situations involving the death of the parent due to violence, substance use, or AIDS.

Another trend caused by rising divorce and remarriage rates is that middle adults are merging with or raising second families or both. Women over 40 years of age comprise a small but significant group of obstetrical clients whose age has classified them as advanced maternal age. Risks of fetal abnormality, particularly genetic deficits, are thought to increase significantly with age. For women in this age group, special counseling and monitoring are needed in the event of planned or unplanned pregnancy. The trend toward childbearing and child rearing in the 40s and beyond is particularly true for men, whose fertility does not diminish in midlife but may continue into older adulthood.

ENVIRONMENTAL DOMAIN

The environment is a crucial factor in health status and health promotion. Many characteristics of the environment contribute to or detract from health, such as air and water pollution, noise, toxic substance exposure, high-stress work situations, economic constraints, and the like. Tobacco use is the single greatest cause of chronic illness, death, and disability in the United States (National Center for Health Statistics, 2010). Although there has been a decline in cigarette smoking in the United States to a current level of about 25% of the population, certain subgroups continue to smoke and use chewing tobacco. The prevalence of tobacco use is inversely related to education and socioeconomic status. See Chapter 18 for further information regarding tobacco and other substance use.

Mortality and morbidity are significantly increased for smokers. Death and disease from tobacco use are seen primarily in the middle and later adult years because of the lag time for the manifestation of harmful effects on the respiratory and cardiovascular systems. Many conditions, including cancer (particularly of the respiratory tract), cardiovascular disease, gastric ulcer, postmenopausal osteoporosis, and low birth weight in offspring of pregnant smokers, are firmly associated with smoking. Each of these conditions is potentially seen in the middle adult. Further, secondhand smoke has been documented to have important health consequences such as chronic lung disease, coronary artery disease in spouses of smokers, and asthma and respiratory infections in children of smokers.

Another important aspect of the environment is the microenvironment consisting of the relationship of humans to certain bacterial or viral organisms. Some communicable diseases have become increasingly significant threats to health due to world travel and increased population concentrations in urban areas. The emergence of resistant strains of organisms compounds the treatment and eradication of some diseases

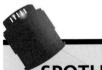

SPOTLIGHT ON

Grandparent Parenting

The American Association of Retired Persons (AARP) has recognized this growing phenomenon by establishing a hotline for assistance to the group of midlife and older individuals who are primary caregivers for a grandchild (www.aarp.org).

such as influenza. Screening for communicable disease is an important function in promoting health, yet economics or policy changes in some areas of the United States and the world can have profound effects on adequate detection of communicable disease.

SEXUAL/GENDER DOMAIN

Despite the physiological changes that occur in middle adulthood, the individual in this age group usually continues to be sexually active and may engage in high-risk sexual practices that could result in the risk for sexually transmitted diseases and acquired immunodeficiency syndrome (AIDS). For this reason, individuals seeking treatment for sexually transmitted diseases (STDs) should also be screened for HIV status using the enzyme immunoassay and confirmed if positive with the western blot. Also in need of HIV screening would be individuals who are past or present injection drug users, persons who exchange sex for money or drugs, sexual partners of HIV-infected persons, injection drug users, or bisexual men, and those who received transfusions between 1978 and 1985 (U.S. Department of Health and Human Services, 2010).

Screening for sexually transmitted diseases such as chlamydia, gonorrhea, and syphilis should be performed on all sexually active women at high risk, which would include those with a history of previous STDs, those with new or multiple sex partners (more than 2 in 6 months), or those who indicate inconsistent use of safe sex practices. A pelvic examination with an endocervical specimen culture for the selected infections should be performed. Pregnant women should also be screened.

Some conditions, such as anemia, are particularly significant in the middle adult years. This is particularly true for females and for members of certain cultural groups, including Blacks or African Americans and those of Mediterranean descent. All menstruating females should receive a determination of hemoglobin and hematocrit levels and more extensive testing if indicated (U.S. Preventive Services Task Force, 2005). Middle-aged males and postmenopausal females need to receive a nutritional assessment and diet analysis as discussed in Chapter 15.

SPIRITUAL DOMAIN

Spiritual health is the integration of each person's mind, body, and soul or inner spirit to form a harmonious whole. Additionally, beliefs of the individual that subscribe to organized religious faiths are important in health maintenance and health promotion. At times, religious beliefs and practices may be contrary to "scientific" medicine. The middle adult and older adult may differ from the child or young adult in their willingness to diversify into prevailing cultural or spiritual norms, preferring instead to retain their individual spiritual or cultural practices. Members of various groups hold certain religious beliefs that may preclude medical practices, such as the use of blood transfusions in a member of the Jehovah's Witnesses. Many middle adults find that spirituality becomes even more important in their lives during this period.

CULTURALLY COMPETENT CARE

Health-promotion attitudes and behavior are influenced by culture. Cultural considerations were discussed in more depth in Chapter 6, but implications for middle adults are briefly discussed here as well. Developing cultural competence to effectively work within the cultural context of a community is crucial to nursing interaction with the multicultural populations that are characteristic of health care settings. In consideration of the general developmental tasks of this age group, concern with family issues and work issues within the context of the culture of the client are important. Does the individual value the well-being of the family or the individual more highly? Are there practices that are dictated by the cultural or ethnic group, such as the avoidance of certain activities, that middle adults will feel they must adhere to despite health advice to the contrary? For example, a 55-year-old Asian woman may be advised and taught to perform breast self-examination as part of her breast health practice. For some Asian subgroups, touching oneself, even for a health-related purpose, is considered inappropriate. An important variable in health-promotion activities and education regarding health promotion with multicultural groups is language. Health professionals need to obtain or consider developing materials in the target language to ensure relevance to the culture and beliefs. The avoidance of stereotyping and generalizing regarding an individual member of an ethnic group is essential to comprehensive assessment and culturally sensitive intervention (Barr & Wanat, 2005; Office of Minority Health, 2011).

GUIDELINES FOR HEALTH PROMOTION AND SCREENING

Within the past few years, national initiatives have taken place for the purpose of highlighting the health-promotion needs of the United States. *Healthy People 2010* was the second of these and represents the results of intense national study. Objectives for the desired health outcomes and health services needed for each population group were outlined. Reduced morbidity, or the effects of disease, from identified chronic illnesses is expected to result from selected preventive and screening activities.

Many publications are helpful in planning health-promotion and screening activities for middle adults. The U.S. Preventive Services Task Force *Guide to Clinical Preventive Services*, first published in 1996, assists clinicians in planning evidence-based preventive and screening services, such as tests, and counseling in risk reduction. The guide, available online, is regularly updated and continues to support the following actions by clinicians in every client encounter (U.S. Preventive Services Task Force, 2010).

- Assess the client's personal health practices.
- Foster shared decision making between clinician and client.
- Use diagnostic and screening services selectively.
- Provide preventive services at every opportunity, particularly for those limited access to health care.

Additionally, the Task Force suggests supporting **community-level interventions** (activities that occur at the community level to promote health or to reduce illness or injury, such as fluoridation of the water supply), rather than just individual efforts for certain health problems, when the comm-level interventsions are effective.

The *Guide to Preventive Services* helps the nurse and other health care providers use a scientific basis for screening and for counseling regarding risk modification. Table 12-3 provides suggested health-promotion actions from these sources that specifically apply to risks in middle adults.

TABLE 12-3 Risk Assessment for the Middle-Aged Adult

RELATED DOMAIN	RISK ASSESSMENT	HEALTH-PROMOTION ACTION
Physical	Nutrition	Assess nutrition status and diet.
		Daily intake should include 25 g of fiber; 30% of total calories from fat; 5–6 servings of vegetables and fruits; 6–11 servings of whole grains, breads, and pasta; limited consumption (2–3 servings) of red meat, poultry, eggs, and dairy products.
Physical	Exercise	Encourage aerobic activity of at least 10 minutes per episode, spread throughout the week resulting in a minimum of 2 hours and 30 minutes (150 minutes) moderate intensity or 1 hour and 15 minutes (75 minutes) vigorous-intensity physical activity.
		Additional health benefits result accrue from 300 minutes of moderate intensity of 150 minutes of vigorous intensity activity spread throughout the week.
		Muscle strengthening activities should be engaged in at least twice/week with attention to safety measures and general health maintenance
Physical Psychological	Tobacco avoidance	Consistently assess regarding tobacco use and interest in cessation, and, if applicable, provide tobacco cessation counseling on a regular basis.
		Advise the use of pharmacological as well as behavioral interventions for smoking cessation.
Physical Environmental Psychological	Accident prevention	Counseling regarding safety for parents of children, for adolescents, and for adults should be provided. Assess individuals for high risk regarding alcohol and substance use.
Physical	Immunizations	Counsel regarding obtaining and maintaining immunizations, including boosters for tetanus and diphtheria. The primary series should be completed for those who have not completed it. Hepatitis A, B, and influenza immunizations should be obtained, as well as pneumococcal vaccination for persons over 65 years of age or those over 50 living in institutional settings.
		Herpes zoster vaccination is recommended in individuals over 60.
Physical Psychosocial	Family history Genetic counseling	The nurse should work with the individual middle adult to complete a 3-generation family history.
		If appropriate, explore the need for further genetic testing or further counseling, regarding genetic/genomic health issues.
Physical Psychological Sociological	Addictive behavior	Assess for signs and symptoms of substance use.
		Advise as to the adverse health consequences associated with alcohol and drug use.
		Monitor through follow-up for problems with alcohol and drug use.
Psychological Sociological Spiritual Physical	Mental health	Assess for positive development and successful passage through the middle years. Screen for depression or counsel regarding stress management, strategies for stress reduction, and resources for assistance with psychosocial issues.
Sociological Environmental	Workplace exposures and injury	Assess for workplace risk factors for injury and exposures to substances, e.g., carcinogens such as benzene, excessive noise.
Physical Environmental	Dental care	Advise regular annual dental care with daily flossing and brushing with fluoridated toothpaste.
Sexual/gender Sociological	Sexuality and family planning	Provide counseling about risk factors for HIV and other STDs and measures to reduce risk.
		Provide information regarding safe sex practice.
		Specifically counsel individuals identified to be injection drug users regarding HIV and STD risk and refer to appropriate treatment facilities.
		Offer testing to individuals at risk for specific STDs.
		Immunize for hepatitis B.
		Provide periodic counseling about effective contraceptive methods.

STRATEGIES FOR ACHIEVING LIFESTYLES THAT PROMOTE HEALTH

Middle-aged adults are becoming increasingly conscious of health and health-promotion issues. Whether they are caregivers for their aging, chronically ill parents, affected by health problems or deaths of family members and friends, or experiencing personal health problem, awareness of the aging process is occurring. Individuals in this age group are usually interested in maintaining health and functional status at optimal levels. Many persons have engaged in certain risk behaviors during their younger years. **Risk factors**, or characteristics associated with increased likelihood of disease or injury, for one condition contribute to the occurrence of other conditions; for example, smokers at risk for lung cancer are also at risk for chronic pulmonary disease. For the middle adult age group, injury, substance abuse, and individual and family violence are important sources of health problems. Middle adults continue to engage in risk behaviors such as tobacco and alcohol use, unprotected sexual activity, lack of seat belt use, and poor nutrition. Primary prevention activities are important because healthier lifestyle changes begun in this period have positive influences on functional ability in later years.

EXERCISE AND NUTRITION

The balance between nutrition and exercise to promote health, maintain cardiovascular fitness, and prevent obesity has been well documented. The U.S. Surgeon General has put forth a vision for a Healthy and Fit Nation to combat the epidemic of overweight and obesity (HHS, 2008). Nutrition is a key element in a healthy lifestyle and is further discussed in Chapter 16. The companion component is exercise, which is further discussed in Chapter 16. A sedentary lifestyle is common in the United Status. Although some improvement in the proportion of men and women who met 2008 guidelines for activity increased in the period 1999–2009, the overall level is below 20% of the adult population (National Health Statistics, 2010). Sedentary lifestyle and concomitant obesity have been linked to cardiovascular disease, cancer, diabetes, and other chronic illnesses. Figure 12-2 illustrates the dramatic increase in overweight and obesity reported in the United States between 1985 and 2009. In the last 20 years, a dramatic rise in obesity and overweight has occurred; in 2009, only the state of Colorado and the District of Columbia noted less than a 20% prevalence of obesity (CDC, 2010). Nine states had a prevalence equal to or greater than 30%: Alabama, Arkansas, Kentucky, Louisiana, Mississippi, Missouri, Oklahoma, Tennessee, and West Virginia (2010).

Thee documented benefits of a regular exercise program include reducing the risks not only of cardiovascular disease and cancer but also of non-insulin-dependent diabetes mellitus, osteoporosis, and mental health disorders. Cardiovascular disease risk could be reduced significantly even in sedentary persons by initiating an exercise program. That the immune system benefits from a regular exercise program has also been suggested. Current guidelines for exercise for adults are suggested per week, with intervals of aerobic activity spread across the time period, and muscle strengthening exercise occurring at least twice per week (Health and Human Services, 2011). Table 12-4 presents selected *HP 2020* objectives related to nutrition, weight, and exercise.

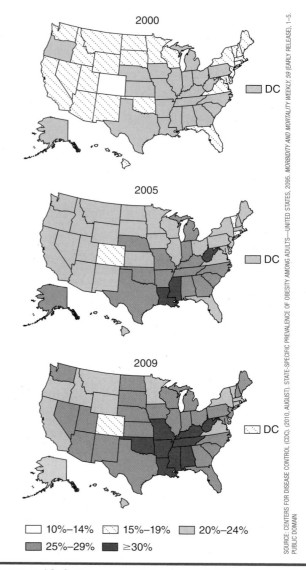

SOURCE: CENTERS FOR DISEASE CONTROL (CDC), (2010, AUGUST). STATE-SPECIFIC PREVALENCE OF OBESITY AMONG ADULTS—UNITED STATES, 2095. *MORBIDITY AND MORTALITY WEEKLY, 59* (EARLY RELEASE), 1–5. PUBLIC DOMAIN

FIGURE 12-2 Percentage of obesity in adults in the United States, 2000–2009.

TABLE 12-4 Selected *HP 2020* Objectives Related to Nutrition, Weight, and Exercise

Increase the proportion of adults who are at a healthy weight.

Reduce the proportion of adults who are obese.

Increase the variety and contribution of vegetables to the diets of the population aged 2 years and older.

Reduce consumption of calories from solid fats and added sugars in the population aged 2 years and older.

Reduce consumption of saturated fat in the population aged 2 years and older.

Reduce consumption of sodium in the population aged 2 years and older.

Increase consumption of calcium in the population aged 2 years and older.

© Cengage Learning 2013

Considering the physiological changes that occur in middle adulthood, exercise functions to maintain bone strength, combat osteoporosis, increase circulation to the periphery, and bolster cardiovascular stamina. The benefits of exercise in lowering the risk of cardiovascular disease and osteoporosis are well established. There is also evidence that exercise decreases the risk of colon cancer as well. Recent studies show that regular moderate exercise can reduce the risk of developing colon cancer through improving digestive function and by maintaining a healthy weight (http://www.cancer.org/Healthy/EatHealthyGetActive/GetActive/make-exercise-work-for-you).

Despite demonstrated benefits, however, it is important to weigh the risks of exercise for certain individuals. Beginning an exercise program, particularly for those who are obese and have known cardiovascular disease or hypertension or both, should be approached cautiously and only after a thorough assessment. Additionally, nurses need to advise those who exercise to use warm-up and stretching activities prior to vigorous workouts, to avoid overexercising to the point of exhaustion or pain, and to take basic safety precautions to avoid injury.

TOBACCO AVOIDANCE

There are several documented benefits of smoking cessation in the middle adult years: immediate cardiovascular reduction in workload, respiratory function improvement with decreased risk of infection, and long-term pulmonary function stabilization and reduction in respiratory cancer risk. Nurses should be knowledgeable about methods that are most effective in helping smokers quit. Health care providers can assist the tobacco user to at least contemplate quitting. If the smoker is already trying to quit, the provider can guide and support this individual in multiple ways to maintain nonsmoking status. Research supports the effectiveness of a combination of gradually tapering nicotine replacement and behavioral approaches to address the psychological addiction. Chapter 18 provides further discussion on smoking cessation.

The Agency for Health Care Policy and Research has developed guidelines for nurses to assist clients in successful cessation approaches (*A Guide for Nurses*, 2008). Support and reinforcement for the smoker must be based on behavioral change principles; long-term follow-up and counseling regarding relapse are essential to successful smoking cessation.

IMMUNIZATIONS

Middle adults should be counseled to keep their immunizations up-to-date. The tetanus-diphtheria-toxoid series should be completed in adults who were not immunized during childhood with the primary series. In adults of any age, regular boosters should be obtained at a recommended interval of every 10 years, barring serious injury during the interval necessitating an additional booster [Advisory Committee on Immunization Practices (ACIP), 2011]. The series of hepatitis B vaccine should be provided to all young adults and any other adults at high risk for infection, including those who are sexually active, are seeking treatment for sexually transmitted disease, are substance abusers, or require blood transfusions or clotting factor concentrates, are health care personnel, and travel to areas high in endemic disease. For hepatitis A, adults should be immunized who travel or work in areas of the world except the United States, Canada, Western Europe, Australia and New Zealand, and Japan; other candidates are those who have chronic liver disease, risk factors related to injectable drug

users, and sexual risk factors, as well as food handlers if deemed appropriate, and those with close contact with international visitors or household contacts. Herpes zoster immunization should be advised for adults who are 60 and older. Meningococcal vaccine is recommended for adults who are traveling to Saudi Arabia during the Haaj (ACIP, 2011).

Annual seasonal influenza vaccination (trivalent inactivated influenza vaccine, TIV) is recommended for all adults, including health adults ages 19–49 years without risk factors,. Family members of individuals in high-risk groups should also be immunized for influenza annually. Nurses should obtain immunization histories on all clients seen in health care settings and inform them of needed boosters of primary immunizations. It is also the nurse's responsibility to be aware of community services providing free or low-cost immunizations to indigent or uninsured clients.

PROMOTING AWARENESS OF GENETIC/GENOMICS ISSUES

A new area of emphasis in *Healthy People 2020* is genetics/genomics. **Genetics** refers to a one-gene disorder, whereas the newer term, **genomics**, refers to the situation in which multiple genes are interacting with each other and with the environment (Calzone, Masny, & Jenkins, 2010). One of the goals of *HP 2020* is "to improve health and prevent harm through valid and useful genomic tools in clinical and public health practices" (U.S. Department of Health and Human Services, 2011). It is imperative that nurses are educated about genetic issues and help achieve the goals of *Healthy People 2020* by informing patients and families about genetic and genomic risks that may affect them.

There is increasing scientific evidence of the benefit in using genetic testing and family health history to guide both individual and community health interventions. These interventions may range from recommendations regarding genetic testing for women with high-risk family histories to those with colorectal cancer to the incorporation of assessment of family history in every clinical encounter. In the past, genetic testing and application of genomic medicine have involved rare diseases, but now they are applied to more common diseases: heart disease, diabetes, Alzheimer's disease, in addition to cancer. Over 1,700 genetic tests are currently available, many available directly to consumers (U.S. Department of Health and Human Services, 2011). Informing the public about the appropriate use of genetic testing and interpretation of results will become more and more the responsibility of nursing.

Additionally, the use of family health history has been shown to be a cost-effective approach to improving health for those at high risk for disease based on family history who are undiagnosed. For instance, a common genetic disorder, familial hypercholesterolemia (FH), causes elevated low-density lipoprotein (LDL), which increases risk for premature cardiovascular disease. Approximately 1/500 have FH, but many are undiagnosed (Genomics and Heart Disease, 2011). A lack of awareness of the disorder prevents appropriate education and counseling for affected individuals and families, as well as the implementation of lifestyle changes to reduce risk.

The Office of the U.S. Surgeon General has developed an online tool, "My Family Health Portrait," which helps users organize family history information into a graphical representation and then print it out in English or Spanish for inclusion in the individual's health record. The user-friendly tool is designed to assist with predicting illness and counseling on intervention and lifestyle changes for the prevention of disease, and it was used in a study of primarily Hispanic working adults in a Southwestern city. Participants were assessed by objective measures (blood lipid testing, BP, weight, waist-to-hip ratio measurement, and BMI calculation) and were assisted in the completion of the family history tool. They were then provided information about their risks associated with both family history and physical findings, and they were counseled on ways to lower their risk. Almost half of this sample had first-degree relatives (FDRs) with cardiovascular disease or hypertension, and over half had FDRs with diabetes. Given the occurrence of individual risk factors (over half were assessed in the overweight and obese category, and about 20% had high blood lipid levels), participants were counseled on nutrition and exercise changes to reduce risk, in addition to referral for appropriate lipid-reducing drug therapy (McNeill, Cook, Mahon, Rauschhuber, Jones, and Estrada, 2008).

The use of family history in wellness and health promotion should become standard practice in nursing. *HP 2020* recommendations for the future include facilitating the use of valid genetic testing and family history tools to guide clinical practice, along with policy and program planning at the local, state, and national levels. Further, family history information needs to be added to electronic health records (HP 2020-Genetics/Genomics, 2011).

SLEEP

Difficulty in falling asleep and staying asleep, known as insomnia, is a commonly occurring problem that can have significant consequences. A recent report noted that one in three Americans are affected by insomnia, at least some of the time and that 9–15% experience resulting function problems during the day (Harvard Health Publications, 2011). Not only does insomnia cause daytime drowsiness, it may impair quality of life in other ways, including reduced concentration or poor work performance. Sleep problems are also frequently associated with other mental health disorders such as anxiety, depression, attention deficit hyperactivity disorder, and bipolar disorder.

Transient insomnia is temporary, lasting less than a month and resulting from a variety of causes such as minor illness; a different sleeping environment; medications for cold, flu, depression, hypertension, and the like; travel or jet lag; physical or emotional stress, and so on. Addressing the cause is key to overcoming transient insomnia. Insomnia becomes chronic when it occurs for longer than 6 months (Harvard, 2011).

It is important to balance rest and sleep with activity to promote overall health. Some individuals begin to experience changes in patterns and requirements for sleep during the middle adult years. Although the number of hours of sleep recommended for adults, 6–8 hours per night, remains unchanged during the middle years, individuals vary in the amount of sleep that helps them feel rested and enables them to maintain their desired level of activity. The changes that may occur include more frequent waking at night, less deep sleep, and increased influence of other factors on sleep quantity and quality.

Middle-aged adults should always be queried about their sleep habits and about their satisfaction with their sleep pattern. The nurse can suggest a variety of cognitive and behavioral interventions, which have been shown through research to be preferable to medication in alleviating insomnia (Harvard, 2011). Cognitive behavioral approaches include setting realistic goals about sleep and the practice of more sleep-promoting habits, including lifestyle changes. Helpful approaches can be recommended, such as relaxation tapes, relaxing baths, massage, increased exercise, and decreased caffeine and heavy food intake, particularly in the evening. Reliance on medication or alcohol to promote sleep should be avoided (Harvard, 2011).

DENTAL HEALTH

Dental caries and periodontal disease are problems for many Americans. The National Center for Chronic Disease Prevention and Health Promotion, Oral Health Division (2006) has identified the following in regard to adult oral health:

1. The baby boomer generation, born between 1946 and 1964, is the first in which the majority will maintain their natural teeth over their entire lifetime, a fact attributed to water fluoridation and fluoride toothpastes.

2. The percentage of adults missing all their natural teeth has declined from over 31% to 25% for those over 60 years of age and from 9% to 5% for adults 40–59 years of age.

3. Most adults show signs of gum disease, with severe gum disease affecting approximately 14% of adults of age 45–54. Further, about 40% of poor adults (20 years or older) have at least one untreated decayed tooth compared with only 16% of nonpoor adults. Non-Hispanic Blacks, Hispanics, and American Indians and Alaska Natives generally have the poorest oral health of any racial and ethnic groups in the United States.

4. Over 70% of adults report visiting a dentist in the past 12 months. Adults with incomes at or above the poverty level are twice as likely as those with lower incomes to report a visit to a dentist in the past 12 months. For every adult without medical insurance, three are without dental insurance.

Dental conditions can result in great economic cost and human suffering. Although fluoridating the water supply and increased usage of fluoridated toothpaste have been effective in decreasing the incidence of cavities, problems persist. However, many population groups, particularly those in underserved

---

?

ASK **YOURSELF**

Enhancing Sleep in the Middle-Aged Adult

You are counseling a 50-year-old male executive who reports that excessive work pressures prohibit restful sleep the night before a big presentation. He states that he was always able to "sleep like a log" despite outside pressures. What would you suggest to aid sleep? What would you advise against using to promote sleep?

GLOBAL HIGHLIGHTS IN HEALTH PROMOTION

Traveling: A Global Health Issue

The world is shrinking, and individuals and families are traveling at an increasing rate. After getting a passport, health concerns should be uppermost in the individual/family considerations and planning. The Centers for Disease Control and Prevention provides a wealth of information for travelers. Information ranging from tips for hygiene and health practices to needed vaccinations by destination can be found at the traveler's health site of the CDC. Yellow fever vaccination is the one required by International Health Regulations for travel to certain countries in sub-Saharan Africa and tropical South America. See www.cdc.gov/travel/content/vaccinations .aspx.

and low socioeconomic areas, lack information regarding ways to maintain oral health and prevent dental problems, and as a result they suffer greater oral health problems (Centers for Disease Control and Prevention, 2011). Nurses can encourage regular dental care and refer low-income clients to available dental services. Regular dental care also accomplishes the goal of routine oral screening, which is important for those at high risk for oral cancer, including smokers, smokeless tobacco users, and heavy alcohol users. Patients with cancer and other immune diseases should be referred for preventive dental care. An estimated 400,000 patients per year undergoing cancer chemotherapy suffer from oral health problems such as mucositis, painful oral ulcers, or dry mouth.

OCCUPATIONAL SAFETY

Occupational issues are important to the middle-aged adult. Work roles remain a primary concern in this age group. Nurses in both primary care settings and occupational health settings share the responsibility for promoting health and safety. The U.S. Department of Labor (2011) reported that there were approximately 4,547 work-related deaths and over 3 million nonfatal illnesses and injuries in private industries during 2009; these numbers represent decreases over the last decade. Workplace homicides accounted for 423 deaths in 2010, approximately 9% of the total for that year. Nonfatal occupational injuries and illnesses requiring days away from work decreased in 2010 to 3.6 per 100 workers (U.S. Bureau of Labor Statistics, 2011).

Primary care providers are in an essential position to assess the effect of the work environment on the middle-aged adult. Some important areas to assess are (1) work-related potential for stress and violence, (2) risk for back injuries due to personal or occupational history, and (3) exposure to environmental carcinogens. Implications for nurses regarding occupational health are to ask clients about their work, the related stresses, and the potential for injury. Occupational exposure to carcinogens or other dangerous substances is an area of concern that nurses should assess in all clients. Nurses in occupational health settings are particularly concerned with these issues.

NURSING ROLE IN HEALTH PROMOTION AND EARLY DETECTION

Pender's Health Promotion Model (2006) has served as a guide for practice and for research into the complex processes—biological and psychosocial—that determine individual health behavior. This model is further discussed in Chapter 3. It is applied here because it explains and gives direction to nursing actions to assist clients with their health-promotion efforts.

The model applies across the life span and effectively guides practice with the middle adult. Important variables include individual characteristics and experience, behavior-specific cognitions and affect, and outcomes. Each of these variables is discussed in the following sections. Table 12-5 depicts these variables within the context of the domains that frame human existence: psychosocial, biological, environmental, and cultural.

- Individual characteristics and experience—Prior related behavior and personal biological, psychological, and sociocultural factors make up these individual characteristics. For example, the middle adult who has abused alcohol (prior behavior that has caused biological changes) also may have had distinct enabling factors, such as a family pattern of alcoholism (psychological and sociocultural), interacting with the biological factors to perpetuate this dangerous health behavior. Health-promotion efforts, to be successful, must include consideration and intervention targeted at each of these areas.

- Behavior-specific cognitions and affect—Perceived benefits and barriers to action, perceived self-efficacy, and activity-related affect are cognitive responses to the known health threat and recommended preventive behavior. These are affected by the individual's characteristics and experiences as well as by other interpersonal influences such as family, peers, role models, and situational influences.

Outcomes, or the results of nursing intervention with clients, consist of observable health-promoting behavior that is influenced by other competing demands and level of commitment to a plan of action.

EDUCATING ABOUT RISK REDUCTION AND HEALTH-PROMOTING ACTIVITIES

Communicating about risk status and risk reduction is a vital role for health care providers, with particular importance for the middle adult. An important component of health promotion is educating the client regarding risk and health-promoting activities for risk avoidance, reduction, or modification. The health risks faced by some middle adults are related to lifestyle and behavior and can be very significant. High-risk behaviors tend to be interrelated, for example, alcohol use with unsafe sexual practices; drug use with poor nutrition; a lack of exercise with high-fat, low-fiber intake. Sharing risk assessment and risk reduction recommendations with clients gives them control. The developmental tasks at this stage influence middle adults to desire control over their lives and the lives of those for whom they feel responsible. The middle adult often perceives a heavy burden of commitment to others, such as aging dependent parents, dependent children, or both. These factors may heighten the

TABLE 12-5 Examples of Risk Factors, Health-Promotion Activities, and Expected Outcomes According to the Health-Promotion Model for Middle Adult with Alcohol Abuse Problem and Obesity

VARIABLE	SPECIFIC RISK FACTOR	HEALTH-PROMOTION ACTIVITY	EXPECTED OUTCOME
Individual characteristics	Alcohol abuse	Assist client in identifying need for health promotion. Explore options such as substance abuse programs or support group for help with alcohol abuse. Include client and family members if possible.	Patient attains sobriety. Family members obtain assistance with coping.
Behavior	Excessive caloric intake, obesity	Assist client in identifying need for health promotion. Explore options such as nutritional counseling, local support group, exercise programs. Assist client to adopt new nutritional habits, develop a food diary, and begin an exercise program. Include family members if possible.	Client exhibits healthy meal planning and caloric intake appropriate for body size and activity. Exercise program is maintained as tolerated.
Outcomes	Lack of commitment to exercise program	Explore incentives to increase commitment to an exercise program. Assist in developing an exercise log. Include family members if possible.	Client maintains regular program, develops a relationship with an exercise buddy to maintain schedule. Client reduces weight gradually to within 10% of ideal body weight (IBW).

© Cengage Learning 2013

client's receptivity to recommendations that will result in decreased risk of illness. Giving individualized feedback regarding risk, rather than routine information about risks, is more likely to result in behavioral change and adherence to recommendations.

The counseling of adults must be based on theories of adult learning, which propose that adults are motivated to learn information and skills that will enhance independence and problem solving, that they can immediately apply to their life situations, and that are congruent with their life experience and role demands (Bastabe, 2008). It is also vital to provide opportunities to practice newly acquired skills immediately, such as doing diabetic foot care, monitoring one's blood pressure, or taking cholesterol-lowering medications.

HEALTH PROMOTION
THEORY LINK

Health Promotion for Middle Adult: Orem's Model of Self-Care

Dorothea Orem's Model of Self-Care defines the concept of self-care as "activities that individuals initiate and perform on their own behalf in maintaining life, health and well being" (Orem, 1991, p. 117). Orem's model has been used as a theoretical support for health-promotion behaviors in various populations, including middle-aged women, and in various ages of women related to breast health and screening practices. By exhibiting Self-Care Agency, a central concept in the model, a person deliberately chooses goal-directed activities that promote or maintain his or her health, such as healthy exercise or nutrition practices, or participation in screening activities. When individuals lack the ability to perform health-promoting or -supporting activities, the theory proposes that they need assistance, which can be provided by the nurse who can help meet the self-care deficit with nursing agency. Nursing agency refers to the nurses' specialized training, obtained through formal education and directed toward serving the patient and helping to meet self-care needs.

Source: Fitzpatrick, J., & Whall, A. (2005). *Conceptual models of nursing: Analysis and application* (4th ed.). Upper Saddle River, NJ: Pearson-Prentice Hall; Orem, D. (1991) *Nursing: Concepts of practice* (4th ed.). St. Louis, MO: Mosby-Yearbook.

SPOTLIGHT **ON**

Occupational Exposure to Carcinogens

Although occupation-related cancers account for 4% of all cancers, they are almost entirely preventable. Nurses cannot keep updated on all carcinogenic agents, but they can assess the client's work history for current and past exposure to metals, dust, chemicals, fumes, radiation, loud noise, heat or cold, and biological agents. The possible exposure of family members, through dust on clothes, chemical residue, and so on, should also be assessed. The nurse should also ask whether protective equipment is available as well as instruction in its use. Although in the United States most sources of occupational exposure to carcinogens are regulated, unplanned exposure can occur due to accidents, breaches in regulations, or unknown hazards. Current research in the area of carcinogenic exposures in occupational settings is currently focused on identifying new sources of exposure and on examining the interaction between the exposure and lifestyle factors. A comprehensive risk assessment includes identification of the person's own health habits, such as tobacco use and diet, as well as occupational hazards to best counsel individuals regarding risk reduction (American Cancer Society, 2007).

Nurses should advise all individuals in the middle adult years to adopt essential health habits: getting regular exercise, reducing the fat and increasing the fiber in the diet, avoiding tobacco and other substance use, and taking measures to prevent accidents. Other health-promotion and screening activities should be targeted on groups at risk for a certain disease or injury, that is, individuals who are more likely to develop the disease or injury or dysfunction than others because of their certain characteristics s. Nurses should be alert for characteristics that may be unique to the person, such as a person who injects IV drugs. Or risk factors can derive from the environment

NURSING **ALERT**

Tips for Teaching the Adult Learner

1. *Make it relate* to the adult's life situation.
2. *Make it fit* the adult's life experience.
3. *Make it work* as the adult carries out old roles or takes on new roles.

of the person, such as a plant worker who is exposed to asbestos. For many conditions, risk factors have been identified. For the first situation, the IV drug user, educational and behavioral interventions to reduce the risk of AIDS and hepatitis need to be instituted. For the second, a job-related situation, broad community-based solutions are needed, such as the safety programs instituted by the Occupational Safety and Health Administration. Thus, a key consideration in prevention and early detection is to target education and screening on the individuals in the population who are at risk.

ASSESSMENT OF THE MIDDLE-AGED ADULT

When deciding on the screening tests to use for middle adults, two questions need to be answered. First, is there a benefit to the early detection of the condition to be screened for? Second, are the available screening tests accurate?

Consider whether early detection leads to intervention to prevent or delay the worsening of the condition. This issue causes one to consider whether treatment for the disease is effective or there is any benefit to early detection versus waiting until symptoms arise. For the middle adult, if early treatment can produce a more favorable long-term outcome, instituting it is important because the expected life span for men and women has lengthened. An example of this situation is prostate cancer, where "watchful waiting" is sometimes advocated when early prostate cancer is found in older men (ACS, 2010). On the other hand, if detection does not affect the effectiveness of treatment, as in the typical case of lung cancer, the cost of screening outweighs its benefit.

When considering the accuracy of screening tests, key issues of sensitivity and specificity are involved. The **sensitivity of a screening test** is the ability of the test to correctly give a positive result when the person has the condition. The **specificity of a screening test** is the accuracy of the test in correctly giving a negative result when the person being screened does not have the disease (Meires & Ledbetter, 2012). If a test has low sensitivity, persons with the disease are missed by the screening procedure. The false-negative results may delay treatment and allow the disease to progress undetected. When a test has low specificity, false-positives result, and persons who do not have the disease have to undergo further testing to determine whether they are disease free. This problem has been identified with fecal occult blood testing for colon cancer. False-positive results can occur unless the individual pays strict attention to the dietary and medication guidelines for the test (for example, no red meat, cruciferous vegetables, aspirin, nonsteroidal anti-inflammatory drugs for 72 hours before the beginning of stool collection and throughout the period needed to collect three stool samples). A positive test necessitates follow-up with a colonoscopy at a significant monetary cost and anxiety for the individual being screened. The cost of false-positives is a problem to the already economically challenged health care system.

There is agreement that, for certain acute and chronic illnesses, periodic evaluation of all clients based on certain age and gender characteristics is justified. These conditions include hypertension; hyperlipidemia; smoking behavior; colon, breast, and cervical cancer; and alcoholism (U.S. Preventive Services Task Force, 2010). Screening for obesity, because of its relationship to both cardiovascular and cancer incidence, is also recommended. The U.S. Preventive Services Task Force has evaluated evidence about screening practices in primary care (U.S. Preventive Services Task Force, 2010). Tables 12-6 and 12-7 represent a compilation of the screening recommendations for middle adult men and women from the Task Force document. The recommendations of the American Cancer Society (2010) have also been added for some cancer sites.

HEALTH-PROMOTION MEASURES FOR MAJOR DEVIATIONS FROM HEALTH

Persons with chronic illnesses, notably diabetes mellitus, cardiovascular diseases, such as angina pectoris and hypertension, and renal and pulmonary disease and cancer, have special health-promotion needs. Although they may be maintained on medications, special regimens, or procedures and live with the threat of disease recurrence or exacerbation, these individuals need health-promotion and health-maintenance activities as do other population groups. Formerly the diagnosis of some diseases such as cancer precluded attention being given to health promotion. These persons may not have been counseled to maintain a more ideal body weight, quit smoking, get regular exercise, maintain sexual function at a level desired by themselves and their partners, or pursue fulfilling career or recreational interests. With the increased

longevity made possible by scientific advances in treatment for many of these illnesses, the nurse must be diligent in providing encouragement and education to chronically ill persons regarding health promotion and health maintenance. Similarly, those with, or at risk for, functional impairments need to be specifically targeted for health-promotion and screening activities.

VISION AND HEARING

Increased IOP, family history, older age, diabetes, severe myopia (nearsightedness), and being of African American descent place an individual at increased risk for glaucoma (U.S. Preventive Services Task Force, 2005). Screening for glaucoma varies among professional groups. The American Academy of Ophthalmology recommends screening for glaucoma as part of the comprehensive adult medical eye evaluation, starting at the age of 20; the Department of Veterans Affairs recommends screening for every veteran over the age of 40 (with frequency depending on age, ethnicity, and family history); and the American Optometric Association recommends annual eye examinations for people at risk for glaucoma. Nonetheless, the U.S. Preventive Services Task Force (2005) concluded that there is insufficient evidence to recommend for or against screening adults not at risk for glaucoma.

Many clinicians in practice conduct hearing screening on adults over age 65, on those with exposure to excessive occupational noise, or on all middle adults who indicate difficulty

TABLE 12-6 Common Screening Tests and Recommended Frequency for Middle-Aged Adult Females

SCREENING TESTS	AGE RANGE	FREQUENCY
BP monitoring	>18 years	Every 1–2 years
Blood cholesterol	>45	Annually
Height and weight measurement	All ages	At health checkup
Assessment of smoking status, interest checkup in cessation if smoker	All ages	At health checkup
	Pregnant women	At every visit
	Mothers	
Mammography	>50**	Every two years***
Clinical breast exam*	>40	Annually
-	-	-
Fecal occult blood (FOB), fecal immunochemical test (FIT), sigmoidoscopy, or colonoscopy	50–75	FOB or FIT annually, sigmoidoscopy every 5 years, and colonoscopy every 10 years
Papanicolaou smear	3 years following beginning sexual activity, or 21 years of age. <70	Three or more normal results can begin screening every two years
History, assess use of tobacco, alcohol, other substances	All ages	At health checkup
	Pregnant women	At every visit

*Although it lacks scientific support, breast self-exam and clinical breast exam continue to be recommended practices by the American Cancer Society.

**The U.S. Preventive Services Task Force (USPSTF) recommends beginning mammography at 50, whereas the American Cancer Society recommends beginning at 40 years of age.

***The UTPSTF recommends mammography at 2-year intervals, whereas the American Cancer Society recommends annual mammography.

Source: U.S. Preventive Services Task Force (2010). *Guide to Clinical Preventive Services*.

TABLE 12-7 Common Screening Tests and Recommended Frequency for Middle-Aged Adult Males

SCREENING TEST	POPULATION GROUP	FREQUENCY
Blood pressure measurement	18 years	Every 1–2 years
Blood cholesterol, fasting or nonfasting	>35 years	Annually
Height and weight	All ages	At health checkup
Assessment of smoking status, interest in cessation if smoker	All ages	At health checkup
	Fathers	Every visit
Fecal occult blood (FOB) Fecal immunochemical test (FIT), sigmoidoscopy, or colonoscopy	50–70	FOB or FIT annually, sigmoidoscopy every 5 years, and colonoscopy every 10 years
	50–70	Recommended informed decision making offered to man in considering personal preference and risk profile in consultation with health care provider
History, questionnaires (CAGE or AUDIT) for alcohol or substance use	All ages	At health checkup

*PSA recommended by ACS, with or without digital rectal exam; PSA not recommended by USPSTF; however, informed decision making regarding prostate screening is recommended.

Source: Adapted from *Guide to Clinical Preventive Services*, U.S. Preventive Services Task Force, 2010.

with hearing upon questioning. The U.S. Preventive Services Task Force (USPSTF) is currently reviewing the evidence for hearing screening and has not made a recommendation as of 2011.

DIABETES MELLITUS

In the United States, Type 2 diabetes mellitus is prevalent in approximately 11% of adults age 20 years and older, with increased rates noted in those 20–44 years and over 65 years in the period 1994–2008 (National Health Statistics, 2010). Some population subgroups among adults have a higher prevalence of diabetes than others: obese men and women over 40 years of age; members of racial or ethnic groups such as Native Americans, Mexican Americans, and African Americans; and those with a family history of diabetes. Other major risk categories are adults with hyperglycemia (elevated blood glucose) and hyperlipidemia (elevated low-density cholesterol and total cholesterol). Although the U.S. Preventive Services Task Force (USPSTF, 2008) concludes that the evidence is insufficient to recommend for or against routinely screening asymptomatic adults for Type 2 diabetes mellitus, it does recommend screening adults who have hypertension or hyperlipidemia.

CANCER

Postmenopausal women who are at high risk for endometrial cancer are Caucasians, obese women over 50 years, and those with abnormal bleeding. Women over 50 years of age should have a regular pelvic exam for early detection of other gynecological cancers, including ovarian and cervical. High-risk groups

for cervical cancer include women with diethylstilbestrol exposure, multiple sexual partners (two or more), AIDS, and human papillomavirus (HPV). The USPSTF strongly recommends screening for cervical cancer in women who have been sexually active and who have a cervix (U.S. Preventive Services Task Force, 2010).

Persons who should be screened for head, neck, and oral cancers include past or current tobacco users, frequent alcohol users, and all with suspicious oral lesions. An oral examination, as well as a physical assessment of the lymph system, should be performed. Those with a history of upper body (head and neck) radiation in childhood should be screened for thyroid cancer with a physical examination and imaging techniques (U.S. Preventive Services Task Force, 2010; American Cancer Society, 2010).

OSTEOPOROSIS

Risk factors include low body weight (<70 kg [154 lb]), no current use of estrogen therapy, and age (55 and older). The USPSTF has confirmed that there is less evidence to support the use of other individual risk factors, such as smoking, weight loss, family history, decreased physical activity, alcohol or caffeine use, or low calcium and vitamin D intake, as a basis for identifying high-risk women younger than 65. All racial groups are at risk with aging; however whites are most commonly affected. The USPSTF (2010) makes no recommendation for or against routine osteoporosis screening in postmenopausal women who are younger than 60 or in women age 60–64 who are not identified as being at risk; also, there is no evidence-based data recommending screening for men.

SUMMARY

This chapter has provided an overview of the physiological and psychosocial changes occurring in the middle adult years and their health-promotion implications. The importance of including genetic and/or genomic risk factors as part of family history was discussed. Recommendations for health-promotion activities were presented, including the gathering of family history data to enable more individualized risk counseling. Specific discussion of recommendations for the special group of chronically ill persons were presented. Finally, screening recommendations were discussed for conditions for which there is agreement regarding recommended screening procedures and intervals. Screening recommendations for individuals at higher-than-average risk for certain conditions were discussed regarding controversies in various standards of practice.

CASE STUDY

Laura Jensen: Promoting Health in the Middle-Aged Adult

OBJECTIVES/GOALS: Through participation in a discussion of this case study, participants will have the opportunity to:

1. Identify factors affecting exercise in middle-aged adults.
2. Describe interventions to facilitate exercise in middle-aged adults.

HEALTH-PROMOTION CONCERN, HISTORY AND PHYSICAL, PRESENT HEALTH STATUS, PAST HEALTH STATUS, FAMILY HISTORY, AND SOCIAL HISTORY

Laura Jensen is a 52-year-old female of German descent who is employed in marketing for a successful advertising firm in a Midwestern city. She is divorced, with two children, ages 20 and 23, who no longer live at home but who are alive and well. Her mother lives in a nursing facility, recovering from a stroke that occurred when she was 67. Her father died at age 52 of a heart attack. She is completing a bachelor's degree in business, and her goal is to be chief executive officer of the advertising firm where she is currently employed. She works 12–14 hours a day. She does not cook for herself and has gained 30 lb in the past 2 years.

REVIEW OF PERTINENT DOMAINS

Biological Domain

PHYSICAL EXAM: Reveals a 5 ft, 5 in. female weighing 155 lb.

CARDIOVASCULAR: Laura has a history of hypertension managed with Captopril 25 mg twice daily.

GASTROINTESTINAL: She rarely eats dinner but tries to eat vegetables twice a week, fruit daily, and snacks often throughout the day just to "keep from getting hungry." Her favorite snack items are granola bars, crackers and cheese, and an occasional cookie.

Psychological Domain

Laura is an intelligent woman completing a bachelor's degree in business. She is an independent and highly motivated person who sets goals and accomplishes them. She denies feeling depressed or sad.

Social Domain

Laura has several friends living in the same apartment building. She rarely socializes due to the time spent on her job.

Environmental Domain

Laura lives in a high-rise apartment located adjacent to a public park. Her employing agency offers discounted memberships to the fitness center located in the same building as the agency.

QUESTIONS FOR DISCUSSION

1. What is Laura's body mass index, and how is this interpreted? (Refer to Chapter 14 for the calculation and interpretation.)

2. Complete a three-generation family history for Laura. Does she have family history–related risk for cardiovascular disease?

3. What goals or outcomes can guide Laura in promoting and improving her health status?

4. Develop a plan to help Laura in achieving her health-promotion goals.

KEY CONCEPTS

1. The middle adult period is characterized by the physiologic changes that accompany menopause and the male climacteric, increasing family and work-related commitments, and beginning concerns regarding retirement and health issues, all of which influence many individuals to adopt more healthy lifestyles.

2. Health-promotion activities, even if only recently begun in the middle adult years, reap benefits in older years when functional status and quality of life are greatly influenced by health status.

3. Environmental influences that affect health include air and water pollution, tobacco use and secondhand smoke, work-related exposure and stress, economic pressures and global health influences.

4. Prevention recommendations for the middle adult include: engaging in a planned exercise program; consuming a nutritionally sound diet that is high in fiber and low in fat; keeping immunizations up-to-date, including flu vaccination; obtaining restful sleep as appropriate to the individual; maintaining dental health; and taking measures to ensure safety at home, in recreational activities, and at work.

5. Nurses are vitally important in assessing risk for middle adults based on their age, gender, past and current medical history, genetic and family history, occupational history, and lifestyle factors and in recommending screening practices specific to the identified risk status and congruent with guidelines established by various national bodies.

CHAPTER REVIEW

Learning Activities

1. Develop a plan to implement a health screening for a group of adults in your community to address the *Healthy People 2020* disease-specific objectives for middle-aged adults. Identify the target population, resources, screening measures to be offered, and health-promotion recommendations related to these objectives.

2. Using the U.S. Surgeon's General's Family Health History site, complete your own family history, and share it with your family members.

3. Use Table 12-3 to perform a health risk assessment on a consenting middle-aged adult relative, friend, or colleague. Develop a health-promotion plan addressing your findings.

Multiple Choice

1. Which of the following accurately represents the change in morbidity and mortality rate for coronary artery disease?
   a. The rate has decreased by 25%.
   b. The rate has decreased by 45%.
   c. The rate has increased by 25%.
   d. The rate has increased by 45%.

2. Which of the following nursing interventions would help to achieve the goals of *Healthy People 2020* related to genetics/genomics?
   a. Gathering family health history from every client
   b. Becoming knowledgeable about referring clients to genetic testing services as appropriate
   c. Counseling individuals about family history and other risk factors to improve their health status.
   d. All of the above

3. Health-promotion actions for risk management in middle age include counseling regarding:
   a. immunizations, including tetanus and diphtheria, only if continually employed.
   b. risk factors for HIV and other STDs as well as practicing safe sex.
   c. the influence of peers on risk-taking activities.
   d. the need for less sleep as one ages.

4. With regard to the accuracy of screening tests for health promotion, which of the following is the ability of the test to correctly give a positive result when the person has the condition being tested for?
   a. Sensibility of a screening test
   b. Sensitivity of a screening test
   c. Significance of a screening test
   d. Specificity of a screening test

5. An important part of assessing family history is to:
   a. evaluate the environment of the individual.
   b. focus on family patterns of accidents and injuries.
   c. interview parents of the patient if possible.
   d. review the family history of three generations.

6. You are counseling Mr. Marks, a 55-year-old truck driver, regarding health-promotion activities he could begin. He does not exercise regularly and has just quit smoking. He mentions that "I guess it is probably too late to make much of a difference for me, but I have a new grandchild and I want to be with him as long as I can." Which of the following responses are based on evidence regarding healthy lifestyle practices and health risks?
   a. He should be engaging in healthy exercise for his own benefit, not someone else's.
   b. Overall fitness has its own health benefits but does not improve life span.
   c. Regular exercise can assist him in remaining a non-smoker, which will improve his health.
   d. Although it might be too late for cardiovascular benefit, he will increase his overall fitness.

7. Ms. Johnson is a 52-year-old woman who cares for three children and aging parents in addition to maintaining a full time position as an automobile parts factory line supervisor. She presents with problems related to her weight management and insomnia. Ms. Johnson is typical of many in the middle adulthood period in which of the following:
   a. The ability to focus efforts on work related achievements
   b. The ability to focus on family life responsibilities
   c. The sandwich effect of parent and child responsibilities
   d. The stability of the life stage related to family responsibilities

ORGANIZATIONS AND WEBSITES

AARP: Organization for mature adults 50 and above in the United States; provides information on health, long-term care, economic security, independent living, consumer affairs, and more: **http://www.aarp.org**

American Cancer Society: Offers a wealth of information on prevention, screening, treatment, and survivorship issues related to cancer; *Learn About Cancer,* and *Stay Healthy* are particularly helpful in terms of health promotion: **http://www .cancer.org**

Centers for Disease Control and Prevention: The most recent report on the nation's health with a specific section on death and dying: **http://www.cdc.gov/nchs/data/hus/hus10.pdf**

HealthyPeople.gov: A government organization that promotes a national health-promotion and disease-prevention initiative with goals to increase the quality and years of healthy life for all people: **http://www.healthypeople.gov**

My Family Health Portrait: A tool from the office of the U. S. Surgeon General for use by individuals and health professionals; a user-friendly site, accommodating Spanish, Portugese, and Italian language users; can be completed in English and printed in one of these other languages. The user is guided to complete a three-generation family history, which can also be saved and added to by other family members: **https://familyhistory .hhs.gov/fhh-web/home.action**

PreventDisease: Offers Health Headlines, with the latest news in prevention and health matters, including weekly wellness facts on diverse health topics that contribute to a happy life during middle age: **http://preventdisease.com**

Seekwellness: Offers practical advice for staying healthy via nutrition, exercise, self-care, humor, play, relationships, and adding meaning and purpose to your life: **http://www .seekwellness.com**

U.S. Department of Health and Human Services. (2010). Human immunodeficiency virus (HIV). Retrieved from **http://www.fda.gov/MedicalDevices/Products andMedicalProcedures/InVitroDiagnostics/ HomeUseTests/ucm125797.htm**

Womenshealth: Offers information on health issues important to women of diverse populations throughout the lifespan. Education, outreach, and policy development are **http:// womenshealth.gov/**

REFERENCES

American Cancer Society (ACS). (2010). Cancer facts and figures, 2010. Atlanta, GA: American Cancer Society. Retrieved from http://www.cancer.org/acs/groups/content/@epidemiologysurveilance/documents/document/acspc-026238.pdf

American Cancer Society (ACS)/ (2007). Occupation and cancer. Retrieved from http://www.cancer.org/acs/groups/content/@nho/documents/document/occupationandcancerpdf.pdf

Advisory Committee on Immunization Practices (ACIP) (2011). *ACIP Recommendations.* Retrieved from http://www.cdc.gov/vaccines/recs/schedules/adult-schedule.htm#hcp

Barr, D. A., & Wanat, S. F. (2005). Listening to patients: Cultural and linguistic barriers to health care access. *Family Medicine, 37*(3), 199–204.

Bastable, S. (2008). *The nurse as educator: Principles of teaching and learning for nursing practice* (3rd ed.). Sudbury, MA: Jones & Bartlett.

Bromberger, J. T., Harlow, S., & Avis, N. (2004). Racial/ethnic differences In the prevalence of depressive symptoms among middle-aged women: The study of women's health across the nation (SWAN). *The American Journal of Public Health, 94*, 1378–1385.

Bureau of Labor Statistics. Injuries, Illnesses and Fatalities (2010). Retrieved from http://www.bls.gov/iif/

Calzone, K. A., Masny, A., & Jenkins, J. (2010). *Genetics and genomics in oncology nursing practice.* Pittsburgh, PA: Oncology Nursing Society.

Carroll, R. (2005). Anatomy and physiology review: The reproductive systems. In J. M. Black and J. H. Hawks (eds.), *Medical-surgical nursing: Clinical management for positive outcomes* (4th ed.). St. Louis, MO: Elsevier-Saunders.

Center for Disease Control and Prevention (CDC). (2009). *The power to prevent, the call to control: At a Glance 2009.* Retrieved from http://www.cdc.gov/chronicdisease/resources/publications/AAG/chronic.htm

Columbia University's Mailman School of Public Health. (October 27, 2005). *Largest survey on depression suggests higher prevalence in U.S.* Retrieved from http://www.brightsurf.com/news/headlines/21612/Largest_survey_on_depression_suggests_higher_prevalence_in_US_reports_Mailman_school.html

Division of Oral Health, National Center for Chronic Illness Control and Prevention. (2006). Oral Health for Adults. Retrieved from http://www.northwestern.edu/observer/issues/2005/11/16/depression.html

Fiandt, K. (2005). Health promotion in middle-aged adults. In J. M. Black and J. H. Hawks (eds.), *Medical-surgical nursing: Clinical management for positive outcomes* (4th ed.). St. Louis, MO: Elsevier-Saunders.

First, M. B., Frances, A., & Pincus, H. A. (2004). Major depressive disorder. *DSM IV TR Guidebook.* Arlington, VA: American Psychiatric Publishing, pp. 186–191.

Fitzpatrick, J., & Whall, A. (2005*). Conceptual models of nursing: Analysis and application,* (4th ed.). Upper Saddle River, NJ: Pearson-Prentice Hall.

Health and Human Services. (2008). At a Glance: Physical Activity Guidelines for Americans. Retrieved from http://www.health.gov/paguidelines/factsheetprof.aspx

McNeill, J. A., Cook, J., Mahon, M., Rauschhuber, M., Jones, M. E., & Estrada, R. (2008). Family history: Value-added information in assessing cardiac health, *American Association of Occupational Health Nursing, 56*(7), 297–306.

Meires, J., & Ledbetter, C. (2012). Screening and prevention of diseases. In Macha, K., & McDonough, J. P, (eds.), *Epidemiology for advanced nursing practice.* Sudbury, MA: Jones & Bartlett Learning.

National Center for Health Statistics. (2010). *Health, United States, 2010: With special feature on death and dying.* Retrieved from http://www.cdc.gov/nchs/data/hus/hus10.pdf#highlights

Office of Minority Health, U.S. Department of Health and Human Services. (2010). *Assuring cultural competence in health care: Recommendations for national standards and an outcomes-focused research agenda.* Retrieved from http://minorityhealth.hhs.gov/Assets/pdf/checked/Assuring_Cultural_Competence_in_Health_Care-1999.pdf

Orem, D. (1991). *Nursing: Concepts of practice* (4th ed.). St. Louis, MO: Mosby-Yearbook.

Pender, N. J., Murdaugh, C. L., & Parsons, M. A. (2006). *Health-promotion in nursing practice* (5th ed.). Upper Saddle River, NJ: Pearson Prentice Hall.

United States-2009 2009 and site is: http://www.cdc.gov/mmwr/preview/mmwrhtml/mm59e0803a1.htm Publication info: http://www.cdc.gov/mmwr/preview/mmwrhtml/mm59e0803a1.htm

U. S. Department of Health and Human Services. (2000). *Healthy people 2010.* Retrieved from http://www.cdc.gov/nchs/healthy_people/hp2010.htm

U. S. Department of Health and Human Services. (2011). *Topics and objectives index-Healthy people.* Retrieved from http://www.healthypeople.gov/2020/topicsobjectives2020/default.aspx

U.S. Public Health Service. Agency for Healthcare Research and Quality. (2008, May). Helping smokers quit: A guide for clinicians. Retrieved from http://www.ahrq.gov/about/nursing/hlpsmksqt.htm

CHAPTER 13
The Older Adult

Karyn Taplay, MSN, RNC, PhD (Student)
Alma Flores-Vela, PhD, MSN, RN

KEY TERMS

ageism

assisted living facility (ALF)

atrophy

baby boomers

centenarians

dementia

dysomnia

elder abuse

empowerment

eustress

geriatrics

gerontology

heterogeneity

polypharmacy

spiritual well-being

OBJECTIVES

Upon completion of this chapter, the reader should be able to:

- Identify nursing responsibilities in promoting the health of older adults.
- Explore demographic trends related to aging.
- Examine developmental theories with respect to aging.
- List health promotion tips for expected physiological changes of aging.
- Identify strategies within the biological domain (nutrition, fitness and exercise, sleep, and sex) to promote health in older adults.
- Relate effects from the socioeconomic domain to the health of older adults.
- Describe issues from the psychological domain (stress, depression, and elder abuse) that contribute to the health of older people.
- Consider the influence of spirituality in promoting the health of older adults.
- Identify environmental influences that contribute to the health of older adults.
- Discuss future research trends that may influence the health of older adults.
- Identify health promotion resources for this age group.

INTRODUCTION

As the new millennium progresses, it is impossible to ignore the fact that an unprecedented number of people are age 65 and over. Increased life span is the direct result of advances in science, technology, and medicine. Unfortunately, living longer does not always mean living healthier. Health problems in the later years of life often are a result of unhealthy or harmful behaviors and events in adolescence and adulthood. Additionally, many seniors need to continue to address and manage age-related conditions or chronic illnesses that are identified in the middle adult years.

Geriatrics is a specialized branch of medicine that focuses on the diagnosis and treatment of diseases affecting the elderly. In contrast, the study of the elderly and the aging process is called **gerontology**. Gerontology, which is studied by a variety of disciplines including nursing, encompasses the concepts of health and wellness. As such, gerontology is concerned with the biological, psychological, socioeconomic, and environmental challenges that older people face. The collective consequences of these challenges form important issues for the older individual, the community, and society at large.

Growing older is not necessarily a downward spiral. It is often viewed positively as a new beginning or an achievement, a time when freedom and recreation can be enjoyed. Successful healthy aging depends on the individual's ability to cope with the effects of aging, to manage chronic illness, and to confront new challenges utilizing personal capabilities and existing resources.

The concept of health promotion embodies the attributes of self-care and **empowerment**. These attributes become highly important in older persons regardless of their health status. To become facilitators of health promotion among older adults, nurses must become more knowledgeable about the issues and needs that affect the health and well-being of these patients.

This chapter is based on a gerontological perspective. It addresses demographic characteristics and developmental theories. Nursing responsibilities are discussed as related to health promotion and aging among the various domains (developmental, biological, socioeconomic, psychological, and environmental).

DEMOGRAPHIC CHARACTERISTICS OF OLDER ADULTS

Older adults represent a special segment of the population. Looking at demographics for this age group is helpful in developing a general profile. Note, however, that, although a general profile is helpful in forming an understanding of the uniqueness of older adults, recognition of the vast differences among individual members of this group is equally important.

WHO ARE THE OLDER ADULTS?

Age identity for older adults has shifted from focusing solely on chronological age to include objective, subjective, and functional perspectives. In other words, an individual's birth date, personal perceptions of age and aging, and ability to function physiologically, psychologically, socially, and economically influence whether that person is considered an older adult. From these perspectives, terms such as *feel-age, cognitive age,*

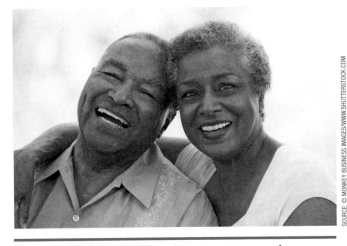

FIGURE 13-1 Young older African American couple.

stereotype age, comparative age, and *self-perceived age* have been identified by gerontologists (Kaufman & Elder, 2002). For legal purposes, such as obtaining Social Security benefits and Medicare, age 65 is recognized as the minimal age for entering the elderly population age group.

The marked increase in the numbers of older people, particularly those over 85, will drive many changes in the near future and beyond. From the perspective of a professional health care provider, remember the **heterogeneity** of the population we call "elderly" because of the differences encountered in the various age groups. For example, people who are 65–74 years old are considered the younger old (see Figure 13-1), 75 to 84 years are considered the older old (Figure 13-2), and people 85+ are considered the oldest old (Figure 13-3) [Center for Addictions and Mental Health, (CAMH), 2009]. Each group should be considered a separate entity with a corresponding collection of unique traits that include culture, geographic location, socioeconomic status, as well as mental and physical health.

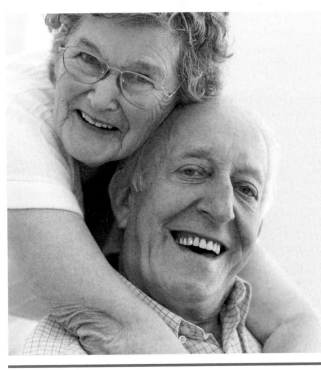

FIGURE 13-2 Older old.

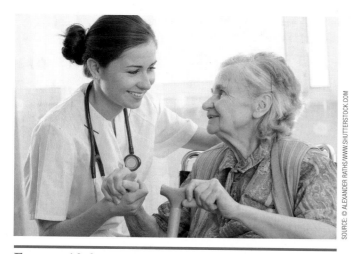

SOURCE: © ALEXANDER RATHS/WWW.SHUTTERSTOCK.COM

FIGURE 13-3 Oldest old (85+).

Because the diversity in the age range of this group is so great, it is easy to see how variations exist. The lifestyles, health, and behaviors of a 65-year-old person can vary significantly from those of a 90-year-old. However, nurses need to avoid stereotyping elderly people because many in the older old and oldest old group can be healthier and more productive than those in the younger old group.

Regarding gender and marital status, there are more elderly women than men and more elderly widowed women than widowed men. When assessing an elderly patient include an assessment of marital status. Being a widow or a widower has a significant impact on all other aspects of life. Table 13-1 demonstrates that the trend of women outliving men is not expected to change in the future. Additionally, Table 13-2 summarizes significant demographic characteristics related to the elderly. These demographics are important considerations in planning and implementing health promotion programs for the geriatric population.

POPULATION TRENDS

In 1776 America celebrated its first Independence Day. A baby born that year could anticipate living to the ripe old age of 35. During the next 125 years, or by 1900, the average life span

SPOTLIGHT **ON**

Facts on Aging

As of January 1, 2011, it is expected that 10,000 people will turn 65 every day and that this trend is expected to continue for 20 years [Alliance for Aging Research (AFAR), 2011]. The number of persons age 65 and older is expected to increase from approximately 40 million in 2010 to an estimated 55 million in 2020, and those age 85 and older are expected to increase from 6.1 million in 2010 to 7.3 million in 2020. The number of centenarians in the United States is anticipated to be 757,000 by the year 2045 (AFAR. 2011).

expectancy had increased to only 47 years of age. By the 1990s, however, with scientific advances, medical breakthroughs, and increased focus on healthy living, people could expect to live about 78.3 years in the United States [Central Intelligence agency, (CIA), 2011]. Life expectancy has increased rapidly in recent years, and a continued, albeit slower, increase is expected. This increase in life expectancy means there are more seniors than ever before.

In 1900 only 4% of the population was over the age of 65. By contrast, in 1996 the percentage of the total population of the United States of people age 65 and over was 13. This rising number of senior citizens is only expected to increase as the first of the **baby boomers**—the large post–World War II generation—reach 65. It is projected that the percentage of persons over 65+ will increase from 12.4% in 2000 to 19.6% by 2030 (Centers for Disease Control and Prevention, 2003).

This expected, dramatic increase in the older segment of the population creates a need for the health care industry to handle tremendous change. The $1 trillion annual expenditure for health care in America currently accounts for 34 million

TABLE 13-1 Projections of Life Expectancy, 1999–2100

YEAR	TOTAL POPULATION		WHITE		BLACK		AMERICAN INDIAN		ASIAN		HISPANIC ORIGIN	
	MALE	FEMALE	MALE	FEMALE	MALE	FEMALE	MALE	FEMALE	MALE	FEMALE	MALE	FEMALE
1999	74.0	79.7	74.7	80.1	68.3	75.1	72.8	82.0	80.8	86.5	77.1	83.7
2025	76.5	82.6	76.9	82.6	72.4	79.3	77.2	85.3	81.5	86.8	79.0	85.1
2050	79.5	84.9	79.5	84.8	76.6	82.7	80.3	87.3	83.2	88.1	81.4	86.8
2100	85.0	89.3	84.8	89.0	83.9	88.4	85.6	90.6	86.6	90.7	85.8	90.1

Note: Census Bureau terms:

"American Indian" includes American Indian, Eskimo, and Aleut.

"Asian" includes Asian and Pacific Islander.

"Hispanic Origin" may be of any race (e.g., "Black-Hispanic," "White-Hispanic"; see Chapter 6).

Source: Hollman, F., Mulder, T. J., & Kallan, J. E. (2000, January). Methodology and assumptions for the population projections of the United States: 1999 to 2100. Washington, DC: Bureau of the Census, U.S. Department of Commerce.

TABLE 13-2 Summary of Current Elderly (55 and Over) Population Characteristics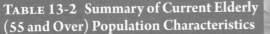

Population size and composition	Total age 55 and over: 59.6 million 26.6 million men and 33.0 million women Ratio of 81 men to 100 women
Married and living with spouse	Age 55–64: 75% men and 63% women Age 65–84: 74% men and 45% women Age 85 and over: 58% men and 12% women
Education High school graduate	Age 55–64: 84% Age 64–84: 71% Age 85 and above: 58%
Bachelor's degree	31% of men and 22% of women
Below poverty level	Total age 55 and over: 5.8 million or 9.8% Age 55–64: 8.4% men and 10.3% women Age 65 and over: 10.3% men and 12.4% women

Source: Smith, D. (2003). The Older Population in the United States: March 2003. U.S. Census Bureau Current Population Reports, P20-546, Washington, DC: U.S. Census Bureau.

GLOBAL HIGHLIGHTS IN HEALTH PROMOTION

The World Health Organization's Guide for Age-Friendly Cities

The World Health Organization (WHO) recognizes the aging population and increasing development of cities and towns as two worldwide developments that will impact our global society. As a response to these trends, the WHO sought information from approximately 1,500 older adults across 33 cities worldwide. As a result of this investigation, the WHO has proposed a guide to enhance active aging through the creation of age-friendly cities. An age-friendly city is based on the philosophy that the entire community benefits from a healthy and active older population. It encourages active living, provides availability and accessibility for health-promotion and wellness activities, and provides the organizational structures and services that support an aging population. The findings from this research indicate that key attributes of an age-friendly city are housing, transportation, and social inclusion. The WHO reports that the guide is already being used to develop age-friendly cities throughout the world [American Association of Retired Persons International (AARPI), 2007].

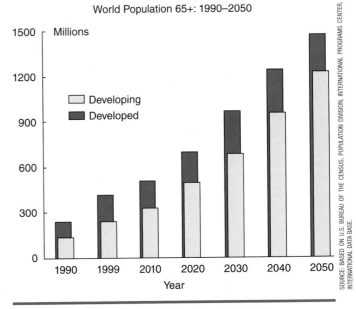

FIGURE 13-4 World Population 65+: 1990–2050.

seniors. With the expected increase in seniors and the reality that older persons typically have at least one chronic condition and that many older persons will have multiple chronic conditions (Larson & Lubkin, 2009), it is likely that if nothing changes there will be significant demand on America's health care expenditures. Modifying the focus of health care from curing or caring for the sick to providing comprehensive health-promotion and disease-prevention strategies is therefore imperative. Several governmental agencies have joined forces to develop the Healthy Aging Project. This is the first step to examining ways to promote healthy behavior and lifestyle choices in the elderly population.

The dramatic rise in the population of seniors is not confined to the United States. The world's population of older people, in both developing and developed countries, increased 159 million or over 60% in the 10-year period 1990–1999 (Figure 13-4). The world's older population is expected to triple by the year 2050 (Figure 13-5). The rapid increase in the

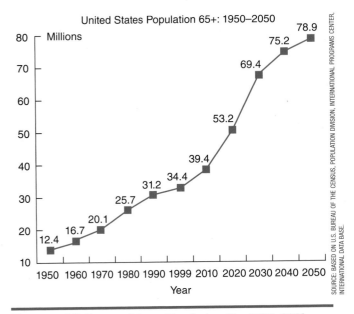

FIGURE 13-5 United States Population 65+: 1950–2050.

numbers of older people worldwide reinforces the concept that improving health in all nations requires the long-term commitment and participation of all involved in their health and well-being.

DEVELOPMENTAL DOMAIN

It has been said that some people grow old gracefully, others gratefully, and then there are those who grow old grudgingly. The older adult is subject to significant developmental age-related transitions that affect health. Having knowledge about developmental tasks and theories of how people age physically and mentally increases the ability of nurses to collaborate with older persons to promote a high level of wellness and successful aging.

DEVELOPMENTAL TASKS OF AGING

To better understand the elderly, several psychosocial theories of aging have been formulated to provide insight into the developmental tasks of the older adult. The psychologist Erik Erikson identified eight stages that cover the life span from infancy to old age. The final stage, which focuses on the older adult, is ego integrity versus despair. Each stage includes specific tasks or challenges that people need to progress through. Older people who are able to look back on their lives with a sense of pride and accomplishment are those who enter the final stage of development with satisfaction and contentment. They are symbolic of Erikson's integrity stage. Unfortunately, this is not the case for everyone. Interestingly, elderly people who exhibit happiness with their younger phase of life usually have the same experience with the older phase of life. As these people age, they accept life and their roles in the world. In doing so, they are better able to handle the concerns that come with aging, including the fear of death (Erikson, 1964).

Erikson's theory, although it covers the life span, offers little differentiation in the older adult stage, integrity versus despair. With the elderly population increasing in number and living even longer, greater detail is needed to sufficiently explore this developmental stage. Robert Peck enhanced Erikson's old-age stage by adding three specific tasks for the elderly, which influence the outcome of ego integrity versus ego despair (Peck, 1968).

1. Ego differentiation versus role preoccupation—to find satisfaction with oneself instead of satisfaction through parental or occupational roles

2. Body transcendence versus body preoccupation—to enjoy life instead of being consumed by age-related physical changes

3. Ego transcendence versus ego preoccupation—to reflect positively on times past rather than obsessing about the limited time remaining

Additionally, Havighurst (1972) delineated six developmental tasks for the older adult. These tasks relate to adjustments needed for physical, social, and environmental effects of aging.

Table 13-3 demonstrates that psychosocial theories of aging, when used in combination, provide a clear, comprehensive perspective on the developmental tasks of the older adult. Although individuals adapt to the aging process in different ways, these psychosocial theories of aging provide a predictable pathway with which to plot progression through various developmental stages or tasks.

THEORIES RELATED TO AGING

Predictably, we all age with time. Less predictable is how we respond physically and mentally to aging. Why and how we age have always been of interest to researchers. There was a surge in the creation of developmental theories in the late 1960s and early 1970s that remain pertinent today in understanding human development. These various theories attempt to explain how adults respond differently to the aging process. These can be categorized as of biological, sociological, psychological, and evolving theories of aging as depicted in Table 13-4. These theories should be kept in mind when reading about the health-promotion domains for the older adult that follow.

BIOLOGICAL DOMAIN

Aging is not a disease. It's a natural process that begins the minute a person is born. The nursing profession has valuable sources of information and research that help with understanding this progression. Providing quality nursing care for patients 65 years or older requires genuine attention to the complex issues that accompany this population. Physiological changes of aging occur in every body system, so it is imperative to understand these changes and how they may impact nursing care. Table 13-5 outlines each body system and highlights some of the expected age-related changes. Nursing considerations and health-promotion tips are also delineated in this table and are categorized by the age-related changes.

TABLE 13-3 Erikson, Peck, and Havighurst: Developmental Tasks of Aging		
ERIKSON	**PECK**	**HAVIGHURST**
Ego integrity versus despair	1. Ego differentiation versus role preoccupation 2. Body transcendence versus body preoccupation 3. Ego transcendence versus ego preoccupation	1. Adjusting to decreasing physical strength and health 2. Adjusting to retirement and reduced income 3. Adjusting to the death of a spouse 4. Establishing an explicit association with one's age group 5. Adapting to social roles in a flexible way 6. Establishing satisfactory physical living arrangements

TABLE 13-4 Theories of Aging

CATEGORY	THEORY	DESCRIPTION
Biological	Genetic Theory	We are programmed to age by a predetermined biological clock.
	Wear and Tear Theory	The body and its cells are damaged by overuse and abuse. Wear and tear is not confined to our organs, however; it also takes place on the cellular level.
	Neuroendocrine Theory	Hormones are vital for repairing and regulating our bodily functions, and when aging causes a drop in hormone production, it causes a decline in our body's ability to repair and regulate itself as well.
	Free Radical Theory	Free-radical damage begins at birth and continues until we die. In our youth, its effects are relatively minor because the body has extensive repair and replacement mechanisms that in healthy young people function to keep cells and organs in working order. With age, however, the accumulated effects of free-radical damage begin to take their toll.
	Cross-Linkage Theory	A chemical reaction that binds molecules attaches itself to a strand of DNA and damages it. Natural defense mechanisms are inadequate to repair the damage.
Sociological	Disengagement Theory	Older people desire to cut back or to stop working, which provides a mutual benefit to society because younger people are ready and willing to assume these roles.
	Activity Theory	This theory reflects the idea that older people can remain psychologically and socially fit if they remain physically active.
	Continuity Theory	A person's characteristics and coping strategies are in place long before old age occurs. How people age depends on how they adjust to changes throughout their life.
Psychological	Human Needs Theory	Uses Maslow's Hierarchy of Basic Needs. For example, safety and security needs must be met before self-actualization can occur.
Evolving	Evolutionary Theory	Evolutionary theories of aging and longevity try to explain the remarkable differences in observed aging rates and longevity records across different biological species.

Source: Based on American Academy of Anti-Aging Medicine (n.d). Theories of aging: retrieved http://www.longevity-and-antiaging-secrets.com/biological-theories-of-aging.html; Birklow, R., & Beers, M. H.(eds.). (2000). *Theories of aging. Merck Manual of Geriatrics.* Whitehouse Station, NJ: Merck Research Laboratories; Gavrilov, L. A., & Gavrilov, N. S. (2002). Evolutionary theories of aging and longevity. *Scientific World Journal, 2*, 339–356; retrieved from http://longevity-science.org/; Powell, J. L. (2005). *Social theory and aging.* Lanham, MD: Rowman and Littlefield.

PHYSICAL ASSESSMENT

Evaluation of a patient's health status requires a systematic approach to the collection of information. Having a solid understanding of age-related physiological changes aids in an accurate evaluation and assessment of the older adult. Comprehensive assessments that address possible functional and mental impairments in older patients are valuable in assuring improved health care outcomes and directing the focus of health promotion (Figure 13-6). Box 13-1 outlines the aspects that should be included in a comprehensive assessment to ensure a holistic approach to nursing the elderly patient.

It is entirely possible that a child born today may expect to live to age 100 or older. It's incredible to think of 60 or 70 as middle age. Since 1900, life expectancy has increased by 30 years, and, according to the U.S. Census Bureau (2006), more than 67,000 **centenarians** are alive today. That is more than double the number of people who were over the age of 100 in 1990 (Kestenbaum & Ferguson, 2006).

People should think of the years remaining in their healthy life span as an open bank account. Each time they exercise, eat nutritious foods, control stress, keep their weight in the normal range, keep regular appointments with their health care provider, and make room for additional types of health-promoting behavior, they are making a sizable deposit into their healthy

? ASK **YOURSELF**

Centenarians

Can you picture yourself celebrating your 100th birthday? Where would you be? Who would be with you? Are you interested in living into triple digits?

TABLE 13-5 Nursing Considerations and Health Promotion Tips for Age-Related Physical Changes

SYSTEM	AGE-RELATED CHANGES	NURSING CONSIDERATIONS	HEALTH-PROMOTION TIPS
Integument	Dry and scaly, decreased elasticity, increased wrinkles and thinning, decreased perspiration. Darker pigmentation spots from sun exposure.	Prone to skin breakdown. Alteration in thermoregularity. Lifelong exposure to sun increases risk for skin cancer.	Use a moisturizer. Drink plenty of water (skin becomes dry when dehydrated). Encourage the use of sunscreen. Decrease temperature on hot water heater to 120° F.
Eyes	Decreased visual acuity. Reduced adaptation to darkness and sensitivity to glare. Increased dryness.	May need corrective lenses. Caution should be exercised while driving. Vulnerable to infection.	Encourage annual eye exams and use of prescription sunglasses. Ask optometrist about the use of saline eye drops. Review driving tips for older adults (see Box 13-2).
Ears	Up to 30% of older persons have significant hearing loss.	Hearing loss may lead to social isolation.	Encourage routine hearing exams. Encourage use of hearing aids.
Nose	Decreased sensitivity to odors.	Potential safety hazard. May not be able to detect smoke or harmful odors.	Install smoke and carbon monoxide detectors strategically throughout the home.
Mouth	Drying of oral mucosa. Absence of teeth or ill-fitting dentures. Decreased sense of taste.	Changes can lead to difficulty chewing or pain that can lead to malnutrition.	Have a dental exam every six months. Ensure that dentures fit properly.
Respiratory	Reduced overall efficiency of oxygen exchange.	Increased susceptibility to infection.	Encourage the patient not to smoke. If patient smokes, provide support and strategies to quit.
Cardiovascular	Thickening of the wall of the left ventricle. Decreased cardiac output.	May have a decreased response to stress and a higher incidence of arrythmias.	Warning signs for heart attack may present differently in women than in men (i.e., women may have indigestion or pressure in the chest). Have cholesterol levels checked yearly, exercise regularly; eat a low-fat diet.
Gastrointestinal	Decreased salivary secretions, reduced intestinal motility.	Swallowing may become difficult. Increased incidence of constipation or hemorrhoids. Increased incidence of colon cancer.	Encourage drinking liquids with meals. Increase daily intake of water and fiber. Encourage elderly to have a yearly physical.
Genitourinary	Reduced renal mass. Decreased renal blood flow and functioning.	Drug dosages and administration may need to be altered due to excretion changes.	Encourage Kegel exercises. Encourage adequate fluid intake.
Reproductive	Women: decreased vaginal wall elasticity and vaginal wall thinning. Reduced lubrication during arousal state. Men: erectile dysfunction. Increased incidence of prostate cancer.	Potential for discomfort during intercourse. Potential for sexual dysfunction. Increased risk for sexually transmitted diseases.	Use a barrier method of contraception if there are multiple partners. Add a water-based lubricant to increase comfort during intercourse. After age 50, men should discuss testing for prostate cancer, this includes a PSA blood test and may or may not include a rectal exam (ACS, 2010).

SYSTEM	AGE-RELATED CHANGES	NURSING CONSIDERATIONS	HEALTH-PROMOTION TIPS
Musculoskeletal	Decreased muscle mass and strength. Bone demineralization. Decreased rate of autonomic reflexes.	Potential for injury related to decreased ROM and joint motion. May need to alter environment to ensure safety and decrease risks.	Encourage use of multivitamin with calcium or a calcium supplement. Exercise regularly.
Neurological	Decreased ability to respond to multiple stimuli. Insomnia.	Potential for injury. Potential alteration in pain response. Possible cognitive and memory changes.	Encourage elderly to implement recommendations for improving home safety.

Source: Based on: Seidel, H. M., Ball, J. W., Dains, J. E., Flynn, J. A., Solomon, B. S., & Stewart, R. W. (20-ii). *Mosby's guide to physical examination* (7th ed.). St. Louis, MO: Elsevier;. Goolsby, J., & Grubbs, L. (2006). *Advanced assessment: Interpreting findings and formulating differential diagnoses*. Philadelphia: F. A. Davis.

life span bank account. These deposits accrue benefits, just as money collects interest. These benefits become increasingly valuable as the years go by. Increased longevity makes attention to health-promotion and disease-prevention strategies for older adults even more important.

NUTRITION

The food consumed each day has a profound and sustained impact on overall health, aging processes, and longevity. Even though good nutrition is so important, it often becomes a progressively lower priority for seniors as they attempt to cope with the demands of daily life. Older people who now live alone sometimes pay little attention to meals or have no interest in

cooking for themselves. Inadequate nutrition among the elderly is not uncommon. Nutritional deficits can result from lack of intake of sources of protein, vitamins, and minerals. These nutritional deficits can result in malnutrition unfortunately, and it is very common for the signs and symptoms of malnutrition to mislead health care professionals. Weight loss, lightheadedness, disorientation, lethargy, and loss of appetite can be misdiagnosed as illness (Saka, et al., 2010).

A survey completed for the Nutrition Screening Initiative, targeted at improving the nutritional health status of older Americans, showed that, although 85% of seniors surveyed believe that

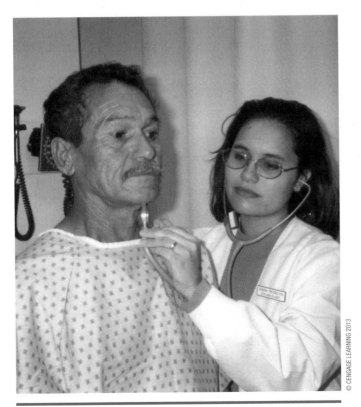

FIGURE 13-6 Comprehensive assessments are important for promoting health in the older adult.

BOX 13-1

COMPREHENSIVE ASSESSMENT FOR THE ELDERLY

A comprehensive assessment for the elderly should include all of the following in order to provide holistic care:

- Complete medical history
- Immunizations
- Vision screen
- Mental status
- Elimination patterns
- Socioeconomic status
- Activities of daily living
- Advance directives
- Sexual assessment
- Comprehensive physical exam
- Sleeping pattern disturbances
- Hearing screen
- Medications (prescription, OTCs, vitamins, herbs)
- Dental health
- Depression screen
- Nutritional status
- Social support systems
- Risk for falls

nutrition is important for their health and well-being, few act on these beliefs [American Academy of Family Physicians (AAFP), 2011]. Furthermore, many older adults frequently skip at least one meal a day. Sound nutrition is important in good health for people of all ages. In response to the prevailing lack of nutritional knowledge, the National Council on the Aging has joined forces with other organizations to promote the Nutrition Screening Initiative. The campaign was initiated to increase awareness not only in the older population but also in the health care community. Since this initiative, the Nutritional Screening tool has been used throughout the United States and other countries as a tool to identify elderly people 65 years and older to assess for risk of malnutrition; it is considered an initial step in the detection of malnutrition (Alvarenga et al., 2010).

Nurses encounter a complex challenge when encouraging older adults to eat well and pay serious attention to sound nutrition. There is no simple solution. As a matter of fact, the aging process itself becomes part of the problem. As many people age, they begin to lose lean body mass, which contributes to a decreased appetite. Consequently, interest in food tends to diminish and caloric intake decreases quickly, leading to nutritional deficiencies. This results in eating less, which quickly leads to deficiencies. Other barriers to eating well include a decline in the sense of smell and drying of the oral mucosa. Both of these age-related changes directly affect a person's ability to taste and enjoy food (Brownie, 2006).

In addition, social isolation can play a contributing role in the nutritional status of seniors. Elderly persons who are living alone and who are retired have less opportunity for social interaction related to food preparation and sharing a meal with another person. This can increase the risk for poor or insufficient nutritional intake (Brownie, 2006).

Financial concerns and loss of independent activities of daily living play a role in the nutritional status of the elderly. As people age, they may have a reduction in income as a result of retirement and cost-of-living increases. This can cause older persons to reduce their monthly expenditures, which may lead to a cut in their food budget. Lack of funds may lead older people to avoid perishable food items like fresh fruits, vegetables, or meat because of higher cost and possible waste. Additionally, as some people age, they may have not have a vehicle, be able to drive any longer, or have a reduced ability to negotiate public transportation resulting in their reliance on others to shop for them (Evans, 2005).

Many community-based and national programs assist the elderly with regard to nutrition. Meals on Wheels and food banks are the primary examples of these programs. These programs provide nutritional support for the elderly and provide an opportunity to socialize. For those who qualify, food stamps are also available. A one-person household can receive up to $155 a month, depending on individual income and living arrangements (Food Stamp Services, 2007).

Proper nutrition in later years can help lessen the effects of diseases prevalent among older Americans, or improve the quality of life for people who have such diseases. This includes osteoporosis, obesity, high blood pressure, heart disease, certain cancers, gastrointestinal problems, and chronic malnutrition. A nutritious diet in later years helps both in reducing the risk of these diseases and in managing their signs and symptoms. Proper nutrition contributes to a higher quality of life and enables older people to maintain their independence by continuing to perform basic daily activities. Poor nutrition, on the other hand, can prolong recovery from illness and lead to a poorer quality of life (Alvarenga et al., 2010). Therefore nurses

must incorporate a nutritional analysis as an integral part of the assessment of the elderly adult. After such an assessment (perhaps a 3-day dietary log or journal), the nurse can identify the underrepresented food group, advise patients accordingly, and offer education regarding available community resources.

FITNESS AND EXERCISE

The world is a dramatically different place for those people who are now 65 or older. Changes in the ways people live and work today may have been impossible to comprehend during the childhood of today's seniors. Scientific knowledge of the advantages of healthy nutrition and regular exercise is growing by leaps and bounds. Many elderly people are not aware of these advantages, and nurses can increase their patients' knowledge base. Research has revealed that only 47% of Americans age 50–79 exercise regularly (American Association of Retired Persons, 2002).

Nurses have an obligation to promote the benefits of exercise and its potential to extend quantity of life and improve quality of life. Additionally, nurses may have an even stronger influence through example, with their own physically active lifestyles.

The human body has remarkable capacity to repair itself, and habitual exercise and excellent nutrition enable it to perform even more efficiently. This is especially true for the lungs, heart, veins, arteries, and capillaries, as well as for the musculoskeletal system. Physical activity during midlife corresponds with maintenance of high physical function during early old age. Loss of physical function could be delayed by being physically active (Hillsdon et al., 2005). Recent studies indicate the importance of physical exercise in the elderly to slow down physical degeneration and improve quality of life (Brach et al., 2003). In the absence of exercise, fat displaces muscle, and the muscles begin to **atrophy** (become smaller and weaker). Many people, especially those who are older, feel that they are out of shape and have absolutely no hope of regaining their physical endurance. Health care professionals know this is not true. It is never too late to begin exercising, and one is never too old to benefit from physical activity.

Research indicates that the combination of weight training for strength; aerobics for strength and endurance; and calisthenics (stretching, moving, bending, twisting) for increased flexibility and balance have improved health benefits for older persons. Exercise may minimize physical frailty in the elderly and produce significant health benefits (Chandler & Studenski, 2010).

The WALC model is an example of an evidence-based nursing intervention that was created to enhance exercise self-efficacy in older adults. A study using this model found that using a walking program (Walk), paying attention to physical and psychological effects (Address sensations), gaining knowledge about exercise (Learn), and having exercise role models (Cues) helped older adults to begin and stay with an exercise program (Resnick, 2002).

Exercise intensity for aerobic conditioning is measured by heart rate. People who are not used to exercise should begin by getting medical clearance from a health care practitioner and be mindful of current health conditions; for instance, a person who suffers from low blood sugar should eat a light snack prior to exercising. The next step is to start slowly and find a type of exercise you like. One suggestion is to space exercising into short segments throughout the day. Finally, be alert to problems (AARP, 2010). If a patient's favorite exercise is not aerobics, suggest walking, swimming, or tai chi, or advise the patient to

HEALTH PROMOTION THEORY LINK

The Elderly, Exercise, and Pender's Health-Promotion Model

Pender's Health-Promotion Model includes theoretical propositions, one of which is that people are more likely to engage in behaviors that they anticipate as being personally beneficial (Rankin, Stallings, & London, 2005). This is a fundamental principle to keep in mind when promoting exercise in the elderly population. Health care professions need to individualize patient teaching and highlight how adopting an exercise regime may result in personal benefits. When people are able to understand how exercise can specifically benefit them and improve their health, they are more likely to adopt and adhere to an exercise regime.

go dancing. Dancing is often a perfect solution for those who habitually avoid exercise. A regular schedule of dancing 30–40 minutes 2–3 times a week can slow the heart rate, reduce blood pressure, improve cholesterol levels, and strengthen the cardiovascular system. Benefits include decreased blood pressure and improved function of all major organs. Sustained aerobic exercise can help control Type 2 diabetes mellitus because it improves insulin sensitivity and aids in the metabolism of glucose (American Diabetes Association, 2007).

SLEEP

Complaints of sleep disturbances rank high among problems reported by the elderly. In a study by Sukying, Bhokakul, and Udomsubpayakul (2003), insomnia was found in 46.3% of an elderly population. Even though older adults spend an increased amount of time in bed, they may have disruptive sleep patterns from a variety of causes that affect the quality of sleep.

Alterations in sleep may be referred to as **dysomnia**. The elderly suffer from these disturbances as a result of age-related and external influences. Anxiety and psychological factors, including **dementia**, depression, and sensory impairments, have been shown to affect the quality and quantity of sleep. Other impacts may include daytime boredom and a lack of social demands. Physiologic reasons such as pain, sleep apnea, periodic limb movements, pathology, altered circadian rhythm, and effects of medication, caffeine, and alcohol also have a strong influence on the elderly and sleep (Miller, 2009).

Commonly reported sleep disturbances are trouble getting to sleep, trouble staying asleep, and early morning awakenings. A combination of physiological, medical, psychiatric, psychosocial, and pharmacologic factors have been found to play a role in sleep disturbances reported in the elderly. Factors associated with sleep problems in the elderly are poor self-rated health, depression, pain, and polypharmacy (Blay, Andreoli, & Gastal, 2008). Health conditions more commonly found along with sleep disturbance include arthritis, incident angina pectoris, myocardial infarction or CHF, respiratory symptoms, and depression. Depression was the most important predictive factor associated with the presence of sleep disturbances (Quan et al., 2005).

Older adults take longer to fall asleep, awaken more easily and more often, and spend more time in the drowsiness stage rather than in deeper sleep referred to as rapid eye movement sleep (Miller, 2009). Disruptions are characterized by a decrease in the amount and amplitude of delta sleep compared to younger persons; in simple terms they spend more time in bed but not sleeping (Miller, 2009). Sleep problems in the elderly may also be explained by their frequent naps during the daytime.

Measures to promote healthier sleep habits should include but are not limited to the following recommendations:

1. Reassure the elderly that alterations in sleep patterns are normal.
2. Establish a bedtime ritual.
3. Avoid food, beverages, and medication that contain caffeine late in the day.
4. Avoid smoking cigarettes, or reduce evening smoking.
5. Avoid alcohol late in the day.
6. Drink milk or chamomile tea, and eat a light snack prior to bedtime.
7. Utilize relaxation methods.
8. Maintain a daily wake-sleep schedule.
9. Perform daily exercise.
10. Sleep in a low-stimulus, dark, cool environment (adapted from Miller, 2009).

Sleep patterns are an integral segment of any health assessment. Dysomnia may provide insight into a biological or emotional problem that may not otherwise be detected.

SEX

Sex and sexuality constitute a basic human need. However, this aspect of health promotion and health functioning is often overlooked in the elderly population by health care professionals, health researchers, and government policy agendas (Bouman, Arcelus, & Benbow, 2006). Sexuality is a multidimensional concept that is vital in a complete assessment of the elderly patient. Sexual expression and meeting sexual needs plays a part in an individual's feeling valuable as a respected human being (Watters & Boyd, 2009). Dysfunction in other areas of the physical domain may disrupt sex and sexuality in the elderly, but it does not obscure sexual desire or needs (Bauer, McAuliffe, & May, 2007). Sexuality in the elderly should encompass aspects of intimacy, love, warmth, sharing, and touching as depicted in Figure 13-7. These activities are meaningful for the well-being of the elderly (Nagaratnam & Gayagay, 2002).

? ASK YOURSELF

Seniors and Their Sex Lives

Should you discuss sex and sexuality with your elderly patients? Would you feel comfortable completing a sexual assessment on a patient over the age of 65?

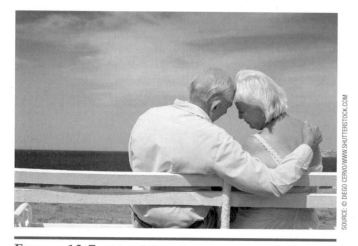

SOURCE © DIEGO CERVO/WWW.SHUTTERSTOCK.COM

FIGURE 13-7 Older adults still experience the need for companionship and intimacy.

Many elderly complain of a less than ideal sex life as well as touch deprivation. This may be a result of physiologic changes of aging. Some of these age-related changes, seen in Table 13-5, include decreased circulation to genitalia, decreased reflex impulses, decreased hormone levels, and alterations in the intactness of genitalia. Therefore, practitioners must incorporate a sexual assessment when doing a comprehensive holistic assessment of an elderly patient. If a patient is dissatisfied with his or her sexual performance, it may be due to medication or some other variable that the nurse may be able to identify. Many patients are willing to discuss issues of sex and sexuality with a health care provider but may be less willing if they sense fear or embarrassment on the part of the health care provider.

Viagra, followed by Cialis and Levitra, became the wonder drugs of the 1990s, creating a media flourish and, more important allowing topics such as erectile dysfunction and impotence to become part of mainstream conversation. Drugs such as these may help provide an erection or sustain an erection for elderly men who were unable to do so in the past. They have provided success and increased sexual satisfaction for a majority of the affected general population. However, health care providers must understand the benefits, side effects, and contraindications of these drugs (Mayo Clinic, 2006). They may be wonder drugs to some, but they may react with many seniors' medications and cause side effects such as headache, runny nose, upset stomach, and diarrhea.

In addition, health professionals must not neglect an awareness of alternative sexual orientations. Homosexuals comprise approximately 10% of the population and so also make up 10% of the elderly population. Many gay and lesbian seniors take a low profile because they were not able to come out in the past. They have suffered discrimination and rejection with 45% experiencing physical abuse and 75% suffering verbal abuse due to their sexual orientation (Heath, 2006). These seniors have families and health concerns common to many others in society. A study by Chamberland (2003) found that aging lesbians suffer social invisibility, which is a major obstacle to accessing health care services to their needs. Families are defined by those within that individual family unit, and therefore nurses must prevent themselves from passing their own judgment on their patients.

SPOTLIGHT **ON**

Alternative Treatment for Erectile Dysfunction

Research supports the effectiveness of traditional pharmacologic methods, such as Viagra, Cialis, and Levitra, in treating erectile dysfunction and validates that these drugs can also produce harmful side effects.

Some men may seek the use of natural supplements or treatments instead. Nutritional supplements such as the amino acid arginine, bioflavonoids, zinc, vitamin C, vitamin E, and flaxseed meal have been used to improve erectile function, as have two herbal supplements, Asian ginseng and ginkgo biloba. Acupuncture has also been known to be helpful. There is insufficient research, however, to support the use of nontraditional or alternative treatments. Future treatment for erectile dysfunction includes the development of oral medications with fewer or no side effects. Gene therapy also has potential in treating this disorder. Men considering the use of an alternative treatment should first seek the advice of their health care provider.

Source: From Erectile Dysfunction: Alternative Treatments. (n.d.). WebMD. Retrieved from http://www.webmd.com/erectile-dysfunction/guide/alternative-treatments-ed.

? ASK **YOURSELF**

AIDS and the Elderly

Should the elderly population be concerned about HIV/AIDS? Is HIV/AIDS something you should consider during your assessment of elderly patients? Should safe sex be added to your list of health-teaching topics with this population?

Human immunodeficiency virus (HIV) and acquired immunodeficiency syndrome (AIDS) in the elderly are an underestimated and unappreciated reality. HIV/AIDS is not exclusively a disease of youth, and it is commonly underreported in the elderly population. Diagnosing HIV/AIDS in older individuals is also complicated because the symptoms—night sweats, chronic fatigue, weight loss, dementia, and swollen lymph nodes—mimic the natural aging process (Anderson, 2005). In addition, the elderly are at a higher risk for contracting HIV/AIDS because they generally have a more compromised immune system. According to the Centers for Disease Control and Prevention, between 2000 and 2003, an estimated 78,118 persons age 55–64 were living with HIV/AIDS. The number of cases in the

65 and over population was estimated to be 21,239 (CDC, n.d.). Fourteen percent of all new AIDS cases are now in people older than 50 years (Janssen, 2005). HIV/AIDS must be considered a differential diagnosis with illness in the elderly, and proper support and education must be provided to prevent the associated depression and isolation. Most important, nurses have an obligation to teach safe sex practices regardless of age, lifestyle, or marital status as they would in any other adult population.

SOCIOECONOMIC DOMAIN

A person's socioeconomic level may affect all other domains pertaining to health promotion. A lower economic status is often related to a lower level of education and less ability to afford health care expenses. Awareness of a patient's socioeconomic status may change the focus of a nurse's health-promotion interventions.

POVERTY

In spite of significant gains in research, the chronic problem of poverty among the elderly remains a daunting challenge. Understanding that there are differences in poverty characteristics among ethnicities, genders, and across geographic locations increases the opportunities for nurses to assist impoverished older Americans. The number of people in poverty age 65 and older was 34 million in 2009. This number would quadruple if Social Security payments would be omitted from money income (DeNavas-Walt, Proctor, Smith, 2010). With regard to gender and ethnicity, statistics show that most elderly poor are women, and higher rates of poverty (7.9%) are found in elderly people of color (Cawthorne, 2008). Rural elderly have been found to have higher rates of poverty, limited transportation, and less access to necessary services. Other issues related to poverty in the elderly include delayed retirement, increased cost of health care, and higher expenditure on health care, utility costs, food insecurity, limited transportation, and predatory lending (Cawthorne, 2008).

Poverty creates a disparity that can severely diminish access to health care and health-promotion education. Nurses need to recognize that the impoverished elderly, as a subgroup of older Americans, have unique strengths as well as challenges in achieving optimal health. Health-promotion programs, including screenings and disease prevention, must be directed at all economic levels without bias.

EDUCATION

Educational levels are increasing in the older population. In 2008, 77% were high school graduates or more, and 21% had achieved a bachelor's degree or higher (Federal Interagency Forum on Age-Related Statistics, 2010). What is known is that people with higher levels of education tend to have a higher functional status and to engage in healthy productive behaviors later in life contributing to enhanced well-being at older ages. Low-income, less-educated, elderly are less likely to enjoy good health, and they have a higher incidence of smoking, obesity, and sedentary lifestyle. This same population is less likely to have health insurance and less likely to seek preventive care (Federal Interagency Forum on Age-Related Statistics, 2010).

Providing affordable or free screening opportunities such as mammograms, blood draws, and diabetic risk profiles allows for the early diagnosis and prevention of complications in an otherwise underserved population. In addition, health care providers must consider that living at poverty level may make compliance with treatment impossible. A simple example of this is the diabetic patient who may not have electricity to operate a refrigerator to cool his insulin. With education levels of the elderly rising, such problems may be decreasing, but they remain valid concerns for health care providers. This is why it is essential for nurses to include socioeconomic status and barriers to health care or health maintenance when assessing the older adult.

HEALTH CARE EXPENDITURES

Between 1998 and 2008, the total percentage of health care expenditures doubled from $1 trillion to $2 trillion. The elderly had the highest rates of emergency room visits (24.9%) in 2009 and the highest use of prescription drugs (90.1%) between 2005 and 2008 (National Center for Health Statistics, 2010).

There has been a significant increase in health care costs incurred by older Americans between 1992 and 2006, with higher costs directly related to increased age. In older Americans, hospital (25%) and physician (35%) services account for the greatest health care costs, followed by prescription drugs (16%) and long-term care facilities (13%) in 2006. Out-of-pocket spending for health care services in older adults increased the most among those in the poor/near poor income category from 12% to 28% between 1977 and 2006. In 2006, more than half of the out-of-pocket spending among persons aged 65 and older was for prescription drugs (Federal Interagency Forum on Aging-Related Statistics, 2010).

Chronic health conditions, hospital stays, and work absences lead to increases in health care expenditures and, in turn, to personal financial loss and a drain on the Medicare system. Prevention costs less than treatment. Therefore, the prevention of complications from chronic disease and the prevention of new disease states can lessen the financial burden. Nurses must encourage annual exams, wellness screening, and healthy lifestyles in the elderly patient.

PSYCHOLOGICAL DOMAIN

Influences within the psychological domain include depression, stress and coping, and issues of abuse. Each of these has a great impact on learning and maintaining healthy behaviors.

DEPRESSION

Depression can occur during any stage of life, but the changes that occur to older people may increase their risk for depression. Some common changes that occur in the elderly population are the loss of loved ones, coping with physical and mental changes, illness, and social isolation. Accurately assessing and treating depression in the elderly is a challenge.

The percentage of people aged 65 or older reporting clinically relevant symptoms of depression was 12% for men and 19% for women in 2006 (Federal Interagency Forum on Aging-Related Statistics, 2010). Sadly, only a small fraction of these are accurately diagnosed and treated (Shear, Roose, Lenze, & Alexopoulos, 2005). Reasons for the lack of identification and treatment in late life include atypical symptoms, body system symptoms, apathetic affect, misrepresentation of the problem, **ageism** among health professionals, and stigma among older adults (to, 2005). It is important to screen for and treat depression in the elderly to prevent self-neglect and to have positivee effects on quality of life (Tanner, 2005). The Geriatric Depression Scale, consisting of 12–15 items, has been the most widely used to assess for depression among the elderly (Holroyd & Clayton, 2002). A short form of this screening tool is available in English, Spanish, and the original translated Latin American Spanish version.

STRESS

Stress is a fact of life for each developmental stage. The elderly, however, have some unique factors that may add to stress and influence coping—specifically, the individual's meaning of life, and his or her collection of life experiences, timing, and anticipation of life events, particularly the death of friends and family. Reactions and coping styles may also be influenced by financial resources, social support, social status, spirituality, and connection with organized religion (Miller, 2009). Stress is viewed as having potential for both positive and negative influences on human behavior. **Eustress** refers to the positive stress that mobilizes us to action. Health teaching and screening are examples of this eustress, which motivates healthier behavior. In addition, many negative stressors accompany the aging process.

When assessing the elderly patient for stress level and stressors, offer creative and individualized stress-reduction techniques. Activities that can reduce stress include but are not limited to the following:

- Physical activity (swimming, dancing)
- Socializing
- Owning a pet
- Listening to music
- Volunteering
- Talking on the phone
- Reading
- Making crafts
- Participating in an organized religion

Complementary modalities, such as massage, healing touch, meditation, guided imagery, and aromatherapy, are other options for reducing and managing stress in older patients. Figure 13-8 depicts a quiet moment in a chapel, which may reduce stress.

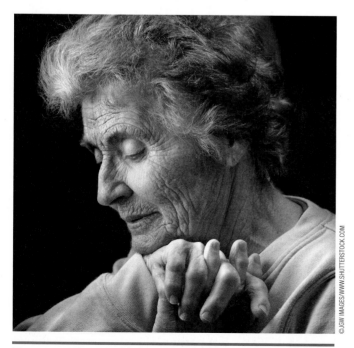

FIGURE 13-8 **Spirituality can help older adults reduce stress.**

ELDER ABUSE

Elder abuse is any knowing, intended, or careless act that causes harm or serious risk of harm to an older person, whether it is physical, mental, emotional, or financial. The term is quite broad and encompasses many different types of mistreatment. No one knows exactly how many elders are victims of abuse, but evidence suggests that many thousands have been harmed. Conservative estimates for the

RESEARCH NOTE

Understanding Elder Abuse

STUDY PROBLEM/PURPOSE

The purpose of this study was to examine factors that influence the identification and assessment of abuse in the elderly.

METHODS

Two hundred thirty-nine participants, aged 18–55, were randomly assigned to review one of four case scenarios. The scenarios were designed to examine the participants' views on elder abuse, acceptability, and justifiability. Because these views contribute to one's perception, they were combined with the administration of perceptions of abuse scale. Additional questions that were asked of the participants were (1) how likely the participant would be to report the actions in the scenarios and (2) whether their own parents had ever cared for an elderly family member.

FINDINGS

The data revealed that the quality of the relationship between caregiver and elder correlates with the perceived level of abuse. If the quality of the relationship is perceived to be poor or difficult, the perception of abuse increased. Conversely, if the relationship is perceived to be supportive and loving, the perception of abuse decreased. Similar findings related to the likelihood of reporting. If the relationship was perceived to be difficult, there was a greater response in the likelihood to report than if the relationship was perceived to be loving. Participants who had experience with caregiving revealed a greater level of sensitivity toward abuse in the elderly population.

IMPLICATIONS

The quality of the relationship abuse that is perceived as out of the norm in a typically loving relationship is less likely to be viewed as abuse or reported as such. Health care workers need to be aware that the perception of and likelihood of reporting of elder abuse can be altered based on the perception of the relationship between caregiver and elder.

Source: Fitzpatrick, M. J., & Hamill, S. B. (2011). Elder abuse: Factors related to perceptions of severity and likelihood of reporting. *Journal of Elder Abuse and Neglect, 23*,1–16. DOI: 10.1080/089465666.2011.534704.

TABLE 13-6 Recognizing Abuse of Older Adults

SIGNS AND SYMPTOMS OF MALTREATMENT OF OLDER ADULTS INCLUDE, BUT ARE NOT LIMITED TO, THE FOLLOWING.

Physical abuse
- Unexplained injuries
- Frequent visits to the emergency department for treatment of traumatic injuries
- Untreated injuries in various stages of healing
- Broken eyeglasses/frames
- Loss of patches of hair, pulling of hair
- Signs of being restrained, including rope marks
- Laboratory findings of medication overdose or underutilization of prescribed drugs
- Elder's report of being hit, slapped, kicked, or mistreated
- Elder's refusal to disrobe for bath; trying to hide injuries
- Caregiver's refusal to allow visitors to see an elder alone

Sexual abuse
- Bruising around the breasts or genitalia
- Unexplained venereal disease or genital infections
- Unexplained vaginal or anal bleeding; torn, stained, or bloody underclothing
- Elder's report of being sexually assaulted or raped

Emotional/psychological abuse
- Emotionally upset or agitated; paranoid
- Extremely withdrawn and noncommunicative or nonresponsive; depressed
- Unusual behavior usually attributed to dementia (e.g., sucking, biting, rocking)
- Elder's report of being verbally or emotionally mistreated

Psychological neglect
- Dehydration or malnutrition
- Untreated health problems
- Poor personal hygiene
- Hazardous or unsafe living environment (e.g., improper wiring, no heat, or no running water)

- Unsanitary living environment (e.g., dirt, fleas, lice on person, soiled bedding, fecal/urine smell, inadequate clothing)
- Social isolation
- Low self-esteem
- Elder's report of being mistreated

Financial or material exploitation
- Sudden changes in bank account or banking
- Unauthorized withdrawal of the elder's funds
- Abrupt changes in a will or other financial documents
- Substandard care or living though adequate financial resources are available
- Elder's signature being forged for financial transactions
- Sudden appearance of previously uninvolved relatives claiming rights to an elder's affairs and possessions
- Purchase of services or supplies that are not indicated
- Elder's report of financial exploitation

Self-neglect
- Dehydration or malnutrition
- Untreated health problems
- Poor personal hygiene
- Hazardous or unsafe living environment (e.g., improper wiring, no heat, or no running water, animal/insect infestation, no functioning toilet, fecal/urine smell)
- Unsanitary living environment (e.g., dirt, fleas, lice on person, soiled bedding, fecal/urine smell)
- Inadequate or inappropriate clothing
- Social isolation
- Lack of the necessary health aids (e.g., eyeglasses, hearing aids, dentures)
- Grossly inadequate housing or homelessness

Source: Adapted from National Center on Elder Abuse (2005a, June). 15 Questions & Answers About Elder Abuse, retrieved, from http://www.scribd.com/doc/38961554/15-Questions-Answers-About-Elder-Abuse; National Center on Elder Abuse (2005b). Types of elder abuse in domestic settings. Elder Abuse Information Series No. 1, retrieved from http://www.elderabusecenter.org/default.cfm?p=statistics.cfm

United States put the number of elders who have been injured, exploited, or otherwise mistreated at about 1–2 million (National Center on Elder Abuse, 2005a). This number is conservative; recent research suggests that only one in 14 domestic elder abuse incidents come to the attention of the authorities (National Center on Elder Abuse, 2005b).

The identification of potential victims and abusers may result as knowledge is gained and as society becomes more aware of the growing problem of elder abuse. Table 13-6 highlights specific signs of elder abuse. Health care professionals need to be able to detect signs of elder abuse and take appropriate and immediate actions.

The physically and psychologically debilitated of any age are especially vulnerable to abuse. Perhaps even more important than identification of abuse is to take a more proactive stance aimed at preventing its development in the first place. The responsibility of caring for any chronically ill person can

become burdensome. Health care professionals, for example, can teach families and caregivers helpful techniques to relieve the stresses that often accompany caring for those with multiple needs.

Understanding the physical, cognitive, social, and economic problems that elderly people face can help focus teaching on promoting their health and alleviating their abuse. The study described in the accompanying Research Note was designed to improve understanding and awareness of the prevalent and increasing problem of elder abuse.

SPIRITUAL DOMAIN

Spirituality is often overlooked as an important dimension for health and well-being. To truly promote health in the holistic sense, facilitating health of the mind and the body is incomplete without facilitating the health of the human spirit. Many people look upon spirituality or religion as a resource for coping or stress reduction. There is considerable research linking prayer and/or belief in a higher power with increased health and healing (Parachin, 2011).

The National Interfaith Coalition on Aging suggests that relationships and friendships can encourage the deepening of spiritual life in the contexts of congregation and community. Close personal ties across the life span may help people find meaning and purpose in their lives and may enable the elderly to maintain independence and cope with change and loss (NICA, 2004). Having had a lifetime of experiences on which to reflect, the older adult has the opportunity to harmoniously connect personal beliefs, faith, and hope with life. This becomes very important in progressing successfully through Erikson's final stage of development, ego integrity versus despair.

Many elderly use a variety of spiritual sources to cope with the stressors of everyday life and respond to illness, the death of loved ones, and anticipation of their own death. Spiritual groups or associations within organized religions may provide an excellent arena for socialization. Additionally, many organized religions offer wellness or health-promotion programs such as weight reduction programs. They offer social and emotional support essential to coping and provide incentive to participate in healthy group activities.

To guide nurses in identifying spiritual needs, the North American Nursing Diagnoses Association (2007–2008) identified two diagnoses related to spirituality: (1) spiritual distress and (2) potential for enhanced **spiritual well-being**. If an elderly patient seems distressed, or is not a part of a spiritual group, or does not see him- or herself as spiritual, the potential for enhanced spiritual well-being could be explored.

CULTURAL DOMAIN

Incorporating cultural considerations is imperative in providing individualized and holistic nursing care for all patients. Population trends and ethnicity related to older adults presented earlier in this chapter highlight a corresponding increase in diversity. In 2008, approximately 19% of persons greater than 65 years of age were members of minorities; by 2050, the older minority population is expected to increase to 20% in Hispanic, 12% in Black, and 9% in Asian populations Among the minority groups, the Hispanic population is projected to grow the fastest, reaching 17.5 million in 2050, from 3 million in 2008 (Federal Interagency Forum on Aging-Related Statistics, 2010).

The increase in elder minorities is accompanied by challenges that create opportunities for health promotion. These challenges are based on the knowledge that the older population at risk for chronic conditions will become more diverse; that disparities exist among ethnicities regarding access to health care; and that literacy, language, and communication problems affect comprehension and adherence to health teaching (Georgetown University, 2004, 2005).

Considering the patient's culture helps the nurse understand the patient's values, attitudes, and behaviors, which also helps to eliminate stereotyping and biases that would undermine health-promotion efforts. Miller (2009) has suggested that nurses perform a cultural self-assessment to gain insight into their own feelings regarding culture and older patients. Nurses who can focus on their own cultural identity and on how that identity influences their attitude toward older adults from diverse cultures and health practices enhance their ability to provide culturally competent care, as discussed in Chapter 6.

ENVIRONMENTAL DOMAIN

Many environmental factors may contribute to, or hinder an elderly patient from, initiating or maintaining a healthy lifestyle. Understanding more about your patient's activities is important when planning health promotion for their safety and enjoyment. The health-promotion focus for this environmental domain is safety on the road, at home, in the use of medications, with respect to health care services and facilities, and disaster preparedness.

SAFETY IN DRIVING

Access to friends, families, employment, shopping, personal care, cultural enrichment, and religious expression depends on one's ability to move from one location to another. A high level of mobility means easy access to choice and opportunity, which can lead to self-fulfillment and enrichment. Low levels of mobility often mean isolation, depression, and social impoverishment.

The rapid growth of our aging population presents special transportation challenges. When people with diminishing capabilities continue to drive, this creates increased safety risks for all members of society. Yet older Americans have grown up in a culture that depends on the ability to drive, and the loss of this option may present a major life crisis.

ASK **YOURSELF**

Elderly Drivers

How do you feel about elderly drivers? Should older adult drivers have mandatory testing to determine whether they are competent to drive?

As the U.S. population ages, a significantly great number of older drivers will be on the road. It is estimated that there will be more than 40 million licensed drivers over the age of 65 by the year 2020 (Dellinger, Langlois, & Li, 2002). The National Highway Traffic Safety Administration (2008) reported that older drivers account for 15% of all traffic fatalities and 14% of all vehicle occupant fatalities. Statistics show that over 80% of traffic fatalities involving older drivers occur during the daytime and that over 72% occur on weekdays (NHTSA, 2008).

Many national and international organizations have developed suggestions to help compensate for the aging effects on driving. Everyone ages differently, so some people are perfectly capable of continuing to drive in their 70s, 80s, and even beyond. Many older adults, however, are at higher risk for road accidents due to loss of hearing acuity, loss of visual acuity, chronic diseases, physical impairment, and medications. When working with elderly patients, it is imperative to assess whether they drive. Box 13-2 suggests driving tips for the elderly that can help accommodate for age-related physical changes. These driving tips can increase the confidence of the driver, make driving less stressful, and make the roads safer for everyone.

<table>
<tr><td>

BOX 13-2

DRIVING TIPS FOR OLDER ADULTS

1. Limit driving to daytime hours if seeing or driving at night is a problem.
2. Turn the head frequently to compensate for diminished peripheral vision.
3. Add a larger rearview mirror.
4. Limit distractions.
5. Keep fit. Physical activity is needed to keep a person strong and flexible for the quick reactions that are needed for driving.
6. Avoid driving for a few days after the start of new medication. Side effects of medication can worsen after a couple of days.
7. If medication causes sleepiness or disorientation, *don't drive.*
8. Attend a driver refresher course for the elderly.
9. Avoid texting or talking on a cell phone while driving.

</td><td>

BOX 13-3

NURSING TEACHING TIPS: SAFETY IN THE HOME

- Ensure that fire detectors and carbon monoxide detectors are in working condition.
- Clear front and back walkways of clutter, snow, and ice.
- Ensure that all entrances inside and out are well maintained.
- Keep flashlights or battery-operated lights handy throughout the house.
- Get to know the neighbors if not already acquainted.
- Consider placing a phone in the bedroom and bathroom.
- Remove scatter rugs.

When using the stairs:
- Provide enough lighting to see steps clearly, and keep them free of clutter.
- Cover stairs with a nonslip surface such as tightly woven carpet.
- Install sturdy handrails on both sides of the stairs.

In the kitchen:
- Avoid climbing and reaching to high shelves.
- Use a stable step stool with handrails, if climbing is necessary.
- Arrange storage at counter level.
- Clean spills as soon as they happen.
- Don't wax floors.

In the bathroom:
- Keep a night light on.
- Use rugs with nonskid backing.
- Install handrails in the bathtub and toilet areas.

</td></tr>
</table>

SAFETY AT HOME

A majority of older Americans are active members of their families and communities and relish the independence of living in their own homes. In many cases, their home is the place where they raised their children and enjoyed the happiest years of their lives. Millions of other seniors, however, are at risk of losing their independence, including 4 million Americans age 85 and older. Many of these people live alone and have no immediate family nearby to give them assistance.

The Centers for Disease Control and Prevention (CDC, 2006) has stated that falls in the home are the leading cause of fatal and nonfatal injuries to people 65 and older. It is predicted that 30% of people 65 or older will fall each year. In fact, statistics suggest that falls led to emergency room visits for an estimated 1.8 million Americans age 65 or older in 2000 (CDC, 2006). Box 13-3 lists important recommendations to keep in mind when teaching the elderly, their caregivers, and their families about home safety.

One way to reduce falls in the home is by modifying homes in order to eliminate or abate common hazards for older persons. Using a relatively new concept known as universal design, AARP (n.d.) advocates for a home that is architecturally designed to allow people to stay in it at any age. As the nation grows older at a record pace, this feature will be increasingly important. The house has step-free front and garage entrances. It features nonslip tile, extra wide doorways and showers, and a barrier-free design. Although people often refer to the safety of home, the home poses many opportunities for injury. Therefore, nurses must promote safety in the home.

A monitoring device can be a helpful safety feature for older adults who live alone. These devices are transmitters that can be worn hanging around the neck or wrist and can even be worn while bathing in a tub or shower. They are connected remotely via telephone service to a 24-hour monitoring center that will know the wearer is in trouble within seconds of pushing a button on the transmitter. Many transmitters have an open voice channel for communication with the elderly person.

MEDICATIONS AND THE ELDERLY

The geriatric population consumes approximately 25% of all medications produced. Approximately 70% of over-the-counter medications are used by people over the age of 65 (Thompson, 2005). The use of multiple medications is called **polypharmacy**. Some elderly people take as many as 15 different medications a day. The risk of drug interaction directly corresponds with the number of drugs being taken. As an example, an elderly person taking five medications has a 50% chance of a drug interaction, and when the number increases to eight medications, there is a 100% chance of a drug interaction (Thompson, 2005). Box 13-4 lists 10 risk questions, any one of which can lead to polypharmacy. It is essential to improve problem-solving abilities in the clinical setting by understanding an elderly patient's medications, including herbal and other nonprescription drugs. Teach elderly patients about their medications, when to take them, how to take them, what the medication is expected to do, and

SPOTLIGHT ON

Facts about Falls, Hip Fractures, and Older Adults

Falls account for 90% of the more than 352,000 hip fractures in the United States each year. It is estimated that by 2050, there will be 1,800 hip fractures daily and 650,000 hip fractures yearly. Hip fractures occur 2–3 times more in women than men. One of every seven White, postmenopausal women will have a hip fracture. Taller women, 5 ft, 8 in. or more, have twice the risk of those under 5 ft, 2 in. Almost half of all women who reach age 90 have suffered a hip fracture. Twenty-five percent of those with hip fracture have a full recovery, and 24% of those over the age of 50 will die within 12 months due to complications. Approximately 220,000 total hip replacements were performed in the United States in 2003. Increased risk factors of an adverse outcome of the surgery include advanced age, male gender, Black race, existing health problems, and a low income.

Source: Adapted from D'Angelo, K., Murena, L., & Cheribino, P. (2008). The unstable total hip replacement. *Indian Journal of Orthopeadics, 42,* 252–259.

BOX 13-5

MEDICATION GUIDELINES FOR THE ELDERLY PATIENT

The following guidelines are helpful for all who take medications and are especially important for older individuals.

1. Know the names of all medications, what they are for, and when to take them.
2. Keep a current medication list with you at all times (sample list, see Table 13-7).
3. Wear a medical alert bracelet for allergies or a chronic health condition.
4. Follow the exact instructions provided by your doctor or nurse practitioner.
5. Never stop taking a medication on your own. Contact your doctor or nurse practitioner first.
6. Have prescriptions filled in advance to prevent running out.
7. Choose over-the-counter (OTC) medications that have only the ingredients you need.
8. Use OTC medication as directed on the label.
9. Keep medications out of the reach of small children.
10. Take only your own medications. Never take medications that have been prescribed for someone else, and never offer your medications to another person.

BOX 13-4

POLYPHARMACY RISK ASSESSMENT QUESTIONS

- Do you take five or more prescription medications?
- Do you take dietary supplements, vitamins, or over-the-counter medications?
- Do you take homeopathic or herbal remedies?
- Do you get your prescription filled at more than one pharmacy?
- Is more than one doctor prescribing your medications?
- Do you take your medications more than once a day?
- Do you have trouble opening your medication bottles?
- Do you have poor eyesight or hearing?
- Do you live alone?
- Do you have a hard time remembering to take your medications?

Source: Based on Peterson, E. A. (2003). Are you at risk for polypharmacy? Health Alliance Plan. Retrieved from http://www.hap.org/info/formulary/polypharmacy_risk.php

potential side effects. Box 13-5 offers additional guidelines to teach the elderly about their medications. Additionally, nurses will want to teach elderly patients to keep a current medication list with them at all times. Keeping an accurate medication record provides many benefits for the elderly patient. It provides a quick, easy reference when meeting with the health care worker and is easier than carrying all of the medication bottles. It may prevent the possibility of duplicate or contraindicated prescriptions from being ordered. Most important, a medication record empowers the elderly by involving them in their own care. Table 13-7 provides a sample medication record.

SAFETY AND ASSISTED LIVING FACILITIES

An **assisted living facility (ALF)** is designed to provide a special combination of personalized care, supportive services, and health-related services for care of the elderly. There are thousands of ALFs in communities across the United States with such names as residential care facility, community-based retirement facility, personal care facility, adult living facility, adult foster care, adult homes, congregate care, supportive care, enhanced care, and elder care facility. Although the types of services and levels of care vary, most facilities provide assistance with bathing, dressing, grooming, personal hygiene, ambulating, and monitoring of medications and dietary intake.

TABLE 13-7 Sample Current Medication List for Elderly Patients

Note: Include all prescription medications, over-the-counter medications, vitamins, minerals, and herbal remedies.
Important: Have all medications reviewed annually by your primary physician.

Name of Patient Carl Daniels   Allergies Penicillin

MEDICATION NAME	DOSAGE	DOSAGE SCHEDULE	PRESCRIBING DOCTOR OR NURSE PRACTITIONER AND SPECIALTY	PURPOSE	SIDE EFFECTS (IF ANY)
Lasix	20 mg (1 tab) twice per day	Take 1 tab at 8:00 a.m. & 1 at 2:00 p.m.	Dr. Brown (cardiologist)	Hypertension	Dizziness, blurred vision, urinary frequency, low blood pressure
Lipitor	10 mg (1 tab) once per day	Take 1 tab at 8 a.m.	Dr. Brown	Lower Cholesterol	Fatigue, muscle and joint pain, diarrhea, urinary tract infection, nausea, insomnia
Ibuprofen	400 mg (2 tabs) twice per day as needed		Beverly Kline (family nurse practitioner)	Joint pain	Nausea, diarrhea, constipation, nose bleed, headache, dizziness, sensitivity to light
Chamomile	Tea bags	As desired	Self prescribed	Indigestion	Drowsiness, rash, stomach irritation

© Cengage Learning 2013

Additionally, meals, transportation, laundry, and housekeeping are usually provided; however, the amount of health care provided varies widely among facilities.

With no common definition, operations of ALFs range from residential retirement homes to nursing homes. Each state has a different set of regulations governing its ALFs, and most, but not all, require some type of licensure, certification, or both. Although nursing homes must operate under strict federal regulation, inconsistency in regulating ALFs has created issues of safety for residents. Having adequate and qualified staff to provide care and to supervise residents is one major area of concern. Some ALFs accept those who are severely ill and who require skilled personnel to prevent development of pressure sores and complications associated with feeding and elimination. ALFs that do not accept severely ill patients must still have adequate personnel to supervise residents who, for example, might have wandering tendencies that could result in tragedy.

The following common criteria have been suggested for state law that would preclude a person's admission to assisted living facilities (Downey, 2004). A person would be excluded if he or she:

- Is a threat to self or others
- Has a contagious or infectious disease
- Requires care beyond the facilities' skill
- Requires physical or chemical restraints or both
- Requires 24-hour nursing or other care
- Is bedridden
- Requires specialized long-term care
- Has stage III/or IV pressure sores or both
- Requires more than minimal assistance in moving to a safe area during an emergency
- Is less than 18 years old
- Requires help with tube feeding

Choosing a quality care facility that is also safe and affordable is an important decision for older persons and their family members. Location or setting, cost, types and extent of services, condition of the other residents, the reputation of the managing company, and the rights of residents are all important considerations. Before making a decision, visit several facilities, talk to the staff, talk to residents, ask to have a meal at mealtime, and check for reviews or comments on the Internet.

In an effort to enhance the safety of older persons living in ALFs, the Joint Commission on Accreditation of Healthcare Organizations (JCAHO) has delineated goals and actions to achieve the goals (Table 13-8).

Goals for the health promotion of older individuals are based on risk assessment. Table 13-9 provides selected risks for older adults arranged according to related domains. Suggested health-promotion actions are provided as a guide.

ELDERLY AND DISASTER PREPAREDNESS

An area in need of more attention to address and promote the well-being of older adults is disaster response and preparedness. The elderly are highly susceptible to the untoward effects of disasters due to several unique characteristics. Three identified issues that increase the vulnerability of the elderly affected by disaster situations are poverty, chronic health conditions, and depression (Evans, 2010). As noted, a great number of older adults are living in poverty, which compromises their ability to prepare for, respond to, repair, and recover after a disaster. Chronic conditions and long-term illness among the elderly place them at further vulnerability during a disaster. Individuals with chronic illness encounter diminishing health as a result of experiencing a disaster. The elderly with preexisting cardiovascular disease, diabetes mellitus, and respiratory diseases show greater deterioration following a disaster

TABLE 13-8 The 2007 Assisted Living National Patient Safety Goals

GOAL	ACTION
Correctly identify residents.	• Use at least two resident identifiers when providing care treatment or services such as the resident's name and date of birth. • Prior to the start of any invasive procedure, conduct a final verification process to confirm the correct patient, procedure, site, and availability of appropriate documents. This verification process uses active—not passive—communication techniques.
Reduce the possibility of harm associated with anticoagulant therapy	• Use unit-dose, prefilled, or premixed types of products when available. • Use approved protocols for initiation and maintenance of anticoagulant therapy. • Establish the resident' baseline coagulation status through laboratory testing or risk factors including age, weight, bleeding tendency, and genetic factors. • Consult resources to manage potential food and drug interactions. • Use programmable pumps for continuously administered heparin.
Use evidence-based practice to prevent central line-associated bloodstream infections.	• Educate staff when hired and annually thereafter about central line-associated infections and prevention. • Use standardized protocol to disinfect catheter hubs and injection ports before accessing ports. • Establish a routine evaluation of central venous catheters and remove all nonessential venous catheters.
Accurately and completely reconcile medications across the continuum of care.	• There is a process for comparing the resident's current medications with those ordered for the resident while under the care of the organization. • A complete list of the resident's medications is communicated to the next provider of service when a patient is referred or transferred to another setting, service, practitioner, or level of care within or outside the organization. The complete list is provided to the resident or family member upon discharge.
Reduce the risk of resident harm resulting from falls.	• Assess each resident's risk for fall. • Implement Interventions to reduce the potential for fall. • Implement a program to include assessment, interventions, and education to with outcome indicators to decrease the number of falls and severity of fall-related Injuries.
Assess, reassess, and act to address each resident's risk for pressure ulcer development.	• Develop a plan to identify and prevent pressure ulcers. • Conduct an initial assessment of each resident and a systematic risk assessment/reassessment using a validated assessment tool such as the Braden Scale or Norton Scale. • Take action to prevent and educate staff.

Source: Based on Joint Commission on Accreditation of Healthcare Organizations (JCAHO). (2011). National Patient Safety Goals Effective July 1, 2011. Retrieved from http://www.jointcommission.org/assets/1/6/NPSG_EPs_Scoring_LTC_20110707.pdf NewsRoom/NewsReleases/nr_npsg_al.htm

(Evans, 2010). Along with physical complications, cognitive and emotional distress is found to occur. Stress, anxiety, emotional exhaustion, and depression are present to a greater degree in the older adult (Evans, 2010). Inversely, practitioners must remember that the elderly have inherent strengths during disasters. The ability to demonstrate resilience and leadership during a crisis places them as a great resource in disaster situations (Deeny et al., 2010). Older adults have been found to identify some disaster preparedness tasks and believe they have the ability to prepare accordingly. They have also expressed mistrust in the ability of the government to aid them during disasters (Duggan et al., 2010). The voice of the elderly must be heard in preparation for disasters and valued as a potential resource in disaster preparedness (Duggan et al., 2010). Acknowledging the complexities of issues related to older adults and disasters, conducting age-specific needs assessments, and integrating the ideas in the planning aspect make for a start in addressing this issue.

TABLE 13-9 Risk Assessment for the Older Adult

RELATED DOMAIN	RISK ASSESSMENT	HEALTH-PROMOTION ACTION
Physical	Nutrition	Recommend a daily caloric intake of 1,600–2,000 for females and 2,000–2,800 for males depending on activity, health status, and metabolism. Consume extra vitamin B_{12} and vitamin D in fortified foods. Daily intake should include 25 g of fiber, < 30% of total calories from fat, 5–6 servings of vegetables and fruits, 6–11 servings of whole grains, breads, and pasta, limited consumption (2–3 servings) of red meat, poultry, eggs, and dairy products.
Physical	Exercise	Advise to stretch every day. Engage in consistent exercise, such as walking or swimming, 30 minutes each time 3–5 times per week. Pay special attention to safety measures and general health maintenance.
Physical Psychological	Tobacco avoidance	Assess use of tobacco, interest in cessation, and, if applicable, provide tobacco cessation counseling on a regular basis. Advise the use of pharmacological as well as behavioral interventions for smoking cessation.
Physical Environmental Psychological	Injury prevention	Counseling regarding safety in the home and while driving. Assess individuals for high risk regarding alcohol and substance use. Evaluate all medications for adverse interactions. Assess for abuse.
Physical	Immunizations	Counseling and intervention regarding the obtaining and maintenance of immunizations, including boosters for tetanus and diphtheria. The primary series should be completed for those who have not completed it. Hepatitis and influenza immunizations should be obtained.
Psychological Sociological Spiritual Physical	Stress and mental health issues	Assess for risk factors for depression or other mental health problems, including suicidal ideation. Counsel regarding prevention or management of depression or both. Discuss preferences on limits of medical interventions and other advance planning needs.
Physical	Oral and skin care	Advise regular annual dental care and daily care of teeth, dentures, or dental appliances. Report any signs of gum disease. Report any changes in skin condition or appearances of lesions.
Sexual/Gender Sociological	Sexuality	Provide counseling about risk factors for HIV and other sexually transmitted infections and about measures to reduce risk.

© Cengage Learning 2013

SUMMARY

Individual development through the stages of the life cycle requires both individual initiative and an enabling environment. An emphasis on wellness is an integral part of many health-promotion programs for all age groups. Health-promotion programs throughout the nation provide a necessary community link with resources and support for acute and chronic disease, and they reassure the elderly with regard to expected age-related changes.

Throughout the nation, wellness programs are in keeping with the agenda of *Healthy People 2020*, whose goal is to "improve the health, function, and quality of life of older adults." This goal is consistent with the goals nurses have for health promotion in the elderly.

The future brings a challenging vision for the health of the aging population. Persons age 65 and older constitute the fastest-growing population worldwide. This unprecedented societal trend places a heavy demand on professionals throughout the health care field. Health care professionals need to become knowledgeable about the developmental tasks and physical changes specific to this age group. Additionally, health care providers must be well informed about programs and resources that exist for health promotion in this population. Older adults should be given every opportunity to age in good health. Healthier aging will contribute to a healthier society.

CASE STUDY

Beatrice Hernandez: Activity Intolerance, Sleep Pattern Disturbance, and Depression

OBJECTIVES/GOALS: Through participation in a discussion of this case study, participants will have the opportunity to:

1. Discuss factors contributing to activity intolerance, sleep pattern disturbance, and depression in an elderly female patient.
2. Identify health risks related to the biological, psychological, cultural, and spiritual domains.
3. Explore health-promotion interventions in increasing exercise and sleep in an elderly female patient.

HEALTH-PROMOTION CONCERN, HISTORY AND PHYSICAL, PRESENT HEALTH STATUS, PAST HEALTH STATUS, FAMILY HISTORY, AND SOCIAL HISTORY

Ms. Hernandez, an 83-year-old female Hispanic and a retired department store clerk, arrives at the rural health clinic requesting to have her blood pressure checked. Her past medical history is significant for mild hypertension, which is being controlled by Bumex 0.5 mg every day. She admits to taking up to six regular-strength aspirin per day for arthritic pain. Ms. Hernandez complains that she is very tired and has no energy. She says she has difficulty walking out to the end of her driveway to get her mail and has been unable to sleep well for the past 3 months, getting 4–5 hours of sleep most nights. She admits to drinking at least two cups of chamomile tea every evening before bedtime but says that she still cannot sleep. She lights a candle by her bed every night and prays for sleep to come. She has not seen a health care provider in the last 12 months.

REVIEW OF PERTINENT DOMAINS

Biological Domain

PHYSICAL EXAM: Reveals a female, 5 ft, 2 in. tall, 135 lb, with a blood pressure of 165/95, pulse 85. Heberden's nodules of arthritis are observed on fingers of both hands. Skin is dry and lacks elasticity. Over her arms are numerous purple lesions, which she says happen with the slightest bump. Eyes have a sunken appearance, and her affect is dull.

GASTROINTESTINAL: Ms. Hernandez admits to snacking because she is too tired to cook. She recalls breakfast as a bowl of instant oatmeal and coffee; dinner yesterday was an apple and four cookies; lunch yesterday was a cold meat sandwich and a glass of tea.

INTEGUMENTARY: Easily bruises.

CARDIOVASCULAR: No chest pain or discomfort.

MUSCULOSKELETAL: States that the arthritis in fingers and knees is sometimes painful.

NEUROLOGICAL: Balance intact, no gait disturbances.

Psychological Domain

COGNITIVE: Completed high school, is coherent, and is fluent in English and Spanish.

EMOTIONAL: Ms. Hernandez reports that she often feels depressed and is currently taking no medication for this. She drinks two cups of chamomile tea every night. She frequently eats only 1–2 times a day and averages 5 hours of sleep at night.

Social Domain

Ms. Hernandez has two sons in their mid-50s and has been divorced for 30 years. Her parents died in their mid-50s of unknown causes. Ms. Hernandez has three brothers, two of whom have undergone open heart surgery.

Environmental Domain

Ms. Hernandez states that her sons have taken away her car because she was having difficulty operating the controls due to arthritis in her hands and knees. Although one son takes her shopping for groceries every Saturday, she reports feeling very lonely.

Cultural/Spiritual Domain

HERBAL REMEDIES: Ms. Hernandez has had problems sleeping before, and she has obtained relief by drinking chamomile tea.

QUESTIONS FOR DISCUSSION

1. List all the possible factors that may contribute to Ms. Hernandez's sleeplessness, activity intolerance, and depression.
2. What health risk factors does she have that are unrelated to her complaints?
3. What risks are specifically related to her cultural and spiritual practices?
4. What measures could be taken to help relieve sleeplessness, increase activity, decrease depression, and promote the general health of an elderly person such as Ms. Hernandez?

KEY CONCEPTS

1. As facilitators of health promotion, nurses must be aware of issues and needs of older adults in order to empower them in self-care, personal health, and well-being.

2. The elderly population is the fastest-growing population worldwide. By the year 2050 there will be more elderly than children.

3. The psychosocial theories of development as perceived by Erikson, Peck, and Havighurst along with theories of aging provide a comprehensive view of the developmental tasks of older adults. These theories can be a helpful guide to understanding how individuals adapt to physical, psychosocial, and environmental effects on aging.

4. Each body system goes through age-related changes. Special nursing consideration needs to be taken and health-promotion tips offered to patients going through these changes.

5. There are many physical, psychological, and environmental challenges to consider when encouraging an older adult to eat a well-balanced diet. Exercise, such as swimming, dancing, and walking, is proven to stop or slow some of the physical changes of aging. There are many simple ideas that can be taught to the elderly that will assist in improving their quality of sleep. Because sex and sexuality are important to the health of the elderly, a sexual assessment should be included in your comprehensive assessment, and teaching should include information on safe sex.

6. Low economic status and low level of education are two socioeconomic influences on health-promoting behaviors in the elderly that affect accessibility to and the availability of health resources.

7. For many elderly, the stresses of living are compounded by physical, psychological, social, economic, and environmental changes. Incidences of stress among the elderly and elder abuse are occurring frequently; research in this area is ongoing.

8. Spiritual well-being is important for many elderly to achieve or maintain harmony as they progress through the later stages of life.

9. The rapid growth of our aging population presents special environmental challenges. There is a disproportional number of accidents involving the elderly compared to the time they spend driving. Many accidents can be the result of age-related physical changes; therefore, teaching driving safety tips is imperative.

10. A multitude of wellness programs and health-promotion resources are available for the elderly within their communities, across the nation, and on the Internet.

11. Health care workers must be knowledgeable in properly identifying and assessing elder abuse and in understanding the warning signs of elder abuse.

12. Assisted living facilities provide a special combination of personalized care for the elderly. These facilities exist throughout the nation, and many different levels of care are provided.

13. The elderly have complex needs during disaster preparedness and response that are often overlooked. During disasters, this population can demonstrate both vulnerability and resilience.

CHAPTER REVIEW

Learning Activities

1. List five of the possible physiologic changes of aging. Suggest creative nursing tips to teach your elderly patients about these changes.
2. Develop a pamphlet for healthy sleep patterns for the elderly.
3. List three signs of elder abuse.
4. Give three examples of simple ways the elderly can make their homes safer.
5. Select an older adult, such as a grandparent or neighbor. Ask the person to list or show the medications being taken. Utilize the suggested medication table.

Multiple Choice Questions

1. In 2008, the percentage of minority persons greater than 65 years of age in the United States was approximately:
   a. 8%.
   b. 19%.
   c. 26%.
   d. 37%.
2. Which of the following is Erikson's developmental stage for the older adult?
   a. Body transcendence versus body preoccupation
   b. Ego differentiation versus role preoccupation
   c. Ego integrity versus despair
   d. Establishing an explicit association with one's own age group
3. Which one of the following theories is based on the concept that humans are programmed to age by a predetermined biological clock?
   a. Free radical theory
   b. Genetic theory
   c. Human needs theory
   d. Neuroendocrine theory

4. Which of the following is the most responsible for fatal and nonfatal injuries to people age 65 and older?
   a. Auto accidents
   b. Cigarette smoking
   c. Falls
   d. Polypharmacy
5. With regard to accessibility to health resources, which of the following is a socioeconomic factor that would have the greatest influence on health-promoting behaviors in the elderly?
   a. Cultural Identity
   b. Gender
   c. Geographic location
   d. Level of education
6. An estimation of the yearly number of cases of elder abuse in the United States is:
   a. 100,00–200,000.
   b. 500,000–750,000.
   c. 1,000,000–2,000,000.
   d. 3,000,000–5,000,000.
7. With regard to gender, which of the following is an accurate characteristic of the population of persons age 55 and over?
   a. There are fewer women in the ratio of women to men.
   b. There are fewer women than men living with a spouse.
   c. More women than men are living below the poverty level.
   d. More women than men have higher education.
8. Elderly patients with sleep pattern disturbance should be advised to:
   a. avoid establishing a bedtime ritual.
   b. consume moderate alcohol intake late in the day.
   c. drink milk or chamomile tea, and eat a light snack prior to bedtime.
   d. seek psychiatric help for this abnormal behavior.

ORGANIZATIONS AND WEBSITES

Administration on Aging: Offers a wealth of information related to health and aging resources for minorities and diverse populations; includes a guidebook for providers of service to elderly patients to promote culturally competent care for the elderly and their families: **http://www.aahf.info/sec_news/ section/real-fountains-of-youth_012507.htm**

Administration on Aging, Dept. of Health & Human Services: Provides access to information, resources, and issues related to aging: **http://www.aoa.gov**

American Association of Retired Persons (AARP): Dedicated to promoting the health and welfare of Americans over the age of 50: **http://www.aarp.org**

National Institute on Aging: Lists more than 300 national organizations that provide help to older people; leads the federal effort on aging research; provides links to health and research information: **http://www.nia.nih.gov/HealthInformation/ ResourceDirectory.htm**

Office of Disease Prevention and Health Promotion: Works to strengthen the disease-prevention and health-promotion priorities of the U.S. Department of Health and Human Services: **http://www.osophs.dhhs.gov**

Red Hat Society: Source to generate connections with women over 50 who want to find some support, camaraderie, and comedy relief associated with the responsibilities of middle and older adulthood: **http://www.redhatsociety.com**

Sanford University: Site for the Geriatric Depression Scale and various interpretations: **http://www.stanford.edu**

Sexuality Information and Education Council of the United States: Serves as the national voice for sexuality education, sexual health, and sexual rights; provides information to the public to promote sexuality education for all ages: **http://www .siecus.org**

U.S. Census Bureau: Provides statistics on the United States population: **http://www.census.gov/**

REFERENCES

Alliance for Aging Research (AFAR). (2011). Chronic disease and medical innovation in an aging nation. Retrieved from http://www.silverbook.org/browse.php?id=.57

Alvarenga, M., Oliveira, M., Faccenda, O., & Amendola, F. (2010). Evaluation of the nutritional risk in elderly assisted by family health teams. *Revista da Escola de Enfermagem da USP, 44*, 1046–1051. DOI: 10.1590/S0080-62342010000400027.

American Academy of Anti-Aging Medicine. (n.d.). Theories on Aging. Retrieved from www.worldhealth.net/p/90,4863.html

American Academy of Family Physicians. (AAFP). (2011). Nutrition and health. Retrieved from http://www.aafp.org/afp/980301ap/edits.html

American Association of Retired Persons. (AARP). (n.d.). Understanding universal design. Retrieved from http://www.aarp.org/life/homedesign/Articles/a2004-03-23-whatis_univdesign.html

American Association of Retired Persons. (AARP) (2002). Exercise, attitudes and behaviors: A survey of midlife and older adults. Retrieved from http://www.aarp.org/research/health/healthquality/aresearch-import-65a.html

American Association of Retired Persons. (AARP), (2010). Senior exercise and fitness tips: How to gain energy and feel stronger. Retrieved from http://www.helpguide.org/life/senior_fitness_sports.htm

American Association of Retired Persons International. (AARPI). (2007). WHO launches age-friendly cities guide. Xinhua News Agency, London. Retrieved from, http://www.aarpinternational.org/news/news_show.htm?doc_id=542993eeeeeee

American Cancer Society (ACS). (2010). American Cancer Society guidelines for the early detection of cancer. Retrieved from http://www.cancer.org/Healthy/FindCancerEarly/CancerScreeningGuidelines/american-cancer-society-guidelines-for-the-early-detection-of-cancer.

American Diabetes Association. (2007). Diabetes mellitus and exercise. *Diabetes Care*. Retrieved from http://care.diabetesjournals.org/content/25/suppl_1/s64.full

Bauer, M., McAuliffe, L., & Nay, R. (2007). Sexuality, health care and the older person: an overview of the literature. *International Journal of Older People Nursing*, 2, 63–68.. DOI: 10.1111/j.1748-3743.2007.00051.x.

Birklow, R., & Beers, M. H. (eds.). (2000). Theories of aging. *Merck Manual of Geriatrics*. Whitehouse Station, NJ: Merck Research Laboratories.

Blay, S. L., Andreoli, S. B., & Gastol, F. L. (2008). Prevalance of self reported sleep disterbances among older adults and the association of disturbed sleep with service demand and medical conditions. *International Pychogeriatrics, 20*(3), 582–595.

Bouman, W., Arcelus, J., & Benbow, S. (2006). Nottingham Study of Sexuality & Ageing (NoSSA I). Attitudes regarding sexuality and older people: A review of the literature. *Sexual & Relationship Therapy, 21*, 149–161. DOI: 10.1080/14681990600618879.

Brach, J. S., Fitzgerald, S., Newman, A. B., Kelsey, S., Kuller, L., VanSwearingen, J. M., & Kriska, A. M. (2003). Physical activity and functional status in community dwelling older women: A 14-year prospective study. *Archives of Internal Medicine, 163*, 2565–2571. DOI: 10.1001/archinte.163.21.2565.

Brownie, S. (2006). Why are elderly individuals at risk of nutritional deficiency? *International Journal of Nursing Practice, 12*, 110–118. DOI: 10.1111/j.1440-172X.2006.00557.x.

Cawthorne, A. (2008). Elderly poverty: The challenge before us. Center for American Progress. Retrieved from http://www.americanprogress.org/issues/2008/07/pdf/elderly_poverty.pdf

Center for Addictions and Mental Health, (CAMH). (2009). Best practice guidelines for mental health promotion programs: Older adults 55+. Retrieved from, http://knowledgex.camh.net/policy_health/mhpromotion/mhp_older_adults/Pages/bkgrnd_older_adults.aspx

Centers for Disease Control and Prevention. (n.d.). Cases of HIV infection and AIDS in the United States, 2003. **HIV/AIDS Surveillance Report** (Vol. 15). Retrieved from http://www.cdc.gov/hiv/stats/2003SurveillanceReport.htm

Centers for Disease Control and Prevention. (2006). Falls among older adults. **National Center for Injury Prevention and Control**. Retrieved from http://www.cdc.gov/ncipe/factsheets/adultfalls.htm

Central Intelligence agency, (CIA). (2011). Life expectancy at birth. **The World Fact Book**. Retrieved from https://www.cia.gov/library/publications/the-world-factbook/fields/2102.html

Chamberland, L. (2003). Elderly women, invisible lesbians. **Canadian Journal of Community Mental Health, 22**(2), 85–103.

Chandler, J., & Studenski, S. (2010). Exercise practice of geriatrics. **Med Text**. Retrieved from http://medtextfree.wordpress.com/2010/09/30/chapter-14-exercise/

D'Angelo, K. (2003). News release: New analysis indicates age, gender, race, income, and coexisting medical conditions affect rates and outcomes of primary and revision total hip replacements. **American Academy of Orthopedic Surgeons**. Retrieved from http://orthoinfo.aaos.org/topic.cfm?topic=A00121

D'Angelo, K., Murena, L., & Cheribino, P. (2008). The unstable total hip replacement. **Indian Journal of Orthopeadics, 42**, 252–259. DOI:10.1093/aje/155.3.234.

Deeny, P., Vitale, C., Spelman, R., & Duggan, S. (2010). Addressing the imbalance: Empowering older people in disaster response and preparedness. **International Journal of Older People Nursing, 5**, 77–80. DOI:10.1111/j.1748-3743.2009.00204.x.

Dellinger, A. M., Langlois, J. A., & Li, G. (2002). Fatal crashes among older drivers: Decomposition of rates into contributing factors. **American Journal of Epidemiology, 155**, 234–241. DOI:10.1093/aje/155.3.234.

DeNavas-Walt, C., Proctor, B. D, & and Smith, J. C. (2010). **U.S. Census Bureau, Current Population Reports, P60-238, Income, Poverty, and Health Insurance Coverage in the United States: 2009.** Washington, DC, : U.S. Government Printing Office

Downey, J. (2004). **Increased safety in assisted living.** Retrieved from http://www.rkmc.com/Increased_Safety_in_Assisted_Living.htm

Duggan, S., Deeny, P., Spelman, R., & Vitale, C. (2010). Perceptions of older people on disaster response and preparedness. **International Journal of Older People Nursing, 5**, 71–76. DOI:10.1111/j.1748-3743.2009.00203.x.

Erikson, E. (1964). **Child and society**. New York, NY: Norton.

Evans, C. (2005). Malnutrition in the elderly: A multifactorial failure to thrive. **The Permanente Journal, 9**(3). Retrieved from http://xnet.kp.org/permanentejournal/sum05/elderly.pdf

Evans, J. (2010). Mapping the vulnerability of older persons to disasters. **International Journal of Older People Nursing, 5**, 63–70. DOI:10.1111/j.1748-3743.2009.00205.x.

Fitzpatrick, M. J., & Hamill, S. B. (2011). Elder abuse: Factors related to perceptions of severity and likelihood of reporting. Journal of Elder Abuse and Neglect, 23,1–16. DOI: 10.1080/089465666.2011.534704.

Federal Interagency Forum on Aging-Related Statistics. **Older Americans 2010: Key indicators of well-being. Federal Interagency Forum on Aging-Related Statistics**. Washington, DC: U.S. Government Printing Office. July 2010.

Food Stamp Services. (2007, January). Applicants & recipients. Retrieved from http://www.fns.usda.gov/fsp/applicant_recipients/default.htm.

Gavrilov, L. A., & Gavrilov, N. S. (2002). Evolutionary theories of aging and longevity. **Scientific World Journal, 2**; 339–356. Retrieved from http://www.longevity-science.org/

Georgetown University (2004). Cultural competence in health care. *Issue briefs on challenges for the 21st century: Chronic and disabling conditions.* Center on an Aging Society. Retrieved from http://hpi.georgetown.edu/agingsociety/pubhtml/cultural/cultural.html

Georgetown University (2005). *Demography is not destiny: Revisited.* Center on an Aging Society. Retrieved from http://hpi.georgetown.edu/agingsociety/pdfs/DINDII.pdf

Goolsby, M. J., & Grubbs, L. (2006). *Advanced assessment: Interpreting findings and formulating differential diagnoses.* Philadelphia: F. A. Davis.

Havighurst, R. J. (1972). *Developmental tasks and education* (3rd ed.). New York, NY: David McKay.

Health Alliance Plan of Michigan. (2011). *Are you at risk for polypharmacy?* Retrieved from http://www.hap.org/prescriptions/polypharmacy_risk.php

Healthy People 2020. (2010). Older adults. Retrieved from http://healthypeople.gov/2020/topicsobjectives2020/overview.aspx?topicid=31

Heath, H. (2006). The gift of understanding: Behind closed doors. *International Journal of Older People Nursing, 1,* 250–251. DOI:10.1111/j.1748-3743.2006.00040.x.

Hillsdon, M. M., Brunner, E. J., Guralnik, J. M., & Marmot, M. G. (2005). Prospective study of physical activity and physical function in early old age. *American Journal of Preventive Medicine, 28,* 245–250. DOI:10.1016/j.amepre.2004.12.008.

Hollmann, F., Mulder, T. J., & Kallan, J. E. (2000). Methodology and assumptions for the population projections of the United States: 1999 to 2100. Washington, DC: Bureau of the Census, U.S. Department of Commerce.

Holroyd, A., & Clayton, A. (2002, March 25). Measuring depression in the elderly: Which scale is best? Retrieved from http://www.medscape.com/viewarticle/430554

Janssen, R. S. (2005). *HIV/AIDS in persons 50 years of age and older.* Testimony presented on May 12, 2005, at the Special Committee on Aging, U.S. Senate. Retrieved from www.hhs.gov/asl/testify/t050512a.html

Joint Commission on Accreditation of Healthcare Organizations (JCAHO). (2011). *National Patient Safety Goals Effective July 1, 2011.* Retrieved from http://www.jointcommission.org/assets/1/6/NPSG_EPs_Scoring_LTC_20110707.pdf

Kaufman, G., & Elder, G. H. (2002). Revisiting age identity: A research note. *Journal of Aging Studies, 16,* 169–176. DOI: 10.1016/S0890-4065(02)00042-7

Kestenbaum, B. & Ferguson, R. B. (2006). The number of centenarians in the United States on January 1, 1990, 2000, and 2010 based on improved Medicare data. *North American Actuarial Journal, 10*(3), 1–6.

Larson, P. D., & Lubkin, I. M. (2009). Chronic illness: Impact and intervention. Sudbury, MA: Jones & Bartlett.

Mayo Clinic. (2006). *Erectile dysfunction: Viagra and other oral medications.* Retrieved from http://www.mayoclinic.com/print/erectile-dysfunction/MC00029/METHOD=print

Miller, C. (2009). *Nursing for wellness in older adults: Theory and practice* (5th ed.). Philadelphia, PA: Williams and Williams.

Nagaratnam, N., & Gayagay, G. (2002). Hypersexuality in nursing care facilities. A descriptive study. *Archives of Gerontology and Geriatrics, 35,* 195–203. DOI:10.1016/S0167-4943(02)00026-2.

NANDA, (2007–2008). NANDA approved nursing diagnosis. Retrieved from http://wps.prenhall.com/wps/media/objects/3918/4012970/NursingTools/koz74686_AppC.pdf

National Center for Health Statistics. (2011).Health, United States, 2010: In Brief. Hyattsville, MD; U.S. Department of Health and Human Services.

National Center on Elder Abuse. (2005a). *15 questions & answers about elder abuse.* Retrieved from http://www.scribd.com/doc/38961554/15-Questions-Answers-About-Elder-Abuse

National Center on Elder Abuse. (2005b). Types of elder abuse in domestic settings. *Elder abuse prevalence and incidence.* Retrieved from http://ncea.aoa.gov/ncearoot/Main_Site/pdf/publication/FinalStatistics050331.pdf

National Highway Traffic Safety Administration (NHTSA). (2008). *Traffic Safety Facts 2008: Older Population.* Retrieved from http://www-nrd.nhtsa.dot.gov/Pubs/811161.PDF

Parachin, V. M. (November-December 2011). Power of prayer. *Vibrant Life, 27*(6), pp. 28–31.

Peck, R. (1968). Psychological developments in the second half of life. In B. Neugarten (ed.), *Middle age and aging.* Chicago, IL: University of Chicago, pp. 88–92.

Powell, J. L. (2005). *Social theory and aging.* Lanham, MD: Rowman and Littlefield.

Quan, S. F., Katz, R., Olson, J., Bonekat, W., Enright, P. L., Young, T., & Newman, A. (2005). Factors associated with incidence and persistence of symptoms of disturbed sleep in an elderly cohort: The cardiovascular health study. *Southern Society for Clinical Investigation, 329,* 163–172. DOI: 10.1097/00000441-200504000-00001.

Rankin, S. H., Stallings, K. D., & London, F. (2005). *Patient Education in Health and Illness.* Philadelphia: Lippincott Williams and Wilkins.

Resnick, B. (2002). Testing the effects of the WALC intervention on exercise adherence in older adults. *Journal of Gerontological Nursing, 28*(6), 40–49.

Saka, B., Kaya, O., Ozturk, G., Erten, N., & Karan, M. (2010). Malnutrition in the elderly and its relationship with other geriatric syndromes. *Clinical Nutrition, 29,* 745–748. DOI: 10.1016/j.clnu.2010.04.006.

Seidel, H. M., Ball, J. W,, Dains, J. E., & Benedict, G. W. (2006). *Mosby's guide to physical examination* (6th ed.). St Louis, MO: Mosby.

Shear, K., Roose, S. P., Lenze, E., & Alexopoulos, G. S. (2005). Depression in the elderly: The unique features related to diagnosis and treatment. *CNS Spectrums, 10*(18), 33–42.

Smith, D. (2003). *The older population in the United States: March 2002.* U.S. Census Bureau Current Population Reports, P20–546. Washington, DC: U.S. Census Bureau.

Stanford University. (n.d.). *Geriatric depression scale.* Retrieved from http://www.stanford.edu/~yesavage/GDS.html

Sukying, C., Bhokakul, V., & Udomsubpayakul, U. (2003). An epidemiological study on insomnia in an elderly Thai population. *Journal of the Medical Association of Thailand, 86*(4), 316–324.

Tanner, E. K. (2005). Recognizing late-life depression: Why is this important to nurses in the home setting? *Geriatric Nursing, 26*(3), 145–149.

Thompson, D. (2005). Exercise and nutrition: The true fountains of youth. Healthfinder. Retrieved from http://www.aahf.info/sec_news/section/real-fountains-of-youth_012507.htm

U.S. Census Bureau. (2006). *Facts for features: Older Americans month.* Retrieved from http://www.census.gov/newsroom/releases/pdf/cb06-ff05.pdf.

Watters, Y., & Boyd, T. (2009). Sexuality in later life: Opportunity for reflections for healthcare providers. *Sexual & Relationship Therapy, 24*(3–4), 307–315. DOI: 10.1080/14681990903398047.

WebMD. (n.d.). Erectile dysfunction: Alternative treatments. Retrieved from http://www.webmd.com/content/article/94/102933.htm

World Health Organization, (WHO). (2007). *Global age-friendly cities: A guide.* WHO Library Cataloguing in Publication Data. Retrieved from, http://whqlibdoc.who.int/publications/2007/9789241547307_eng.pdf

CHAPTER 14
Health Promotion through End-of-Life

Beatriz Nieto, PhD, RN

KEY TERMS

advance directive	environmental loss	loss
ambiguous loss	grief	loss of aspect of self
bereavement	hospice	mourning
diagnosing dying	illness trajectory	palliative care

OBJECTIVES

Upon completion of this chapter, the reader should be able to:

- Describe the relationship between health-promotion concepts and end-of-life care.
- Identify a variety of end-of-life issues and challenges facing those who are dying.
- Compare and contrast between palliative care and hospice.
- Formulate ways to help the patient and family facing the end-of-life.
- Familiarize self with the different theories on grief and loss.
- Define loss, grief, bereavement, and mourning.
- Reflect on own feelings, thoughts, and beliefs about death, dying, and the end-of-life.

INTRODUCTION

Death is a topic very few individuals have come to terms with, yet the most obvious truth of our existence is based on the fact that, because we are alive, all of us will eventually die (Gyatso, 2011). We can be sure that death is occurring somewhere around the world every second of every day. In fact, it has been approximated that 146,357 people die each day, 6098 people die each hour, 102 people die each minute, and about 2 people die each second (Central Intelligence Agency, 2011; Wholesome Words, 2011). The universal reality of life is that it will come to an end, and its only uniqueness is that we do not know how, when, and where we will die.

Over the course of the past century, the demographics of death in terms of age profile, cause of death, and place of death have changed tremendously. For example, in the 1900s, most people died in their own homes. The major cause of death back then was acute infection, and the majority of all deaths occurred in childhood or early adult life. Around the start of the twenty-first century, the major causes of death are chronic illnesses, such as heart disease, cancer, stroke, chronic respiratory disease, neurological disease, or dementia, with most deaths occurring in hospitals. As a result of such historical changes, familiarity with death in today's society as a whole has decreased. Many people do not experience the death of someone close to them until they themselves are well into midlife. Many others have never seen a dead body, except perhaps on television. As a society, we do not discuss death and dying openly (Department of Health, 2008).

Death, dying, end-of-life, loss, and grief—all extremely powerful words, with as many meanings and connotations as there are people. Thinking about dying or the end-of-life is not a topic many people embrace easily, even though the end-of-life is something we all will encounter. Throughout history, theologians, scientists, and philosophers have tried to understand people's fears of death. A variety of reactions is not unusual when people are facing death, whether someone else's or their own. Those who have been long suffering may respond to the thought of death with acceptance or even a welcoming plea, while others may do everything within their power to avoid acknowledging the final termination of life (Richardson, Berman, & Piwowarsk, 1983; Routledge, Ostafin, Juhl, Sedikides, Cathey, & Liao, 2010). Many others view the end-of-life as a separate entity, apart from the rest of life's stages, experiences, trips, and journeys. These views of death often arise from anxiety and/or fear of the unknown, and they may also be due to one's not coming to terms with death's inevitability and finality, as well as its universality and humanness.

Whatever prevents us from transcending our fears and anxiety about death and dying, we need to continue to develop an awareness of our own mortality in order to help others promote health and achieve wellness even at the end-of-life. We can do so by continuing to dialogue, train, conduct research, educate others, and incorporate all aspects of best practices in promoting the health of those journeying toward the end of their lives.

The primary focus of this chapter is to enlighten the reader in matters concerning health promotion and the end-of-life. This will be done by providing an overview of various health-promotion and end-of-life issues—as well as thoughts and concepts related to loss, palliative care, hospice, pain management, spirituality, communication, decision making, among other topics—that will help the reader promote health and wellness as they continue life's journey toward its end.

HEALTH PROMOTION AND THE END-OF-LIFE

The fairly recent movement in nursing that focuses on addressing end-of-life issues has been instrumental in bringing this important concept to the forefront. Professional health care providers and their patients now have the opportunity for a long overdue dialogue, but much work remains to be done. Taking on such a taboo topic has not been easy, but the task has to start somewhere. One of the best places to begin is by examining one's own feelings, thoughts, and beliefs about death and dying, as well as all that is associated with the end-of-life, in order to be instrumental in helping others. Nurses are very used to dealing with health-promotion issues and strategies, but they find it difficult to see that health promotion may also play a role when people are nearing the end-of-life. Talk about health promotion and dying in the same breath may seem oxymoronic. However, if we know where we stand personally on these issues, we can become an essential part in helping others to deal with what can be one of the most difficult journeys of life, all while focusing on promoting health, hope, and dealing with every aspect of the patient and the patient's family.

Nurses are often in a prime position to help others because of the intimate nature of the nurse-patient relationship, which enhances trust. Without a doubt, nurses can be particularly effective at such times if they are willing to prepare themselves to take on the challenges and opportunities that arise when providing care to those facing the end of their lives. Therefore, nurses must keep abreast of the latest trends and findings associated with end-of-life issues in order to be of benefit when promoting health and wellness to those entrusted to our care. We should know where our fears and anxieties about death lie in order for us to conquer them, and we need to be instrumental in helping others journey toward the end. How we care for the dying is an indicator of how we care for all sick and vulnerable people. It is not only a measure of society as a whole, but a litmus test for all health and social services (Department of Health, 2008).

END-OF-LIFE ISSUES

Several issues and challenges have been affecting—and continue to affect—end-of-life care. Some of the major issues that relate to the biological, psychological, spiritual, and environmental domains are:

- Making an accurate diagnosis of dying.
- Pain and symptom control.
- Shared decision making.
- Choosing alternative sites of care

References: Singer, Martin, & Kelner, 1999; Billing, 2007; Yeolekar, Mehta, & Yeolekar, 2008.

It is imperative that nurses do everything within their power to help the patient and the family get through what may be one the most difficult times in a person's life. Therefore, making a diagnosis of dying is imperative so that treatment may be tailored appropriately and, most importantly, so that patients may be made aware of the stage of their illness and be empowered to make choices about how the last phase of their lives are managed (Sykes, 2008). In other words, to facilitate the effective care of dying patients, staff needs to recognize the onset of the dying process, not only to make symptom control provisions, but also so that appropriate communication can occur with patients and those close to them (Sykes, 2008, p. 1157).

Some believe that the end-of-life phase can be marked as a time of shifting and evolving hope (Fredriksson & Eriksson, 2001; Kissane, Clarke, & Street, 2001; Kissane, 2002) and that, like any other life stage, its many essential issues compel us to face the reality of our being. The patient, as well as his or her family, are confronted by many emotions, feelings, questions, as well as decisions that need to be made during the end-of-life phase. Issues that they may face include supporting the dying person, dealing with the health care system, managing pain and discomfort, interacting with caregivers, managing stress and coping, preparing for death, and saying goodbye (Baird & Rosenbaum, 2003; Canadian Hospice and Palliative Care Association [CHPCA], 2006; Gibson & Gorman, 2010). Other possible issues are the impact of the actual end-of-life journey on the family, ongoing care issues for the dying person, decisions on where to die, and, of course, actual **bereavement** (Gibson & Gorman, 2010). Nurses, along with the physicians and other health care providers, must be willing to identify those approaching the end-of-life and to take on the challenging and emotional task of helping them. Taking on that challenge can be perhaps one of the most important and rewarding areas of care one can be involved with. However, it can also be demanding and emotionally draining. That is why nurses must understand that a variety of circumstances may arise when someone is journeying through to the end and be willing and prepared to take on this very important challenge.

DIAGNOSING DYING

It is imperative that we acquire the necessary knowledge, skills, and attitudes to ensure that we deliver optimal care to our patients. **Diagnosing dying** requires recognizing some of the major symptoms that one who is dying may exhibit. Some key symptoms at the end-of-life include restlessness, agitation, breathlessness, pain, and noisy respirations from retained airway secretions (Glare, Virik, Jones, Hudson, Eychmuller, Simes, & Christakis, 2003; Sykes, 2010). Predictors of life expectancy have also been identified in a systematic review of literature (Maltoni, Caraceni, Brunelli, Broeckarert, Christakis, Eychmuller, Glare, Nabal, Vigano, Larkin, De Conno, Hanks, & Kassa, 2005; Sykes, 2010) (see Box 14-1). Some prognostic factors identified are a poor functional status, signs and symptoms of the cancer anorexia-cachexia syndrome, the presence of breathlessness or delirium, and the so-called death rattle (Wildiers & Menten, 2002; Maltoni, Caraceni, & Brunelli, et. al., 2005; Sykes, 2010). Being bedridden, semicomatose, able to take only sips of fluids, and no longer able to swallow tablets were found to be predictive factors for life expectancy as well (Ellershaw, Sutcliffe, & Saunders, 1995; Sykes, 2010). Also, on average, patients dying of cancer may develop respirations with jaw movements, peripheral cyanosis, loss of the radial pulse, and diminished consciousness (Morita, Ichiki, Tsunoda, Inoue, & Chihara, 1998; Sykes, 2010).

Unfortunately, health care providers consistently overestimate the patients' survival time (Glare, Virik, Jones, Hudson, Eychmuller, Simes, & Christakis, 2003; Sykes, 2010), but familiarizing oneself with these findings can be useful when caring for people facing the end of their lives. Although deaths do not all occur exactly in the same way, knowing that some

BOX 14-1
PREDICTORS OF LIFE EXPECTANCY FOR PEOPLE IN END-STAGE CANCER

PROGNOSTIC FACTORS	LIFE EXPECTANCY
Declining functional status Signs and symptoms of the cancer Anorexia-cachexia syndrome Presence of breathlessness Increasing delirium	< 90 days

Two or more of the following:
   Being bedridden
   Semicomatose
   Able to take only sips of fluids
   No longer able to swallow tablets
	~ 2 days

Increased secretions retained in airway	Within 48 hours
Decreased ability to cough and clear the airway Death rattle	seen in ~50% of patients
Diminishing consciousness	~ 24 hours
Respirations with jaw movements	~ 8 hours
Peripheral cyanosis	~ 5 hours
Loss of radial pulse	~ 3 hours

© Cengage Learning 2013

patients will experience and exhibit similar signs and symptoms may help guide us in providing effective, meaningful care. We must pay careful attention to the individual who is near the end of the life. Otherwise, we will not be able to provide the best care possible.

PAIN

Both patients and those close to them often fear a painful death more than death itself (Knaus, Harrell, Lynn, Goldman, Phillips, Connors, Dawson, Fulkerson, Califf, Desbiens, Layde, Oye, Bellamy, Hakim, & Wagner, 1995). Unfortunately, the fear of unrelieved pain is a reality for many individuals facing a life-threatening illness. In fact, for many Americans, pain is vastly undertreated, even for those facing the end of their lives (American Pain Foundation, 2010).

The American Pain Foundation (APF) (2010) has found that most pain problems can be managed to a reasonable comfort level through the use of pain-relieving medications provided by knowledgeable health care professionals. Advances in pain treatment, including new drugs, injections, infusions, implantable devices, radiation treatments, and surgical techniques, have enabled many difficult pain problems to be alleviated and managed. It has been predicted that close to 98% of all pain problems can be relieved or reduced (American Pain

Foundation, 2010). The availability of pain specialists, pain management teams, and/or health care professionals willing to work together with people living with pain are key to successful pain relief (American Pain Foundation, 2010). The use of holistic and health-promoting approaches can also provide some measure of pain relief.

Pain during the final stages of life is no different. Whether the length of life is projected in days, weeks, months, or years, relief of a dying person's pain must be a priority. Moderate to severe pain interferes with the ability to perform daily activities and lowers quality of life. Unrelieved pain also interferes with one's dignity. The person living with pain should determine the level of comfort desired, and pain relief should continue until life has ended. When dying persons are no longer able to make their wishes known, their appointed representative (proxy) has the responsibility to honor those wishes (American Pain Foundation, 2010). Contrary to what people might believe about pain and the related fears, if pain is managed well before the end-of-life, then it should not be of a concern at the end-of-life. In fact, pain may diminish in the last days to weeks of life (Fainsinger, Miller, Bruera, Hanson, & Meceachem, 1991; Mercadante, Casuccio, & Fulfaro, 2000; Ellershaw, Smith, Overill, Walker, & Aldrige, 2001; Sykes, 2010).

END-OF-LIFE CARE DISCUSSIONS

Communication is the essence of the nurse-patient relationship. It is therefore important that all people who are approaching the end-of-life have their needs fully assessed. An assessment of their needs can be an excellent opportunity for them to express their thoughts, wishes, and preferences about how they are cared for and where they wish to die. For greater effectiveness, an agreed-on set of actions reflecting their choices should be recorded in a care plan, which should be available to all who have a legitimate reason to access the information (Department of Health, 2008).

Little data is available regarding when physicians and their terminally ill patients typically discuss end-of-life issues (Foley & Gelband, 2001; Earle, Neville, Landrum, Avanian, Block, & Weeks, 2004; Wennberg, Fisher, Goodman, & Skinner, 2008; Keating, Landrum, Rogers, Baum, Virnig, Huskamo, Earle, Kahn, 2010). National guidelines recommend advance care planning for patients with terminal illnesses and life expectancies of less than 1 year (National Consensus Project for Quality Palliative Care, 2004–2011; National Cancer Clinical Practice Guidelines in Oncology, 2011; Keating et al., 2010). Some health care providers have a difficult time discussing end-of-life issues with their patients. In fact, they may assume that patients facing these issues will be reluctant to think about or discuss the issues at hand, including whether patients have advanced directives and, if so, with whom they have discussed their written plans. An **advance directive** consists of written instructions on the specific procedures to be followed if a person becomes incapacitated. The directive describes a person's desire for medical treatment used in cases where the person is no longer capable of making decisions. Examples of advance directives are living wills and durable power of attorney (Legal Explanations.com, 2004–2007). A study focusing on women with metastatic breast cancer and their providers from two academic medical centers in the United States showed that, although the majority of the patients gathered information about advance directives and had made written plans regarding their care, only a few had discussed these plans with their providers (Ozanne, Partridge, Moy, Ellis, & Sepucha, 2009). The researchers concluded that explicit discussion of advance directives and patient preferences regarding end-of-life care are definitely lacking and a fertile ground for future growth and improvement. Open communication between health care providers and their patients is extremely important and imperative in order to provide quality care and meet the needs of the patients at this time of their life (Ozanne, Partridge, Moy, Ellis, & Sepucha, 2009).

Deciding when and how to discuss end-of-life issues with a person can be daunting for all involved. In serial interviews of 20 people with lung cancer, nearly all of them stated that they would have liked to talk about the future and how their illness would pan out right from the time of diagnosis (Murray, 2005). Unfortunately, the odds of this happening are small. When someone is diagnosed with a terminal illness, they often begin considering the meaning and purpose of life as well as their impending death. The reality, however, is that they may feel unable to vocalize this with either their family or with their health care provider. It is often toward the latter stage of the illness that clinicians may raise the issue about end-of-life (Murray, 2005). Although clinicians may feel ill prepared and find it difficult to initiate the needed dialogue with their patients, the patients and all health care providers involved must do so in order to plan the best possible care.

? ASK YOURSELF

End-of-Life Conversations

Murray (2005) identifies possible questions to start the supportive care/end-of-life conversation with patients facing their end-of-life:

- What's the most important issue in your life right now?
- What helps you keep going?
- What is your greatest problem?
- How are you feeling within yourself today?
- You usually seem quite cheerful, but do you ever feel down?
- If things got worse, where would you like to be cared for (p. 38)?

Think about these questions, and ask yourself if you could answer them honestly.

Other key components that may be incorporated in the end-of-life discussion are the concepts of loss and meaning for the person with advanced disease, the timing of the discussion, the use of active listening, and ways to encourage disclosure and handle silences (Edwards, 2005). However we choose to address the issues, we must remember to avoid raising the subject insensitively or right out of the blue. Give the patient and family an opportunity to plan for a good death. This is more fulfilling for all involved than just focusing on a set of downward physical trends until death occurs (Murray, 2005, p. 38).

SPOTLIGHT **ON**

Delivering Bad News

Delivering bad news is very stressful for health care providers with the aftereffects lasting for hours to days. Here are some things to remember when delivering bad news:

- Competence is a great stress reliever. The clinician who is adequately trained in communication skills is more likely to break bad news both sensitively and efficiently.

- Hearing bad news is very stressful and distressing to patients. Patients with a previous history of mental illness and those with poor social and financial support systems are especially vulnerable to the aftereffects of bad news.

- Ask before you tell. First ask the patient, "What is your understanding of your illness?"

- Deliver the bad news in simple clear sentences. Avoid using medical jargon.

- Arrange for follow-up care.

- Allow time for debriefing your staff and for self-reflection (Periyakoil, 2008).

Source: Adapted from End-of-life Curriculum Project Funded by a grant to the Veterans Administration Nationwide Palliative Care Network by the National Library of Medicine, 2008. Retrieved from http://endoflife.stanford .edu/index_dev.html

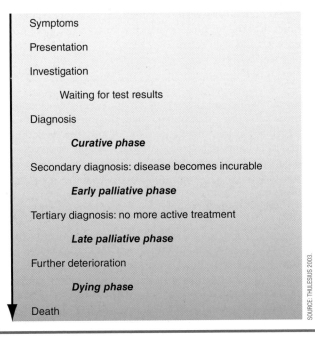

FIGURE 14-1 **Illness trajectory: Example of a cancer journey.**

Thulesius et al. (2003) point out that palliative care is divided into an early and a late stage, often divided by an event such as termination of chemotherapy and/or other treatments. They further describe an illness trajectory where the patient moves through a curative phase during which the aim is to cure the disease, an early palliative phase during which the goal is increased survival, and then a late palliative phase that focuses on maintaining quality of life (see Figure 14-1). Illness trajectories are not all the same; many may not have a curative phase, and some illnesses may contain several transitory phases. What is important to remember is that looking at illness trajectories serves to demonstrate how some terminal illnesses, like cancer, are often made up of long plateau periods, punctuated by episodes when abilities and symptoms change rapidly (Thulesius, Hakansson, & Petersson, 2003; Edwards, 2005). Moreover, these illness trajectories can be applied to other life-limiting illnesses, such as motor neuron disease (MND) (MND Association, 2000) or end-stage heart disease (Walden-McBride & McBride, 2000; Edwards, 2005).

TIMING AND PLANNING FOR THE END-OF-LIFE DISCUSSION

Exquisite planning can help make the most of an end-of-life discussion. When planning a discussion with a patient, take into consideration the time of day when the patient is strongest or less likely to have visitors or other engagements. Arranging a time with the patient can, in itself, demonstrate respect, and a compromise may need to be made between the wishes of the patient and the demands of the unit (Edwards, 2005, p. 22). The hospital environment is notoriously nonconducive to good communication (Edwards, 2005; Robinson & Watters, 2010), mainly due to distractions such as noise, other patients, and nursing activities. For the most part, a curtain around a bed does not provide enough security to ensure confidentiality and often is a barrier for a patient wanting to talk. It may be more appropriate to use a lounge or vacant single room when planning for a discussion.

The timing of an end-of-life discussion is an essential tool and the key to palliative care (Edwards, 2005; Baker et al., 2009). An end-of-life discussion is believed to have great value following the major transitional periods of a patient's illness. This brings into play the **illness trajectory**, which includes the phases of the illness itself and the two major stages of palliative care (Thulesius, Hakansson, & Petersson, 2003).

LOSS, GRIEF, MOURNING, AND BEREAVEMENT

Loss, grief, mourning, and *bereavement* are words commonly used interchangeably. However, each is unique in its meaning and use in describing different aspects of emotions, feelings, and behaviors exhibited when someone is deprived of a loved someone or a valued something. Often these words are used when the end-of-life is approaching or when actual death occurs. According to *Merriam-Webster* (2011), *loss* is defined as the act of losing possession, and *grief* is the cause of suffering or a deep and poignant distress. **Mourning** is an outward sign of grief for a person's death or a period of time during which signs of grief are shown. It can also be defined as the actual feeling or expression of sorrow, such as lamentation over someone's death (Dictionary.com, 2011). *Bereavement* is the state of being deprived of something or someone (*Merriam-Webster,* 2011). One can see from these definitions how closely related these concepts are and therefore why they are used interchangeably at times. For the purpose of this chapter, loss and grief are differentiated and elaborated.

Loss

Loss can be defined as the state of being deprived of or being without something that one has had: the undesired change or removal of a valued object, person, or situation (Dictionary. com, 2011; Lamanna, 2011). Although people often associate loss with losing a loved one through death, we actually experience loss on a daily basis, mainly because our life is full of changes and with change comes loss.

From the moment of birth, we begin our journey filled with change and new experiences, including loss. The first time we all experience loss is when we arrive in this world and lose the warmth and security of our mother's womb. After that, our life is a series of ebbs and flows, losses and gains, until we reach the end of our life—the ultimate loss, the death of self (Lamanna, 2011). Each developmental stage of life brings many changes and losses. For example, in childhood and adolescence, someone may experience a loss due to changing schools. In young and older adulthood, losses may include getting or changing jobs, facing retirement, a change in location, and altered living arrangements. Losses dealing with job-retirement-location-etc., can also be classified as an **environmental loss** because it involves a change in the familiar, even if the change is perceived as positive.

The essential point is that we can classify or categorize a loss in a variety of ways. Getting a good grasp of these concepts can help guide us as we confront caring for those experiencing loss. The most common ways of categorizing loss are:

- Actual loss
- Perceived loss
- Physical loss
- Psychological loss
- Anticipatory loss

Some losses may fit into more than one category

Actual Loss

An actual loss is one that can be seen or identified by others, not just by the person experiencing the loss. Actual loss may include, but is not limited to, the death of a loved one; the loss of a significant relationship (e.g., spouse, sibling, family member, or significant other through death, divorce, or separation as in times of war); the loss of an object through theft, deterioration, destruction, and/or natural disaster. The loss of an object can also be classified as an external loss, that is, actual losses of objects that are significant because of their cost or sentimental value. Examples of objects in this category are jewelry, a pet, a home, and, for a child, perhaps a special toy, blanket, etc. (Lamanna, 2011).

Perceived Loss

Perceived loss, on the other hand, is an internal, personal type of loss that can be identified only by the person experiencing the loss. Others may not be aware of this type of loss unless they are made aware of the person's perspective. An example of perceived loss is a woman who has been sexually assaulted and who, because of that assault, might perceive herself as having lost her purity. Other examples of perceived losses are youth, beauty, strength, and independence. Because we live in a society that values youth, beauty, vitality, and the like, persons may perceive themselves as no longer being beautiful because of the natural aging process. It is no wonder that so many seek ways to retain their youthful look through cosmetic surgery, botox injections, and other means. In fact, according to the American Society for Aesthetic Plastic Surgery (2010), Americans spent nearly $10.7 billion on cosmetic procedures in 2010. Further, of all the cosmetic procedures performed, people between 35 and 50 years of age had the most—more than 4 million procedures and 44% of the total; people ages 19 to 34 had 20%; those ages 51 to 64 had 28%; those 65 and over had 7%; and individuals 18 and younger had 13%.

Physical Loss

A physical loss is perhaps one of the easiest to identify, such as the loss of limb(s) due to amputation. Other examples of a physical loss are the removal of body organs (e.g., hysterectomy, mastectomy, etc.), and/or loss of a body function, such as mobility and flexibility. These types of losses can also be classified as a **loss of aspect of self**. Within this category, there could also be psychological and perceived losses, including aspects of one's personality, developmental change, as in the aging process, as well as the loss of hopes, dreams, and faith (Lamanna, 2011).

Psychological Loss

Psychological loss challenges our belief system. These types of losses are often seen in the areas of sexuality, control, fairness, meaning, and trust. Some losses bring with them a plethora of mixed emotions and feelings. For example, after the removal of a breast, a woman may feel both the physical and psychological loss of sexuality; it may be the same for a man after removal of the prostate gland.

In the categories of physical and psychological loss, one can also find another type of loss, known as **ambiguous loss**. Ambiguous loss, for families, involves physical or psychological losses that are not as concrete or identifiable as traditional losses, such as death. Ambiguous loss can include anything from miscarriage to losing one's spouse to Alzheimer's disease while he or she is still living. Another type is not knowing whether a loved one is living or dead, as in cases of child abduction or military personal who are missing in action. Ambiguous loss is inherently characterized by the lack of closure and clear understanding (Betz & Thomgren, 2006).

Anticipatory Loss

Family members or caregivers commonly anticipate how they will feel, react, or cope when the person's death finally occurs. In fact, many try to envision their life without that person and mentally play out possible scenarios, which may include grief reactions and ways they will mourn and adjust after the death. Anticipatory loss is often seen as a natural process that enables the family more time to prepare for the reality of the loss. People can often complete unfinished "business" with the dying person (for example, saying their good-byes, letting the person know they are loved, or even asking for forgiveness) (Assist-Guide Information Services, 2009).

Grief

Grief is a natural response to a loss and can be defined as the emotional suffering someone feels when a valued something

BOX 14-2
MYTHS AND FACTS ABOUT GRIEF

Myth:	Fact:
The pain will go away faster if you ignore it.	Trying to ignore the pain or keep it from surfacing will only make it worse in the long run. For healing to occur, it is necessary to face your grief and actively deal with it.
Myth:	Fact:
It is important to "be strong" in the face of loss.	Feeling sad, frightened, or lonely is a normal reaction to loss. Crying does not mean you are weak. You don't need to "protect" your family or friends by putting on a brave front. Showing your true feelings can help them and you.
Myth:	Fact:
If you do not cry, it means you are not sorry about the loss.	Crying is a normal response to sadness, but it is not the only response you may feel. Those who don't cry may feel the pain just as deeply as others. They may simply have other ways of showing it.
Myth:	Fact:
Grief should last about a year.	There is no right or wrong time frame for grieving. How long it takes can differ from person to person.

Source: Adopted from Hospice of the North Shore & Greater Boston: The Bertolon Center for Grief and Healing (2011), www.griefandhealing.org.

or a loved someone is taken way, dies, or is no longer accessible (Helpguide, 2001–2011). One of the most important aspects of grief is that it is a personal and highly individualized experience. Although it is a universal experience, no two people grieve in the same way. In fact, there is no right or wrong way to grieve a loss; healing from a loss, however, takes time and cannot be forced or hurried. Nurses need to remember that there is no "normal" timetable for grieving. Some individuals will begin to feel better in weeks or months, while others may grieve for years. Many factors play a part in how an individual responds to a loss. The factors may include a person's personality and coping style, life experiences, faith, conflicts existing at the time of death, previous loss, the amount of support for the bereaved, the timeliness of death, and the nature and significance of the loss. Whatever the grief experience, the person simply has to be patient and allow the grieving process to take its natural course. Nurses need to be aware of the many myths (see Box 14-2) regarding grief and loss. Remember that the more significant the loss is, the more intense the grief will be; so teaching others about grieving and loss is important in order for them to get the help they need when they need it the most (Hospice of the North Shore and Greater Boston, 2011).

THEORIES AND MODELS OF GRIEF

Many theories and models have been developed focusing on the stages or steps people encounter when experiencing and working through their grief (see Box 14-3). One of the most well-known writers on the processes involved in grief and grieving is George Engel. Engel (1961) wrote that uncomplicated grief has a clear onset and a predictable course, modified mainly by the abruptness and significance of the loss and the preparedness of the bereaved person. In the description of his biopsychosocial model, he asked whether grief was actually a disease. In further exploring the topic of grief, he stated that

uncomplicated grief is universal and does not require any form of treatment. According to Engel, grief basically has three major stages: (1) shock and disbelief, (2) developing awareness of the loss and (3) restitution and recovery (see Table 14-1).

On the other hand, Bowlby (1982) explored the concept of grief and grieving and, drawing from attachment theory, suggested that grief occurs when the bereaved learn that the object of their attachment is lost. Although some experts assert that Bowlby's theory does not take into account the individual nature of grief, implying that loved ones can be replaced, it can be argued that one's understanding of grief can be broadened by Bowlby's idea that grief is a mature way of dealing with loss of attachment. Bowlby describes the cycle of grief in the following phases: (1) shock and numbness, (2) yearning and searching, (3) disorganization and despair, and (4) reorganization.

Another well-known theorist on grieving is Rando (1984), who identified three major processes of grieving in

TABLE 14-1 Theories of Grief	
THEORIST	**THEORY/MODEL**
Engel	Biopsychosocial Model: Theory of Grief and Mourning
Bowlby	Attachment, Loss and Grief Theory
Rondo	Stage of Grief Model
Worden	Four Tasks of Grieving
Kübler-Ross	Model of Coping with Dying: Five Stages of Grief

© Cengage Learning 2013

BOX 14-3

MAJOR THEORIES AND MODELS OF GRIEF

THEORIST	DESCRIPTION	COMPONENTS
George Engle (1961)	Focused on processes involved in grief and grieving. Identified grief as having 3 major stages.	1. Shock and disbelief 2. Developing awareness of the loss 3. Restitution and recovery
Elisabeth Kübler-Ross (1969)	Based on her studies of patients facing terminal illness. Introduced what became known as the Five Stages of Grief.	1. Denial 2. Anger 3. Bargaining 4. Depression 5. Acceptance
John Bowlby (1982)	Draws from attachment theory and suggests that grief occurs when the bereaved learns that the object of attachment is lost.	1. Shock and numbness 2. Yearning and searching 3. Disorganization and despair 4. Reorganization
Therese Rando (1984)	Identified 6 stages of grieving, commonly referred to as the Six Rs of grieving.	1. Recognizing the loss 2. Reacting to the separation 3. Recollecting memories of the deceased 4. Relinquishing the old attachment 5. Readjusting to the new environment 6. Reinvesting self
William Worden (2002)	Developed a theory of grief that involves recognizing the tasks of grieving.	1. Accepting the reality of the loss 2. Working through the pain and grief 3. Adjusting to an environment in which the deceased is missing 4. Emotionally relocating deceased and moving on with life

the Stages of Grief Model: (1) avoidance, (2) confrontation, and (3) accommodation. The stages of grieving described by Rando are commonly referred to as the "Six Rs" of grieving: (1) recognizing the loss (awareness), (2) reacting to the separation (feeling the emotions), (3) recollecting memories of the deceased (remembering, reliving), (4) relinquishing the old attachment (finding new ways of living without the deceased), (5) readjusting to the new environment (developing new coping skills), and (6) reinvesting self (energy, once turned inward on grief, begins to be focused outward again).

Several others describe theories of grief. Worden (2002), for example, developed a theory of grief that involves recognizing the tasks of grieving, and he was instrumental in describing these tasks: (1) accepting the reality of the loss, (2) working through the pain and grief, (3) adjusting to an environment in which the deceased is missing, and (4) emotionally relocating the deceased and moving on with life (Lammana, 2011). Perhaps the most well-known psychiatrist and author on grieving is Elisabeth Kübler-Ross. Kübler-Ross introduced what became known as the "five stages of grief." Based on her studies of the feeling of patients facing terminal illness, Kübler-Ross (1969), outlined the five stages of grief as (1) denial, (2) anger, (3) bargaining, (4) depression, and (5) acceptance.

One can see many similarities among these theories and models and the stages or phases of grief. As nurses, we need to

use these as guides to promote healing and wellness in those who are experiencing a loss or have experienced one. Experiencing grief is like a roller coaster ride with many dips and turns, and the reactions associated with grief are natural and unique to every person. It takes time to heal. Further, a person need not go through every stage or phase or go through them in any particular sequence in order to heal. Nurses need to convey understanding and provide support in a nonjudgmental way. In her book before her death in 2004, Kübler-Ross said that the stages of grief were never meant to tuck messy emotions into neat packages. Grief stages, in fact, are responses to loss that many people experience. Of utmost importance is that there is not a typical response to loss because there is no typical loss; our grieving is as individual as our lives (Kübler-Ross & Kessler, 2005, p. 7).

EXPERIENCING AND REACTING TO GRIEF

People who are grieving a loss are affected in a variety of ways; however, certain reactions are common among those who are grieving. Almost anything that people experience in the early stages of grief may be considered normal, including feeling as though you are losing your mind or living in a nightmare. Some may begin questioning their religious beliefs, asking how or why this happened to them.

Other common reactions or feelings are shock and disbelief, especially right after a loss. It is often difficult to accept what has happened. The person may feel numb, have trouble believing the loss really occurred, and at times even deny that it happened. Sadness is probably the most universally experienced symptom of grief. Sadness is often accompanied by feelings of emptiness, despair, yearning, or deep loneliness. Crying and feeling emotionally unstable are not uncommon at this point.

Another common feeling is guilt, which arises from feelings of regret about things said or unsaid, done or left undone. Guilt may be due to feeling relieved when the person dies after a long, difficult illness. A person may feel guilty for not doing something to prevent the death, even if nothing could have been done.

Anger after a loss is also common. Even if no one is to blame for the loss, an individual may feel angry and resentful. Often, bereaved persona may turn their anger toward God, the physician, the person who died, or even toward themselves.

A significant loss can trigger a host of worries and fear. Because of these overwhelming feelings, some individuals may even experience panic attacks. The loss of a loved one can produce fears about your own mortality, about facing life without that person, or about the responsibilities you now face alone. Often people also experience physical symptoms including fatigue, nausea, lowered immunity, weight loss or weight gain, aches and pains, and insomnia (Helpguide.org, 2011). Nurses need to understand the whole gamut of emotions and reactions that might occur after individuals experience a loss.

ASK **YOURSELF**

Experiencing Personal Loss

How do you react to a personal loss or death of a loved one? Do you experience physical symptoms such as inability to sleep or eat? Do you respond with psychological symptoms, such as anger or denial? Do you express regret? What can you do to help accept your loss?

PALLIATIVE AND HOSPICE CARE

According to the World Health Organization (WHO) (2011), **palliative care** is an approach that improves the quality of life of patients and their families facing the problems associated with life-threatening illness. This is achieved through the prevention and relief of suffering by means of the early identification and impeccable assessment and treatment of pain and other problems, whether physical, psychosocial, or spiritual. The WHO further describes other components or goals of palliative care that are outlined in Box 14-4.

HOSPICE

The word *hospice* is derived from the Latin word *hospitium*, meaning guesthouse. It was originally used to describe a place of shelter for weary and sick travelers returning from religious pilgrimages. During the 1960s, Dr. Cicely Saunders, a British physician, began the modern hospice movement

HEALTH PROMOTION THEORY LINK

Health Promotion and the End-of-life: Reed's Self-Transcendence Theory

Reed's theory of self-transcendence incorporates three basic concepts: vulnerability, self-transcendence, and well-being (Reed, 1997, 2003, 2008; Coward, 2010). Reed defines vulnerability as the awareness of personal mortality that arises with aging and other life or health events (Reed, 2003; Coward, 2010). Vulnerability serves to clarify the context in which self-transcendence is realized when confronting not only end-of-life issues but also life crises. *Self-transcendence* refers to the pandimensional fluctuations in perceived boundaries that extend persons beyond their immediate and constricted views of self and the world. *Well-being* means "feeling whole and healthy, in accordance with one's own criteria for wholeness and well-being" (Reed, 2003, p. 148; Coward, 2010). Research studies have used Reed's theory of self-transcendence and have provided evidence supporting the association between self-transcendence and increased well-being in populations that are typically confronted with an awareness of their own personal mortality (Coward, 2010).

by establishing St. Christopher's Hospice near London. At St. Christopher's, a team approach to professional caregiving was organized, and the hospice is also known to be the first program to use modern pain management techniques to compassionately care for the dying. The first hospice in the United States was established in New Haven, Connecticut, in 1974 (Hospice Foundation of America [HFA], 2011). Today there are more than 4700 hospice programs in the United States, and it is estimated that hospice programs cared for 1.4 million people in 2008 (National Hospice and Palliative Care Organization [NHPCO], 2009; HFA, 2011).

A **hospice** is considered the model for quality compassionate care for people facing a life-threatening illness. Hospice provides for all aspects of patient care: expert medical care, pain management, emotional support, as well as spiritual support. All the care provided is specifically tailored to the patient's needs and wishes. An essential component of the hospice's support is that it is provided to the patient as well as to the family and loved ones. The major focus of hospice is caring, not curing. In most cases, care is provided in the patient's home but may also be provided in freestanding hospice centers, hospitals, nursing homes, and other long-term care facilities. It has been estimated that about 80% of hospice care is provided in the patient's home, family member's home, and nursing homes. Inpatient hospice facilities are sometimes available to assist with caregiving as well. Hospice services are available to patients with any terminal illness of any age, religion, or race. Hospice, it has been said, is not a place but a concept of care (NHPCO, 2009, p. 3).

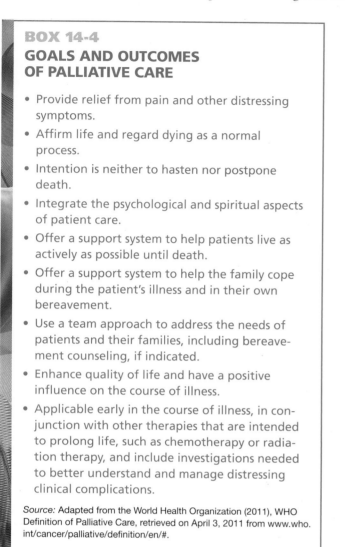

GOALS AND OUTCOMES OF PALLIATIVE CARE

- Provide relief from pain and other distressing symptoms.
- Affirm life and regard dying as a normal process.
- Intention is neither to hasten nor postpone death.
- Integrate the psychological and spiritual aspects of patient care.
- Offer a support system to help patients live as actively as possible until death.
- Offer a support system to help the family cope during the patient's illness and in their own bereavement.
- Use a team approach to address the needs of patients and their families, including bereavement counseling, if indicated.
- Enhance quality of life and have a positive influence on the course of illness.
- Applicable early in the course of illness, in conjunction with other therapies that are intended to prolong life, such as chemotherapy or radiation therapy, and include investigations needed to better understand and manage distressing clinical complications.

Source: Adapted from the World Health Organization (2011), WHO Definition of Palliative Care, retrieved on April 3, 2011 from www.who.int/cancer/palliative/definition/en/#.

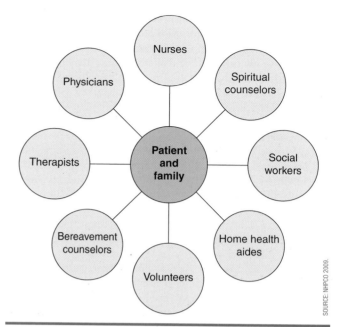

FIGURE 14-2 Hospice interdisciplinary team.

Hospice is based on comfort-oriented care. Referral into hospice is a movement into another mode of therapy, which may be more appropriate for terminal care. Hospice provides a less high-cost technology because family, friends, and volunteers provide 90% of the day-to-day patient care at home. Additionally, patients eligible for Medicare or Medicaid will pay few out-of-pocket expenses for their hospice care. Most private insurers also cover some or most hospice-related expenses.

Nurses must understand the concept of hospice to relay the appropriate and correct information to patients who are facing a life-threatening illness. Effective communication skills are imperative when caring for this population of patients. We need to remember not to be judgmental and that patients have every right to refuse any type of care that they might deem inappropriate for them. They also have the right to effective, efficient, compassionate care by qualified health care providers.

END-OF-LIFE: THE GOOD DEATH CONCEPT

Every human being on this earth has one thing in common: We all experience loss, and we all experience death sooner or later, whether it is someone else's or our own. What differs is where and how we die. Once an individual is diagnosed with a life-threatening illness, such as cancer, the diagnosis definitely changes the life of everyone involved, including the patient and the patient's family. The illness typically becomes the focal point of all involved. Because of the uncertainty involved with a life-threatening illness, caring for a dying person also requires the involvement of physicians, nurses, and others, depending on the wishes and needs of the patient. Nurses must understand that, even if people prefer to die at home and be cared for by family members, they still need the support and assistance of their physician as well as other health care professionals (Proot, Abu-Saad, Crebolder, Luker, & Widdershoven, 2003; Iranmanesh, Hosseini, & Esmaili, 2011).

Anyone who has ever been involved with caring for someone who has a life-threatening illness or who is dying knows

The hospice team consists of a group of specialized individuals dedicated to the care of those facing a life-threatening illness. Their primary goal is to develop a health-promotion plan of care that meets each patient's individual needs, whether for pain management or symptom control. The hospice team is interdisciplinary (see Figure 14-2), usually consisting of the patient's personal physician, hospice physician or medical director, nurses, home health aides, social workers, bereavement counselors, clergy or other spiritual counselors, trained volunteers, as well as speech, physical, and occupational therapists, as needed. Usually, a family member serves as the primary caregiver and, when appropriate, helps make decisions for the terminally ill individual. Once an individual is admitted into hospice, members of the hospice staff make regular visits to assess the patient and to provide additional care or other services, as needed. It is comforting to know that the hospice staff is on call 24 hours a day, seven days a week (Hospice Foundation of America, 2011).

Although hospice care has been around for over 30 years, many individuals and their family members do not take advantage of this type of care, mainly due to misconceptions about what hospice is and what it is for. Although many have taken advantage of hospice care, others are still misled by the concept. Several myths need to be addressed in order to educate others regarding the use of hospice (see Box 14-5).

BOX 14-5
HOSPICE: MYTHS AND REALITY

Myth:	Reality:
Hospice is where you go when there is "nothing else to be done."	Hospice is the "something more" that can be done for the patient and the family when the illness cannot be cured.
Myth:	Reality:
Families should be isolated from a dying patient.	When family members (including children) experience the dying process in a caring environment, it helps counteract the fear of their own mortality and the mortality of their loved one.
Myth:	Reality:
Hospice care is more expensive.	Studies have shown hospice care is no more costly. Frequently it is less expensive than conventional care during the last six months of life.
Myth:	Reality:
You can't keep your own doctor if you enter hospice.	Hospice physicians work closely with your doctor of choice to determine a plan of care.

Source: Adopted from Hospice Foundation of America (HFA), 2011.

that a tremendous amount of compassion, time, and effort is required. Although much has been done to improve the care of those facing loss and death, much work still has to be done. Improving the quality of death has become an important issue not only for patients, their families, and loved ones, but also for health care professionals, researchers, and policy makers who organize and provide care (Patrick, Engelberg, & Curtis, 2001; Iranmanesh, Hosseini, & Esmaili, 2011).

To improve the quality of death and end-of-life care, nurses can learn about the concept of the so-called good death from family members who have faced the death of their loved ones. Family members can evaluate the quality of end-of-life care received and convey valuable information to the nurse and other health care givers. The concept of a good death is culturally perceived, although usually factors in a good death include the importance of respect and communication. The concept of a good death is not easily defined; however, 12 principles of a good death have been identified:

- To know when death is coming and to understand what can be expected
- To be able to retain control of what happens
- To be afforded dignity and privacy
- To have control over pain relief and other symptom control
- To have choice and control over where death occurs (at home or elsewhere)
- To have access to information and expertise of whatever kind is necessary
- To have access to any spiritual or emotional support required
- To have access to hospice care in any location, not only in the hospital
- To have control over who is present and who shares the end
- To be able to issue advance directives that ensure wishes are respected
- To have time to say good-bye and to have control over other aspects of timing

- To be able to leave when it is time to go, and not to have life prolonged pointlessly

(Debate of the Age Health and Care Study Group, 1999; Smith, 2000, p. 129).

INTERNATIONAL PERSPECTIVES ON THE GOOD DEATH

Although what constitutes a good death varies among cultures and populations throughout the world, literature exists to support the concept of a good death; many studies have

GLOBAL HIGHLIGHTS IN HEALTH PROMOTION
World Cultures and Good Death

Griggs (2010), in a qualitative study, analyzed perceptions of a good death among community nurses in England. The nurses identified several key themes for a good death (see Box 14-6). They concluded that when these components are in place, a good death is possible. Other factors, such as lack of necessary medication or resources, unsuccessful interprofessional relationships, and lack of teamwork, were significant determinants of less successful care. The study concluded that a good death can be provided in the community, although many challenges are associated with such care. Due to the unpredictability of death, challenges may always be a threat to effective anticipatory care planning; thus, it is important to recognize that patients need and are entitled to specialist care. In so doing, many of these difficulties can be overcome (Griggs, 2010, p. 139).

BOX 14-6

KEY COMPONENTS FOR A GOOD DEATH

Symptom control	Spirituality
Patient choice	Interprofessional relationships
Honesty	Effective preparation
Organization	Provision of seamless care

Source: Adapted from Griggs (2010).

---

produced findings related to the international perspective on a good death. For example, a study focusing on evaluating the concept of a good death was on the views of a representative sample of bereaved family members in Iran. It was concluded that it is important for "professional caregivers to be sensitive and pay attention to the preference of each unique person's perceptions through his or her senses. This includes views, tastes, sounds, smells, and bodily contact. They also point out that it is imperative to also pay attention to the patients' spiritual needs, if we are to implement holistic care" (Iranmanesh et al., 2011, p. 62).

Americans' perception of what constitutes a good death has also been studied. In a study focusing on Americans and their perception of a good death, it was concluded that a good death involved respect for the individual's autonomy with open communication among family members (Winland-Brown, 2001). Vig and Pearlman (2004) concluded that a good death has an individual meaning for Americans and does not have a consensual meaning (Iranmanesh et al., 2011). Interestingly, the study findings supported the notion that a good death does not have the same meaning to everyone; it is individually perceived.

The good death concept has also been evaluated in other cultures including studies in Japan (Hattori, McCubbin, & Ishida, 2006), Norway (Ruland & Moore, 1998), Thailand communities (Kongsuwan & Locsin, 2009), Muslim society (Tayeb, Al-zamel, Fareed, & Abouellail, 2010), and Ghana (Van der Geest, 2004). In the Japanese culture, Hattori, McCubbin, & Ishida (2006) found that a good death is seen as a multidimensional, individual experience based on personal and sociocultural domains of life that incorporate the person's past, present, and future. The research in Norway, focused on the theory of a peaceful death, which is believed to have five major aspects: not being in pain, experience of comfort, experience of dignity/respect, being at peace, and closeness to significant others and/or persons who care (Ruland & Moore, 1998). People in Thailand used the term "peaceful death" instead of "good death." Intensive care unit nurses in Thailand defined a peaceful death as awareness of dying, creating a caring environment, and promoting end-of-life care (Kongsuwan & Locsin, 2009). Three domains related to a good death were identified in the study focusing on the Muslim society: religion and faith, self-esteem and personal image, and satisfaction about family security (Tayeb, Al-zamel, Fareed, & Abouellail, 2010). Finally, in a study done in Ghana, it was determined that a good death was integrated with a peaceful death, meaning peace with others, being at peace with one's own life and soul, dying in

---

RESEARCH NOTE

A retrospective survey of the care of adults in Alice Springs Hospital

STUDY PROBLEM/PURPOSE

There are varying levels of responsiveness from health care providers to the end-of-life needs of hospitalized patients and their families. The main purpose of this study was to explore end-of-life issues and differences in the services provided to people of Aboriginal and non-Aboriginal backgrounds in a busy regional hospital serving remote Australia.

METHODS

A consecutive cohort case-note survey was conducted of adult deaths in Alice Springs Hospital (ASH) over an 18-month period. The exclusion criteria were people younger than 18 years, death in less than 48 hours after admission, any coroner's cases, and any individuals who died and had no case notes. Data on whether a diagnosis of dying was made were recorded as not-for-resuscitation status, intensive care unit (ICU) admission, social worker input, referral to the palliative care service, and documented comfort at the end-of-life.

FINDINGS

Of the 128 admissions, 55 cases were excluded based on predetermined exclusion criteria, and 73 cases were reviewed. Of the 73 deaths surveyed (33 men), 47 (64%) were Aboriginal. Of the 73 cases of death reported in the study, a diagnosis of dying was made in 84% of them. Eighty-eight percent of the deaths had a not-for-resuscitation order, 48% were admitted to ICU during their last admission, 66% were referred to social workers, 68% were referred to palliative care, and 85% of people were documented to be comfortable during the dying process. There were no differential outcomes for Aboriginal and non-Aboriginal decedents except age ($P < 0.0001$).

IMPLICATIONS

For 33% of deaths reported, the diagnosis of dying was made in the last 48 hours of life. The findings support the idea that the training and support of clinical staff to proactively make the diagnosis of dying is needed across the health system. Clinicians need to use objective thresholds for referral to palliative care by identifying the people with the most complex needs.

Nadimi, F., & Currow, D. C. (2011). As death approaches: A retrospective survey of the care of adults in Alice Springs Hospital. *Australian Journal of Rural Health, 19,* 4–8.

the fullness of time, dying at home, and being surrounded by relatives and loved ones (Van der Geest, 2004; Iranmanesh et al., 2011, pp. 59–60).

As noted in these studies, there is no universal definition of a good death. The definition of a good death is for the most part based on the sociocultural context and religious background. Because nurses come across a variety of people with different backgrounds, cultures, and religions, they must be sensitive to their uniqueness in perceiving and experiencing death in order to provide the best end-of-life care possible and to help patients journey to a good death.

DEATH WITH DIGNITY: PROMOTING WELLNESS AT THE END-OF-LIFE

Nurses are in a prime position to employ a health-promotion perspective in helping a patient die with dignity. However, nurses must develop and enhance their ability to help those approaching the end of their lives. According to Mathiews (2010), the concept of dying with dignity is a dynamic process; it takes time to develop and continuously evolves over a nurse's career. A novice nurse, for example, may focus, most assuredly, on the patient as a person. As nurses mature and gain experience, they attain insight into facilitating family grieving. As seasoned professionals, nurses emphasize the dignity that, through effective nursing, can be restored to those dying. Preservation of dignity is found in the way we honor death (p. 185). The following Spotlight On illustrates how a nurse can be instrumental in preserving dignity at the end of a patient's life.

KNOWING YOURSELF: ASSESSING YOUR FEELINGS

A major area in which we need to invest time is self-awareness. As nurses, we often find ourselves caught up in caring for others, not realizing that how we respond to certain situations may have an everlasting impact on those under our care. Therefore, we need to take time to contemplate our thoughts, feelings, beliefs, biases, prejudices, and fears about dying and death. Many nurses are uncomfortable and perhaps feel inadequate in caring for those facing the end-of-life. Many times, patients who are facing the end of their lives are usually left to deal with the reality of facing their deaths alone. Often, the end of someone's life brings with it great turmoil, fear, and uncertainty for all

those involved. Conducting a self-assessment on our perceptions and feelings about the end-of-life and death is an essential task for nurses or anyone entering health care. If we are not able to deal with all these feelings and issues, how can we help others? When confronted with the dying patient, we need to remember what we do best: care for those in need regardless of circumstances. A good place to start is learning about the needs of those facing the end-of-life, advocating for them, and educating others.

SPOTLIGHT ON

Facilitating Dying with Dignity

Melie was diagnosed with metastatic breast cancer. She did not have surgery but agreed to an oral antineoplastic medication and radiation treatments. Her husband and her daughter were her primary caregivers. The cancer caused much devastation, and her body weight dropped to less than 100 lb. Melie told her family that she didn't want any heroics performed and that her biggest fear was dying in agony. The family decided to engage a hospice to help care for Melie. The hospice provided the family with services that included emotional and spiritual support. When Melie died, the nurse took care to prepare her body and allowed her daughter to help. She also let each family member spend a few minutes with Melie before calling the funeral home. The nurse asked her daughter whether she wanted them to cover Melie's face when taken to the funeral home. The daughter told the nurse that Melie should have her face covered because she wouldn't want others to see her without her makeup. Melie cared about how she looked, and both the nurse and the daughter recognized the need to preserve Melie's dignity. Melie's daughter never forgot the nurse who had provided her mother the dignity that she deserved.

SUMMARY

The main purpose of this chapter was to highlight important issues and challenges facing those at the end-of-life. It also brought to light how health-promotion concepts can be incorporated into the nursing practice to enhance the quality of care for all individuals facing death. As health care practitioners, we need to be willing to step up to the challenge and advocate for

those who are at what may be the most vulnerable time of their lives. We also need to be aware of our perceptions about death and where we stand on the related issues. By knowing ourselves first, we can acquire the needed enthusiasm and openmindedness to work with not only individuals facing the end-of-life but also their family and loved ones.

Maria Alanis: Grieving Anticipatory/Anxiety, Death; Ineffective Health Maintenance, Powerlessness; Ineffective Family Coping; Activity Intolerance; Imbalanced Nutrition: Less Than Body Requirements

OBJECTIVES/GOALS: Through participation in discussion of this case study, participants will have the opportunity to:

1. Identify specific factors and/or issues that may affect a nursing student caring for a patient at the end-of-life.
2. Discuss how a nursing student's health-promotion practices can influence the outcomes and quality of a patient's end-of-life care.
3. Identify positive health-promotion strategies that can be incorporated into curricular activities focusing on the end-of-life.

HEALTH-PROMOTION CONCERN, HISTORY AND PHYSICAL, PRESENT HEALTH STATUS, PAST HEALTH STATUS, FAMILY HISTORY, AND SOCIAL HISTORY

Maria Alanis is a 58-year-old white, Mexican-American female. She has been married to her husband for 40 years and has a 37-year-old son. She has a fifth-grade education and is a stay-at-home mom.

Maria has three brothers and two sisters. Her eldest brother suffers from diabetes and chronic renal failure; her younger brothers suffer from hypertension that is controlled with medication. Maria's sisters are both healthy with no major problems. Both of her parents are deceased; her father died at the age of 80 from metastatic prostate cancer, and her mother died at 75 from metastatic breast cancer.

Maria has been healthy for the majority of her life, has helped her husband maintain their family ranch, and is an active member of her local parish. She was diagnosed with breast cancer at age 50 and opted for a double mastectomy. Maria was given chemotherapy and radiation therapy. She had been doing well for the first 5 years after her diagnosis and was determined to be cancer-free. Her health started deteriorating shortly after the start of her sixth year postmastectomy when she started experiencing fatigue, lack of appetite, weight loss, and general aches and pains. Maria also started having difficulty sleeping at night, sleeping only approximately 3–4 hours per night, waking early, and being unable to go back to sleep. She has lost approximately 50 lb within a 2-month period and is no longer able to participate in her normal daily activities.

After several diagnostic exams, Maria was diagnosed with stage IV breast cancer with metastases to her spine, lungs, and brain. Her health has deteriorated, and she is now bedridden and requires a g-tube to be placed for nutrition and medication administration. She requires assistance for all ADLs, provided mainly by her husband and a home health aide. Because of her rapidly deteriorating health and decreased treatment options, her physician has recommended placing her into hospice, but unfortunately none provided service to her place of residence, which is in a rural area. The family decided to admit Maria into a long-term, rehabilitation facility. One week after being admitted, Mrs. Alanis was assigned to a first-year nursing student.

REVIEW OF PERTINENT DOMAINS

Biological Domain

Physical exam reveals a 5-in., 5½-ft female who weighs 105 lb.

GASTROINTESTINAL: She is currently NPO (nothing by mouth) and is on continuous tube feeding with Jevity (½ cal/mL) at 25 mL/hour via PEG tube. She has been having small amounts of loose stools 2–3 times a day and is now using adult diapers. Normal bowel sounds present to all 4 quadrants.

GENITOURINARY: Maria has an indwelling 16 French Foley catheter in place to bedside drainage. Urine is dark amber, and output is approximately 800 mL per shift.

INTEGUMENTARY: Maria's skin is pale, cool, and moist with even pigmentation and turgor with delayed recoil. She has short gray hair and it is evenly distributed and dry. Nails are pale, thick, and firm without ridges and of normal length.

Psychological Domain

Maria is a pleasant, motherly, intelligent woman who enjoyed taking care of her family and being involved in church activities and in helping others. She grew up on a ranch with five siblings, enjoyed being busy, and takes pride in her work. Maria is quiet and has a sad demeanor. She answers questions readily but requires extra time due to extreme fatigue.

Her main concern, she states, is that she is ready to die and that her family is not ready to accept her wishes. They insist on her participating in rehabilitation activities on a daily basis. She continuously asks anyone who walks into her room to "please tell them to stop" and "I can't do this anymore."

Maria does not have a living will or advance directive, and, because of her poor health, her family took it upon themselves to make the decisions regarding her care. Whenever her son was present and heard her say this, he would just tell her that it was for her own good and that he wanted "everything done for his mother, because she would want to give up." Her husband was told of her wishes but was offended that someone was telling him that his wife was getting weaker and that the family should consider a facility providing hospice care. He stated, "My wife is OK; all she needs is to eat and keep moving." Currently she is a full code with no do-not-resuscitate (DNR) order. Her son and her husband visit her as often as possible, usually 1–2 times a week.

Social Domain

Since the reoccurrence of her cancer, Maria's health has taken a rapid turn for the worse, leaving her with very little energy and totally dependent on others for assistance. She participates as much as possible in the rehab activities but would rather be left alone. She is visited only by her son and husband because her siblings live in other states. Her immediate family is having difficulty accepting her deteriorating health and impending death, as they insist that everything be done for her.

Environmental Domain

Maria spends most of her time in her hospital room except for when she is taken to participate in prescribed occupation and physical therapy twice a day. She is bedridden and totally dependent on others for all her needs. Maria is not able to ambulate, turn, or get into and out of bed on her own. She requires total patient care, including frequent oral suctioning because of increased respiratory secretions. She has a Foley catheter to bedside drainage, PEG for tube feeding and medication administration, and an IV of normal saline at KVO (keep vein open).

Epilogue

The following week, Maria's health condition worsened to the point that she had to be taken to the emergency room of a local hospital. While there, she arrested, was resuscitated, and admitted to the intensive care unit (ICU), where she arrested and was resuscitated two more times. She was then on a ventilator and IV fluids, and she was being monitored continuously. She improved enough to be transferred to the step-down unit, where she arrested one more time, and resuscitation was not successful. She died after the fourth resuscitation attempt failed.

QUESTIONS FOR DISCUSSION

1. What health-promotion issue most stood out?
2. Did her family have the right to make decisions for her?
3. What role, if any, should the physician and nurses have played in this situation?
4. Would a living will and/or advance directive have made a difference? If yes, how?
5. Did Maria experience a good death?
6. Would hospice care have been beneficial? If yes, how?

KEY CONCEPTS

1. Health care professionals have to become aware of a variety of end-of-life issues and challenges in order to ensure health promotion and quality of care to those journeying to the end of their lives.

2. Although at times the terms are used interchangeably, *loss, bereavement,* and *mourning* have distinct meanings.

3. Theories and stages of grief are guidelines that nursing students, as well as all other health care professionals, can use to assess others' reaction to loss and grieving.

4. Although loss is universal, the reactions, emotions, and feelings a person displays are individualized.

5. Communication is the essence of a therapeutic relationship. Nurses and all health care professionals must acquire the required skills in order to facilitate an end-of-life discussion.

6. The initiation of palliative and hospice care at the appropriate time is essential for promoting quality patient care for those with life-threatening illnesses.

7. Each illness follows a trajectory; knowing this allows one to assist patients and family in making important decisions.

8. Diagnosing dying requires that health care professionals have the necessary assessment skills to recognize the common signs and symptoms of a person who is dying.

9. Self-reflection enhances the care we can provide to those facing the end-of-life.

10. Health care providers are in a unique position to ensure dignity for those who are dying.

CHAPTER REVIEW

Learning Activities

1. Contemplate the last time you experienced a loss. How did you react to the loss? What kinds of emotions did you display? Were you aware of your grieving?

2. Interview a peer, and discuss personal feelings about end-of-life.

3. Discuss the importance of advance planning for end-of-life care.

Multiple-Choice Questions

1. An elderly woman who is no longer able to tend to her flower garden might experience which type of loss?
   a. Actual
   b. Perceived
   c. Anticipatory
   d. External

2. The type of loss that challenges our belief system is known as a:
   a. physical loss.
   b. actual loss.
   c. psychological loss.
   d. none of the above.

3. Major issues affecting end-of-life care include which of the following?
   a. Communication
   b. Symptom management
   c. Decision making
   d. All of the above
   e. a and b only

4. This phenomenon occurs about 50% of the time and is predictive of death occurring within 48 hours.
   a. Delirium
   b. Restlessness
   c. Death rattle
   d. Anorexia

5. True or false: When someone is diagnosed with a terminal illness, it is not uncommon for them to begin considering the meaning and purpose of life, as well as impending death.

6. You have a patient who has been ill for many years with prostate cancer and is now facing the end of his life. You wish to initiate a conversation about his plans, wishes, and thoughts. Which of the following questions would be best to initiate the conversation?
   a. "Have you thought about you want?"
   b. "How do you feel within yourself today?"
   c. "Does your family know you don't have long to live?"
   d. All of the above.

7. There are many theories on loss and grief. As nurses we need to understand that:
   a. it normally takes a few months to get over the grief.
   b. a person should experience all the stages of grief in order to heal.
   c. theories are guides that help nurses promote healing and wellness.
   d. people usually experience and respond to a loss in the same way.

8. It is not uncommon for a person to feel a variety of emotions during the early stages of grief, including:
   a. feeling numb.
   b. questioning your religious beliefs.
   c. feeling like you are not in control of the situation.
   d. all of the above.
   e. b only.

9. The most universally experienced symptom of grief is said to be which of the following?
   a. Guilt
   b. Anger
   c. Frustration
   d. Sadness

10. To be an effective provider of care to someone facing the end-of-life, which of the following attributes is the most important for a nurse to possess?
    a. Knowing where one stands regarding end-of-life issues
    b. Avoiding being judgmental
    c. Using therapeutic communication skills
    d. Being familiar with the theories of loss and grief

ORGANIZATIONS AND WEBSITES

AARP: Advance Directives: Planning for the Future: **http://assets.aarp.org/external_sites/caregiving/multimedia/EG_AdvanceDirectives.html**

AARP: Talking About Your Final Wishes: **http://www.aarp.org/relationships/grief-loss/info-2003/endoflife-finalwishes.html**

Agency for Healthcare Research and Quality: Advance Care Planning: Preferences for Care at the End-of-life: **http://www.ahrq.gov/research/endliferia/endria.htm**

Aging with Dignity: Five Wishes: **http://www.aging-withdignity.org/five-wishes.php**

American Bar Association's Commission on Law & Aging: Consumer's Tool Kit for Health Care General Medical Counsel: Information on Treatment and care towards the end-of-life: Good practice in decision making: **http://www.gmc-uk.org/End_of_life.pdf_32486688.pdf**

Helpguide.org: A trusted nonprofit resource with information to help empower people with knowledge, support, and hope: **http://www.helpguide.org**

National Hospice and Palliative Care Organization: Caring Connections: **http://www.caringinfo.org/**

National Long Term Care Ombudsman Resource Center: Helpful contacts: **http://www.ltcombudsman.org/contact**

REFERENCES/RESOURCES

American Pain Foundation. (2010). *End-of-life.* Retrieved on June 8, 2011, from http://www.painfoundation.org/learn/living/end-of-life/

American Society for Aesthetic Plastic Surgery. (2010). *Quick facts: Highlights of the ASAPS 2010 statistics on cosmetic surgery.* Retrieved on April 28, 2011, from www.surgery.org

AssistGuide Information Services. (2009). *Types of grief and loss.* Retrieved on May, 1, 2011, from www.agis.com

Baird, R. M., & Rosenbaum, S. E. (eds). (2003). *Caring for the dying: Critical issues at the edge of life.* Amherst, NY: Prometheus Books.

Baker, J. N., Rai, S., Liu, W., Srivastava, K., Kane, J. R., Zawistowski, C. A., Burghen, E. A., Gattuso, J. S., West, N., & Althoff, J. et al. (2009). Race does not influence do-not- resuscitate status or the number or timing of end-of-life care discussions at a pediatric oncology referral center. *Journal of Palliative Medicine,* 12(1), 71–76.

Betz, G., & Thorngren, J. M. (2006). Ambiguous loss and the family grieving process. *Family Journal,* 14(4), 359–365. DOI: 10.117/1066480706290052.

Billing, J. A. (2007). Care of the dying patients and their families. In L. Goldman & D. Ausiello (eds.), *Cecil medicine* 23rd ed, Philadelphia, PA: Saunders Elsevier, pp. 11–16.

Bowlby, J. (1982). *Attachment and loss.* New York, NY: Basic Books.

Canadian Hospice and Palliative Care Association. (2006). *The pan-Canadian gold standard for palliative home care: Towards equitable access to high quality hospice, palliative and end-of-life care at home.* Ottawa: CHPCA.

Central Intelligence Agency (CIA). (2011). *The world factbook.* Retrieved on April 13, 2011, from www.cia.gov/libraries/publications/the-world-factbook/geos/xx.html

Coward, D. D. (2010). Pamela Reed: Self-transcendence theory. In M. R. Alligood & A. M. Tomey (eds.). *Nursing theorists and their work* (7th ed.). Maryland Heights, MI: Mosby-Elsevier, pp. 618–637.

Debate of the Age Health and Care Study Group. (1999). *The future of health and care of older people: The best is yet to come.* London: Age Concern.

Department of Health. (2008). *End-of-life care strategy: Promoting high quality of care for all adults at the end-of-life.* Retrieved on April 22, 2011, from www.dh.gov.uk/publications

Dictionary.com. (2011). Retrieved on April 22, 2011, from www.dictionary.reference.com/browse/mourning

Earle, C. C., Neville, B. A., Landrum, M. B., Ayanian, J. Z., Block, S. D., & Weeks, J. C. (2004). Trends in the aggressiveness of cancer care near the end-of-life. *Journal of Clinical Oncology,* 22(31), 315–321.

Edwards, P. (2005). An overview of the end-of-life discussion. *International Journal of Palliative Nursing,* 11(1), 21–27.

Ellershaw, J. E., Sutcliffe, J. M., & Saunders, C. M. (1995). Dehydration and the dying patient. *Journal of Pain Symptom Management,* 10, 192–197.

Ellershaw, J., Smith, C., Overill, S., Walker, S. E., & Aldridge, J. (2001). Care of the dying: Setting standards for symptom control in the last 48 hours of life. *Journal of Pain and Symptom Management,* 21, 12–17.

Engel, G. L. (1961). Is grief a disease? A challenge for medical research. *Psychosomatic Medicine,* 23(1), 18–22.

Fainsinger, R., Miller, M. J., Bruera, E., Hanson, J., & Meceachem, T. (1991). Symptom control during the last week of life on a palliative care unit. *Journal of Palliative Care,* 7, 5–11.

Foley, K. M., & Gelband, H. (eds.) (2001). *Improving palliative care for cancer.* Washington, DC: National Academy Press.

Fredriksson, L., & Ericksson, K. (2001). The patient's narrative of suffering: A path to health? *Scandinavian Journal of Caring Science,* 5(1), 3–11.

Gibson, M., & Gorman, E. (2010). Contextualizing end-of-life care for aging veterans: Family members' thoughts. *International Journal of Palliative Nursing,* 16(7), 339–343.

Glare, P., Virik, K., Jones, M., Hudson, M., Eychmuller, S., Simes, J., & Christakis, N. (2003). *British Medical Journal,* 327(7408), 195–200.

Griggs, C. H. (2010). Community nurses' perceptions of a good death: A qualitative exploratory study. *International Journal of Palliative Nursing,* 16,140–149.

Gyatso, G. K. (2011). *Modern Buddism—The path of compassion and wisdom.* Glen Spey, NY: Tharpa Publications.

Hattori, K., McCubbin, M. A., & Ishida, D. N. (2006). Concept analysis of good death in the Japanese community. *Journal of Nursing Scholarship,* 38, 165–170.

Helpguide.org. (2001–2011). *Coping with grief and loss: Support for grieving and bereavement.* Retrieved on April 30, 2011, from www.helpguide.org

Hospice Foundation of America (HFA). (2011). *What is hospice?* Retrieved on June 5, 2011, from http://www.hospicefoundation.org/pages/page.asp?page_id=47055

Hospice of the North Shore and Greater Boston. (2011). *Myths and facts about grief.* Retrieved from http://www.hns.org/Bertolon_Center_for_Grief_Healing/The_Grieving_Process.aspx

Iranmanesh, S., Hosseini, H., Esmaili, M. (2011). Evaluating the "good death" concept from Iranian bereaved family members' perspective. *The Journal of Supportive Oncology, 9*(22), 59–63.

Keating, N. L., Landrum, M. B., Rogers, S. O., Baum, S. K., Virnig, B. A., Huskamo, H. A., Earle, C. C., & Kahn, K. L. (2010). Physician factors associated with discussions about end-of-life care. *Cancer,* February 15, 2010, 998–1006. DOI: 10.1002/cncr.24761

Kissane, D. W. (2002). *Family focused grief therapy: A model of family centered care during palliative care and bereavement.* Philadelphia: Open University.

Kissane, D. W., Clarke, D. M., & Street, A. F. (2001). Demoralization syndrome: A relative psychiatric diagnosis for palliative care. *Journal of Palliative Care, 17*(1), 12–21.

Knaus, W. A., Harrell, F. E., Lynn, J., Goldman, L., Phillips, R. S., Connors, A. F., Dawson, N. V., Fulkerson, W. J., Califf, R. M., Desbiens, N., Layde, P., Oye, R. K., Bellamy, P.E., Hakim, R. B., & Wagner, D. P. (1995). The SUPPORT prognostic model. Objective estimates of survival for seriously ill hospitalized adults. Study to understand prognoses and preferences for outcomes and risks of treatments. *Annals of Internal Medicine, 122*(3), 191–203.

Kongsuwan, W., & Locsin, R. C. (2009). Promoting peaceful death in the intensive care unit in Thailand. *International Nursing Review, 56,* 116–122.

Kübler-Ross, E., & Kessler, D. (2005). *On grief and grieving: Finding the meaning of grief through the five stages of loss.* New York: Scribner

Lamanna, S. J. (2011). Loss, grief & dying. In J. Wilkinson & L. Treas, *Fundamentals of nursing: Theory, concepts, and applications,* Vol. 1 (2nd ed.). Philadelphia, PA: F. A. Davis.

Legal Explanations.com. (2004–2007). *Advance directive.* Retrieved on June 5, 2011, from http://www.legal-explanations.com/definitions/advance-directive.htm

Maltoni, M., Caraceni, A., Brunelli, C., Broeckaert, B., Christakis, N., Eychmuller, S., Glare, P., Nabal, M., Vigano, A., Larkin, P., De Conno, F., Hanks, G., & Kassa, S. (2005). Prognostic factors in advanced cancer patients: Evidence-based clinical recommendations—A study for the Steering Committee of the European Association for Palliative Care. *Journal of Clinical Oncology, 23*(25), 6240–6248. DOI: 10.1200/JCO 2005.06.866.

Mathiews, A. K. (2010). Death with dignity. *Creative Nursing, 16*(4), 185–187. DOI: 10.1891/1078-4535.16.4.135.

Mercadante, S., Casuccio, A., & Fulfaro, F. (2000). The course of symptom frequency and intensity in advanced cancer patients followed at home. *Journal of Pain and Symptom Management, 20,* 104–112.

Merriam-Webster. (2011). Retrieved on May 1, 2011, from www.merriam-webster.com

MND Association. (2000). *MND resource file.* Northhampton, MA: MND Association.

Morita, T., Ichiki, T., Tsunoda, J., Inoue, S., & Chihara, S . (1998). A prospective study on the dying process in terminally ill cancer patients. *American Journal of Hospice and Palliative Care, 15,* 217–222.

Murray, S. (2005). Broaching the subject of end-of-life. *Pulse,* July 16, 2005, 38.

Nadimi, F., & Currow, D. D. (2011). As death approaches: A retrospective survey of the care of adults in Alice Springs Hospital. *Australian Journal of Rural Health, 19,* 4–8.

National Cancer Clinical Practice Guidelines in Oncology (2011). Retrieved November 7, 2011, from http://www.nccn.org/

National Consensus Project for Quality Palliative Care. (2004–2011). Retrieved November 7, 2011, from http://www.nationalconsensusproject.org/

National Hospice and Palliative Care Organization. (2009). *NHPCO facts and figures: Hospice care in America.* Retrieved November 7, 2011, from http://www.nhpco.org/files/public/Statistics_Research/NHPCO_facts_and_figures.pdf

Ozanne, E. M., Partridge, A., Moy, B., Ellis, K. J., & Sepucha, K. R. (2009). Doctor-patient communication about advance directives in metastatic breast cancer. *Journal of Palliative Medicine, 12*(6), 547–553. DOI: 10.1089/jpm.2008.0254.

Patrick, D. L., Engelberg, R. A., Curtis, J. R. (2001). Evaluating the quality of dying and death. *Journal of Pain and Symptom Management, 22,* 717–726.

Periyakoil, V. J. (2008). *End-of-life online curriculum.* End-of-life Curriculum Project, a joint project of the U.S. Veterans Administration and SUMMIT, Stanford University Medical School. Funded by a grant to the Veterans Administration Nationwide Palliative Care Network by the National Library of Medicine. Retrieved on June 8, 2011, from http://endoflife.stanford.edu/index_dev.html

Proot, I. M., Abu-Saad, H. H., Crebolder, H. F. J. M., Luker, K. A., Widdershoven, G. A. M. (2003). Vulnerability of family caregivers in terminal palliative care at home; balancing between burden and capacity. *Scandinavian Journal of Caring Science, 17,* 113–121.

Rando, T. (1984). *Grief, dying, and death: Clinical interventions for caregivers.* Champaign, IL: Research Press.

Reed, P. G. (1997). The place of transcendence in nursing's science of unitary human beings: Theory and research. In M. Madrid (ed.). *Patterns of Rogerian knowing.* New York, NY: National League for Nursing, pp. 187–196.

Reed, P. G. (2003). The theory of self-transcendence. In M. J. Smith & P. R. Liehr (eds.). *Middle range theory for nursing.* New York, NY: Springer, pp. 145–165.

Reed, P. G. (2008). The theory of self-transcendence. In M. J. Smith & P. R. Liehr (eds.). *Middle range theory for nursing,* 2nd ed. New York, NY: Springer, pp. 163–200.

Richardson, V., Berman, S., & Piwowarski, M. (1983). Projective assessment of the relationships between the salience of death, religion, and age among adults in America. *The Journal of Psychology, 109,* 149–156.

Robinson, K. L., & Watters, D. (2010). Bridging the communication gap through implementation of a patient navigator system. *Pennsylvania Nurse, 65*(2), 19–21.

Routledge, C., Ostafin, B., Juhl, J., Sedikides, C., Cathey, C., & Liao, J. (2010). Adjusting to death: The effects of mortality salience and self-esteem on psychological well-being, growth motivation, and maladaptive behavior. *Journal of Personality and Social Psychology, 99*(6), 897–916.

Ruland, C. M., & Moore, S. M. (1998). Theory construction based on standard of care: A proposed theory of the peaceful end-of-life. *Nursing Outlook, 46,* 169–175.

Singer, P. A., Martin, D. K., & Kelner, M. (1999). Quality end-of-life care: Patient's perspective. *JAMA, 2*(19), 163–168.

Smith, R. (2000). A good death. An important aim for health services and for us all. *BMJ, 320,* 129–130.

Sykes, N. (2008). End-of-life issues. *European Journal of Cancer, 44,* 1157–1162.

Tayeb, M. A., Al-zamel, E., Fareed, M. M., & Abouellail, H. A. (2010). A "good death" perspective of Muslim patients and health care providers. *Annals of Saudi-Arabia Medicine, 30,* 215–221.

Thulesius, H., Hakansson, A., & Petersson, K. (2003). Balancing: A basic process in end-of-life cancer care. *Qualitative Health Research, 13*(10), 1353–1377.

Van der Geest, S. (2004). Dying peacefully: Considering good death and bad death in Kwahu-Tafo, Ghana. *Social Science Medicine, 58,* 899–911.

Vig, E. K., & Pearlman, R. A. (2004). Good and bad dying from the perspective of terminally ill men. *Archives of Internal Medicine, 164,* 977–981.

Walden-McBride, D., & McBride, J. (2000). Listening for the patient's story. The psychosocial story of a patient with end-stage heart disease. *Journal of Psychosocial Nursing and Mental Health Services,* 38(11), 26–31.

Wennberg, J. E., Fisher, E.S., Goodman, D. C., & Skinner, J. S. (2008). *Tracking the care of patients with severe chronic illness/The Dartmouth atlas of health care 2008.* Lebanon, NH: Dartmouth Institute for Health Policy and Clinical Practice. Available at http://www.dartmouthatlas.org/downloads/atlases/2008_Chronic_Care_Atlas.pdf

Wholesome Words. (2011). *The harvest fields: Statistics—2010 edition.* Retrieved on April 13, 2011, from www.wholesomewords.org/missions/greatc.html

Wildiers, H., & Menten, J. (2002). Death rattle: Prevalence, prevention and treatment. *Journal of Pain Symptom Management, 23,* 310–317.

Winland-Brown, J. E. (2001). Public's perceptions of a good death and assisted suicide. *Issues in Interdisciplinary Care, 3,*137–144.

Worden, J. W. (2002). *Grief counseling and grief therapy: A handbook for the mental health practitioner,* 3rd ed. New York, NY: Springer.

World Health Organization (WHO). (2011). *WHO definition of palliative care.* Retrieved on April 3, 2011, from www.who.int/cancer/palliative/definition/en/#.

Yeolekar, M. E., Mehta, S., & Yeolekar, A. (2008). End-of-life care: Issues and challenges. *Journal of Postgraduate Medicine, 54*(3), 173–175.

BIBLIOGRAPHY

Addicott, R. (2011). Supporting care home residents at the end-of-life. *Journal of Palliative Care, 17*(4), 183–187.

Crippen, D. (2008). *End-of-life communication in the ICU: A global perspective.* New York, NY: Springer.

Fleming, D. A., & Hagan, J. C. (2010). *Care of the dying patient.* Columbia: University of Missouri Press.

Lansdell, J., & Mahoney, M. (2011). Developing competencies for end-of-life care in care homes. *International Journal of Palliative Nursing, 17*(3), 143–148.

Lynn, J. (2004). *Sick to death and not going to take it anymore: Reforming health care for the last years of life.* Berkeley, CA: University of California Press.

Wilson, B. A., & Wilson, M. (2004). *The first year, the worst year coping with the unexpected death of our grown up daughter.* Hoboken, NJ: John Wiley.

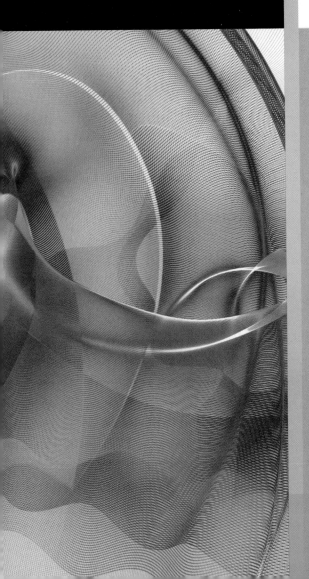

Section IV

Health-Promotion Strategies and Interventions

CHAPTER 15
Embracing Proper Nutrition

Carolina G. Huerta, EdD, MSN, RN

KEY TERMS

anorexia nervosa
basal metabolic rate
bulimia
determinants of
  health (DOH)
Dietary Guidelines
dietary reference intakes (DRIs)

essential nutrients
estimated safe and adequate daily
  dietary intake (ESADDI)
exchange system
Food Guide Pyramid
MyPlate
MyPyramid

nonessential nutrients
nutrients
nutrition
phytochemicals
recommended dietary
  allowance (RDA)

OBJECTIVES

Upon completion of this chapter, the reader should be able to:

- Recognize those nutrients that are essential to maintaining health.
- Identify the major goals of *Healthy People 2020*.
- Describe how the biological, psychological, sociocultural, spiritual, and environmental domains influence eating behaviors.
- Develop an awareness of how nutritional excesses and deficits affect health promotion.
- List dietary strategies that promote a healthful diet.
- Utilize the food guide pyramid in planning a healthy diet.
- Recognize how the exchange system and/or My Plate can be utilized as a tool for menu planning.
- Recognize how the nursing process may be utilized in developing a nutritionally balanced health-promotion plan.

INTRODUCTION

Obesity among the U.S. population has become a significant social as well as health problem. Obesity rates have increased over the past decades, and obesity is partly to blame for soaring health care costs. Spending on obesity-related illnesses has increased in the United States and accounts for a large percentage of the national health budget. It is estimated that the United States spent over $147 million in medical care costs associated with obesity in 2008 (Finkelstein et al., 2009). Health problems associated with overweight and obesity have a major impact on the United States health care system In fact, recent data indicates that 72% of U.S. men and 64% of U.S. women are overweight or obese. These obesity rates are major causes of morbidity and mortality (Fiegel et al., 2010). Yet, as is evident by the growing number of health-food stores, nutritional supplements, and vitamins, the public obviously continues to be obsessed with controlling weight, dieting, and knowing what foods actually promote good health, to little or no avail.

Everyone wants to have a healthy, long, and productive life and delay the onset of chronic diseases. It is also apparent that eating patterns and the knowledge of a balanced diet are essential to maintaining the quality of life, especially when entering the senior years. What is not as well understood or accepted is the ease with which diet-related health problems, due to excess, lack, or inappropriate amounts of the essential nutrients, can be alleviated.

Nursing and health care professionals recognize an awareness that nutrition plays a major role in disease prevention and health promotion. Nurses are thus an important asset to patients who are intent on achieving a nutritionally balanced diet in addition to their other health-promotion goals. The previous chapters have addressed the conceptual foundations of health promotion and described various factors that are related and that impact individual health promotion throughout the life cycle. This chapter presents the concepts of nutrition and nutrition's role in maintaining health. General nutritional guidelines will be emphasized as well as the role of the nursing process and health-promotion model in meeting nutritional needs.

IMPORTANCE OF NUTRITION IN HEALTH PROMOTION

Nutrition is the study of food substances essential for health. Nutrition is also the study of how the body uses these substances to promote and support growth and to maintain health throughout the life cycle. It includes the study of digestion, absorption, transportation, metabolism, and storage of nutrients, as well as excretion of waste products.

Foods contain **nutrients** that our bodies can use for the maintenance of body functions throughout life. Nutrients may be essential or nonessential. A variety of health problems can occur when persons lack **essential nutrients** or consume excessive or inappropriate nutrients. A nutrient is considered essential when the body requires it for growth or maintenance, but it is not manufactured in sufficient amounts to meet the body's needs. It must be supplied by foods in our diet. Nutrients that the body can make are considered **nonessential nutrients**.

The nutrients are classified into six categories: water, carbohydrates, lipids, proteins, vitamins, and minerals. Only carbohydrates, lipids, and proteins provide energy. Vitamins and minerals do not provide energy but are essential nutrients, required in very small amounts for specific metabolic function, health promotion, and disease prevention. Table 15-1 provides

---

SPOTLIGHT ON

Dietary Reference Intakes (DRIs)

DRIs is a general term for a set of reference values used to assess and plan nutrient intakes of normal, healthy individuals. These values vary by age and gender and include:

- Recommended dietary allowance (RDA)—average daily level of intake sufficient to meet the nutritional requirements of nearly all the people (97–98%).
- Adequate intake (AI)—established when evidence is insufficient to develop an RDA and is set at a level assumed to ensure nutritional adequacy.
- Tolerable upper intake level (UL)—maximum daily intake unlikely to cause adverse health effects.

DRIs are established for calcium, vitamin D, folate, other B vitamins, vitamins A, C, K, and E, selenium, and carotenoids. There are also established DRI recommendations for trace elements and macronutrients such as protein, fat, and carbohydrates, and water and electrolytes (National Institutes of Health, 2011b).

HEALTH PROMOTION THEORY LINK

Labeling Dietary Reference Intakes in Europe

In 2008, the European Commission requested that the Panel on Dietary Products, Nutrition and Allergies review and provide advice on labeling reference intakes on energy, fat, saturated fat, carbohydrate, sugar, and salt. These were presented for inclusion in the proposal for the Regulation of the European Parliament and the Council on the Provision of Food Information to the Consumer. This advice was solicited to make information available to consumers so that they may compare nutritional value of the various food products.

European Food Safety Authority. (2009). Review of labeling reference intake values. Retrieved from http://www.efsa.europa.eu/de/scdocs/doc/nda_op_ej1008_labelling_reference_intake_values_en.pdf

---

a list of the most well-known vitamins and mineral supplements and their health-promotion implications.

Water is a major part of every tissue of our bodies. It functions as the fluid in which substances are dissolved, broken down, and reformed for use by our bodies. Tables 15-2 and 15-3

TABLE 15-1 Vitamins, Mineral Supplements, and Health-Promotion Implications

VITAMINS AND MINERALS	DIETARY USE	HEALTH-PROMOTION IMPLICATIONS
Beta carotene	Antioxidant nutrient that neutralizes harmful substances called free radicals, resulting from body cells' normal metabolism.	Damage from free radicals may contribute to cardiovascular disease and cancer: Some studies have found that beta carotene increases risk of lung cancer in smokers.
Folic acid	Involved in protein synthesis and participates in the reproduction of every cell; found to prevent spinal cord birth defects during pregnancy.	The Food and Drug Administration has mandated that all breads, cereals, pasta, and grain products be fortified with folic acid; recommended that all women capable of becoming pregnant consume 400 mcg of folic acid from supplements or fortified food. UL set to prevent masking a vitamin B_{12} deficiency that may occur in the elderly
Vitamin C (ascorbic acid)	Essential for formation of collagen and fibrous tissue, teeth, bone, cartilage, connective tissue, skin, and capillary walls.	Studies have found that people who have high vitamin C intakes have lower cardiovascular disease and cancer. A total of 75–90 mg/day is recommended for all adults. This recommendation is achieved with five servings of fruits and vegetables.
Vitamin D and calcium	Vitamin D and calcium work together. Vitamin D helps in absorbing dietary calcium and depositing it in the bones. Studies show that people who supplement their diets with Vitamin D and calcium experience slower bone loss and reduced number of fractures.	The Institute of Medicine (2010) recommends that children consume 500–800 mg of calcium daily; adolescents are to consume 1,300 mg daily, and adults are recommended to consume between 800 to 1,000 mg daily. Because Vitamin D comes from the diet and synthesis through sunlight exposure, the recommended vitamin D daily intake is on average 400 international units. Age affects the ability to use vitamin D and calcium. Supplements may be appropriate for those who do not get enough of this vitamin and mineral in their foods or who live in cloudy areas or rarely go outside.
Vitamin E	Fat-soluble antioxidant that protects against cardiovascular disease. Thought to prevent or slow progression of atherosclerosis. Also thought to prevent or slow progression of side effects associated with psychotropic drugs. Acts as an antihemolysis and is essential for reproduction and muscle development.	Vitamin E may affect prostaglandins that regulate a variety of body processes. Available data does not support supplementation to prevent cardiovascular disease, cancer, Parkinson's, or Alzheimers.
Selenium	Antioxidant thought to prevent cancer and cardiovascular disease.	More research is needed on this trace mineral. Taking excessive amounts of selenium may cause hair and nail loss.
Vitamin A	Necessary for vision, healthy epithelial tissue, proper bone growth, and energy regulation.	Dietary deficiencies may produce night blindness or impaired dim-light vision. Long-term intake of large amounts of vitamin A may lead to bone abnormalities. Fetal malformations can be caused by either deficiency or excess of vitamin A.
Vitamin B complex (thiamine, riboflavin, B6, B12, folic acid, niacin, pantothenic acid, biotin)	Function as oxidative coenzymes by joining with enzymes to activate them. Group of vitamins essential for carbohydrate, fat, and protein metabolism and for nerve conduction; also participates in the synthesis of fatty acids; B_{12} is essential for normal red blood cell formation.	Deficiencies in B complex vitamins may cause peripheral neuropathy. Increased risk of deficiency found among those who smoke, miss meals, drink excessive alcohol, lose weight, or consume excessive sugars. Deficiencies may cause dermatitis, oral lesions, and anemias.
Vitamin K	Active role in blood clotting. Recently has been identified as needed for regulation of serum calcium levels.	Use may affect action of prescribed anticoagulants. Instructions regarding vitamin K intake should be provided to those taking warfarin.

Source: Based on Lutz, C., & Przytulski, K. (2011). *Nutrition and diet therapy* (5th ed.), Philadelphia: F. A. Davis; Katz, D. L. (2008). *Nutrition in clinical practice* (2nd ed.), Philadelphia: Wolters Kluwer/Lippincott Williams & Wilkins.

TABLE 15-2 Energy Nutrients and Vitamins: Their Functions and Food Sources

NUTRIENTS	FUNCTIONS	FOOD SOURCES	DEFICIENCY	TOXICITY	RDA*
Water	Body fluids—blood, saliva, digestive juices; urine	Water, beverages, foods	Dehydration: thirst, loss of appetite, nausea, headache, lightheadedness, fatigue, low blood pressure, low pulse, shock	Water intoxication: loss of appetite, edema, loss of consciousness, increased blood pressure	Adults 19–30 years: 3.7 L for men and 2.7 L for women; 30+ monitored individually Infants: 1.5 mL/kcal ingested
Energy nutrients Carbohydrates: (glucose)	Provides energy; protein sparing	Cereals, fruits, vegetables, milk	Protein store breakdown, fat breakdown, ketosis, fatigue, nausea, lack of appetite	None	45–65% of kcal consumed
Lipid (fat) (essential lipid: linoleic acid)	Provides essential fatty acids and energy; absorbs and transports fat-soluble vitamins (A, D, E, and K); protects vital body tissues; insulates body	Fats and oils, meats, fish, nuts, some seeds, dairy products	Increased hunger, inadequate minerals, vitamins, and fatty acids	Increased cardiovascular risk, obesity, diabetes	Children: 25–40% of kcal ingested Adults: 20–35% of kcal ingested
Protein (essential amino acids: histidine, isoleucine, leucine, lysine, methionine, phenylalanine, threonine, tryptophan, valine)	Growth and repair of tissues; maintains fluid and acid-base balances; provides energy	Meats, fish, dairy products, eggs, nuts, legumes, cereals	Lack of energy, poor wound healing, thinning hair, marasmus, kwashiorkor, muscle wasting, mental retardation, albumin, deficiency, edema, lower immunity levels	None	Men: 56 g Women: 46 g Lactating women: 71 g
Vitamins Fat-soluble A	Affects vision; health of skin; growth of hair, nails, bones, and glands; prevents infections	Dairy products; liver; green, yellow, and orange fruits and vegetables; dairy products	Night blindness, xerophthalmia, poor growth, dry skin	Fetal malformations, hair loss, skin changes, bone pain	Females >19 years: 700 mcg/d Males > 19 years: 900 mg/d
D	Calcium and phosphorus absorption; bone mineralization	Dairy products, egg yolks, fatty fish	Rickets, osteomalacia	Growth retardation, kidney damage, calcium deposits in soft tissue	> 1 year: 600 IU/d Adults > 19 years 15 mcg/d
E	Antioxidant—prevents cell damage	Vegetable oils, nuts, seeds, whole grains	Red blood cell destruction, nerve destruction	None: no supplements with anticoagulant drugs	Adults > 19 years: 15 mg/d
K	Blood clotting	Green vegetables	Hemorrhage	Anemia, jaundice	Females > 19 years: 90 μg/d Males >19 years: 120 mcg/d

(Continues)

TABLE 15-2 Energy Nutrients and Vitamins: Their Functions and Food Sources (*Continued*)

NUTRIENTS	FUNCTIONS	FOOD SOURCES	DEFICIENCY	TOXICITY	RDA*
Water-soluble C	Antioxidant—prevents cell damage; causes collagen formation; affects health of teeth and gums	Citrus fruits, green peppers, broccoli, cantaloupe, kiwi fruit, cabbage, strawberries	Scurvy, poor wound healing, pin point hemorrhages, bleeding gums	>2 g can cause diarrhea, kidney stone formation	Females > 19 years: 75 mg/d Males > 19: 90 mg/d
B complex thiamine (B$_1$)	Muscle nerve function; coenzyme for energy metabolism	Whole grains and enriched cereals, pork, legumes, seeds, nuts	Beriberi, poor coordination, edema, weakness	None	Females > 19 years 1.1 mg/d Males > 19 years 1.2 mg/d
Riboflavin (B$_2$)	Coenzyme for energy metabolism	Whole grains and enriched cereal products, eggs, meats, fish, green leafy vegetables	Ariboflavinosis, cheilosis, glossitis, seborrheic dermatitis, pellagra	None	Females > 19 years: 1.1 mg/d Males > 19 years: 1.3 mg/d
Niacin	Coenzyme for energy metabolism	Meats, fish, nuts, whole grains, eggs	Pellagra, dermatitis, diarrhea, dementia	Vasodilation, liver damage	Females > 19 years: 14 mg/d Males > 19 years: 16 mg/d
Pyridoxine (B$_6$)	Metabolism of amino acids and protein, neurotransmitter synthesis	Whole grains, most high-protein foods, spinach, broccoli	Headache, anemia, convulsions, nausea	Nerve destruction > 2 g daily	Females > 19 years: 1.3 mg/d >70 years: 1.5 mg/d Males > 19 years: 1.3 mg/d Males > 51 years: 1.7 mg/d
Folate/Folic acid (folacin)	Involved in protein synthesis; Aids metabolism of DNA and RNA (genetic material); red blood cell maturation	Green leafy vegetables, nuts, legumes, grain products	Megaloblastic anemia, poor growth, birth defects	None	Adults > 19 years: 400 mcg/d
B$_{12}$	Coenzyme in synthesis of DNA and RNA Folate metabolism, nerve function	Foods of animal origin; microorganisms in fermented foods	Megaloblastic anemia, poor nerve function	None	Adults > 19 years: 2.4 mcg/d
Pantothenic acid	Coenzyme for energy metabolism	Most foods of plant and animal origin	Fatigue, headache, nausea	None	Adults > 19 years: 4–7 mg/d
Biotin	Coenzyme for energy metabolism	Most foods of plant and animal origin	Dermatitis, anemia	None	Adults > 19 years: 30 mcg/d

*RDAs and DRIs (specifically, AIs) may both be used as goals for individual intake.

Sources: National Academies of Sciences, Institute of Medicine, Food and Nutrition Board. (2010). Dietary references intakes: RDA and AI for vitamins and elements; National Academies of Sciences, Institute of Medicine, Food and Nutrition Board. (2010). Dietary.reference intakes: Macronutrients; Institute of Medicine of the National Academies. (2010). Dietary reference intakes for calcium and vitamin D; Lutz, C., & Przytulski, K. (2011). *Nutrition and diet therapy*. Philadelphia: F. A. Davis.

TABLE 15-3 Minerals: Their Functions and Food Sources

NUTRIENTS	FUNCTIONS	FOOD SOURCES	DEFICIENCY	TOXICITY	RDA*
Macrominerals Calcium	Forms bones and teeth; blood clotting, nerve function, muscle contraction	Dairy products, dark green vegetables, salmon, sardines, fortified orange juice	Poor bone and tooth development, osteoporosis	Potential calcification of soft tissue May cause kidney stones in susceptible people;	Males > 19 years: 1,000 mg/d > 51 years: Females > 19 years: 1,200 mg/d Adults > 70 years 1,200 mg/d
Phosphorus	Forms bones and teeth; part of some coenzymes; major ion of intracellular fluid	Dairy products, meats, processed foods, soft drinks	Impaired growth; osteomalacia; arrhythmias,	None	Adults >19 years: 700 mg/d
Magnesium	Nerve and muscle function; part of some coenzymes; bone strength; ADP and ATP energy metabolism	Green vegetables, whole grain cereals, nuts, chocolate, legumes	Weakness, muscle pain, poor heart function	Weakness in people with kidney failure	Females >19 years: 310 to 320 mg/d Males >19 years: 420 mg/d
Sodium	Nerve and muscle function and body fluid balance	Salt (sodium chloride), soy sauce, processed foods, cheese, chips	Muscle cramps, diarrhea, vomiting	Hypertension, thirst, fatigue, agitation, coma	Adults > 19 years: 1.5 g/d
Potassium	Nerve and muscle function and body fluid balance	Dairy products, fruits and vegetables (especially bananas), whole grains, legumes, meats	Irregular heartbeat, appetite loss, muscle cramps	Slow heart rate, skeletal muscle weakness	Adults >19 years: 4.7 g/d
Chloride	Nerve and muscle function, body fluid balance; forms hydrochloric acid in the stomach	Salt, soy sauce, salted foods, cheese, processed foods	Convulsions in infants	Hypertension in susceptible people when combined with sodium	Adults >19 years 2.3 g/d > 70 years 1.8 g/d
Microminerals (trace minerals) Iron	Transports oxygen (in hemoglobin in blood)	Meats, legumes, cereals, eggs	Low blood hemoglobin levels	Seen in people with hemochromatosis	Females: > 19 years: 18 mg/d Males: > 19 years: 8 mg/d Adults > 70: 8 mg/d
Zinc	Coenzyme; heals wounds; affects taste, sexual development	Whole grains, seafood, tea, meats, greens	Skin rash, loss of taste, hair loss, poor wound healing, poor growth and development	Decreased immune function, diarrhea, cramps	Females > 19 years: 8 mg/d Males > 19 years: 11 mg/d

(Continues)

TABLE 15-3 Minerals: Their Functions and Food Sources (*Continued*)

NUTRIENTS	FUNCTIONS	FOOD SOURCES	DEFICIENCY	TOXICITY	RDA*
Iodine	Part of thyroid hormones	Seafood, iodized salt, dairy products, some breads	Goiter, poor growth in infancy	Acne-like lesions, inhibits thyroid function	Adults > 19 years: 150 mcg/d
Selenium	Part of antioxidant system, glutathione peroxidase; acts with vitamin E	Seafood, whole grains, meats	Muscle pain and weakness, poor growth	Nausea, vomiting, hair loss, weakness	Adults > 19 years: 55 mcg
Fluoride	Affects tooth and bone structure	Fluoridated drinking water, seafood, tea, seaweed	Increased risk of dental caries	Mottling of teeth during development, bone pain	Females > 19 years: 3 mg/d Males > 19 years: 4 mg/d
Copper	Coenzyme involved in hemoglobin synthesis	Cocoa, seafood, nuts, legumes, liver	Anemia, poor growth	Vomiting, nervous system disorders	Adults > 19 years: 900 mcg/d
Chromium	Glucose and energy metabolism	Brewer's yeast, seafood, meat, liver	High blood glucose, weight loss	Anemia, liver dysfunction, kidney failure	Females: > 19 years: 25 mcg/d > 70 years: 20 mcg/d Males: > 19 years: 35 mcg/d > 70 years: 30 mc/g
Manganese	Involved in bone formation and amino acid, cholesterol, and carbohydrate metabolism	Whole grains, fruits, nuts, vegetables	Dermatitis, decreased hair and nail growth, changes in hair color	Seizures	Females: 280 mg Males: 350 mg Females > 19 years: 1.8 mg/d Males > 19 years: 2.3 mg/d
Molybdenum	Coenzyme	Cereals, legumes, some vegetables	Tachycardia, headache, mental disturbances	None	Adults > 19 years: 45 µg/d

*RDAs and DRIs (specifically AIs) may both be used as goals for individual intake.

Sources: National Academies of Sciences, Institute of Medicine, Food and Nutrition Board. (2010). Dietary references intakes: RDA and AI for vitamins and elements; National Academies of Sciences, Institute of Medicine, Food and Nutrition Board. (2010). Dietary reference intakes: Macronutrients; Institute of Medicine of the National Academies. (2010). Dietary reference intakes for calcium and vitamin D; Lutz, C., & Przytulski, K. (2011). *Nutrition and diet therapy.* Philadelphia: F. A. Davis.

list the nutrients, their functions, food sources, and deficiency and toxicity symptoms as well as the **recommended dietary allowance (RDA)** for each nutrient and/or the **estimated safe and adequate daily dietary intake (ESADDI)**. RDA is the daily dietary intake that is sufficient to meet the nutrient requirements of 97–98% of all healthy individuals in the specific life-stage and gender groups (NIH, 2011b). ESADDI provides a range of recommended intake for some nutrients because not enough information is available to set a specific RDA.

Dietary reference intakes (DRIs) have also been established as bases for the amount of dietary intake that is sufficient to meet the nutritional requirements of the body. DRIs are four reference values that include the estimated average requirements, recommended dietary allowances, adequate intake levels (AI), and tolerable upper intake levels (UL). RDAs and DRIs may both be used as goals for individual dietary intake (Lutz & Przytulski, 2011).

HEALTHY PEOPLE GOALS AND NUTRITIONAL HEALTH

The goal of health promotion is to improve the overall health of all individuals. The United States has been actively pursuing this goal for almost four decades. National objectives related to health and health promotion have been established and serve as the basis for development of a framework for public health-prevention priorities and actions (USDHHS, 2010a). *Healthy People* is a national health initiative under the jurisdiction of the U.S. Department of Health and Human Services (USDHHS) that identifies the most significant preventable threats to health and focuses efforts toward eliminating them. The *Healthy People* process began in 1979, and at the start of each decade the program sets goals for improving the nation's health during the following 10 years. In the last decade, preliminary analysis has indicated that the United States has met 71% of the *Healthy People 2010* targets (USDHHS, 2010c). The nation has made progress toward the goal of reducing health disparities for more than one-half of the special population identified to be at increased risk.

An important development for the next decade is the publication of *Healthy People 2020* (USDHHS, 2010). As the fourth generation of 10-year goals for the nation, it builds on initiatives pursued over the past three decades. *Healthy People 2020* has identified four overarching goals, which challenge the nation to (1) attain high-quality, longer lives free of preventable disease, disability, injury, and premature death; (2) achieve health equity, eliminate health disparities, improve health for all; (3) create social and physical environments that promote health for all; (4) promote quality of life, healthy development, and healthy behaviors across all life stages. Like its predecessors, *Healthy People 2020* is the product of an extensive cooperative national process involving both the public and private sectors and reflects input from a diverse group of individuals. Many national organizations, as well as state public health, mental health, substance abuse, and environmental agencies, provided input in the development of the *Healthy People 2020* goals. *Healthy People 2020* builds on the previous 2010 objectives and provides a renewed focus on identifying, measuring, tracking, and reducing health disparities. In addition, it provides a focus on the importance of the determinants of health. **Determinants of health (DOH)** are factors—biological, social, personal, environmental, and economic—that influence a person's health status. DOH can be classified under several broad categories that, when interacting with each other, form the basis of individual and population health. The broad DOH categories include policy making, social factors, health services, individual behaviors, and biology and genetics (USDHHS, 2010b). Box 15-1 provides a description of *Healthy People 2020* Nutrition and Overweight Objectives. Box 15-2 provides a listing of *Healthy People 2020* focus areas.

DOMAINS INFLUENCING EATING BEHAVIOR

Good health depends on many factors, such as adequate diet, family health history, level of physical activity, and other lifestyle behaviors. Adequate nutritional status is not only important in maintaining structural integrity but also adds to our quality of life. Our food choices as well as food-related activities are usually associated with pleasurable events, social and cultural interactions, and caring and comfort (Miller, 2012). Although healthy eating can be simple, eating behaviors can be influenced by multiple factors. These multiple factors can be categorized in terms of the biological, psychological, sociocultural, spiritual, and environmental domains previously identified as influencing health promotion. Technology has also affected eating behavior as well as food preparation.

BIOLOGICAL DOMAIN

Energy requirements affect eating behavior. Infants, children, and adolescents, for example, require a high caloric intake that should contain adequate amounts of the recommended nutrients. Older adults, too, have special nutritional needs. Evidence indicates that older adults require an increased intake of several nutrients because of diminished absorption and utilization of nutrients. In addition, food interactions with multiple medications must be considered and adjustments made. Medications can affect food consumption through adverse effects such as anorexia, constipation, and chewing discomfort (Miller, 2012). If caloric intake is inadequate to meet energy needs, fatigue, listlessness, and apathy can result. If the body's energy requirements are not met, growth retardation may occur in children.

Biological changes can also affect the eating behaviors of people in all age groups, especially as a person gets older. Changes that occur as a result of aging include diminished taste and smell acuity, which, as might be suspected, contribute to a decreased enjoyment of food. Other changes that occur as a result of aging may contribute to nutritional deficiencies. Energy requirements depend on age and body size. A major threat to the older adult is physical inactivity, which can lead to obesity and overweight. Nutritional deprivation in the older adult, on the other hand, can also lead to a major loss of body mass in terms of muscle mass. Because muscle is more metabolically active tissue than fat, a person's energy needs decline with diminished muscle mass (Lutz & Przytulski, 2011). This loss of muscle mass leads to a decrease in the body's basal metabolic rate and composition. **Basal metabolic rate** is the rate at which the body uses energy to support its involuntary activities that are necessary to life, such as breathing and digestion. The biological domain is quite important when considering nutrition and its implications for health promotion. The ease with which our bodies burn energy determines whether we gain or lose weight. Adjustment in caloric intake is essential to maintaining a healthy weight. Other biological factors that influence our energy requirements include gastrointestinal motility and caloric absorption. If there is a decreased gastrointestinal motility, constipation may result. A high intake of high-fiber foods, such as fruits, vegetables, and whole wheat grains, and

---

BOX 15-1

HEALTHY PEOPLE 2020 NUTRITION AND WEIGHT STATUS OBJECTIVES

- Increase the number of states with nutrition standards for foods and beverages provided to preschool-aged children in child care.
- Increase the proportion of schools that offer nutritious foods and beverages outside of school meals.
- Increase the number of states with state-level policies that incentivize food retail outlets to provide foods that are encouraged by the *Dietary Guidelines.*
- Increase the proportion of Americans who have access to a food retail outlet selling a variety of foods that are encouraged by the *Dietary Guidelines for Americans.*
- Increase the proportion of primary care physicians who regularly measure the body mass index of their patients.
- Increase the proportion of physician office visits that include counseling or education related to nutrition or weight.
- Increase the proportion of worksites that offer nutrition or weight management classes or counseling.
- Increase the proportion of adults that are at a healthy weight.
- Reduce the proportion of obese adults.

- Reduce the proportion of obese children and adolescents.
- Prevent inappropriate weight gain in youths and adults.
- Eliminate very low food security among children.
- Reduce household food insecurity and in so doing reduce hunger. Increase the contribution of fruits to the diets of the population aged two years and older.
- Increase the variety and contribution of vegetables to the diets of the population aged two and older. Increase the contribution of whole grains to the diets of the population aged two years and older.
- Reduce the consumption of calories from solid fats and added sugars in the population two years and older.
- Reduce the consumption of saturated fat in the population two years and older.
- Reduce the consumption of sodium in the population two years and older.
- Increase the consumption of calcium in the population two years and older.
- Reduce iron deficiency among young children and females of childbearing age.
- Reduce iron deficiency among pregnant females.

Note: "Nutrition and Weight Status" is one of 42 focus areas, each with numerous objectives.

Source: Healthy People 2020. http://*www.healthypeople.gov*

---

an increase in fluids increase motility. Likewise, a decrease in hydrochloric acid may result in decreased absorption of some nutrients such as iron, calcium, and vitamin B_{12}.

Psychological Domain

In American society, the media bombard us with images of what constitutes the ideal body image. We are led to believe that the average person is eternally young, slim, and, of course, beautiful. The supermodels with their waiflike appearance and ultraslim bodies encourage an anorexic, unhealthy weight and look. Our goal, it seems, should be to lose weight and eat as if we are on a perpetual weight-reduction diet. Many of the programs on television and radio, as well as all of the literature available to our communities, stress dieting as the ultimate goal. Television programs, advertisements, magazines, newspapers, and movies are proponents of this ultraslim body that is presumed to bring fame, success, and happiness. Unfortunately, young people are especially susceptible to these messages and are more likely to alter their eating behaviors to maintain slim bodies. Researchers have reported that as much as 1% of the adolescent female population has anorexia. That means that one out of every 100 females between the ages of 10 and 20 is starving herself, sometimes to death. Other statistics reveal that an estimated 0.5–3.7% of all women experience anorexia nervosa in their

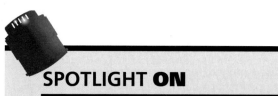

SPOTLIGHT **ON**

Psychological Influences and Food

Parents and other family members have the potential to positively influence children's eating habits. Family meals have been found to influence improved dietary intakes. Research has found that parents can influence their children's eating choices by deciding when the family meals will be, who will be included at the meal, what food choices will be provided, who will provide the food (home or restaurant), and what the atmosphere is where the food is provided. Although families today live in such a complex and at times hectic world, family meals have a profound influence on children's eating habits. (Woodruff & Hanning, 2008).

BOX 15-2

***HEALTHY PEOPLE 2020* FOCUS AREAS**

- Access to health services
- Adolescent health
- Arthritis, osteoporosis, and chronic back conditions
- Blood disorders and blood safety
- Dementias, including Alzheimer's disease
- Early and middle childhood
- Older adult
- Preparedness
- Sleep health
- Social determinants of health
- Genomics
- Global health
- Health care–associated infections
- Injury and violence prevention
- Lesbian, gay, bisexual, and transgender health
- Maternal, infant, and child health
- Cancer
- Medical product safety
- Chronic kidney disease
- Mental health and mental disorders
- Diabetes
- Nutrition and weight status

- Disability and health
- Occupational safety and health
- Educational and community-based programs
- Oral health
- Environmental health
- Physical activity
- Family planning
- Health-related quality of life and well-being
- Public health infrastructure
- Food safety
- Respiratory diseases
- Health communication and health information technology
- Sexually transmitted diseases
- Heart disease and stroke
- Substance abuse
- HIV
- Tobacco use
- Immunization and infectious diseases
- Vision
- Hearing and other sensory or communication disorders

Source: Department of Health and Human Services. (2010c). *Healthy People 2020.* http://www.healthypeople.gov/.

---

lifetime, and an estimated 1.1–4.2% of women have experienced bulimia nervosa in their lifetime as well. No reliable figures for younger children and older adults exist, but cases are not very common. Anorexia nervosa has a higher mortality rate than any other cause of death in females 15–24 years of age. For each decade that an individual has the disorder, mortality rates increase by 5%; the mortality rate increases by 20% in individuals who have had the disorder for 20 years (National Association of Anorexia Nervosa and Associated Disorders [ANAD], 2011a). Many people such as models, actresses, ballet dancers, figure skaters, and gymnasts, whose professions require slim bodies, have longstanding histories of anorexia nervosa or bulimia.

Food is also linked with personal emotional experiences. Many of our memories may be closely associated with foods. Food is a source of both comfort and pleasure. Eating certain foods can have the ability to stimulate the release of certain substances, called opioids, that produce a sense of calm and euphoria in the human body. Some foods, such as those that contain chocolate, have been found to produce these effects and thus may be overconsumed.

SOCIOCULTURAL, RELIGIOUS, AND SPIRITUAL DOMAINS

The United States is considered the melting pot of the world because its people come from many different cultural and ethnic backgrounds. The different types of foods found in this country reflect the intermingling of cultures. It is not unusual to walk or drive on a main street and see restaurants offering foods, even fast foods, from many ethnic origins. Some of the ethnic foods featured in restaurants include Mexican tacos, Chinese egg rolls, Italian lasagna and pizzas, Greek gyros, and French croissants. The choices are endless and usually restricted only by what the consumers can afford.

Ethnic, religious and spiritual, and cultural backgrounds influence eating behaviors, as do a person's parents' beliefs and knowledge about what constitutes a healthy diet. Consequently, the foods people eat may be totally different from the foods recommended by scientific organizations and dietary associations. Many food habits are culturally based. One example of foods that are firmly intertwined with culture is the inclusion of tortillas and beans as a staple in the diet of the Mexican American. These foods in combination, fortunately, provide sufficient nutritional benefits. Neither corn nor beans alone supply the essential amino acids to maintain optimum health. Combined, they provide a complete protein. Culturally based dietary customs are usually not a source of concern in health promotion. The primary concern, however, is whether the foods usually eaten are nutritious and do not aggravate any underlying health conditions. For example, some foods enjoyed by Mexican Americans are loaded with saturated fats and may not be suitable eating choices for those who are overweight or who have diabetes or high levels of blood cholesterol. Examples are tamales (lard and corn dough filled with a variety of meats or fruit or both) and menudo (tripe).

A limited income may also influence food choices and food purchases. If nutrient intake is inadequate due to financial limitations, the nutritional status of the individual may be affected. This may be especially true in older adults who may have age-related changes in nutritional needs (Miller, 2012). Also, in certain parts of the world, some foods may not be available to or accessible by the general population. In some countries, people may have a narrower choice of food selection. In many countries, some of the staples that make up sound nutritional choices may be simply unattainable.

Although religious and spiritual beliefs are not necessarily synonymous, they may play a part in a person's eating behaviors. Some individuals belonging to a particular religious sect, for example, may have certain food restrictions. Others may follow food regimens that are based on spiritual beliefs. Seventh-Day Adventists, for example, have guidelines about what their congregational members can eat. Orthodox Jews require that some foods be consumed only in certain combinations. Spiritual beliefs can also guide food preferences. Followers of the Indian Ayurvedic principles, for instance, focus on a holistic approach that involves the entire body, including spiritual fulfillment. According to Ayurveda, all foods have their own heating or cooling energy and a postdigestive effect. Food combinations are also of great importance in Ayurveda. If two or more foods have different energies, tastes, and postdigestive effects, they can overload the stomach and inhibit enzymes, resulting in toxin production. If these same foods are eaten separately, they may stimulate digestion and help to burn energy. Poor food combinations can result in indigestion, fermentation, and putrefaction, and, if eaten on a regular basis, they can lead to toxemia and disease (Lad & Lad, 2006). Geographical location, as well as whether an individual lives in the city or the country, also influences what foods are consumed.

ENVIRONMENTAL DOMAIN

The American food environment is increasingly encouraging healthier eating behavior. Currently, thousands of low-fat products are sold in grocery stores, and these foods continue to increase. New mandatory food labels on all packaged foods

? ASK YOURSELF

Environmental Influences and Eating Behavior

Do you have a tendency to overeat at festive occasions or holidays? Do your friends' or family's eating behaviors at these social functions contribute to your eating behavior? Our immediate environment can certainly influence our nutritional health and weight gain. What can you do to resist overeating at festive occasions such as parties or other social events?

⚕ HEALTH PROMOTION THEORY LINK

Importance of Environment to Health and Well-Being

Nurses and nurse theorists are always referring to the link between the environment and the health and well-being of people. Nurse theorist Rosemarie Parse's awareness of the environment's influence on health has led to her creation of the word *human-universe* in lieu of the noncombined words *human* and *universe.* In referring to the metaparadigm of nursing, she uses the word *human-universe* to describe the connection between the concept of person and the environment. In doing so, she has made explicit the idea of the concepts' indivisibility.

Source: Morrow, M. (2011). Ecological intelligence and nursing: What is the connection? *Nursing Science Quarterly, 24*(2), 172–173.

contain useful and accurate information to assist individuals and families in making healthy food choices.

Despite the more health-minded American food environment, lifestyle behaviors are still largely responsible for the decreased energy expenditures that ultimately lead to weight gain. Factors such as eating out, eating fast or convenience foods, skipping breakfast, and consuming sweetened sodas are known to increase calorie consumption (Lutz & Przytulski, 2011). The nutrient quality of many fast foods is questionable. Such foods are usually high in fat, salt, and refined carbohydrates and low in dietary fiber and important nutrients. With the increased awareness of a healthful diet, fast-food restaurants are now providing lower-fat food choices for consumers. Ease of preparation also plays an important role in food selection. Quick preparation techniques appeal to families who have busy schedules.

TECHNICAL DOMAIN

The food environment has changed throughout the world as a result of revolutionary technology that affects food production, food preparation, safety, and composition. Food engineering has resulted in bigger, more attractive, and better-tasting crops. It has also been used to develop the type of nutrition needed by livestock so that these animals are bigger and produce better tasting and more tender meats. Technology has also changed the landscape of food preparation. Foods can be prepared faster, for example, in convection ovens and can be made to taste and look like the foods that previously took hours to cook, broil, or brown. These foods are more visually appealing when prepared that way and may be more likely to be eaten than when prepared in a microwave or conventional oven.

Technology has also been used to protect foods and make them safer for consumption. For example, synthetic cysteine, used to condition dough and to produce meat flavors, replaces natural cysteine derived from hair or feathers. On the other hand, technology has also been responsible for imposing an industrialized approach to food production, causing an imbalance in the intricate biological processes required to produce nutritious and healthy foods. This experimental industrialized approach to our food system has resulted in antibiotic-resistant bacteria, morbidity and mortality from nutrition-related diseases, and water and air pollution. According to some, from a public health perspective, the technological influences on food production have failed (Harvie, Mikkelsen, & Shak, 2009).

? ASK YOURSELF

Dietary Supplements and Safety Concerns

The Food and Drug Administration has no authority to regulate the safety of nutritional supplements before they are on the market. It can intervene only after an illness or injury occurs. Therefore, nurses should not automatically assume that all nutritional supplements sold today are safe and effective. Nurses involved in patient teaching should encourage patients to discuss all of the nutritional supplements that they have taken or are taking.

NUTRITIONAL EXCESSES, DEFICITS, FADS, AND HEALTH PROMOTION

Nutritional excesses, as well as nutritional deficits, can affect the health of individuals young and old. These nutritional states, known commonly as overnutrition (obesity) and undernutrition (anorexia) are quite prevalent in the United States and the world today. Popular nutritional fads capitalize on our need to be thin, beautiful, and active. Many nutritional fads exist and influence our consumption, whether the fad is to eliminate excess weight or to provide for optimal energy. All nursing professionals who are involved in patient teaching should be aware of the impact of nutritional excesses and deficits and of nutritional fads on health-promotion and health-promoting behaviors.

OVERNUTRITION

Although hunger still exists in the United States, a more significant problem is overnutrition rather than undernutrition. Of the leading causes of death in the United States, several are associated with dietary excesses and with excessive alcohol consumption (National Center for Health Statistics, 2010). It has been noted that an increase in chronic diseases is associated with an excessive intake of certain nutrients such as saturated fats, cholesterol, sodium, and sugars. Government agencies, voluntary health associations, and scientific associations have made dietary recommendations to address the problem of increases in diet-related diseases such as heart disease, hypertension, cancer, diabetes, osteoporosis, and obesity. There is consensus among these agencies that dietary

SPOTLIGHT **ON**

Overweight and Diabetes

Type 2 diabetes is a disease in which blood sugar levels are elevated. High blood sugar is a major cause of early death, heart disease, kidney disease, stroke, and blindness. The World Health Organization states that in just 5 years (2015), more than two billion people will be overweight and 700 million will be classified as obese. Individuals who are overweight have a four-fold increased risk of developing diabetes in their lifetime (Voice of America, 2010). Why people who are overweight are more likely to suffer from diabetes is not exactly known. Perhaps being overweight causes cells to change, making them less effective at using sugar from the blood. This then puts stress on the cells that produce insulin (a hormone that carries sugar from the blood to cells) and makes them gradually fail. Individuals can lower their risk for developing Type 2 diabetes by losing weight and increasing the amount of their physical activity. If they have Type 2 diabetes, losing weight and becoming more physically active can help control blood sugar levels. Losing weight and exercising more may also increase self-esteem, increase physical fitness, and reduce the amount of medication needed to control diabetes.

guidelines are essential for the maintenance of good general health. Recommendations from these groups have been issued as national goals. There is agreement that obesity is of national concern and that the intake of total fat, saturated fat, cholesterol, and sodium should be reduced, starting at about 2 years of age. Further recommendations include the avoidance of excessive caloric intake and increased intake of dietary fiber, complex carbohydrates, fruits, and vegetables. These goals are the basis of health-promotion efforts for chronic disease prevention.

UNDERNUTRITION

It may seem that overnutrition and obesity are the primary problems facing U.S. citizens, but many people in the United States are going hungry today. Some reasons for the incidence of undernourishment in our population may include poverty, ignorance of what constitutes a healthy diet, and eating disorders, such as anorexia nervosa and bulimia.

ANOREXIA NERVOSA

Anorexia nervosa may be defined as the relentless pursuit of thinness or a prolonged refusal to eat or maintain normal body weight for age or height. This condition is seen primarily in adolescent girls, although it is also found to occur in males, young children, and the elderly (National Association of Anorexia

SPOTLIGHT **ON**

Bulimia and Binge Eating Disorder

Bulimia is known as a diet-binge-purge disorder, which is different from a binge eating disorder. Individuals with a binge eating disorder do not regularly vomit, exercise excessively, or abuse laxatives, as bulimics do. They diet, make themselves hungry, and then binge in response to that hunger. Bulimics may also eat for emotional reasons such as to comfort themselves, avoid threatening situations, and numb emotional pain.

and Associated Disorders [ANAD], 2011c). Approximately 10–15% of individuals who are anorexic are male (ANAD, 2011a). The disorder is thought to originate from emotional or stress-related conflicts such as anger, irritation, body-image disturbance, and fear of losing control. Anorexia nervosa often includes depression, irritability, withdrawal, and peculiar behaviors such as compulsive or strange eating habits (ANAD, 2011c). The goals of treatment are to help the patient achieve emotional as well as physical health.

NURSING **ALERT**

Physical Damage in Anorexia

If left untreated, anorexia nervosa may lead to irreversible physical damage and even death. Eating disorders are serious and can affect all parts of the body. The assessment of an individual suspected of being anorexic reveals irregular heartbeat, liver damage, swollen glands in the neck, salivary duct stones, anemia, dry blotchy skin, and permanent bone damage (ANAD, 2011a).

BULIMIA

Bulimia is an eating disorder that is also referred to as the diet-binge-purge disorder (ANAD, 2011b). A food-gorging binge is followed by a period where the individual feels out of control and purges the food. These episodes usually involve the uncontrolled, rapid ingestion of large quantities of food and usually begin in adolescence or early adult life. The typical bulimic is white, single, female, and college-aged or in her early twenties (Bulemia Nervosa—Eating Disorder, 2011). Research suggests that about 4%, or four out of 100, college-age women have bulimia. Anorexics can also develop bulimia. In fact, 50% of people who have been anorexic develop bulimia or bulimic patterns. Because people with bulimia are secretive, it is difficult to know how many older people are affected. The goal of

treatment in bulimia is similar to that of anorexia. The patient is helped to focus on resolving psychological issues that may have precipitated the eating disorder and to progress to a state of physical health.

? ASK **YOURSELF**

Gender, Anorexia, and Bulimia

Only about 10–15% of people with anorexia or bulimia are male. Is this gender difference a reflection of society's opposite body expectations for males and females? Is it that men do not feel powerful if they are small? Or is it because men feel ashamed of a skinny body?

NUTRITIONAL FADS

Nutritional fads and myths abound in today's media and literature. These fads and nutritional myths can be costly in terms of money and in terms of impact on a person's health. Thousands of health claims are associated with what we eat. These health claims or myths are frequently taken as truth. For example, there are claims that organically grown fruits and vegetables are superior to those that are not grown organically. Studies have repeatedly found that no scientific evidence for the claims that organic food is nutritionally superior to conventional food. Although these claims are popular, the truth is that many of them have not proven to be clinically significant (Rosen, 2010).

Individuals are always looking for quick results. Normally what is proposed to be the wonder solution for making us lean or more energetic is a very ordinary, everyday item that will neither kill us nor make us better (Godfrey & Dansinger, 2009). Daily, every magazine or newspaper on the newsstand proposes a new magical diet plan, food, or nutrient that can make us thinner, younger, healthier, and probably more beautiful. The truth is that certain foods are good for us and that a balanced diet and activity plan are essential to maintaining health. A variety of nutritious foods can replace fad diets and supplements. See Chapter 17 for more information on different fad diets and issues surrounding weight control.

Fad diets have been around for decades. These diets have included drinks that increase physical endurance, vitamins and herbs that improve physical stamina, and protein and amino acids that supposedly build muscle and improve the immune response. The latest and hottest nutritional fads include a wide variety of energy drinks. These drinks are used as nutritional supplements and usually contain high concentrations of carbohydrates and amino acids and some caffeine. These substances have not proven to have any noticeable effect on performance, and, in fact, they might pose a threat to teenagers and young adults who report mixing these energy drinks with alcohol (Ballistreri & Corradi-Webster, 2008). Because there is little or no regulatory control on these products, they can pose a potential health risk and in some cases may be fatal.

NURSING ALERT

Nutritional Supplement Concerns

Many nutritional supplements have not been clinically proven to work, so caution should be used in determining whether the supplement is of value. Remember that there is little regulatory control on some of these products and that this may cause lack of product standardization or purity or both. Some nutritional fads propose supplements that may have serious side effects. Some nutritional supplements have potentially life-threatening side effects, such as heart attack and serious psychiatric illness. For example, dietary supplements, such as ephedra (also known as ma huang), have major adverse effects that have included stroke, myocardial infarction, seizures, and, in some cases, death (National Institutes of Health, 2011a).

DIETARY STRATEGIES TO PROMOTE A HEALTHFUL DIET

A healthful diet consists of the essential nutrients and calories needed to prevent nutritional deficiencies and excesses. Nurses are increasingly responsible for determining appropriate strategies to assist patients to select healthy diet choices. These strategies should ensure that the diet selected provides the right balance of carbohydrate, fat, protein, vitamins, and minerals. Such a diet is not difficult to achieve because a large variety of foods are available and enjoyable. The following sections describe dietary guidelines that are necessary in promoting wellness and healthful eating.

DIETARY GUIDELINES FOR AMERICANS 2010

By law, *Dietary Guidelines for Americans* is reviewed and updated and published jointly every 5 years by the U.S. Department of Health and Human Services (USDHHS) and the U.S. Department of Agriculture (USDA). The *Dietary Guidelines* provide authoritative, science-based advice for people 2 years and older on how to promote health, reduce overweight and obesity, and lower the risk for major chronic diseases through improved nutrition and physical activity (USDHHS, 2011). The purposes of the *Guidelines* are to summarize and synthesize knowledge regarding individual nutrients and food components and to make recommendations for a pattern of eating that can be adopted by the public. Key recommendations are grouped into interrelated focus areas (see Table 15-4). These recommendations are based on the preponderance of scientific evidence for lowering the risk of chronic disease and promoting health by eating fewer calories, being more active, and making wise food choices. Taken together, the guidelines' recommendations encompass two overarching concepts: (1) Maintain calorie balance over time to achieve and sustain healthy weight; (2) focus on consuming nutrient-dense foods and beverages (U.S. Department of Agriculture & U.S. Department of Health and Human Services, 2011a).

Nutrient needs should be met primarily through the consumption of foods. Foods that provide an array of essential nutrients have a beneficial effect on individual health. Fortified foods and dietary supplements may be useful sources of one or more nutrients that otherwise might be consumed in less than recommended amounts. Dietary supplements, while recommended in some cases, cannot replace a healthful diet.

One example of an eating plan that is based on the premises of the *Dietary Guidelines* is the DASH (Dietary Approaches to Stop Hypertension) Eating Plan. This plan is designed to assist adults in making healthy lifestyle choices to include foods that speed the rate of sodium excretion and help in avoiding high blood pressure (Lutz & Przytulski, 2011). DASH

RESEARCH NOTE

Diabetes Self-Management Activities of African American (AA) Grandmothers

STUDY PROBLEM/PURPOSE

African American females experience a greater burden of diabetes and its complications, with twice the mortality rates of their white female counterparts. The study had two purposes: (1) to compare the diabetes self-management activities of AA primary caregiving grandmothers before and after the initiation of caregiving and (2) to compare the diabetes self-management of AA primary caregiving grandmothers to diabetic women who were not caring for grandchildren.

METHODS

Using a cross-sectional, descriptive design, 68 AA women 55–75 years of age were recruited to participate. Participants were asked the frequency of their performance of six self-management activities. Caregiving grandmothers were asked about their activities before and after the initiation of caregiving.

FINDINGS

Statistically significant differences were noted in diet and the self-monitoring of blood glucose before and after the initiation of caregiving. For the caregiver versus the noncaregiver, significant differences were noted in the self-monitoring of blood glucose and eye examinations.

IMPLICATIONS

The findings provided preliminary data to support further research examining the self-management of diabetic AA caregiving grandmothers. AA primary caregiving grandmothers were found to have more difficulty performing some of the self-management activities, which may severely impact their overall health.

Source: Carthron, D. L., et al. (2010). "Give me some sugar" The diabetes self-management activities of African-American primary caregiving grandmothers. *Journal of Nursing Scholarship, 42*(3), 330–337.

TABLE 15-4 *Dietary Guidelines for Americans* Focus Areas and Selected Recommendations

FOCUS AREA	RECOMMENDATIONS
Balance calories to manage weight.	Consume a variety of nutrient dense foods.
	Limit fats, sugars, salt, and alcohol.
	Control total calorie intake to manage body weight.
	Increase physical activity.
	Decrease time spent in sedentary behaviors.
	Maintain appropriate calorie balance during each stage of life.
Reduce foods and food components that include: • Sodium • Solid fats • Cholesterol • Added sugars • Refined grains • Alcohol	Reduce sodium intake to < 2,300 mg.
	Reduce sodium intake to 1,500 mg among persons 51 and older and those of any age who are African American or have hypertension.
	Consume less than 10% of calories from saturated fatty acids, and replace with mono- and polyunsaturated fatty acids.
	Use oils to replace solid fats.
	Consume < 300 mg of dietary cholesterol per day.
	Limit foods with trans fatty acids by limiting foods that contain synthetic sources of trans fats.
	Reduce intake of calories from solid fats and sugars.
	Consume no more than one drink of alcohol per day for women and two per day for men.
Increase foods and nutritents that include: • Vegetables • Fruits • Whole grains • Fat-free or low-fat dairy • Protein, lean meats • Poultry, seafood • Eggs • Unsalted nuts • Legumes	Increase vegetable and fruit intake.
	Eat a variety of vegetables.
	Consume half of all grains as whole grains.
	Increase intake of fat-free or low-fat dairy products.
	Eat a variety of protein foods, including eggs, poultry, seafood and lean meats, and legumes and unsalted nuts.
	Consume foods that provide more potassium, fiber, calcium, and vitamin D.
	If you are a woman of childbearing age, consume 400 mcg of synthetic folic acid.
Build healthy eating patterns.	Select an eating pattern that meets nutrient needs over time at an appropriate calorie level.
	Account for all food and beverages consumed, and assess how they fit into a total healthy eating pattern.
	Follow food safety recommendations when preparing and storing foods.

Source: United States Department of Agriculture & United States Department of Health and Human Services. *Dietary Guidelines for Americans 2010* (7th ed.). Washington, DC: U.S. Government Printing Office. Retrieved from http://www.health.gov/dietaryguidelines

recommendations include foods low in total fat, saturated fat, and cholesterol, and foods such as fruits, vegetables, and low-fat dairy products. The diet is constructed across a range of calorie levels to meet the needs of the various age and gender groups. The DASH diet recommends that people make healthy changes in their lifestyle to avoid developing high blood pressure and its complications (LeMone, Burke, Bauldoff, 2011).

In describing the *Dietary Guidelines*, one must understand how culture affects individual dietary plans. It is important to incorporate the food preferences of different racial/ethnic groups, vegetarians, and other groups when planning diets and developing educational programs and materials. Cultural sensitivity in relation to types of foods eaten and meaning of foods for ethnic populations is essential when counseling people about dietary and nutritional needs.

MYPYRAMID

MyPyramid replaced the Food Guide Pyramid introduced in 1992 by the U.S. Department of Health and Human Services and the U.S. Department of Agriculture (U.S. Department of Agriculture [USDA], 2011). The **Food Guide Pyramid** was designed to help in following the *Dietary Guidelines for Americans* by providing a guide to the amounts and kinds of foods that we should eat daily to maintain health and to reduce the risks of developing diet-related diseases. The guiding principles for MyPyramid are the same. The principles focus on overall health, are based on up-to-date research, and focus on an individual's total dietary needs. The main goals of MyPyramid are to (1) improve its effectiveness in motivating consumers to make healthier food choices and (2) ensure that

Find Your Balance Between Food and Physical Activity

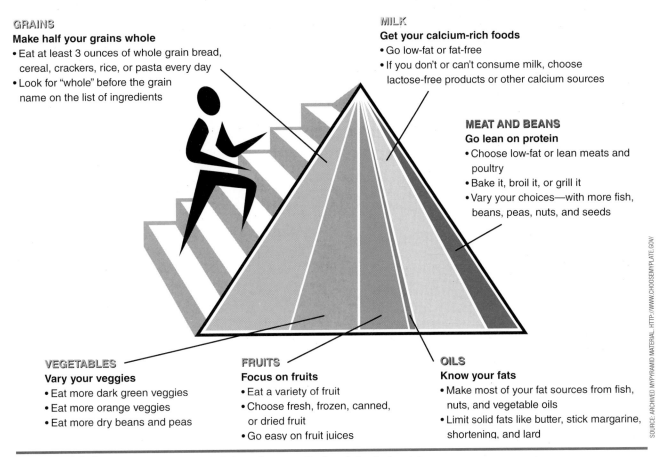

GRAINS
Make half your grains whole
- Eat at least 3 ounces of whole grain bread, cereal, crackers, rice, or pasta every day
- Look for "whole" before the grain name on the list of ingredients

MILK
Get your calcium-rich foods
- Go low-fat or fat-free
- If you don't or can't consume milk, choose lactose-free products or other calcium sources

MEAT AND BEANS
Go lean on protein
- Choose low-fat or lean meats and poultry
- Bake it, broil it, or grill it
- Vary your choices—with more fish, beans, peas, nuts, and seeds

VEGETABLES
Vary your veggies
- Eat more dark green veggies
- Eat more orange veggies
- Eat more dry beans and peas

FRUITS
Focus on fruits
- Eat a variety of fruit
- Choose fresh, frozen, canned, or dried fruit
- Go easy on fruit juices

OILS
Know your fats
- Make most of your fat sources from fish, nuts, and vegetable oils
- Limit solid fats like butter, stick margarine, shortening, and lard

SOURCE: ARCHIVED MYPYRAMID MATERIAL. HTTP://WWW.CHOOSEMYPLATE.GOV/

FIGURE 15-1 **MyPyramid: Find your balance between food and physical activity.**

the USDHHS/ USDA food guidance system reflects the latest nutritional science. MyPyramid incorporates recommendations from the *Dietary Guidelines for Americans 2010* and makes Americans aware of the vital health benefits of simple and modest improvements in nutrition, physical activity, and lifestyle behavior (Figure 15-1). Although MyPyramid's approach is still relevant, the United States Department of Agriculture has decided to substitute the MyPlate icon and wording for the MyPyramid icon. The justification for this substitution is that MyPlate is easier for the consumer to understand than MyPyramid (United States Department of Agriculture & United States Health and Human Services, 2011b). Please note that MyPlate is discussed later in this chapter, but because MyPyramid is still of use to consumers, it is discussed here.

MyPyramid's approach to nutrition is not one-size-fits-all. Instead, it demonstrates an individualized, personalized recommendation about daily food intake. Physical activity as well as dietary planning are emphasized and represented by the steps found on the pyramid graphic. Variety of the food groups is symbolized by the six color bands representing the five food groups and oils. Foods from all six groups are needed each day for good health. Moderation is one of the key messages of MyPyramid. Moderation is represented by the narrowing of each food group from top to bottom. The wider base stands for foods with little or no solid fats, added sugars, or caloric sweeteners. These should be selected more often to get the most nutrition from calories consumed. Proportionality is also shown by the different widths of the "good" group bands.

The width suggests how much food a person should choose from each group. Caution should be taken, however; the widths are just a general guide and not exact proportions.

NURSING ALERT
Maintaining a Healthy Diet

When counseling patients regarding the maintenance of a dietary balance, nurses should point out that variety, moderation, and proportion are the keys to adopting a healthy diet. In addition, patients should be informed that, if they do the following, they will attain their dietary goals:

- Eat moderately, and opt for lower-fat alternatives whenever possible.
- When choosing a higher-fat food, eat a moderate portion, and balance the food choice with a lower-fat food some other time during the day.
- Choices within the food groups should be varied regularly. Follow the recommended number of servings for each food group daily.
- Make sure that all the nutrients needed for good health become a part of the daily diet.

The website Choosemyplate.gov describes activities that make it easy for individuals to personalize their diet. The site also provides motivational tools and educational resources for consumers. Individuals can find general food guidance and suggestions for making smart choices from each food group.

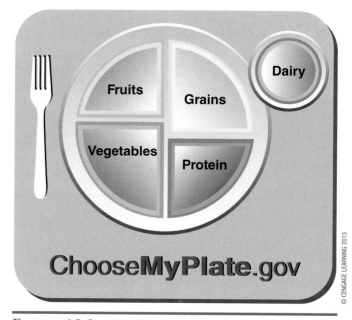

FIGURE 15-2 MyPlate.

NURSING **ALERT**

Fat in the Diet

High dietary fat intakes are associated with certain diseases such as heart disease and some types of cancer. It is recommended that fat intake for adults should be 20–35% of the total daily calorie intake. The following are fat reduction tips to be shared with your patients:

- Choose lean cuts of meat, and trim visible fat before cooking.
- Broil, bake, or roast meats instead of frying.
- Choose low-fat, nonfat or reduced-fat foods as listed on the package.
- Use herbs, spices, and lemon juice on vegetables instead of butter or margarine.
- Use skim or 1% milk instead of whole milk.

Because the previous one-size-fits-all approach is no longer appropriate, it is difficult to determine the number of daily servings needed according to food groups in relation to gender, physical activity, and age. Instead, personalized and individualized food group information is provided, including daily amounts in commonly used measures like cups and ounces. Examples and everyday tips are also included. Downloadable suggestions on all of the food groups and required physical activity are also available.

MyPlate

Because some consumers find the food pyramid too complex, the United States Department of Agriculture has unveiled a new icon called **MyPlate** that is simple to understand and represents the new U.S. Dietary Guidelines (USDA, 2011a). This icon consists of a colorful plate split into four sections (Figure 15-2). Each colored section of the plate represents one of the food groups: fruits, vegetables, grains, and proteins. The largest section on the plate represents the vegetable group. The next largest sections are grains and proteins, followed by a smaller section representing the fruit group. The icon makes very clear that fruits and vegetables should make up half of your meal, while protein should be the smallest part of the plate. A separate section resembling a glass represents the dairy group on the side.

The MyPlate icon is thought to be the visual cue to a unified nutrition message to all Americans. According to the USDA, the food pyramid provides much information, and this icon can change American eating patterns by using tools of modern persuasion (WebMD, 2011). At this point, the food pyramid can still be used because of the useful online tools that are a part of the MyPyramid. However, MyPlate is preferred.

THE EXCHANGE SYSTEM: A MENU PLANNING TOOL

The **exchange system** is another valuable tool for quickly estimating the energy, protein, carbohydrate, and fat content of a meal. It was developed by the American Dietetic Association and the American Diabetes Association (2011). It is a system for classifying foods into numerous lists based on their macronutrient composition and for establishing serving sizes so that one serving of each food on a list contains the same amount of carbohydrate, protein, fat, and energy (calories). By using the exchange system, people may plan daily menus without having to look up the nutrient values of numerous foods.

The meal planning exchange lists have been expanded to include a greater variety of commonly consumed foods, carbohydrate counts for each food portion, portion weights in ounces, reduced-fat and fat-free foods, and vegetarian alternatives as well as fast foods. The revised exchange system remains the same in many ways, but new food groups have been added, thus allowing more flexibility in choosing foods (American Diabetes Association, 2011).

Exchange lists are designed so that when the proper serving size is used, each food on a list provides about the same amount of carbohydrate, protein, fat, and energy. This equality allows the exchange of foods on each list. Thus an individual is able to choose favorite foods from each list while controlling the amount and kind of carbohydrates consumed throughout the day. Because the exchange lists encourage variety while helping to control calories and grams of carbohydrates, protein, and fats, these lists have been adapted to meet the needs of weight reduction programs and medical nutrition therapy planning. See Chapter 17 for other weight control strategies.

Nutrition Facts

Serving Size 1/2 cup (114g)
Servings Per Container 4

Amount Per Serving

Calories 90	Calories from Fat 30

	% Daily Value
Total Fat 3g	**5%**
Saturated Fat 0g	**0%**
Cholesterol 0mg	**0%**
Sodium 300mg	**13%**
Total Carbohydrate 13g	**4%**
Dietary Fiber 3g	**12%**
Sugars 3g	
Protein 3g	

Vitamin A	80%	•	Vitamin C	60%
Calcium	4%	•	Iron	4%

• Percent Daily Values are based on a 2,000 calorie diet. Your daily values may be higher or lower depending on your calorie needs:

	Calories	2,000	2,500
Total Fat	Less than	65g	80g
Sat Fat	Less than	20g	25g
Cholesterol	Less than	300mg	300mg
Sodium	Less than	2,400mg	2,400mg
Total Carbohydrate		300g	375g
Fiber		25g	30g

Calories per gram:
Fat 9 • Carbohydrate 4 • Protein 4

© CENGAGE LEARNING 2013

FIGURE 15-3 Sample food label.

FOOD LABELS

Food labels are the best way for consumers to see how individual foods fit their own nutritional needs. In 1993, the Food and Drug Administration made it easier to figure out serving sizes by improving the nutrition labels that appear on food packages. An example of a label for processed foods is shown in Figure 15-3.

The nutrition facts panel lists the quantities of energy (calories), fat, and specific other nutrients in a serving: total food energy, food energy from fat, total fat, saturated fat, cholesterol, sodium, total carbohydrates, dietary fiber, sugars, protein, vitamin A, vitamin C, calcium, and iron. The information on the label is not based on the entire contents of the package. It is calculated for a typical portion, or serving, of that food.

Paying attention to serving sizes can help an individual make informed choices about what to eat. However, labels are not available in a restaurant. About a third of all meals are eaten at restaurants today, and many entrees can contain up to a day's worth of servings from several food groups. Although the cooking method or the serving size in a restaurant cannot always be controlled, a person can always request a take-home container if there is too much food on the plate. This will reduce the serving size of a meal and, perhaps, allow for continued enjoyment of the food at a later time.

Fruits and Veggies—More Matters

The CDC and the Produce for Better Health Foundation have partnered with several organizations, such as the

National Cancer Institute and the Department of Health and Human Services, to launch a public health initiative called Fruits and Veggies– More Matters. This initiative takes the place of the previous campaign focusing on the 5 a Day Program. The partnership is intended to improve our health (Centers for Disease Control and Prevention, 2011). The purpose of the program is to increase our consumption of fruits and vegetables because a growing body of research shows that fruits and vegetables are beneficial to our health. By doing so, the goals of the *Dietary Guidelines for Americans 2020, Healthy People 2020* and other dietary recommendations may be achieved.

Focusing on fruits and vegetables, is an easy way to decrease the intake of fats because fruits and vegetables are naturally low in fat. A variety of chemical compounds are present naturally in foods that include some of the well-known vitamins and other food components: carotenoids such as beta-carotene, vitamins C and E, selenium, dietary fiber, and other substances such as dithiolthiones, isothiocyanates, indoles, phenols, and phytoestrogens. These are known as **phytochemicals**, which are bioactive compounds of plant origin that can provide protection against heart disease, arthritis, and some types of cancer (Phytochemicals, 2011). A daily diet rich in fruits and vegetables ensures that increased consumption of these phytochemicals also occurs.

The National Cancer Institute (2011) has spent a lot of effort researching the anticancer constituents of plant foods. Those foods and herbs found to possess anticancer activity include garlic, soybean, ginger, and cruciferous vegetables (broccoli, cabbage, and Brussels sprouts) (American Cancer Society, 2011). Other plant foods are currently being evaluated to determine their safety, efficacy, and applicability for preventing and treating cancer.

NUTRITIONAL ISSUES AND HEALTH-PROMOTION STRATEGIES

Nutrition is very important not only for those deemed healthy, but also for those who might have life-limiting illnesses. For those with life-limiting illness, nutrition is important for meeting the body's physical requirements and also for its associated social, cultural, and psychological benefits (Holmes, 2010). Nutritional health is an important health-promotion focus area. Adequate nutritional status is dependent on a whole array of contributing factors and issues that can impact nutritional outcomes. These may include such factors as amount and type of dietary intake, quality of life issues, economic concerns, emotional issues, poor eating behaviors, structural defects, and underlying diseases and conditions. Poor nutritional status and substantial dietary inadequacy may result from poor self-esteem; for example, anorexia is typically seen in adolescent girls and is considered to be related to self-esteem issues.

Depression may also play a part in poor eating habits. The elderly, for example, frequently experience malnutrition that can be attributed to depression, lack of social support, or eating-related disabilities. The effects of mood and social support are well recognized, and intervention in these areas might achieve improvements in nutritional health and quality of life. Several conditions such as menopause and inherited factors have also been noted to impact nutritional status. See Box 15-3 for a listing of some factors that can impact nutritional health.

BOX 15-3
SELECTED FACTORS IMPACTING NUTRITIONAL HEALTH

Age-related changes and conditions

    Calcium deficit in menopause

    Anorexia, bulimia in adolescence

    Malnutrition in the elderly

Hereditary conditions

    Diabetes

    Cardiovascular disease

    Hypercholesterolemia/lipidemia

Disease conditions

    Cancer

    Diabetes

    Obesity

    Heart disease

    HIV

Lifestyle behaviors

    Overindulgence

    Alcoholism

    Smoking

    Eating patterns/cultural eating habits

    Workaholic behavior

✲ NURSING **ALERT**
Foods Rich in Phytochemicals

In providing nutritional information to individuals regarding foods that can protect against heart disease and certain types of cancers, the following phytochemically rich foods should be encouraged:

- Cereals and grains, e.g., barley, brown rice, oats, whole grain bread
- Dry beans, e.g., black beans, kidney beans, pinto beans, soybeans, soy products such as tofu
- Fruits such as apples, apricots, berries, cantaloupe and other melons, citrus (oranges, grapefruit), and grapes
- Vegetables, e.g., broccoli, Brussels sprouts, cabbage, carrots, cauliflower, celery, collard greens, cucumber, eggplant, garlic, kale, leeks, onions, peppers, tomatoes, and turnips

THE NURSING PROCESS IN PROMOTING NUTRITIONAL HEALTH

The role of the nurse in promoting a nutritionally balanced health-promotion plan cannot be overemphasized. As described in Chapter 4, the nurse utilizes the nursing process in identifying the health needs of patients and determines an appropriate plan for addressing the identified needs. Likewise, the nurse involved in the care of a patient carefully assesses the patient's nutritional health and devises a plan to ensure optimal nutritional health. The following nursing process steps are useful in promoting a patient's nutritional health: assessment, diagnosis, planning, implementation, and evaluation.

ASSESSMENT

Assessment is the key step in determining a patient's nutritional health needs. This very important step is quite complex and involves the initial recognition of those factors that might affect nutrition and lifestyle. Each of the domains previously described as influencing eating behaviors should be identified and considered in this phase of the nursing process. Assessment of the biological domain, for example, demonstrates the importance of gender and age in determining nutritional requirements. The body's actual energy requirements as well as the body's ability to absorb nutrients are also essential assessment considerations. The psychological domain assessment may reveal emotional issues that are affecting a person's appetite. How persons interact with others, as well as their interpersonal relationships, can reveal much about eating habits and should not be overlooked. A patient's sociocultural and religious beliefs related to foods, as well as the impact of the environment, are important areas to be assessed when determining nutritional health. Table 15-5 identifies specific domain areas to be assessed when utilizing the nursing process to determine a nutritionally balanced health-promotion plan.

Refer to Chapter 17 for a sample assessment form that can be used in the nutritional screening of adults and children.

CRITICAL ANALYSIS OF DATA

As explained in Chapter 4, collecting data is not enough. The next crucial step after the collection and assessment of the data is analysis in order to arrive at an accurate nursing diagnosis. This step involves the synthesis of data, which requires that the data be sorted and grouped according to its commonalities. For example, a positively worded nursing diagnosis that relates to health promotion and the fact that the patient might be ready to learn about nutrition is *readiness for enhanced nutrition*. The assessment data for this diagnosis might be sorted according to the domains. If the data is sorted and grouped using the biological domain, for example, it will include age, gender, height, and body mass index. The data sorted and grouped under the psychological domain might include information related to the patient's self-esteem, history of depression, and attitudes toward food and nutrition. Sorting data according to the sociocultural domain might also include data like cultural background, financial status, and influences of food choices (Sparks-Ralph & Taylor, 2011). Once sorted and grouped, the data is then analyzed, and the nurse arrives at a plausible diagnosis for the patient. Obviously, the critical analysis and synthesis of data are very important in formulating a nursing process plan.

NURSING DIAGNOSIS

The next step in the nursing process is the identification of the nursing diagnosis or diagnoses. Nursing diagnoses are based on the thorough analysis of data obtained through the nursing assessment. According to NANDA (2007), a number of nutrition-related nursing diagnoses could be applicable in a patient situation. These can usually be classified as:

- Imbalanced nutrition—less than body requirements.
- Imbalanced nutrition—more than body requirements.
- Risk for imbalanced nutrition—more than body requirements.

TABLE 15-5 Assessment of Domains Influencing Nutritional Health

DOMAIN	SPECIFIC ASSESSMENTS
Biological	Patient's age, weight, and height
	Weight changes
	Problems or conditions affecting nutritional status
	Caloric intake, number of meals, servings per day
	Oral health
	Allergies
	Alcohol, caffeine, and sugar consumption daily
	Physical activities and exercise
	Patient 24-hour diet recall
	Laboratory values indicative of nutritional problems: e.g., hemoglobin, hematocrit, lymphocytes, red blood cells, globulins, blood urea nitrogen, fasting blood sugar, and electrolytes (Pagana & Pagana, 2010)
Psychological	Family issues affecting nutrition
	Interpersonal relationships
	Emotional disorders
	Self-esteem issues
	Aversion to specific foods
Sociocultural	Lifestyle
	Ethnic food preferences
	Meal preparation by whom?
	Regular meals eaten at home or out
	Number of snacks per day and type
Spiritual/religious	Feelings regarding certain foods
	Foods related to religious or spiritual events (e.g., Lent, Passover)
	Religious food prohibitions
	Meaning of foods
Environmental	Eats alone or with others
	Lives alone
	Salt readily available
	Other condiments used in food preparation
	Comfort foods, favorite snacks
Technological	Patient's age
	Educational status
	Economic status
	Computer literacy
	Availability of technology
	Comfort level with technology

© Cengage Learning 2013

ASK **YOURSELF**

Goal Setting

Does the setting of short-term goals help a patient feel more self-confident when the goals are accomplished? Is it more realistic to set short-term goals rather than focus on the long-term nutritional behaviors that must be changed?

Selection of the actual nursing diagnosis rests on what is causing the alteration or risk for alteration of the nutrition status. In other words, the nursing diagnosis is always stated as in the following examples, to indicate the cause for the alteration:

- Imbalanced nutrition—less than body requirements related to anorexia or insufficient intake.
- Imbalanced nutrition—more than body requirements related to a decline in basal metabolic rate and physical inactivity (Sparks-Ralph & Taylor, 2011).

The nutrition-related nursing diagnoses can, for the most part, be classified according to the domains covered in this chapter. For example, an alteration in nutrition may be related to the biological domain in that it is caused by a physiological problem such as painful ulcers, or it could be related to the environmental domain if the cause of the nutritional alteration is related to a change in diet. The psychological domain can also have a major influence in nutritional alterations. Note that some nursing diagnoses related to nutritional needs can be stated positively and requires setting positive goals. The nursing diagnosis *readiness for enhanced nutrition related to met metabolic needs* indicates that the nutritional status of the patient is positive but can be strengthened. Although adequate food and fluids are consumed, the goal set for the patient can relate to the patient's ability to articulate the personal value of practicing positive behaviors.

PLANNING

Following the determination of the appropriate nursing diagnoses, the next step of the nursing process is to develop a plan of care. The planning phase includes a careful identification by both the patient and the nurse of the goals, outcomes, or both that will assist both the patient and the nurse in resolving the problems identified. The goals identified are mutually established and should be measurable and, above all, realistic. For example, it is not enough to state that the patient will recognize the reasons for weight loss. Realistic and measurable objectives may include goals or outcomes such as, "The patient will identify five factors that contribute to weight loss," or, "the patient will identify four situations that lead to a decreased appetite." The planning phase is extremely important because this sets the stage for implementation of those measures that will promote the patient's health.

The planning phase arises from the nursing diagnoses and must be congruent with them. So, if a diagnosis is *imbalanced nutrition: Less than body requirements related to decreased appetite due to anorexia nervosa*, the nursing plan should focus on measures that address the cause of the decreased appetite such as, perhaps, low self-esteem and poor interpersonal relationships. Additionally, the plan could address the need for consultation with a nutritionist and the need for an increase in the patient's knowledge base relative to nutritional information. Refer to Chapter 17 for further information on planning care for a patient with nutritional alterations.

IMPLEMENTATION

Though the previous phase of the nursing process, established goals or outcomes or both related to nutritional health and identified a plan of action to achieve these goals, the implementation phase actually attempts to put the identified plan into action. The implementation phase is the most dynamic aspect of the nursing process since it determines which interventions relative to the nutritional goals are appropriate and which are not. This constant evaluation of interventions can subsequently lead to a modification of the plan and perhaps even a reassessment of the patient situation and the identification of new nursing diagnoses.

While the implementation phase is the most dynamic, it is also the most difficult phase because it involves considerable effort in motivating individuals to make changes and perhaps even adopt a healthier lifestyle that will lead to a positive nutritional status. The domains previously identified as influencing nutritional health can be utilized in determining which interventions are necessary to achieve the patient goals. For example, interventions directed toward the biological domain

are useful and can include a monitoring of the patient's weight, a continued assessment of dietary status, and identification of any abnormal lab values that are influenced by nutritional status. Likewise, interventions directed to the sociocultural domain may include dietary counseling for both the patient and the family members affected by needed dietary changes. The environmental domain is also a major consideration when implementing a nutritional plan that might require lifestyle changes. Table 15-6 identifies some specific nutrition-related interventions according to domain areas.

Later chapters also provide useful information on the implementation of interventions for promoting nutritional health.

HEALTH-PROMOTION MODEL AND NUTRITIONAL STATUS

Pender's revised Health-Promotion Model (HPM) is also a useful tool that can be utilized to determine and implement actions to direct behaviors that enhance health (Pender, Murdaugh, & Parsons, 2011). As described in Chapter 3, the HPM focuses on motivation for health behaviors, identifies interactions among cognitive, behavioral, and environmental factors that influence health behaviors, and does not use fear or threats to effect change. Thus, according to this model, interventions implemented to achieve nutritional health will not be effective if the patient is threatened with dire outcomes such as obesity-related consequences or even death. Rather, the nurse works with the patient in determining which required patient actions and behaviors have positive personal value and assists in identifying the motivational significance for successfully achieving these changes. An assessment of the patient's perceived self-efficacy or ability to carry out the required actions and identification of competencies required in achieving goals is essential in establishing a health-promoting plan for the individual.

For example, if the nurse is establishing a plan for Larry, an extremely obese individual weighing 100 lb over the weight limit, it is important to determine whether he believes that a 100-lb weight loss is achievable. Larry's physical abilities, cognitive and individual characteristics, and external influences must be considered in establishing a realistic nutritional health-promoting plan. The biological, psychological, sociocultural, spiritual, and environmental domains, previously described as influencing eating and nutritional behaviors, are also essential components to be considered in utilizing the HPM in achieving adequate nutritional status in all patients.

EVALUATION

The evaluation phase of the nursing process focuses on goals that were established initially in the planning phase. Any unforeseeable changes that have caused the plan to be unworkable must be evaluated and the plan must be modified. A nursing plan, for example, that includes teaching the patient about the need to eat two 5-oz servings from the meat group daily must be based on an awareness of the patient's food preferences. If the nurse is unaware that the patient is a strict vegetarian, the plan must be evaluated and then modified to include foods that are acceptable as meat substitutes. All patient preferences, behaviors, and attitudes must be noted when thoroughly evaluating the patient's progress in achieving the goals set out in the nursing process plan. Table 15-7 provides an example of a nursing process plan that focuses on a patient's nutritional status. A case study for an individual at risk for malnutrition is included at the end of this chapter.

TABLE 15-6 Nutrition-Related Nursing Interventions Categorized by Domain Areas

DOMAIN	INTERVENTIONS
Biological	Monitor patient's weight. Assess patient's dietary intake. Modify dietary intake if necessary. Identify abnormal laboratory values and report. Monitor energy levels and expenditure. Encourage moderate levels of physical exercise.
Psychological	Encourage patient to evaluate the meaning of foods and situations where too much or too little food is eaten. Refer patient for psychological counseling if needed.
Sociocultural	Refer patient for dietary counseling by licensed nutritionist. Provide information on dietary guidelines, low-fat foods, exchange system as needed. Include cultural or ethnic-specific food choices or both in meal planning. Include individual who cooks for the patient in the dietary counseling and exchange of nutrition-related information.
Spiritual/religious	Incorporate specific spiritual or religious beliefs in menu planning.
Environmental	Encourage and support needed lifestyle changes. Include patient's lifestyle in planning of menus. Provide patient education regarding the needed environmental changes to positively influence nutritional health.

© Cengage Learning 2013

TABLE 15-7 Nursing Process for a Slightly Below-Weight Adolescent

Assessment: Medium-Framed 18-Year-Old Active Female; weight = 108 lb; height = 5 ft, 6 in.; average caloric intake = 1,600; ideal body weight = 120 lb

NURSING DIAGNOSIS(ES)	GOALS/OUTCOMES	INTERVENTIONS
Imbalanced nutrition: Less than body requirements related to stressful adolescent relationships evidenced by loss of appetite.	Will consume a daily balanced diet as determined by activity level and metabolic needs. Will gain 2 lb/month until ideal weight is achieved. Will verbalize stress-provoking situations.	Establish patient goals. Consult dietitian on the appropriate dietary intake. Provide diet high in complex carbohydrates and fiber and low in sugar, fats, and salt. Weigh monthly. Encourage patient to verbalize stress-provoking situations. Provide support.
Deficient knowledge related to inadequate understanding of what constitutes a well-balanced diet.	Will verbalize foods needed for a well-balanced diet. Will describe possible causes of dietary inadequacy.	Inform patient on five food groups, food pyramid, diet guidelines, and the importance of well-balanced diets. Reinforce the information both in writing and orally. Have patient list possible causes of poor appetite. Work with patient in developing plan that includes food preferences. Discuss need for moderate exercise as way to promote health and to stabilize weight.

© Cengage Learning 2013

SUMMARY

Nutrition is essential for health promotion. The role of nutrition in health promotion is to maintain health through the consumption of an adequate diet containing the essential nutrients and calories to prevent nutritional deficiencies. Several tools can guide us toward healthful eating: *Dietary Guidelines for Americans 2010*, MyPyramid, exchange system, food labels, and the *Fruits & Veggies—More Matters* program. By utilizing these tools, nurses can plan a balanced diet containing a variety of foods that supply nutrients essential to life, health, maintenance, and prevention of diet-related chronic diseases.

CASE STUDY
Monica Avery: Imbalanced Nutrition—Less Than Body Requirements

OBJECTIVES/GOALS: Through participation in a discussion of this case study, participants will have the opportunity to:

1. Discuss factors that impact nutritional status in the elderly.
2. Discuss the relationship between these impacting factors and the risk for malnutrition in the elderly patient.

HEALTH-PROMOTION CONCERN, HISTORY AND PHYSICAL, PRESENT HEALTH STATUS, PAST HEALTH STATUS, FAMILY HISTORY, AND SOCIAL HISTORY

Monica Avery is a Black, 72-year-old widowed female who lives alone in her own home, although she has a housekeeper who cleans her house and who buys and prepares food for her twice a week. On the other days, Monica is responsible for preparing her own meals. Her two children live more than 100 mi away and can visit only every 2–3 months. Her past medical history includes a broken left hip, which occurred 4 months ago and required surgery. She is on several medications for her hypertension and cardiovascular insufficiency, takes oral hypoglycemic agents for her Type 2 diabetes mellitus, and takes multiple vitamins and fiber supplements. Monica has always engaged in physical activity until recently when she fell and broke her hip. Her family history is positive for diabetes on both sides of her family, and both her father and mother died of a massive heart attack in their early 60s. Her mother also had a positive history for depression.

Monica is visited once a week by a home health nurse who notices that Monica has been losing weight gradually since her dismissal from the hospital. She appears to have lost interest in eating and exercises infrequently. Her primary mode of entertainment is watching soap operas on television.

REVIEW OF PERTINENT DOMAINS

Biological Domain

Physical exam reveals an underweight individual who is 62 in. tall and weighs 105 lb. She has kyphosis, which is evidence of osteoporosis in her back and shoulders. She has full range of motion in her right leg but not in her left leg or arms.

GASTROINTESTINAL: Reports no problems in this area. She has regular bowel movements. The fiber supplement helps in regulating her bowel movements. Her dietary pattern consists of eating three meals only when the housekeeper cooks. Usually she eats one egg and two slices of bread for dinner and supper when she is alone. Occasionally she will eat a sandwich with lean ham and a slice of processed cheese. She will eat a banana or fruit when offered. She drinks black caffeinated coffee without sugar, 2–4 cups a day.

GENITOURINARY: Nonremarkable. Urinates frequently with no discomfort. Urine is clear, straw colored, with no foul odor.

DIAGNOSTIC TESTING: Glucose readings have been slightly below normal for the last 2 months.

Psychological Domain

Psychologically she appears to be slightly depressed. Monica states that she has felt very "down" since she broke her hip.

Social Domain

Cognitively she is alert and oriented. She is able to verbalize her understanding of her current physical condition. She gets along well with her children and other family members. Monica enjoys visiting with family and friends. She was a member of a church club but has not been able to participate recently due to her physical condition.

Environmental Domain

Because she lives alone, Monica does not interact with anyone on a regular basis. She does see her housekeeper twice a week and has a pleasant relationship with her. Monica needs information on the importance of a balanced diet and moderate exercise. She needs to know what foods she should include in her diet and what foods to avoid. She also needs information on health care activities and resources in her community.

QUESTIONS FOR DISCUSSION

1. What foods should Monica include in her diet?avv
2. What are some lifestyle modifications for Monica in relation to food choices?
3. Which of Monica's medicines can affect her appetite?
4. What community resources might be helpful to Monica?

KEY CONCEPTS

1. The essential nutrients to maintain health are water, carbohydrates, protein, lipids, vitamins, and minerals.
2. *Healthy People 2020,* a document by the U.S. Public Health Service, provides health-promotion and disease-prevention objectives for Americans that include a reduction in the incidence of heart disease, cancer, overweight, and growth retardation, an improvement of nutritional health, and the delivery of nutrition services to be achieved by the year 2010.
3. The biological, psychological, sociocultural, environmental, and technological domains can influence eating behavior and can also affect caloric and nutrient intake of an individual.
4. Nutritional excesses such as obesity and deficits, such as anorexia or bulimia, significantly affect the nutritional status of all Americans.
5. Eating a variety of foods such as grain products, vegetables, fruits, lean meats, and fish will ensure provision of essential nutrients for health maintenance and prevention of diet-related chronic diseases.
6. Following MyPyramid guidelines daily is the key to a healthy diet.
7. The food exchange list is a valuable guide that can be used in menu planning.
8. Paying attention to food labels can help an individual choose foods lower in fat so as not to exceed the recommended intake.
9. The nursing process and Pender's HPM can be effectively used to plan strategies to improve a patient's nutritional status.

CHAPTER REVIEW

Learning Activities

1. Record all the foods you eat and all the beverages you drink in one typical 24-hour period. Include items such as the amount of sugar or cream in coffee, sugar in iced tea, and so forth.
2. Record the number of servings you obtained from each food group. Estimate the amount of your intake (use ounces for meat serving; cups for vegetables, potatoes, beverages; small, medium, large for fruits).
3. How does your diet compare to the MyPyramid recommendations? Which food groups are underrepresented in your diet?
4. If you did not follow MyPyramid guidelines for each food group, list the reasons.
5. List six strategies you can use to improve your diet.

Multiple Choice

1. Which of the following factors directly contributes to the development of Type 2 diabetes?
   a. Age
   b. Anorexia
   c. Depression
   d. Obesity
2. Which of the following nutrients has been found to prevent spinal cord birth defects during pregnancy?
   a. Beta carotene
   b. Folic acid
   c. Vitamin C
   d. Selenium
3. Vitamin D is necessary because it does which of the following?
   a. Affects vision
   b. Affects gums and teeth
   c. Helps in the absorption of calcium and phosphorus
   d. Protects vital body tissue

4. Anorexia nervosa primarily affects which of the following?
   a. Adolescent girls
   b. Mature males
   c. Elderly females
   d. Young children

5. Which of the following is the typical bulimic?
   e. Child in elementary school
   f. College-educated female
   g. Male in his early 40s
   h. Senior citizen

6. Phytochemicals:
   a. are nonessential amino acids.
   b. are found primarily in seafood, poultry and lean meats.
   c. provide protection against arthritis, heart disease, and cancer.
   d. prevent malnutrition.

7. The Food and Drug Administration:
   a. assures the public that new food supplements are safe.
   b. establishes the *Guidelines for Americans 2010*.
   c. intervenes to assure food supplement safety after an illness/injury occurs.
   d. regulates the safety of nutritional supplements prior to the marketing phase.

8. The next step in the nursing process plan after sorting and grouping of data is:
   a. evaluation.
   b. goal setting.
   c. implementation.
   d. nursing diagnosis.

ORGANIZATIONS AND WEBSITES

Academy for Eating Disorders: An international transdisciplinary professional organization that promotes excellence in research, treatment, and prevention of eating disorders; provides education, training, and a forum for collaboration and professional dialogue: **http://www.aedweb.org**

American Dietetic Association (ADA): The nation's largest organization of food and nutrition professionals; serves *the* public by promoting optimal nutrition, health, and well-being: **http://www.eatright.org**

American Obesity Association: Offers the most comprehensive site on obesity and overweight on the Internet:

8630 Fenton Street, Suite 918
Silver Springs, MD 20910
Phone: (301) 563-6526 / Fax: (301) 563-6595
http://www.obesity.org

Food and Nutrition Service Assistance Program: This program provides children and low-income people access to food, a healthful diet, and nutrition education: **http://www.fns.usda.gov**

National Association of Anorexia Nervosa and Associated Disorders: The oldest eating disorder organization in the nation; assists individuals and their families to find resources and provides referrals to professionals:

P.O. Box 640,
Naperville, IL 60566
Phone: (630) 577-1333
http://www.anad.org

National Cancer Institute: The National Cancer Institute website provides a comprehensive site for information on cancer, including latest cancer-related news, research, and cancer statistics: **http://www.cancer.gov**

Obesity Society: The leading scientific society dedicated to the study of obesity. Since 1982 NAASO has been committed to encouraging research on the causes and treatment of obesity and to keeping the medical community and public informed of new advances:

8757 Georgia Avenue, Suite 1320
Silver Springs, MD 20910
Tel: (301)-563-6595
Fax: (301) 563-6505
http://www.obesity.org

Western Psychiatric Institute and Clinic: A national leader in the diagnosis, management, and treatment of mental health and addictive disorders: **http://www.upmc.com/HospitalsFacilities/Hospitals/wpic/Pages/default.aspx**

REFERENCES

American Cancer Society. (2011). *Broccoli.* Retrieved from http://www.cancer.gov

American Diabetes Association. (2011). Do you know what you are eating? Retrieved from http://www.diabetes.org

Ballistreri, M. C., & Corradi-Webster, C. M. (2008). Consumption of energy drinks among physical education students. *Revista Latino-Americana de Enfermagem, 16,* 558–564.

Bulemia Nervosa—Eating Disorder. (2011). Information on bulimia, nervosa, causes, consequences and treatment of bulimia nervosa. Retrieved from http://www.annecollins.com/eating-disorders/bulimia.htm

Carthron, D. L., Johnson, T. M., Hubbart, T. D., Strickland, C., & Nance, K. (2010). "Give me some sugar" The diabetes self-management activities of African-American primary caregiving grandmothers. *Journal of Nursing Scholarship, 42*(3), 330–337.

Centers for Disease Control and Prevention. (CDC). (2011) Fruits and vegetables benefits. Retrieved from http://www.fruitsandveggiesmatter.gov

European Safety Authority. (2009). *Review of labeling reference intake values.* Retrieved from http://www.efsa.europa.eu/en/publications.htm

Fiegel, K. M., Carroll, M. D., Ogden, C. L., & Curtain, L. R. (2010). Prevalence and trends in obesity among U.S. adults, 1999–2008. *Journal of the American Medical Association, 303*(3), 235–241.

Finkelstein, E. A., Trogdon, J. G., Cohen, J. W., & Dietz, W. (2009). Annual medical spending attributable to obesity: Payer-and service-specific estimates. *Health Affairs, 28*(5), 822–825.

Godfrey, J. R., & Dansinger, M. L. (2009). Toward optimal health: Sorting out the dietary approaches to achieve a healthy weight. *Journal of Women's Health, 18*(4), 435–438. DOI:10.1089/jwh.2009.1364.

Harvie, J., Mikkelsen, L., & Shak, L. (2009). A new health care prevention agenda: Sustainable food procurement and agricultural policy. *Journal of Hunger and Environmental Nutrition, 4*(3,4), 409–429. DOI: 10.1080/19320240903329055.

Holmes, S. (2010). Importance of nutrition in palliative care of patients with chronic disease. *Nursing Standard, 25*(1), 48–56.

Institute of Medicine of the National Academies. (2010, November). Dietary reference intakes for calcium and vitamin D. *Report Brief.*

Katz, D. L. (2008). *Nutrition in clinical practice.* Philadelphia, PA: Wolters Kluwer/Lippincott Williams & Wilkins.

Lad, U., & Lad, V. (2006). Food combining. In U. Lad & V. Lad. *Ayurvedic cooking for self-healing* (2nd ed.). Albuquerque, NM: The Ayurvedic Institute.

LeMone, P., Burke, K., & Bauldoff, G. (2011). *Medical-surgical nursing: Critical thinking in patient care* (5th ed.). Boston: Pearson Education.

Lutz, C., & Przytulski, K. (2011). *Nutrition and diet therapy.* Philadelphia, PA: F. A. Davis.

Miller, C. A. (2012). *Nursing for wellness in older adults.* (6th ed.). Philadelphia, PA: Wolters Kluwer/Lippincott Williams & Wilkins.

Morrow, M. (2011). Ecological intelligence and nursing: What is the connection? *Nursing Science Quarterly, 24*(2), 172–173.

NANDA. (2009). *NANDA international nursing diagnoses: Definitions and classification 2009–2011.* Oxford: Wiley-Blackwell.

National Academies of Science, Institute of Medicine, Food and Nutrition Board. (2010). Dietary reference intakes: Macronutrients. Retrieved from http://iom.edu/Activities/Nutrition//SummaryDRIs/

National Academies of Science, Institute of Medicine, Food and Nutrition Board. (2010). Dietary reference intakes: RDA and AI for vitamins and elements. Retrieved from http://iom.edu/Activities/Nutrition//SummaryDRIs/.

National Association of Anorexia Nervosa and Associated Disorders (ANAD). (2011a). Eating disorders statistics. Retrieved from http://www.anad.org/get-information/about-eating-disorders/

National Association of Anorexia Nervosa and Associated Disorders (ANAD). (2011b). *Bulimia nervosa.* Retrieved from http://www.anad.org/get-information/about-eating-disorders/

National Association of Anorexia Nervosa and Associated Disorders (ANAD). (2011c). General information. Retrieved from http://www.anad.org/get-information/about-eating-disorders/

National Cancer institute (2011). Antioxidants and cancer prevention: National Cancer Institute Facts Sheet. Retrieved from http://www.cancer.gov

National Center for Health Statistics. (2010). *Health, United States, 2010: With special feature on death and dying.* Library of Congress Catalog Number 76-641496. Washington, D.C.: U.S. Government Printing Office.

National Institutes of Health. (2011a). Ephedra. Office of Dietary Supplements. Washington, D.C. Retrieved from http://ods.od.nih.gov/.

National Institutes of Health (NIH). (2011b). Nutrient recommendations: Dietary reference intakes (DRIs). Office of Dietary Supplements. Washington, D.C. Retrieved from http://ods.od.nih.gov/.

Pagana, K. D., & Pagana, T. J. (2010. *Mosby's manual of diagnostic and laboratory tests* (4th ed.). St. Louis, MO: Mosby-Elsevier.

Pender, N. J., Murdaugh, C. L., & Parsons, M. A. (2011). *Health promotion in nursing practice* (6th ed.). Upper Saddle River, NJ: Pearson Education.

Phytochemicals. (2011). Retrieved from http://www.phytochemicals.info

Rosen, J. D. (2010). A review of the nutrition claims made by proponents of organic food. *Comprehensive Reviews in Food Science and Food Safety, 9*(3), 270–277.

Sparks-Ralph, S., & Taylor, C. (2011). *Sparks and Taylor's nursing diagnosis reference manual* (8th ed.). Philadelphia, PA: Wolters Kluwer/Lippincott Williams & Wilkins.

U.S. Department of Agriculture (USDA), Center for Nutrition Policy and Promotion. (2011a). MyPyramid: Steps to a healthier you. Retrieved from http://www.mypyramid.gov

U.S. Department of Agriculture & U.S. Department of Health and Human Services (USDHHS). (2011a). USDA and HHS announce new dietary guidelines to help Americans make healthier food choices and confront obesity epidemic. Washington, DC: HHS Press Office. Retrieved from http://www.hhs.gov/news/press/

U.S. Department of Agriculture & U.S. Department of Health and Human Services. (2011b). *Dietary guidelines for Americans 2010* (7th ed.). Washington, DC: U.S. Government Printing Office. Retrieved from Http://www.health.gov/dietaryguidelines.

U.S. Department of Agriculture & U.S. Department of Health and Human Services, (2011b). First Lady, Agriculture Secretary launch "MyPlate" icon as a new reminder to help consumers make healthier food choices. Press Release. Washington, DC. Retrieved from http://www.cnppusda.gov

U.S. Department of Health and Human Services (USDHHS). (2010b). Determinants of health. Washington, DC. Retrieved from http://www.hhs.gov

U.S. Department of Health and Human Services (USDHHS). (2010c). Healthy people 2020. Washington, DC. Retrieved from http://healthypeople.gov/2020

Voice of America. (2010, June 2). *Diabetes risk higher among overweight.* Retrieved from http://www.voanews.com

WebMD. (2011). USDA ditches food pyramid for a healthy plate. Retrieved from http://www.webmd.com

Woodruff, S. J., & Hanning, R. M. (2008). A review of family meal influence on adolescents' dietary intakes. *Canadian Journal of Dietetic Practice and Research, 69*(1), 14–22.

BIBLIOGRAPHY

Byers-Kregg, C. M., & Schlenk, E. A. (2010). Implications of food insecurity on global health policy and nursing practice. *Journal of Nursing Scholarship, 42*(3), 278–285.

Duyff, R. L. (2008). *American Dietetics Association: Complete food and nutrition guide* (3rd ed.).Hoboken, NJ: American Dietetic Association.

Ford, J. (2006). *Diseases and disabilities caused by weight problems: The overloaded body.* Philadelphia, PA: Mason Crest.

Inglis, V., Ball, K., & Ctawford, D. (2008). Socioeconomic variations in women's Diets: What is the role of perceptions of the local food environment? *Journal of Epidemiology and Community Health, 62,* 191–197.

Nord, M., Andrews, M., & Carlson, S. (2008). Household food security in the United States, 2007. *Economic Research Report No.* (ERR-66). Retrieved from http://www.ers.usda.gov/Publications/ERR66/.

CHAPTER 16
Engaging in Physical Fitness

Carolina G. Huerta, EdD, MSN, RN
Janice Maville, EdD, MSN, RN

KEY TERMS

ballistic stretching
body composition
body mass index (BMI)
cardiovascular fitness
cooldown
flexibility
heart rate reserve
intensity
maximum heart rate

muscular endurance
muscular strength
overload principle
performance-related fitness (PRF)
physical fitness
plantar fasciitis
principle of progression
principle of specificity
rate of perceived exertion

RICE
social determinants of health
sprains
static stretching
strains
target heart rate
warm-up

OBJECTIVES

Upon completion of this chapter, the reader should be able to:

- Explain why exercise is important in health promotion.
- Define physical fitness, including health-related fitness and motor-performance fitness.
- Assess the various components of health-related fitness.
- Identify the general principles of fitness training.
- Plan a fitness program using the FITT Model.
- Understand the principles and concepts of cardiovascular fitness.
- Describe the essential elements of training.
- Identify frequent problems related to exercise.
- Describe the RICE concept for injury treatment.
- Identify myths and fallacies about exercise.
- Describe how the health-promotion model is useful in developing a fitness program.
- Recognize how the nursing process may be utilized in developing a physical fitness plan.
- Identity practical tips for increasing physical activity.

INTRODUCTION

Nike's slogan "Just do it!" is one of the most recognized slogans focusing on physical fitness. The campaign, which began in the 1980s, is still relevant today and has been credited with embracing not just the resolve and purpose associated with engaging in physical fitness but also the beauty and the emotional uplifting experience associated with it. Implied in Nike's slogan is that physical fitness is necessary to achieve health and that the healthier one is, the more completely one achieves personal potential. This chapter is about achieving physical fitness goals by adopting a "Just do it!" attitude and becoming healthy and physically fit individual.

Many Americans today are emphasizing **physical fitness**, which is the ability to be physically active on a regular basis. People are more aware of the role of fitness in achieving a healthy lifestyle and are inundated from many sources such as TV, magazines, books, and even the Internet about how to include some form of exercise in their busy schedules.

Each day more and more people are choosing to take responsibility for their own well-being by becoming physically active through health-promoting behaviors. Unfortunately, the majority of people are not. For example, despite the proven benefits of physical activity, more than 60% of American adults do not engage in the recommended amount of physical activity, and 25% of all adults are not active at all. It is also a fact that activity decreases with age. Physical activity is less common among women than men and among Hispanics and African Americans. Those with lower incomes and affluence are less likely to engage in physical activity as well (U.S. Department of Health and Human Services [USDHHS], 2011b). Chapter 15 presented the concepts of nutrition and nutrition's role in maintaining health. This chapter focuses on the importance of physical fitness in health promotion. The relationships among physical fitness and health, benefits of exercise, development of a fitness program, and the role of the nurse in promoting health through physical fitness are emphasized.

SPOTLIGHT **ON**

Physiological Benefits of Cardiovascular and Strength-Developing Exercise

There are numerous physiological benefits to cardiovascular and strength-developing exercises. These exercises increase oxygen uptake, cardiac output, stroke volume, heart rate recovery after exercise, blood flow, pulmonary ventilation, metabolic rate, and lean muscle mass. They also increase secretion of specific hormones such as catecholamines and growth hormone and increase certain components of the immune system. Cardiovascular and strength-developing exercises also lower systolic and diastolic blood pressure and resting heart rate, decrease hypertension, and decrease body fat.

EXERCISE AND HEALTH PROMOTION

It is not unusual for a patient to ask a health care professional "Why should I exercise?" Although the immediate response might be "Because it is good for you," most people are not necessarily interested in finding out what is good for them. Rather, they are interested in engaging in activities that feel good. An ideal response to this question is that physical activity or exercise is fun, feels good, and is in fact beneficial. All three of these general reasons are true, and people who agree and respond to this rationale have made a commitment to fitness and are actively pursuing their commitment.

In *Healthy People 2020* (USDHHS, 2010a) a major goal is to improve health, fitness, and quality of life through daily physical activity. The benefits of a fitness program that involves cardiovascular and strength-developing exercises, then, are physiological as well as psychological, such as improvement in one's self-perception. In fact, a health-promoting fitness program may have multiple benefits that can be categorized according to the domains listed in Chapters 4 and 15. As previously indicated, physical exercise has multiple physiological benefits and psychological benefits. The sociocultural domain may also be influenced by physical activity in that physically fit individuals are more likely to exude confidence and engage in social activities, making them well-rounded persons.

The Surgeon General's Vision for a Healthy and Fit Nation 2010 (USDHHS, 2010b) recommends that American adults should engage in 150 minutes of moderate-intensity physical activity per week. Aerobic activity is recommended and includes activities such as a brisk walk or general gardening. According to the Surgeon General, these activities should be done in episodes of at least 10 minutes and should be spread throughout the week. The recommendation for children and teenagers is 60 minutes of physical activity per day most days of the week that includes vigorous activities and activities to strengthen the bones. More exercise may be needed to prevent weight gain, to lose weight, or to maintain weight loss. To promote health, cardiovascular endurance activities should be included, and these should be supplemented with strength-developing exercises at least twice per week.

Healthy People 2020 also focuses on the benefits of physical activity and the acquisition of physical fitness. In fact, *Healthy People 2020* includes four overarching goals that, together, address the importance of physical fitness. These goals are (1) to "attain high quality, longer lives free of preventable disease, disability, injury and premature death; (2) to "achieve health equity, eliminate disparities. . ."; (3) to "create social and physical

ASK **YOURSELF**

Role-Modeling Health-Promoting Behaviors

As a health care provider, should you maintain a physical fitness and exercise routine? Do you practice what you preach regarding health promotion and exercise? Can you influence others if you are not willing to invest time in making yourself as physically fit as possible?

environments that promote good health"; and (4) "to promote quality of life, healthy development, and healthy behaviors" (USDHHS, 2010a). In keeping with these goals, *Healthy People 2020* emphasizes physical activity and fitness.

The development of modern technology such as cellular telephones, computers, riding lawn mowers, even automatic garage door openers provides numerous opportunities for individuals to develop chronic conditions attributed to lack of physical activity. Being physically fit can help to reduce these chronic conditions such as heart disease, diabetes, osteoporosis, hypertension, low-back pain, and obesity.

Members of the health professions can make a difference, both a personal difference and a difference in others. Health care professionals have an opportunity to counsel adults and young people about physical activity as well as other healthful behaviors such as nutrition and stress management. Patient education is an integral part of nursing practice. It is a primary focus for nurses regardless of the setting. Nurses can certainly influence, though not control, a person's health-promotion outlook through education and by following healthy practices and serving as a role model (LeMone, Burke, & Bauldoff, 2011).

PHYSICAL FITNESS

The term *physical fitness* means different things to different people. To some people fitness may mean having a good figure or physique. To a runner, fitness may mean the ability to run a 10K, a common racing distance of 10.2 miles, in a given amount of time. To a teenager, it may mean the ability to perform at a high, sustained athletic level. A college student may deem fitness to be looking good and being free of stress. To an elderly adult, being physically fit may mean being able to complete housework and walk the pet without feeling physically exhausted. All these descriptions can apply to a definition of fitness (Figure 16-1).

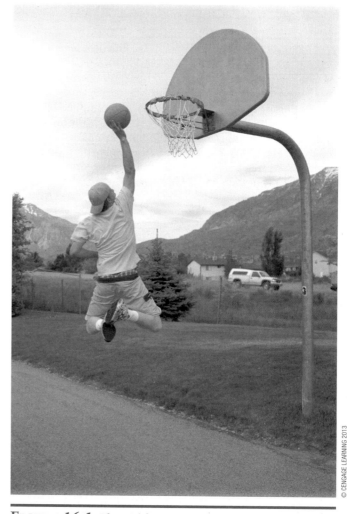

FIGURE 16-1 Physical fitness means many things to many people. What does it mean to you?

© CENGAGE LEARNING 2013

are necessary in determining the physical fitness of an individual. For example, to compete in selected sporting activities, one must have a high level of health-related fitness plus performance-related fitness. PRF components include agility, reaction time, power, coordination, balance, and speed and, most often, also includes the health-related components (ExRx.net, 2011). The health-related components have significance for everyone, not just for the athletically inclined. Although health-related fitness and performance-related fitness often overlap, the goal of the individual determines which component of fitness to pursue.

? ASK YOURSELF

Skill Performance or Health Benefit?

Why would an athlete who is striving for maximum performance in achieving a performance goal train differently than the individual who is seeking a change in lifestyle to improve and maintain a healthy lifestyle? Does a person's physical fitness performance goal affect the type of activities needed to achieve the goal?

Because physical fitness is defined in numerous ways and may include attributes that contribute to skill or athletic performance versus health-related components, a distinction is made between performance-related fitness and health-related fitness. As indicated in Box 16-1, health-related fitness pertains to the health and well-being of the individual and is necessary to maintain a healthy lifestyle. It includes the components of cardiovascular fitness, strength and muscular endurance, flexibility of the lower back and hip region, and body composition (TeachPE.com, 2011).

Performance-related fitness (PRF) components are associated more with performance than good health. Both

---

BOX 16-1

HEALTH– AND PERFORMANCE-RELATED FITNESS

HEALTH-RELATED FITNESS	PERFORMANCE-RELATED FITNESS
Cardiovascular strength, muscular strength, muscular endurance, flexibility, body composition	Strength, power, agility, balance, coordination speed, reaction time

COMPONENTS OF HEALTH-RELATED FITNESS

Health is often based on a continuum, with the extreme ends consisting of positive and negative poles (refer to Chapters 2 and 3 for a review of the health-illness continuum). Health is no longer considered merely absence of disease but a capacity to enjoy life and meet challenges. In addition to the ability to function physically, cognitively, and socially, the concept of health is impacted by what are called the **social determinants of health**. The social determinants of health are the conditions or environment under which people live, their socioeconomic level, geographic location, and the political and cultural factors that influence their health (Pender, Murdaugh, & Parsons, 2011). The health-related components contribute to the overall well-being of the individual without any specific skill-related or motor-performance expertise. The four components of health-related fitness—cardiovascular fitness, muscular strength/endurance, flexibility, and body composition—are described in the following sections.

CARDIOVASCULAR FITNESS

Cardiovascular fitness is synonymous with cardiorespiratory fitness, aerobic fitness, or cardiorespiratory endurance. All are terms that commonly refer to the circulatory system and respiratory system and how effectively and efficiently they function to transport oxygenated blood to working muscles for an extended period of time. The function of these two systems must be efficient to allow the body to perform more effectively during physical activity. Perhaps the most important benefit of cardiovascular fitness is that it is a deterrent to chronic heart disease (CHD).

To develop cardiovascular fitness, large muscle groups must work together in the form of contractions during a relatively long period of time while the cardiovascular components make adjustments to the activity as necessary. For example, the more efficient the heart, lungs, and blood vessels are in transporting the air we breathe to the contracting muscle fibers, the easier it is to walk, run, swim, study, and concentrate for longer periods of time. Activities conducive to developing cardiovascular fitness include walking, running, swimming, stair-stepping, rowing, cycling, step aerobics, low-impact aerobics, hiking, cross-country skiing, in-line skating, cross-country ski simulator, and rowing machines. All are commonly labeled aerobic activities.

MUSCULAR STRENGTH AND ENDURANCE

Muscular strength is the ability to exert force with a muscle against resistance, under maximal conditions in a single effort. For example, being able to lift an object or patient without undue stress or suffering sprain, strain, or muscular difficulties requires a certain amount of muscular strength. Muscular strength, such as that of the abdominal muscles, helps to maintain proper posture and prevents lower-back problems.

Muscular endurance is the ability of a muscle or group of muscles to perform or sustain a muscle contraction over an extended period of time. With good muscular endurance, a person can carry something over a long period of time as well as repeat a movement without becoming tired. It is recommended that individuals incorporate some form of resistance training, such as weight lifting, in their fitness programs to promote muscular strength and endurance. Furthermore, resistance training helps maintain or develop muscle mass and bone strength.

Females typically have lower levels of upper body strength than of lower body strength. Therefore, in general, females should engage in a program of regular, upper body strength development.

FLEXIBILITY

Flexibility is the ability of a joint or group of joints to move freely through a range of motion (ROM). The ROM for a joint may be restricted by the shape of bones and cartilage of the joint, as well as by the muscles, tendons, ligaments, and fascia that cross the joint. On a continuum, an extreme lack of flexibility would be the knee of a person with arthritis and on the extreme other end would be the individual with knees that hyperextend.

? ASK **YOURSELF**

Changing Lifestyle Behaviors

Jennifer is a 42-year-old female 5 ft, 3 in. tall and weighing 167 lb. She is employed as chief nurse executive at a large hospital. Jennifer is feeling stressed at having to perform her duties at work and also handle her young children, husband, and home responsibilities. She is always complaining of being fatigued and overworked. She has never played any sports and feels too time-constrained to start a physical fitness and exercise program sponsored by her employer. As the employee health nurse at the hospital where Jennifer works, what would you recommend to promote a change in her health status?

BODY COMPOSITION

Body composition refers to the relative amount of fat in the body compared to fat-free weight such as muscle, bone, and other elements in the body. In terms of health-related fitness, an excessive amount of fat or being overweight is unhealthy because it requires more energy for movement, may reflect a diet high in saturated fat, and places numerous demands on the cardiovascular system.

A major health problem in the United States is overweight or obesity. Statistics indicate that more than one-third of U.S. adults and 17% of U.S. children are obese. These statistics show that overweight and obesity have tripled in the American population over the last three decades and that overweight and obesity cut across all ages and racial and ethnic groups as well as both genders (Centers for Disease Control and Prevention [CDC], 2011). Many of the leading causes of death can be linked to obesity. For example, cardiovascular disease, stroke, and even cancer may be more prevalent among the obese. As a result of this close link, an economic cost is obviously associated with obesity. In 2008, for example, the United States incurred $147 billion in economic costs associated with obesity (CDC, 2011). That is about $20 billion more than a decade ago. In addition, the latest figures show that obese individuals spent $1,400 more in medical care costs than people of normal weight (CDC, 2011).

ASSESSING HEALTH-RELATED FITNESS

Although starting a fitness program early in life is wise, a person is never too old or too sedentary to begin. The key is realizing that success is gradual and that the present state of fitness or lack of fitness did not occur overnight. A common question a nurse hears is, "Where do I begin?" The appropriate response is determined after conducting an individual fitness assessment.

One of the first things to be assessed is the individual's desire and/or reasons for wanting to become fit. Is it to feel better, look better, join a group, or play on the company's softball team? Fitness requires effort and the fuel for effort is motivation. Determining the reason and goal is essential.

As difficult as it may sound, a person cannot sit and become fit. Before recommending that an individual engage in exercise, the nurse needs to know as much about the person as possible. A fitness program should start with an inventory of the individual that includes the current level of fitness and medical history. Prevailing factors such as age, previous medical conditions, pregnancy, and present medication may necessitate a physical examination. People are often unaware of preexisting conditions that might pose a risk when participating in new or

SPOTLIGHT ON

Obesity-Related Complications

Many physically debilitating diseases can be prevented by following a sound diet and exercising regularly. Being overweight contributes to the prevalence of high blood pressure, diabetes, heart disease, high blood cholesterol, depression, and cancers of the breast, ovary, uterus, prostate, colon, and rectum. Greater risks for complications occur the longer in life an individual remains overweight.

vigorous physical activity programs. A sample of preliminary questions that may be answered by a yes or no can be a starting point for a preexercise program inventory.

CARDIOVASCULAR FITNESS

Prior to beginning a cardiovascular or aerobic fitness program, the present condition of the individual must be assessed. The level of cardiovascular fitness is determined by the maximal amount of oxygen the human body is able to use per minute of physical activity. The greater the oxygen consumption, the more efficient the cardiovascular system will be. Tests for levels of cardiovascular fitness may include maximal or submaximal measures.

Submaximal tests do not require the individual to "gut it out" or push to the limit of exercise tolerance. These tests are a good alternative to the maximal oxygen consumption laboratory tests. By performing these activities periodically, individuals can assess how well they are doing on the road to a healthier lifestyle.

MUSCULAR STRENGTH

Several methods can be used to measure muscular strength, or the ability to exert force against resistance, under maximal conditions in a single effort. The most common way to measure muscular strength is by using a one maximum repetition (1-RM) to determine how much weight one can lift in a single effort. How much weight to use initially for testing purposes must be safely estimated by trial and error. Caution must be exercised for the beginning individual because injury from maximum lifting may occur. It is recommended that inexperienced individuals estimate maximal strength by using a 6-RM—the amount of weight lifted six times and no more and no less.

MUSCULAR ENDURANCE

Muscular endurance allows the individual to repeat a movement over a period of time without getting tired. When muscles become fatigued, they do not relax after each contraction, and the potential for injury increases. Prior to assessing muscular endurance, a person should perform a 5- to 10-minute warm-up using large-muscle groups such as in walking and calisthenics.

A muscular endurance assessment may be done by having the individual lift a certain amount of weight for as long as possible. An example is the bicep curl—lifting a weight toward the chest using the arm flexors—counting the number of completed times the weight is lifted and returned to the starting position.

ASSESSING FLEXIBILITY

Flexibility in an individual can vary throughout the body depending on the specific body part. Maintaining flexibility is essential for healthy aging. To develop and maintain flexibility and ROM, one must continually do flexibility exercises. Stretching exercises are best for improving flexibility and can be performed in two ways: **ballistic stretching** (repeated bouncing) and **static stretching** (slow and deliberate). Caution should be used when performing ballistic stretches because these are prone to cause injury or soreness. Static stretching is preferred, is considered safer, and involves using a slow and gradual lengthening of the muscle. An example is sitting on the floor with one leg extended and the other bent at a 45° angle and slowly moving forward toward the wall, bending at the waist, and extending the hands in a forward position.

Testing for flexibility may involve the sit-and-reach test. The sit-and-reach test as well as other versions provides essentially the same information: the ability to sit on the floor and bend forward at the waist. Good flexibility in the joints can help prevent injuries through all stages of life. Activities that lengthen the muscles such as swimming or a basic stretching program are excellent ways to increase flexibility.

ASSESSING BODY COMPOSITION

There are several methods for assessing body composition: height-weight tables, body mass indexes, and laboratory methods such as bioelectrical impedance, BOD POD, and underwater weighing. In laboratory settings, hydrostatic weighing (underwater) is often done rather than skinfold measurement, although hydrostatic weighing is more time-consuming.

Hydrostatic weighing involves applying Archimedes' principle to determine the body's density. The person is weighed outside water, then submerged and weighed again accounting for air in the lungs. The density is determined, which in turn allows for the total body fat to be calculated.

Skinfold calipers (Figure 16-2), used by a trained person, can give a good estimate of body fat. Although body fat

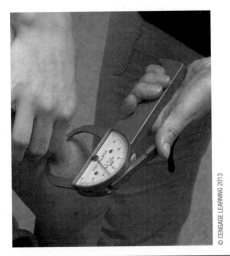

FIGURE 16-2 Fat measurement using calipers.

© CENGAGE LEARNING 2013

BOX 16-2
CALCULATING BODY MASS INDEX

1. Divide your weight in pounds by 2.2 to convert weight to kilograms.
2. Multiply your height in inches by 0.0254 to convert height to meters.
3. Square your height in meters.
4. Divide weight in kilograms by height in meters squared.
5. Use the rating scale for BMI to obtain your BMI rating.

Body Mass Index Rating

CLASSIFICATION	WOMEN	MEN
High risk	27.3	27.8
Marginal	24.5–27.2	25.0–27.7
Good fitness	18.0–24.4	19.0–24.9
Low	15.0–17.9	17.9–18.9

is located throughout the body around organs, muscles, and under the skin, measuring thickness of skinfolds at certain multiple locations provides a good estimate of total body fatness. However, skinfold measurements are not accurate with the obese.

Body mass index (BMI) is a convenient tool and relatively easy to calculate (Box 16-2). It is used to relate height and weight to determine whether the individual is considered overweight or obese. Caution is required when using BMI as well as height-weight tables in that BMI cannot distinguish how much weight fat contributes to the total weight of the individual. The National Institutes of Health have set more stringent BMI guidelines for men and women. A value of 25–29.9 is considered overweight, and a value of 30 or greater is considered obese.

STARTING A FITNESS TRAINING PROGRAM: MAKING THAT DECISION

Once the decision to improve fitness is made and assessments are completed, regular training or work must begin. Starting and maintaining a fitness program is a conscious choice, one that requires planning, goal setting, and executing the plan. Motivation is one of the key ingredients. A fundamental reason to start a program and continue is simple: fun and enjoyment. If a person does not like the workout, does not think he or she can perform the exercises, is not having fun, is getting overly sore, or if exercising is becoming a chore, then the individual probably will not continue regardless of the benefits to be reaped.

A fitness program does not have to be confined to a gym. People do not have to hurt when they train. Patients should be encouraged to exercise with others or make a new friend who has an interest in exercising. Individuals who exercise with others are more inclined to continue the regimen.

GENERAL PRINCIPLES OF FITNESS TRAINING

Three general principles must be applied in a fitness program to reap the benefits from the effort expended: (1) the principle of overload, (2) the principle of specificity, and (3) the principle of progression.

ASK **YOURSELF**

Psychological Benefits of Exercise

Have you ever had trouble dealing with a big worry? Perhaps you became slightly depressed worrying over it. Have you noticed that when you engage in physical activity, you are not able to concentrate on those worries? Exercise has many physiological benefits. Physical conditioning can be effective in preventing high levels of stress. Do you think that exercise can provide psychological benefits for you?

PRINCIPLE OF OVERLOAD

For a muscle, including the heart muscle, to get stronger, the **overload principle** must be applied. Overload means that the body is being forced to do more than it normally does. An overload stimulus can be applied to any muscle or body part for a specific component of fitness: lifting weights for improving strength, walking for cardiovascular endurance, or stretching to improve flexibility. The body may adapt to the overload or higher level of work, in which case fitness improves, or it may fail to adapt and injury may occur.

PRINCIPLE OF SPECIFICITY

The **principle of specificity** applies to all types of training and states that one must overload the body systems or the specific fitness component to achieve a specific outcome. Different methods of exercise place specific demands on the body, and an individual must participate in a specific program to develop each of the four components of fitness. Stretching is specific to flexibility and does not improve cardiovascular endurance. Overload is specific also to each body part. To develop upper body strength, the muscles involved improve only when they are used in the specific way they are trained. A vertical press lift makes it easier to lift heavy objects up to the top shelf of an equipment stand but does not make it easier to carry objects in front of the body. Aerobic exercises concentrate on the cardiovascular system, whereas resistance training is more effective in developing muscular strength. Flexibility exercises are low-energy activities but are the most effective way to develop joint ROM. The overload principle does not imply that spot reducing can be achieved (see Myth 3 in Box 16-4).

RESEARCH NOTE

Health-Related Physical Fitness and Weight Status

STUDY PROBLEM/PURPOSE

Overweight in children and adolescents are increasingly common, whereas physical fitness is declining. Lower fitness in adolescents may track into adulthood. The effects of overweight on health-related physical fitness vary. This study's purpose was to investigate the relationship between health-related physical fitness, body mass index (BMI), and weight among Chinese adolescents.

METHODS

Participating in the Hong Kong Student Obesity Surveillance project were 3,204 students aged 12–18 years. Anthropometric measures (height, weight) and health-related fitness (push-up, sit-up, sit-and-reach, 9-minute mile) were assessed. BMI was calculated, and participants were classified according to normal weight, underweight, overweight, and obese groups. The associations between health-related physical fitness, BMI, and weight status were examined.

FINDINGS

More boys than girls were overweight or obese, and more girls were underweight. Boys performed significantly better in sit-ups and the 9-minute mile. All four physical fitness tests were significantly positively correlated with each other for both genders. The BMI was weakly correlated with sit-up and sit-and-reach tests in boys. Decreasing performance occurred in overweight- and obese-status adolescents. Decreasing performance also occurred in those who were underweight.

IMPLICATIONS

The study results indicate that the relationship between BMI and health-related physical fitness in adolescents were nonlinear. The study found that overweight/obese and underweight adolescents had poorer performance in push-up and sit-up tests than those of normal weight. The findings suggest that different aspects of health-related physical fitness may serve as immediate indicators of potential health risks for underweight and overweight adolescents.

Mak, K., Ho, S., Lo, W., Thomas, G., McManus, A., Day, J., & Lam. (2010). Health-related physical fitness and weight status in Hong Kong adolescents. *BMC Public Health, 10,* 88.

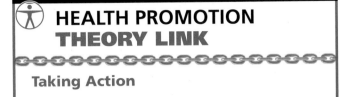

HEALTH PROMOTION THEORY LINK

Taking Action

A concept that is very important in Pender's Health-Promotion Model is that of self-efficacy. Self-efficacy plays a role in personal change and is the foundation for human motivation and action. Taking action on a desired change, such as engaging in a physical fitness program, requires individuals to believe that they have control (self-efficacy) to change behaviors. Health behaviors are also influenced by personal expectations and the goals set by the individual. Perceived personal outcomes and goals serve as incentives for change and taking action.

Source: Pender, N., Murdaugh, C., & Parsons, M.A. (2011). *Health promotion in nursing practice* (6th ed.). Upper Saddle River, NJ: Pearson Education.

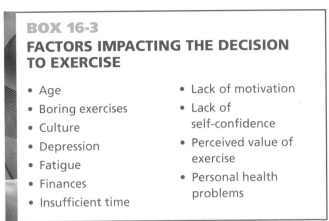

BOX 16-3

FACTORS IMPACTING THE DECISION TO EXERCISE

- Age
- Boring exercises
- Culture
- Depression
- Fatigue
- Finances
- Insufficient time
- Lack of motivation
- Lack of self-confidence
- Perceived value of exercise
- Personal health problems

PRINCIPLE OF PROGRESSION

Principle of progression implies that gradually the overload stimulus is increased as adaptations to the existing workload occur. As the body adapts to one level of exercise, a new overload must be applied to stimulate improvements in physical fitness. For positive fitness results, the progression principle should not be increased too slowly or too rapidly. Minimum and maximum levels of training are based on the progressive exercise principle.

PLANNING A FITNESS PROGRAM

Questions such as "How often should I exercise?" and "What type of exercise is the best for achieving fitness?" and "How hard should I work?" are often asked of health care professionals. Once again, the individual's goal for fitness must be clear. Does the individual want to achieve overall fitness such as a change in cardiovascular endurance, muscular strength and endurance, flexibility, and body composition or concentrate on one or a combination of the various components? Remember that the greater the number of large muscles involved in an exercise regime, such as a cardiovascular program, the greater the return on additional health-related benefits will be.

Physiological, behavioral, and psychological variables impact a person's decision to become physically fit and active. The maintenance of physical fitness and regular physical activity depends on the sources of personal and social motivation within a person's day-to-day environment (Pender, Murdaugh, & Parsons, 2011). Part of the planning procedure to enlist a person in a physical fitness program is to determine variables impacting exercise ability, as well as the frequency, intensity, time involved, and type of training (FITT) to incorporate into the fitness program.

Frequently, when planning an exercise or fitness program, variables such as culture or lack of personal motivation are not taken into account. These variables are quite obvious, yet health-promotion planners may not be aware of their impact on the decision to exercise. For example, people may be motivated to exercise to music if the type of music is relevant to their age group, lifestyle, or culture. An older American may adhere to an exercise plan using Golden Oldies, while younger adults may prefer rap.

Research has found that exercise programs that take culture into account create personal interest and increased adherence. One study conducted by researchers from Lewis University in Illinois found that a culturally focused exercise program for Hispanic adults with Type 2 diabetes was very successful. The results showed an 84% completion rate and a 75% attendance rate when a community-based, culturally focused exercise program was used among Hispanic adults. The researchers concluded that a culture-focused exercise program can be very successful in increasing participation among Hispanic groups (Martyn-Nemeth, Vitale, & Cowger, 2010). Incorporating culture into exercise routines may prove beneficial in other ethnic populations. For example, use of salsa music in an exercise regimen may spark the interest of Hispanic. Box 16-3 identifies factors that impact a person's decision to participate in exercise.

FREQUENCY

Frequency is how many times per week a person is physically active or participating in an exercise program. The more often a person exercises during the week, the greater the caloric expenditure will be. A good practice is to establish a pattern for training such as exercising at the same time each day. Patients should be encouraged to write the times on their calendar; that is, plan time into their schedule that suits them.

INTENSITY

Intensity describes how hard a person must work to improve physical fitness. The intensity of exercise is determined by the maximum heart rate of the individual. In the beginning stages of a fitness program, the intensity should be kept low. High-intensity can often lead to soreness, injury, and frustration.

TIME

Time indicates how long the individual should work out during an exercise session and how often a person should work out during a given time in a week. It is recommended that workout sessions are 20–60 minutes each and that a time pattern for training be set, such as the same time on a specified day (USDHHS, 2011b).

TYPE OF TRAINING

The last element of the FITT model is the type of training a person plans to do for each fitness component. For cardiovascular fitness, the training should be some type of aerobic exercise, such as walking, running, swimming, hiking, and so on. Weight lifting for muscular strength and endurance may include working with free weights, such as barbells and dumbbells, weight machines, or some other type of weight resistance. Flexibility training should involve some type of stretching. Making a change in body composition necessitates a combination of aerobic exercise, weight resistance, flexibility, and good daily nutrition.

ASK **YOURSELF**

Exercise-Related Muscle Soreness

Delayed muscle soreness may occur days after exercising and usually follows vigorous or unaccustomed exercise. How can a person prevent delayed muscle soreness? What are some of the proper training techniques that can be used to prevent this occurrence?

PRINCIPLES AND CONCEPTS OF CARDIOVASCULAR FITNESS

Prior to undertaking an aerobic or a cardiovascular fitness program, an individual must first understand the concepts of resting, target, and recovery heart rates and the rate of perceived exertion. Each of these components is integral for determining the intensity of the workout and is discussed next.

RESTING HEART RATE

Resting heart rate can be an initial indicator of a person's fitness level. An active lifestyle tends to produce a lower resting heart rate, whereas a sedentary lifestyle is associated with a higher resting heart rate.

The resting heart rate is best determined by counting the pulse either at the carotid artery or the radial artery for 1 minute upon awakening in the morning. For best results, several resting heart rates should be taken, and then the average should be determined. When taking the carotid pulse, care should be taken to use only two fingers (the index and middle fingers), to press lightly at the carotid artery and to count the pulse. Be sure that the thumb is not used because it has a beat of its own. The radial pulse is taken, by means of the two-finger method, at the radial artery on an upturned wrist below the heel of the hand, as per usual. Some people have a difficult time taking the radial pulse when at rest and when exercising.

TARGET HEART RATE

The **target heart rate** is the level or zone one should attain during aerobic activity to receive any training benefit. During exercise, the heart rate increases, and immediately after exercise the heart rate gradually decreases. The better the cardiovascular

condition of the individual, the quicker the recovery time for the heart rate to return to its resting rate. The age and heart rate of the individual determine the intensity at which the person should exercise, especially for cardiovascular endurance. The intensity of the workout uses the **heart rate reserve**, which is the difference between the resting heart rate and the maximum heart rate. The **maximum heart rate** is the fastest rate the heart can attain under maximal exercise conditions and still receive benefit. The target heart rate zone is 55–85% of the maximum heart rate. Staying within this range when exercising is ideal (American Heart Association, 2011).

To calculate a target heart rate (THR) zone, determine the maximum heart rate (MHR) and the heart rate reserve (HRR). To calculate the MHR, subtract the person's age from the constant 220. The HRR is then calculated by subtracting the resting heart rate from the MHR. For example, a 30-year-old with a resting pulse of 65 beats per minute would have a 190 MHR (220 – 30 years). The same individual would have an HRR of 125 (190 – 65). The THR zone can then be calculated as either a minimal target heart rate (50% heart work intensity) or a maximal target heart rate (85% heart work intensity). To determine the minimal target heart rate, add 50% of the HRR to the resting heart rate. To calculate MHR, add 85% of the HRR to the resting heart rate. The 30-year-old with a resting pulse of 65 would thus have a minimal target heart rate of 127 beats per minute (50% of 125 HRR plus 65) and a maximal target heart rate of 171 (85% of 125 HRR plus 65).

Frequency and time are important components for increasing the body's response to cardiovascular fitness. Beyond the recommended frequency and time, exercise does not benefit the individual and injury may result. The guidelines previously discussed should be achieved gradually over several months.

Once people become experienced exercisers, they perceive or have a feeling for the amount of intensity or exertion that they are achieving (their **rate of perceived exertion**). Perceived exertion calls on individuals to be in tune with their bodies physiologically and psychologically during exercise. Essentially they are using their sensory information to predict their working capacity.

ASK **YOURSELF**

Intensity

You are engaged in a walking program. How fast should you walk? How do you know you are within your target zone? Can you carry on a normal conversation with your exercise partner, or are you gasping for breath?

Exertion ranges from very, very light to very, very hard, with very light, somewhat hard, hard, and very hard categories in between. If you are walking on a treadmill for 20–30 minutes, for example, you might perceive your workout to be between mildly hard and somewhat hard. However, if you struggled to complete the 30 minutes on the treadmill, you might judge your workout to be extremely hard. It is recommended that you try to maintain your workout somewhere between *somewhat hard* to *hard*.

In the FITT model, frequency and intensity are directly related. The less intense the workout, the longer an individual must work to achieve the same benefit as if the workout were more intense and the duration shorter. When starting a program, exercisers can accomplish their goals by working at the minimum threshold target or submaximally for a longer period of time. Gradual progression is key to remaining motivated and enjoying a fitness program.

A BALANCED FITNESS PROGRAM

A well-balanced fitness program includes achieving and maintaining good body composition, which includes the relative amount of fat in the body compared to fat-free weight, such as that of muscle, bone, and similar elements. Rather than be consumed with weight-measuring scales, a different set of scales can be used—one focused on energy consumption. This set of scales depends on a person's energy expended versus energy consumed. A balanced fitness program includes both physical activity and change in food consumption. To change or decrease weight, lower food intake must be accompanied by more energy output, such as exercise. Exercise can burn calories and helps in achieving weight loss depending on its intensity. For example, high-impact aerobic exercises burn 511–763 cal depending on the person's starting weight. Less intense exercise, such as ballroom dancing, can burn 219–327 cal/hour (Mayo Clinic, 2011). There are numerous activities that can be incorporated into a fitness program that is designed to achieve the person's specific goal.

RESULT EXPECTATIONS

How soon can results be expected from a fitness program? To experience change such as feeling or seeing results, one has to not only actively engage in physical activity but continue in physical activity as well. Immediate results are unrealistic for people just beginning an exercise program. When counseling patients, remind them that results take time and that they should not be discouraged if their results from the fitness program are slow. All changes toward a healthy behavior take time.

> ## NURSING ALERT
>
> ### Reaching Fitness Goals
>
> A well-rounded fitness program should include cardiovascular work, resistance training, and flexibility exercises, all incorporated with a sound nutritional plan. Reaching a patient's fitness goals requires a multidisciplinary approach that includes a professional nurse, trainer, and nutritionist.

During the initial two weeks of an organized physical activity program, people express that they feel better and experience a sense of accomplishment. The actual physiological improvements usually take 6–12 weeks. The key is progression: not to do too much, too soon, and not to expect too much, too soon. Caution should be taken when recommending the type of activity and prescribing an exercise program for the novice exerciser. People new to exercise should be told to start slow, stay with it, and have fun. A good suggestion is to tell individuals to keep their fitness goals on the refrigerator or some other prominent location.

IMPLEMENTATION OF FITNESS PROGRAM: ESSENTIAL ELEMENTS OF TRAINING

Once the assessments are complete and the goal and plan are determined, it is time to begin the actual program. Individuals should be encouraged to dress comfortably, favoring clothing such as loose shorts and T-shirts, socks, and appropriate shoes. Although image may be important, comfort when exercising is more important.

Athletic shoes for the specific types of exercise are important, and certainly an abundance of sport shoes are manufactured. The essential characteristics of the appropriate training shoe are proper support and cushion, the fit, and shoe performance specific to the activity such as running, walking, aerobics, or cross-training.

The essential elements of a training program include the warm-up, workout, and cooldown. The **warm-up** consists of stretching and mild exercise to gradually increase the heart rate, circulation, and body temperature. It occurs prior to the actual workout and should be gradual. An increase in body temperature is essential for a better workout. For some people, stretching is done after the initial 10–15 minutes of slow walking, jogging, or some other large-muscle activity. For others, stretching may be done prior to and at the conclusion of the exercise session.

> ## NURSING ALERT
>
> ### Essential Elements for Training
>
> In preparing individuals for participation in a fitness program, they should be told to include 10–15 minutes of warm-up, 20–30 minutes of workout in the THR zone, and 10–15 minutes of cooldown.

The actual cardiovascular workout should be 20–30 minutes, depending on the initial assessment, present physical condition, and fitness component. It may take a period of time to reach the initial minimum 20 minutes of involvement, depending on the condition of the patient. Benefits such as a sense of accomplishment and feeling better can be immediate. Starting a program, or taking the first step, often requires the most determination.

The **cooldown**, or warm down, is gradual and should be the last 5–10 minutes of the completed workout. Slow jogging or walking (cardiovascular workout), followed by static stretching, helps the body to readjust to a resting phase without abruptly coming to a halt. The heart rate should be monitored during the actual workout and after completing the workout.

This provides immediate feedback for intensity purposes such as staying within the THR zone. After completing the workout and cooldown, the quickness with which the heart rate returns to a resting phase is an indicator of the condition of the individual.

COMMON PROBLEMS RELATED TO EXERCISE

Individual can become discouraged when they begin an exercise program only to become injured because of doing too much too soon or because of an improper exercise technique. Understanding potential dangers as well as listening to the body's various aches and pains can prevent many of the typical injuries. Several frequent injuries may occur, and there are ways to prevent and treat each. Environmental conditions, including warm or cold weather and pollution, also affect exercise.

SIDE STITCH

The exact cause of the sharp pain that occurs in the side during exercise or in the shoulders or upper back is unknown. Some experts suggest that it relates to a lack of blood flow to the respiratory muscles during exercise. Usually it occurs with novice exercisers, particularly in the beginning stages, and with experienced exercisers when their activity reaches higher intensities than usual. The remedies are to slow down, breathe deeply and slowly, or stop altogether, if it persists. When exercising, give particular attention to breathing in a slow rhythmic pattern. This is a reminder to warm up prior to exercising.

MUSCLE SORENESS

Exercising when not accustomed to exercise tends to produce muscle soreness. Usually the soreness subsides gradually and disappears within several days. This soreness is different from the burn felt when doing extreme and heavy workouts or total fatigue. Lactic acid is a byproduct of heavy exercise and can cause pain that is different from the usual soreness. Careful and deliberate warm-ups plus exercising within the THR zone should help in preventing extreme muscle soreness. Remember to apply the principle of progression.

STRAINS AND SPRAINS

Strains, which are injuries to muscles, and **sprains**, injuries to ligaments, can occur during exercise. Without a proper warm-up and cooldown and with overloading body parts, strains most often occur in the quadriceps, hamstring muscles, and back (from improper lifting techniques). **Plantar fasciitis**, or arch pain, most often occurs in walkers and runners. Shin splints, which occur in the front and sides of the tibia, can be extremely painful.

WARM WEATHER CONDITIONS

Whether the individual is a beginner or already an experienced exerciser, extreme caution must be taken when exercising in hot, humid weather. Prolonged exposure to extreme heat as well as high humidity can result in heat cramps, heat exhaustion, or heatstroke. To exercise in heat, a person must gradually acclimatize to the environment and then take certain precautions.

The time of day to exercise is important, and the hottest parts of the day should be avoided at all times. Exercising either in early morning or late afternoon or in an air-conditioned facility is recommended. The type of clothing is also important and should be adjusted to accommodate the heat. A change in the intensity and duration of time during workouts helps to accommodate the environment.

During a workout, it is essential to replace fluids lost through evaporation by drinking large quantities of fluids whether thirsty or not. Individual water needs vary widely based on the level of physical activity and age groups. The average daily fluid intake for an adult is 3.7 L/day for males and 2.7 L/day for females over 19 years of age (Institute of Medicine of the National Academies, 2010). Water can be obtained through consumption of drinking water and beverages, as well as from foods such as fruits and vegetables. To prevent dehydration, weigh yourself before and after exercising, and replenish the weight loss with fluids, preferably water.

NURSING ALERT

Dehydration and Exercise

Dehydration occurs when you lose more water than you take in. If you do not replace the fluids, you become dehydrated. Several common causes of dehydration are diarrhea, vomiting, and fever. Another cause of dehydration is not drinking enough water or fluids when engaging in exercise. Young children, older adults, and those with chronic illness are most at risk. If you engage in intense exercises, monitor your fluid loss, and drink enough liquids to replace the fluids lost.

EXERCISING IN COLD WEATHER

Conserving heat becomes a major concern when exercising in cold weather. Additional problems occur when cold weather is accompanied by wind or wet conditions or both creating, a windchill factor. Dress in thin layers that can be altered as the body temperature rises. Avoid using cotton next to your skin because it stays wet. Protect your hands and feet by wearing gloves and thermal socks. Protect your head by wearing a cap, earmuffs, or headband.

POLLUTION PROBLEMS

Exercising in polluted conditions or smoggy weather warrants the same caution as exercising during extreme weather conditions. Avoid exercising outdoors, particularly in urban areas where pollutants such as carbon monoxide, ozone, and others adversely impact the body. Like heat, pollution levels are often at their highest during mid afternoon.

The nurse involved in promoting health through exercise should stress to all patients that they must learn to self-monitor their bodies during exercise. The fatigue and discomfort that accompany training are often foretelling an injury. Progressive pain during and after exercising is an alert that something is wrong and that the patient should slow down and rest.

RICE CONCEPT FOR INJURY TREATMENT

Minor injuries are not uncommon for anyone who exercises. The RICE method is a good modality to use with muscle sprains or strains or other minor discomforts. The first onset of pain or injury indicates an immediate reduction from the exercise routine; therefore, *rest* the body for a day or more, depending on the extent of the injury. Immediately after an injury, apply *ice* to decrease pain and promote vasoconstriction. It is widely accepted that ice packs should be applied to the injured area for no longer than 30 minutes at a time for 72 hours after an acute injury. A light covering such as a dry-cloth towel should be applied next to the skin prior to applying the ice pack to prevent cold burn.

Compression is vitally important in conjunction with the application of ice to control swelling. Right after apply ice, reduce the amount of space available for swelling by applying an elastic wrap firmly and evenly around the injury.

The fourth aspect of the RICE model is *elevation* of the injured part to assist in controlling swelling. To provide a decrease in the swelling, the injured part must be elevated above the heart. The greater the degree of elevation above the heart, the more effective the control is for the swelling. Elevate as much as possible during the first 72 hours of the injury. The goal is to return to exercise and use the injured part as soon as possible; thus the treatment must be aggressive.

MYTHS ABOUT EXERCISE

The enthusiasm for fitness and exercise seems to be at an all-time high. Yet this enthusiasm is puzzling in that the latest survey by the Gallup Healthways Well-Being Index found that more than 31% of Americans report that they do not exercise on any given day of the week. In fact, only about one-half of Americans reported that they exercise on a regular basis (Wilbert, 2010). People who do not engage in physical activity often succumb to the myths or fallacies about exercise, which are quite difficult to dispel and must be addressed by all health care professionals if fitness and exercise are the national goal. Box 16-4 provides a description of the myths and facts related to exercise and physical activity. These should be shared with all individuals who express an interest in physical fitness or who are in dire need of a physical fitness program.

HEALTH BELIEF AND HEALTH-PROMOTION MODELS

Changing behavior, particularly in promoting health, involves choices and decisions. Having the required information, such as knowledge about health-related fitness components, is insufficient and incomplete for achieving fitness. Daily, choices must be made about how to live a life to influence overall health. Several conceptual frameworks can provide a basis for building a successful fitness program that nursing's patients will adhere to. These frameworks indicate that people are more likely to change their health-related behavior when they believe that there are benefits to doing so or that they can, in fact, effect their own health outcomes.

The Health Belief Model, for example, assumes that everyone wants to achieve well-being and that the person's belief that health is attainable is critical in attaining this well-being (Rosenstock, 1990). Additionally, Pender's (1996) Health-Promotion Model proposes that health-promoting behavior is related to an individual's perceptions of health and perceived control over health status. Essential components of this model are the individual's belief that a certain behavior is possible, that benefits are associated with this behavior, and recognition of the perceived barriers in achieving the health-promotion outcomes. The health care professional establishing a physical fitness program should recognize that patients are more likely to change health-related behavior if the current behavior is perceived to be detrimental to their health status. Behavior may also change if the patient becomes aware that considerable unpleasantness affecting work, family, and health can occur if there are no changes. In educating clients, nurses need to recognize that the patient must believe that the benefits of the new behavior are achievable and worth the effort.

UTILIZING THE NURSING PROCESS IN DEVELOPING A PHYSICAL FITNESS PLAN

As noted, the nursing process can be utilized in developing a health-promotion plan. The nursing process is an appropriate planning tool for nurses involved in addressing physical

---

☀ NURSING **ALERT**

Things to Remember When Exercising

In talking to individuals who are contemplating exercising daily, emphasize the following:

1. Select an activity or sport that you enjoy.
2. Muscle soreness gradually subsides—don't quit.
3. Acclimatize when exercising in heat; use common sense.
4. Drink plenty of water prior to and after exercise.
5. When exercising in cold temperatures, wear a hat and gloves.
6. Dress in thin layers when exercising in cold temperatures.

☀ NURSING **ALERT**

RICE for the Treatment of Injuries

Nurses may have the opportunity to provide information to patients who are embarking on a new physical fitness program. Nurses need to stress that injuries associated with exercise do occur and may require a quick response. The RICE method should be shared with all individuals who are starting an exercise program:

1. *R*est the body or body parts.
2. *I*ce the injured area.
3. *C*ompress the injury.
4. *E*levate the area as high as possible.

BOX 16-4

MYTHS AND FACTS ABOUT EXERCISE

Myth 1: Exercise is too hard and time-consuming.

Fact: An investment of 60 minutes per week divided into bouts of 20 minutes three times per week and working at a minimum of 60% of maximum heart rate can yield healthy benefits.

Myth 2: Exercise is not a quick way to lose weight; you have to do so much to lose even 1 lb of fat.

Fact: Walking at 60% of maximum heart rate, people weighing 120–150 lb can expend 258–318 kcal/hour, respectively. Good nutrition and exercise can lead to loss of about 1 lb per week (Corbin & Lindsey, 2007).

Myth 3: Passive or no-sweat exercise is effective in losing fat in specific areas of the body and can increase fitness.

Fact: Examples of ineffective passive exercise equipment are vibrating belts, muscle stimulators or vibrators, rubber "fat" belts, and body fat-suction suits. Exercise involving large muscle groups stimulates the entire body, including fat deposits.

Myth 4: Exercise causes an increase in appetite and therefore weight gain.

Fact: In a weight-lifting program, an increase in fat-free weight occurs, and there is a possible weight gain because lean muscle mass weighs more than fat. Fat-free tissue expends more energy than fat tissue. A decrease in appetite occurs with moderate exercise. A balanced nutrition plan, combined with exercise, is effective in sensible weight reduction.

Myth 5: If I stop exercising, all my muscle will turn to fat.

Fact: Exercise increases fat-free tissue. Inactivity decreases fat-free tissue and increases fat tissue. The positive health benefits gained from exercise are reversed with inactivity.

---

activity and fitness needs. Frequently, the nurse is the primary health care provider, working with patients who are experiencing health problems related to obesity, high blood lipid levels, nutritional deficiencies, or all three, requiring interventions, possibly including those in the area of physical fitness. In determining physical fitness and activity interventions, a complete assessment must be done, followed by the appropriate nursing diagnosis(es). Once this is done, the planning, implementation, and evaluation phases logically follow.

ASSESSMENTS

The assessment phase is critical to the establishment of a physical fitness plan for any patient. The assessment phase explores all the areas that have a direct bearing on the person's ability, motivation, or both to consistently follow through with the physical activity as designated. The domains described in this textbook and found to influence the attainability of physical fitness must be assessed in order to individualize the health-promotion plan for the patient. For example, some specific assessments that pertain to the biological domain may be the identification of medical conditions that affect or limit physical activity. The person's age, weight, and height, as well as body fat composition and current levels of physical activity, are also important areas to include in the assessment of the biological domain.

An assessment of the patient's mental status, levels of alertness, and motivation are crucial aspects of the psychological domain that must also be included in a thorough assessment. A person's lifestyle and cultural beliefs related to physical activities might also be part of the assessment in the sociocultural domain. Certainly religious beliefs might influence whether a person embarks on a physical fitness plan and when the actual activities will take place. The environmental domain and its influence on physical fitness have been described previously in this chapter and must, of course, be assessed. Table 16-1 identifies the specific assessments that need to be made and that may influence the physical fitness plan, according to the domains.

CRITICAL ANALYSIS OF DATA

As explained, the next step after assessment of the data and prior to developing a nursing diagnosis involves critical thinking, analysis, and synthesis of the data collected during the assessment phase. This step requires that the data be analyzed and grouped according to commonalities in order to arrive at a nursing diagnosis. For example, the analysis of the assessment data might be sorted and grouped according to commonalities related to the different domains. Collected patient data such as "positive attitude related to exercise, appropriate weigh for height, motivated to participate in exercise, and family support" might be grouped under the psychological domain. The sorting and grouping of this data obviously provide support for arriving at the positively worded health promotion-related diagnosis of *readiness for enhanced physical fitness activities.*

NURSING DIAGNOSIS

Next, the appropriate nursing diagnosis(es) must be identified. For the most part, physical fitness and activity are considered interventions rather than problem areas. With the exception of the positively worded nursing diagnosis, many of the possibly applicable nursing diagnoses do not always directly relate to physical fitness, though several may. For example, some nursing diagnoses relate to a person's mental outlook and indirectly influence a person's desire to perform physical activity. Physical

TABLE 16-1 Assessment of Domains Influencing Physical Fitness

DOMAIN	SPECIFIC ASSESSMENTS
Biological	Person's age, weight, and height
	Caloric intake, basal metabolic rate
	Problems or conditions affecting physical activity
	Medical conditions affecting exercise limitations
	Medications that might influence energy levels and heartbeat
	Respiratory conditions such as allergies
	Blood flow to extremities
	Heartbeat, respiration, and blood pressure
	Laboratory values indicative of problems associated with obesity or other diseases such as diabetes mellitus and heart: e.g., cholesterol levels, triglyceride levels, fasting blood sugar, high-/low-density lipoproteins
	Body fat composition
	Current and past level of physical fitness and activity
	Muscular strength and flexibility
Psychological	Individual's desire for fitness
	Motivation level, mental status, mood
	Person's self-perception
	Current stress levels
	Beliefs regarding benefits of physical fitness
Sociocultural	Lifestyle
	Self-confidence levels, attitude toward exercise
	Patient's social activities
	Cultural beliefs regarding physical activities
	Exercise preferences
Spiritual/religious	Patient's introspection
	Meaning of exercise and fitness for the individual
	Religious prohibition of exercise on certain days
Environmental	Lives alone
	Work environment conducive to exercise
	Environmental influences affecting ability to exercise
Technological	Patient's technological competence
	Ability to adapt to new technology

© Cengage Learning 2013

impediments, attributes, or both may also indirectly relate to physical activity and fitness nursing diagnoses.

Some nursing diagnoses might be appropriate for problems associated with physical fitness and activity. These are usually classified as activity intolerance and risk for activity intolerance (Sheila-Sparks & Taylor, 2011). Another nursing diagnosis that may fit with the area of physical fitness might be a diagnosis related to a patient's sedentary lifestyle; for example, *sedentary lifestyle related to physical deconditioning*. Other nursing diagnoses are specific to problems with mobility that may be a consequence of a poorly implemented physical fitness plan (impaired physical mobility). These diagnoses, however, do not seem to fit in as well with the area of physical fitness and activity, as does the diagnosis of activity intolerance or sedentary lifestyle.

The determination of the nursing diagnosis always reflects the actual cause for the alteration or impairment or both. For example, the nursing diagnosis may be stated as risk for activity intolerance related to the presence of circulatory or respiratory problems or activity intolerance related to immobility (Sheila-Sparks & Taylor, 2011). The domains described throughout this textbook are useful in determining the contributing cause of the alteration. Activity intolerance, for example, may be related to psychological problems such as major depression or poor self-concept. The actual cause of the alteration must be determined and is important in implementing appropriate interventions in the health-promotion plan. Table 16-2 presents select nursing diagnoses that may affect physical activity and fitness potential categorized according to domains.

TABLE 16-2 Selected Nursing Diagnoses Related to Physical Activity and Fitness Potential According to Domains

DOMAIN	NURSING DIAGNOSES
Biological	• Activity intolerance related to imbalance between oxygen supply and demand • Risk for activity intolerance related to circulatory problems • Decreased cardiac output related to altered heart contractility • Impaired physical mobility related to obesity
Psychological	• Ineffective coping related to personal vulnerability • Fatigue related to poor physical condition • Hopelessness related to lost belief in transcendent values
Sociological	• Ineffective health maintenance related to lack of resources
Cultural	• Noncompliance related to cultural values • Impaired physical mobility related to cultural beliefs regarding age-appropriate activity
Environmental	• Risk for disuse syndrome related to prescribed immobilization • Sedentary lifestyle related to deficient knowledge
Spiritual/religious	• Spiritual distress related to situational crisis • Risk for spiritual distress related to sociocultural deprivation
Technological	• Impaired wheelchair mobility related to impaired ability to operate wheelchair

Source: Sheila-Sparks-R., & Taylor, C. (2011). *Sparks and Taylor's nursing diagnosis reference manual* (8th ed.). Philadelphia: Wolters Kluwer/Lippincott Williams & Wilkins.

PLANNING

The planning phase is crucial in establishing a realistic physical fitness plan. This phase determines the proposed course of action that will ultimately lead to the patient's success in initiating and maintaining physical fitness. Goals and expected outcomes should be mutually established between the nurse and the patient. In addition to being realistic, the goals should be measurable and based on sound rationale. Realistic and measurable outcomes may include goals such as, "The patient will engage in physical exercise, such as walking, for 30 minutes three times a week," or "The patient will progressively increase current level of activity by adding five extra minutes to her physical activity routine."

The planning phase arises from the establishment of nursing diagnoses and should be in congruence with them. For example, if the cause of the lack of physical activity or activity intolerance is related to fatigue or another biological condition, then the planning phase should address the cause. Refer to Chapters 15 and 17 for information on how physical fitness is used as a strategy in planning care for individuals with nutritional and weight control problems.

IMPLEMENTATION

The implementation phase determines which interventions are more likely to resolve the problems identified and achieve expected outcomes. It is an always changing, dynamic phase that is one of the most difficult in determining a nursing process plan. Knowledge of the Health-Promotion Model is essential for establishing a plan that will lead to positive improvements in physical fitness and activity. The nurse or health care worker has to make considerable efforts to motivate the patients to effect these positive changes.

To succeed, patients must decide how they want to look and feel, not how they think someone wants them to look and feel. Nurses need to design an exercise program with a goal to achieve the maximum health benefit at the lowest risk. The program should emphasize regular physical activity and, more than likely, a change in lifestyle.

The various domains described earlier and throughout this text as influencing health promotion can be utilized in determining an appropriate plan necessary to achieve the established goals. For example, interventions related to the psychological domain may include referral for counseling if the patient is unable or unwilling to engage in physical fitness due to depression. Interventions that address the environmental domain can, likewise, be determined and may include educating the patient on appropriate clothing and gear for strenuous physical activity. Table 16-3 describes some specific physical fitness-related interventions according to the domain areas.

EVALUATION

The evaluation phase is ongoing once the actual interventions are implemented. This phase focuses on outcomes and goals and determines whether these have been met. In the event that the various interventions are not working or addressing the identified nursing diagnoses, the evaluation phase leads to a modification of the plan and reevaluation phase. An example of an evaluation and modification of the plan could be one in which the nurse determines that the patient must walk vigorously three times a week and is unaware that the patient has a painful heel spur on his right foot. The plan must be modified to include other types of exercise that will not cause physical stress on the right foot. Table 16-4 describes a nursing process plan that focuses on establishing a physical fitness program for a patient in a deconditioned status. A case study focusing on physical fitness or activity or both is included at the end of this chapter.

TABLE 16-3 Physical Fitness-Related Nursing Interventions Categorized by Domains

DOMAIN	INTERVENTIONS
Biological	Monitor patient's activity levels.
	Identify abnormal lab values and report.
	Determine plan for intensity level of activity.
	Start fitness program gradually, according to the individual's ability.
	Determine fitness program using FITT model.
	Educate patient on proper activity equipment, including appropriate attire and shoes.
	Specify importance of warm-up and cooldown exercises.
	Set up self-monitoring diary.
	Establish exercise contract.
Psychological	Refer to appropriate counseling if stress levels are high.
	Set up fitness plan utilizing small, attainable goals.
	Refer to kinesiology specialist, if necessary.
Sociocultural	Encourage involvement with formal and informal fitness groups.
	Involve significant others in the fitness plan.
	Encourage and support needed lifestyle changes.
Spiritual/religious	Encourage patient to discuss spiritual/religious needs that may be influential in setting up fitness program.
	Include specific spiritual/religious beliefs in the fitness plan.
Environmental	Include environmental conditions affecting activity and fitness plan.
	Counsel patient to be cognizant of environmental influences on exercise, e.g., excessively hot or cold temperatures, pollution levels.
	Educate the patient on the appropriate clothing to wear when exercising.
Technological	Educate patient on new exercise machinery.
	Monitor patient's use of exercise equipment.

© Cengage Learning 2013

TABLE 16-4 Nursing Process for an Inactive Adult Male

Assessment: A heavy-set, 40-year-old male; weight = 200 lb.; height = 5 ft, 9 in.; is a smoker with a sedentary lifestyle. The only daily exercise routine consists of parking his vehicle and climbing a flight of stairs to his office.

NURSING DIAGNOSIS	GOALS/OUTCOMES	INTERVENTIONS
Risk for activity intolerance, related to deconditioning	Will describe five reasons for participating in progressive physical activity. Increase current activity level as evidenced by participation in a progressive fitness program.	Educate patient on the importance of physical activity. Refer to the benefits of exercise according to the identified domain areas. In consultation with exercise expert, determine activity regimen using FITT. Set attainable goals. Determine what motivates person. Monitor activity level. Increase activity level according to patient tolerance. Educate on the appropriate clothes to wear when exercising. Encourage use of self-monitoring diary.

© Cengage Learning 2013

GETTING STARTED AND STICKING TO IT

The most difficult aspect of becoming physically fit is getting started. As explained, a person's motivation level for engaging in a physical fitness program or activity is crucial to success.

The nurse and health-promotion expert can share several helpful hints with patients that will help them build or maintain motivation. Participation in a fun exercise program reaps many healthful benefits, and nurses should encourage this behavior. Box 16-5 describes helpful training tips that you can share with your patients. Box 16-6 provides some practical tips for increasing activity.

BOX 16-5
HELPFUL TRAINING TIPS

- Take the right step—get out the front door.
- Select activities for the program based on the four components of fitness.
- Set aside time for exercising. Make it a part of your daily schedule.
- Select the proper equipment for exercising, and have it gathered in an accessible place.
- Set your goals and plan of action, and let everyone know; this helps with motivation.
- Locate a friend or group to exercise with. Quitting is more difficult if someone else depends on you.
- Don't overdo it. Listen to your body, and be gradual in progression.
- Work out in different locations and facilities.
- Keep a record of your physical activities, and monitor your progress.
- Reward yourself upon reaching a goal, no matter its size.
- Determine fitness goals; establish a plan incorporating the principles of overload, progression, and specificity; and act on the plan gradually.
- Resistance training should be rhythmical, performed at slow speed through a complete ROM, and with normal unforced breathing.

BOX 16-6
PRACTICAL TIPS FOR INCREASING PHYSICAL ACTIVITY

- Choose activities that you like.
- Make exercise fun, not exhausting.
- Join a neighborhood gym.
- Park your car as far away from where you are going as possible.
- Add variety to your routine.
- Find a convenient time and place to exercise.
- Dance to music you enjoy.
- Walk with a friend.
- Make Saturday family biking day.
- Spend an afternoon in a park with a playground.
- Register for a fun run or walk.
- Share activity time with the family.
- Make walking before or after dinner your family routine.
- If you have a toddler, use the stroller to walk briskly, or push your toddler on a swing.
- Go swimming; don't just soak up the sun.
- Work in the yard raking leaves, planting flowers, and trimming trees.

SUMMARY

Exercise and physical activity are essential to the achievement of health and wellness. Although the public in general recognizes that fitness is important to achieving a healthy lifestyle, far too many people are choosing to remain physically inactive. Physical fitness has been defined in numerous ways, and, for the most part, people think of fitness in terms of athletic performance. As a health care worker, the nurse recognizes that there are different types and levels of physical fitness. Physical fitness may be described as health-related fitness or as performance and motor-skill fitness. Not all patients will achieve motor-skill fitness; however, health-related fitness is achievable.

Cardiovascular fitness, muscular strength and endurance, flexibility, and body composition are all components that must be assessed in developing a realistic physical fitness plan. The general principles of overload, specificity, and progression must also be incorporated in a physical fitness plan. Part of the planning process must include a determination of the frequency, intensity, time, and type of training that the individual is capable of. Many feel incapable of performing any type of physical activity because they succumb to myths or fallacies related to exercise. It is the responsibility of the nurse to work through these myths to help dispel them. The Health Belief and Health-Promotion Models are conceptual frameworks that can be utilized in building a successful fitness program that patients will adhere to.

Marguerite Brown: Physical Fitness Challenges

OBJECTIVES/GOALS: Through participation in a discussion of this case study, participants will have the opportunity to:

1. Describe factors that impact a patient's ability to engage in a physical fitness program.
2. Discuss the relationship between these impacting factors and Marguerite's physical fitness status.

HEALTH-PROMOTION CONCERN, HISTORY AND PHYSICAL, PRESENT HEALTH STATUS, PAST HEALTH STATUS, FAMILY HISTORY, AND SOCIAL HISTORY

Marguerite Brown is a 68-year-old divorced Caucasian female who lives alone in her own home in a retirement park. She is new to the area and is eager to meet people in her community. She is sedentary now because she has osteoarthritis in her knees and slight emphysema. Marguerite is considered overweight at 5 ft, 4 in. tall and 165 lb. Her past medical history includes a right knee replacement approximately 6 years ago. Her right knee is painful at times, but she is able to control the inflammation with nonsteroidal anti-inflammatory medicines. She has been a smoker since she was in her early 20s and is on several medications for her chronic bronchitis, emphysema, and hypertension. She sees her nurse practitioner every 12 months for her checkups or more often if she needs to. Marguerite's family history is negative for any major illnesses. Both of Marguerite's parents lived well into their 80s and did not suffer from anything other than slight hypertension. Marguerite is eager to get involved with the activities enjoyed by her neighbors in the retirement park. Although she recognizes that she is out of shape at this point, she wants to play tennis, join a yoga program, and go dancing like the others in her retirement community.

REVIEW OF PERTINENT DOMAINS

Biological Domain

Physical exam reveals a well developed, overweight individual. She has no major structural disabilities that prevent her from exercising. She does smoke a pack of cigarettes a day, and as a result she has a chronic cough with lung congestion and some difficulty breathing. She has some mobility problems due to osteoarthritis in her right knee.

GASTROINTESTINAL: Reports no problems. She has regular bowel movements. She loves to eat fruits and vegetables and gets her fiber from them.

GENITOURINARY: Nonremarkable. Urinates frequently with no discomfort. Urine is clear, straw colored, with no foul odor. She eats a light breakfast and makes lunch and dinner for herself. She loves to bake and enjoys eating what she bakes as dessert. She drinks Coca-Cola with her lunch and dinner and caffeinated coffee with breakfast.

DIAGNOSTIC TESTING: Marguerite's blood tests are normal with the exception of an elevated cholesterol reading.

Psychological Domain

Cognitively she is alert and oriented. Loves to read the latest news and enjoys reading novels regularly. Although she is divorced, she is happy to be able to travel and enjoy her retirement.

Social Domain

Marguerite wants to meet her neighbors. She is very sociable and eager to get involved. She loves to spend time outdoors and used to engage in a physical fitness routine. She enjoys dancing and playing tennis and hopes to find people with similar interests in her retirement community.

Environmental Domain

Marguerite lives alone in a middle-class retirement park. She has adequate financial resources and is able to perform all activities of daily living without assistance. Marguerite's retirement park has a recreation room with several exercise machines.

(Continues)

CASE STUDY *(Continued)*

Technological Domain

Some of the exercise machines in the park's recreation room are brand-new and computerized. Marguerite needs to have someone show her how to use the machines. She is feeling technologically incompetent and has hesitated to exercise with the rest of her neighbors. Marguerite needs information on how to go about increasing her physical fitness so that she may resume some of the physical activities she enjoys. She also needs information on physical fitness activities and resources in her community.

QUESTIONS FOR DISCUSSION

1. What should Marguerite do initially to improve her physical fitness status?
2. What types of activities can Marguerite engage in when she is alone or at home?
3. Can any of Marguerite's physical problems or medicines affect her ability to do physical activity?

KEY CONCEPTS

1. More people are choosing to take responsibility for their own well-being by becoming physically active through health-promoting behaviors.
2. Health-related fitness includes the cardiovascular, muscular strength and endurance, flexibility, and body composition components.
3. Motor-skills–related fitness, which is associated with athletic endeavor, includes power, speed, agility, balance, and reaction time.
4. Cardiovascular fitness requires large muscle groups to work together in the form of contractions during a relatively long period of time while the cardiovascular components of the heart, lungs, and vessels make adjustments to the activity as necessary.
5. Muscular strength is the ability or capacity to exert force against resistance under maximal conditions in a single effort, whereas muscular endurance sustains a muscle contraction over an extended period of time.
6. The general principles of fitness that should be applied to a fitness program are the overload principle, the principle of progression, and the principle of specificity.
7. For exercise to be effective, the FITT model should be employed: frequency, intensity, time, and type of training.
8. The heart rate reserve is used to determine the intensity of a cardiovascular workout.
9. The essential elements of a training program include the warm-up, workout, and cooldown.
10. Understanding potential danger as well as listening to the body's various aches and pains can prevent many of the injuries that occur during exercise.
11. The RICE method is a good modality to use with muscle strains or sprains or other minor discomforts.
12. People who do not engage in physical activity often believe or adhere to myths and fallacies about exercise.
13. The Health-Promotion and Health Belief Models can be influential in helping people make choices and decisions about engaging in health-promoting behaviors.

CHAPTER REVIEW

Learning Activities

1. Calculate your threshold of training and target heart rate zone using the method described in this chapter.
2. Select either yourself or a patient; Assess the health-related components, and design a walking program as the primary form of exercise for a novice exerciser using the following suggestions. The program is only a guideline for six weeks and is not engraved in stone. It is progressive in nature and should include the essential elements of training with the FITT model.

a. Determine your goals and plan your action. For example, begin walking at a comfortable pace (conversation oriented and walking with a friend) for 12–15 minutes each session, three times per week, with a day of rest in between each session. Distance is less important than the actual time involved in walking. Continue with the following plan.

b. Week 1: Walk 15 minutes each day, 3×/week for a total of 15 minutes each day.

c. Week 2: Increase 3 minutes each day, 3×/week for a total of 18 minutes each day.

d. Week 3: Increase 3 minutes each day, 3×/week for a total of 21 minutes each day.

e. Week 4: Increase 3 minutes each day, 3×/week for a total of 24 minutes each day.

f. Week 5: Increase 3 minutes each day, 3×/week for a total of 27 minutes each day.

g. Week 6: Increase 3 minutes each day, 3× week for a total of 30 minutes each day.

This program does not have to be completed in six weeks. It is merely a guideline for a basic beginning program. If you cannot carry on a normal conversation, slow down. Use the rate of perceived exertion (RPE) to help indicate the intensity of the workout. Monitor your heart rate based on your calculations in Learning Activity 1. Record your progression, and reward yourself upon completion of your goals.

Multiple Choice

1. The *Surgeon General's Vision for a Healthy and Fit Nation* recommends that American adults exercise at least:
   a. 30 minutes per day.
   b. 45 minutes per day.
   c. 60 minutes per week.
   d. 150 minutes per week.

2. Statistics indicate that in the United States, approximately what percentage of adult individuals are overweight or obese?
   a. 25%
   b. 33%
   c. 50%
   d. 75%

3. Muscular endurance refers to which of the following?
   a. The ability of the muscle to perform or sustain a muscle contraction
   b. The capacity of a muscle to exert force against resistance
   c. The relative amount of fat in the body needed to sustain exercise
   d. The ability of a joint and muscle to move freely

4. Which of the following is a technique used for rehabilitative purposes as well as in clinical settings?
   a. Ballistic stretching
   b. Body mass indexing
   c. Flexibility stretching
   d. Proprioceptive neuromuscular facilitation

5. Which of the following is a general principle of fitness training?
   a. Principle of exercise behavior
   b. Plantar fasciitis principle
   c. Principle of specificity
   d. Strength and sprain principle

6. The target heart rate is which of the following?
   a. The level or zone that one should attain during aerobic activity
   b. The same as the resting heart rate
   c. The maximum heart rate reserve
   d. The rate of perceived exertion

7. Social determinants of health refers to:
   a. the conditions or environment under which people live.
   b. the need by all to achieve well-being.
   c. physical fitness needs.
   d. poverty levels in a rural area.

ORGANIZATIONS AND WEBSITES

American Academy of Pediatrics: Organization dedicated to the welfare of all children: **http://www.aap.org**

Fifty-Plus Lifelong Fitness: Formerly Fifty-Plus Fitness Association, a nonprofit organization whose mission is to promote an active lifestyle for older people; publishes a newsletter, distributes books and videos, and sponsors physical activity events for midlife and older adults: **http://www.nia.nih.gov/health/resources/fifty-plus-lifelong-fitness**

Medline Plus: Provides information from the National Library of Medicine and the National Institutes of Health: **http://medlineplus.gov**

Office of Disease Prevention and Health Promotion, Office of Public Health and Science, Office of the Secretary, U.S. Department of Health and Human Services: Works to strengthen the disease-prevention and health-promotion priorities of the department within the collaborative framework of the HHS agencies: **http://www.osophs.dhhs.gov**

Partnership for Prevention™: A national membership organization dedicated to building evidence of sound disease-prevention and health-promotion policies and practices and advocating their adoption by public and private sectors: **http://www.prevent.org**

Partners in Information Access for the Public Health Task Force: A collaboration of U.S. government agencies, public health organizations, and health sciences libraries focusing on health objectives: **http://phpartners.org**

To Be Physically Fit: Website emphasizing physical fitness for Cub Scouts, Boy Scouts, venturers, and leaders: **http://www.scouting.org**

REFERENCES

American Heart Association. (2011). Target heart rates. Retrieved from http://www.americanheart.org

Centers for Diesease Control and Prevention. (2011). Obesity: Halting the epidemic by making health easier: At a glance 2010. Retrieved from http://www.cdc.gov/chronicdisease/resources/publications/AAG/obesity.htm

Corbin, C., & Lindsey, R. (2007). *Fitness for Life* (5th ed.). Champaign, IL: Human Kinetic Publishers.

ExRx.net. (2011). Fitness components. Retrieved from http://www.exrx.net/ExInfo.html

Institute of Medicine of the National Academies (IOM). (2010). Dietary reference intakes for electrolytes and water. Retrieved from http://iom.edu/Activities/Nutrition/DRIElectrolytes.aspx

LeMone, P., Burke, K., & Bauldoff, G. (2011). *Medical-surgical nursing: Critical thinking in patient care* (5th ed.). Boston, MA: Pearson Education.

Mak, K., Ho, S., Lo, W., Thomas, G., McManus, A., Day, J., & Lam, T. H. (2010). Health-related physical fitness and weight status in Hong Kong adolescents. *BMC Public Health, 10,* 88.

Martyn-Nemeth, P.A., Vitale, G. A., & Cowger, D. R. (2010). A culturally focused exercise program in Hispanic adults with type 2 diabetes: A pilot study. *Diabetes Educator, 36*(2). 258–267.

Mayo Clinic. (2011). Exercise for weight loss: Calories burned in 1 hour. Retrieved from http://www.mayoclinic.com.

Pender, N. J. (1996). *Health promotion in nursing practice* (3rd ed.). Norwalk, CT: Appleton & Lange.

Pender, N. J., Murdaugh, C. L, & Parsons, M. A. (2011). *Health promotion in nursing practice* (6th). Upper Saddle River, NJ: Pearson Education.

Rosenstock, I. M. (1990). The health belief model: Exploring health behaviors through expectancies. In K. Glanz, F. M. Lewis, & B. K. Rimer (eds.), *Health behavior and health education: Theory, research, and practice*. San Francisco: Jossey-Bass.

Sheila-Sparks-R., & Taylor, C. (2011). *Sparks and Taylor's nursing diagnosis reference manual* (8th ed.). Philadelphia, PA: Wolters Kluwer/Lippincott Williams & Wilkins.

TeachPE.com. (2011). Health related fitness. Retrieved from http://www.teachpe.com/fitness/health.php

U.S. Department of Health and Human Services. (2001). The surgeon general's call to action to prevent and decrease overweight and obesity. Retrieved from http://www.surgeongeneral.gov/reportspublications.html#public

U.S. Department of Health and Human Services. (2010b). The surgeon general's vision for a healthy and fit nation 2010. U.S. public health Service. Retrieved from http://www.surgeongeneral.gov

U.S. Department of Health and Human Services. (2011a). A report of the surgeon general physical activity and health adults. The President's Council on Physical Fitness and Sports. Retrieved from http://www.fitness.gov.

U.S. Department of Health and Human Services. (2011b). Fitness fundamentals: Guidelines for personal exercise programs. The President's Council on Physical Fitness and Sports. Retrieved from http://www.fitness.gov

U.S. Department of Health and Human Services, Office of Disease Prevention and Health Promotion. (2010a). *Healthy People 2020.* Washington, DC. Retrieved, from http://www.healthypeople.gov/2020

Wilbert, C. (2010). Are Americans backing off exercise? Percentage of Americans getting regular exercise declines, survey finds. *WebMD Health & Fitness.* Retrieved from http://www.webmd.com

BIBLIOGRAPHY

Azevedo, L. F., Perlingeiro, P. S., Brum, P., Braga, A., Negrao, C., & De Matos, L. (2011). Exercise intensity optimization for men with high cardiorespiratory fitness. *Journal of Sports Sciences, 29*(6), 551–5561.

Brumitt, J. (2010). *Core assessment and training: Human kinetics with Jason Brumitt.* Champaign, IL: Human Kinetics.

Buchholz, S. W., & Kark, D. L.(2009). Physical fitness assessment of older adults in the primary care setting. *Journal of the American Academy of Nurse Practitioners, 21*(2), 101–107.

Buchholz, S. W., & Purath, J. (2007). Physical activity and physical fitness counseling patterns of adult nurse practitioners. *Journal of the American Academy of Nurse Practitioners, 19*(2), 86–92

Karper, B. (2011). Deconditioning and fibromyalgia: A pilot study. *Activities, Adaptation, and Aging, 35*(1), 55–65.

CHAPTER 17
Controlling Weight

Carolina G. Huerta, EdD, MSN, RN
Janice A. Maville, EdD, MSN, RN

KEY TERMS

balance
basal metabolic rate
body image disturbances
central obesity
desirable body weight
ideal body weight

negative energy balance
obesity
optimal body composition
overweight
positive energy balance
set-point of weight control theory

severe obesity
sleep apnea
weight control
weight cycling

OBJECTIVES

Upon completion of this chapter, the reader should be able to:

- Identify physiological, psychosocial, and economic consequences of obesity.
- Recognize obstacles encountered in weight control.
- Identify theories associated with obesity.
- Describe how the domains fundamental to health promotion influence weight.
- Describe how the biological/physiological domains influence obesity.
- Recognize the role of heredity in obesity.
- Describe environmental domain influences on obesity.
- Identify biological theories that influence weight control.
- Describe how the sociocultural domain influences weight control.
- Recognize how the nursing process may be utilized in developing a weight control health-promotion plan.
- Utilize nursing's health-promotion model in determining strategies for weight control.
- Explain ways to help promote lifestyle changes and successful weight control.

INTRODUCTION

Prosperous, highly mechanized, technologically advanced societies are continuing to be burdened with the effects of obesity among their populations. With economic growth and prosperity comes a parallel rise in obesity and obesity-related problems. Recent statistics for adults show that 34.4% of the U.S. population and 24.1% of the Canadian people are obese. In 2007–2008, the prevalence of obesity was 24.3% for Canadian men, compared to 32.2% among U.S. adult men; it was 23.9% for Canadian women, compared to 35.5% among U.S. adult women (Statistics Canada, 2011; Flegal, Carroll, Ogden, & Curtin, 2010). Rates of obesity are climbing in these countries and in industrialized countries around the world. Overweight and obesity statistics are found not only in adult populations. Obesity now affects 17% of all children and adolescents in the United States—triple the rate from just one generation ago—and 26% of those in Canada [Centers for Disease Control and Prevention [CDC], 2011a; Childhood Obesity Foundation, n.d.).

A number of health care problems can be linked to overweight and obesity. Most experts conclude that many of these problems are a result of individual lifestyle choices. Lack of activity and obesity and their consequences are correlated with increased incidence of cardiovascular diseases, diabetes mellitus, and other general problems that may be life-threatening and could also lead to immobility. Through the use of weight control health-promoting strategies, many of the health care problems that are associated with a sedentary and technologically enhanced lifestyle may be prevented.

The two previous chapters addressed the importance of nutrition and physical fitness in health promotion. This chapter focuses on the physiological, psychosocial, and economic consequences of obesity and highlights weight control

as a strategy for health promotion. The nursing process and health-promotion model is also emphasized.

CONSEQUENCES OF OBESITY

The prevalence of **obesity**, or being above ideal body weight by 20% or more, among adults living in the United States is at an all-time high. According to the National Heart, Lung, and Blood Institute (2011), it is estimated that about 68% of adults in the United States are overweight, with 75 million considered to be obese (Shields, Carroll, & Ogden, 2011). Obesity and overweight substantially increase the risk of morbidity from hypertension, dyslipidemia, Type 2 diabetes, coronary heart disease, stroke, gallbladder disease, osteoarthritis, sleep apnea and respiratory problems, and endometrial, breast, prostate, and colon cancers (CDC, 2011b). Higher body weights are also associated with increases in all-cause mortality (Shields, Carroll, & Ogden, 2011).

Americans are increasingly becoming **overweight**, defined as being above body weight by less than 20%, but the verdict is still out on whether this trend applies to clinically **severe obesity**. Severe obesity refers to being 100 lb or more (45 kg) over normal body weight (Sturm, 2003), which equates with being approximately 200%, or twice, a person's ideal body weight. Severe obesity may have different causes than overweight and creates different challenges for the health care system. Severe obesity is not that easy to explain. It is considered a complex disorder that has been linked to biochemical, physiologic, genetic, or inherited influences on weight maintenance. Other domains, such as environmental, cultural, socioeconomic, and psychological, are thought to be contributing factors associated with obesity. Box 17-1 describes one way in which obesity has been defined.

A variety of medical problems, including high blood pressure, heart problems, diabetes, sleep apnea, depression, and arthritis, have been associated with being overweight. Numerous physiological consequences are associated with obesity. Cardiovascular problems, for example, are common among obese people. High blood pressure is also associated with obesity, and it can lead to heart problems, kidney failure, and stroke as well. Severely obese people are six times more likely to develop heart disease because the heart in an obese person is required to work harder, which can lead to early development

GLOBAL HIGHLIGHTS IN HEALTH PROMOTION

Worldwide Levels of Overweight in Adults

Data for those over age 15 in over 177 nations worldwide show that the number of adults who are overweight increased from 1.454 billion in 2002 to 1.934 billion in 2010, an increase of 25% in eight years. In that same time period, the percentage of individuals age 15 or older who were overweight jumped from 23% to 38%, whereas the number of adults in the general population increased by only 11% during that time span. These changes are attributed largely to economic, cultural, and possibly genetic factors in the industrialized world. Data showed that in the 10 richest countries in the world, 75% of adults are overweight, with only 18% in the 10 poorest. Regardless of the cause, all countries experienced an increase in preventable medical problems indicative of a major global health issue for health promotion.

Source: Weil, R. H. (2011, June 14). Levels of overweight on the rise. Vital Signs, WorldWatch Institute. Retrieved from http://vitalsigns.worldwatch.org/vs-trend/levels-overweight-rise

BOX 17-1
OBESITY DEFINED

Overweight: Above ideal body weight by less than 20%

OBESITY:	
Mild	15%–30% above ideal body weight
Moderate	30%–100% above ideal body weight
Morbid	50%–100% above ideal body weight
Severe	200% or more above ideal body weight

of congestive heart failure. Severely obese people often have elevated cholesterol levels, which can also contribute to heart disease and the hardening of blood vessels. Diabetes, which frequently strikes the obese, is another risk factor for developing coronary heart disease and is 10 times more likely to develop in overweight individuals. Respiratory problems are also a consequence of obesity because the chest wall is heavier to lift than in the normal weight person. Obesity can aggravate a previously diagnosed condition, such as asthma, and may also cause **sleep apnea**, a condition that is characterized by recurrent periods of absence of breathing for 10 seconds or longer, occurring at least five times per hour (American Sleep Apnea Association, 2006).

? ASK **YOURSELF**

Psychosocial Consequences of Obesity

How many people are not employed because of their appearance? Are obese persons more likely to suffer from some form of discrimination by their employers because they are viewed as less healthy, less intelligent, weak, or lazy? Are obese persons frequently subjected to disapproving looks or comments? Because we equate being slender with power, control, beauty, happiness, goodness, and fitness, are those who are obese viewed as helpless, ugly, unhappy, and lazy?

The location of body fat appears to be of particular importance in determining risk factors. **Central obesity** is a pattern of obesity in which a high proportion of body fat is localized around the abdomen and upper body. Central obesity is associated with a higher probability of developing plasma lipid disorders, abnormalities of insulin action (insulin resistance), increased insulin production, polycystic ovary syndrome, and syndrome X (Parikh, Shashank, & Kirti. P., 2009).

In addition, obesity has important psychosocial and economic consequences. Obesity-related diseases create a huge financial burden to taxpayers as the result of increased health, life, and disability insurance premiums, as well as increased sick leave coverage. According to Finkelstein and colleagues (2009), it is identified that medical costs associated with being overweight or obese accounted for 9.1% of the total U.S. medical expenditures and were 42% higher for obese adults compared to expenses for those of normal weight. Approximately half of these costs were paid by the taxpayer through Medicare and Medicaid. As was seen in Chapter 4, the psychosocial domain also plays a significant role in promoting wellness and preventing disease. The psychosocial impact of obesity, though difficult to measure, can create major obstacles in achieving optimal health. These obstacles will greatly challenge nursing skills in caring for obese patients.

Unfortunately, there is very little information about the psychological impact that obesity may have on severely obese persons. Most studies have been limited to severely obese persons seeking treatment and therefore may not be representative of the general population. From knowledge of

SPOTLIGHT **ON**

Feeling Isolated Because of Obesity

How many times have you seen severely obese persons and either commented about their weight or heard others laugh at their size? Severely obese persons, including children, are likely to feel unattractive and even repulsive to others. Many times severely obese persons are discriminated against due to their size. They frequently cannot enjoy a simple outing such as going to the movies or even flying to a destination because they are afraid that the movie theatre seats or airline seats will not accommodate them. This may cause them humiliation or embarrassment.

the importance of the concept of person in nursing's metaparadigm, however, it is easy to recognize the importance of self-concept and self-esteem to all people. Chapter 2 describes Maslow's hierarchy of needs, which includes the need for self-esteem. This need for self-esteem also incorporates the need for approval and feelings of self-worth. It stands to reason, then, that an obese person who is the subject of disapproval by society because of an overweight condition will probably suffer from low self-esteem.

Given the magnitude and seriousness of obesity, nurses should address weight control in promoting the health of their patients. **Weight control** involves the change, acquisition, and maintenance of a desirable body weight, whereas a **desirable body weight** entails achieving a balance among adequate nutrition, proper body fat, and physical activity (Craven & Hirnle, 2007). The key word is **balance**, which implies that the total energy intake in the form of nutrient calories does not exceed the body's expenditure of energy. As discussed in Chapter 14, food intake and energy needs are met in a way that reduces the risk of disease and promotes the overall stability between the body and mind.

HEALTH PROMOTION AND WEIGHT CONTROL

Current emphasis has been placed by the U.S. government on health promotion and disease prevention. Since the late 1980s the Public Health Service of the U.S. Department of Health and Human Services (USDHHS, 2011) has set forth 22 health-promotion objectives in *Healthy People 2020*, arranged in six categories: healthier food access, health care and worksite settings, weight status, food insecurity, food and nutrition consumption, and iron deficiency. The USDHHS promotes efforts to maintain a healthy weight and emphasizes the need for regular physical activity. Over time, even a small decrease in calories eaten and a small increase in physical activity can help prevent weight gain and facilitate weight loss.

Although nurses may be viewed as pioneers addressing potential health problems and needs, the future of the

SPOTLIGHT **ON**

Food and Social Interactions

Many Americans use food as a means of social interaction. Many of our social gatherings are centered around food. Thanksgiving, for example, is a holiday that Americans seem to have set aside just for eating.

profession may hinge on nurses' ability to take an active role in guiding patients to increase self-understanding and to learn new skills that promote the adoption of sound dietary practices and increased physical exercise. Nurses practicing both in a hospital setting and outside have a unique opportunity to implement a variety of preventive interventions to assist patients in gaining control of their weight and promoting their overall health and well-being.

OBSTACLES TO WEIGHT CONTROL

Finding the necessary balance to achieve weight control is difficult for many. No theory fully explains the nature and causes of obesity. Obesity is a complex phenomenon involving the interaction of multiple factors, including genetic susceptibility, diet composition, inactivity, psychological influences, culture, and physiologic mechanisms.

Although some Americans realize that their dietary habits and inactivity are adversely affecting their health, problems resulting from existing behaviors frequently may not be manifested for decades. Adopting sound nutritional habits is a lifestyle choice. Because many of the diseases that affect individuals as they age are related to their food consumption, dietary modifications may decrease overweight and obesity-related diseases. People who are knowledgeable about the type of health problems they may acquire may be more willing to modify their diets to maximize health (Lutz & Przytulski, 2006). Educating individuals about lifestyle choices may be costly for society but is less costly than treating diseases in the long run.

Our culture and values impact our choices of foods and nutritional patterns. Ethnic identity, nationality, and even educational preparation and religion are factors that influence food choices. Some aspects of culture related to food choices are passed on from birth (Lutz & Przytulski, 2006). Other food patterns and choices are learned, and differences may exist among cultures.

Other cultural factors may also be important determinants of eating and physical activity. Within our society, certain groups may place a greater emphasis on patterns of eating and less importance on physical activity and weight control, which may predispose them toward obesity. Attitudes about specific food preferences and physical size may also contribute to obesity.

Ideal body weight is what a person should reasonably weigh as compared to height. It results from a balance between adequate nutrition, proper body fat, and physical activity. This

definition, as well as definitions for beauty and health, has changed over time. In the 1950s, the Rubenesque, or well-rounded, body was desired. The anorexic look (the thinner, the better), led by the English model Twiggy, dominated the 1960s. Today, the thinness mania is waning. Looking fit and muscular is more popular. It seems that the most realistic approach, then, is to assist people in achieving a balance between food intake and activity and to encourage them to focus on the total consumption of food rather than individual foods. Thinking of foods as either good or bad is not as important as eating a variety of foods in moderate amounts and including regular physical exercise.

Nevertheless, most Americans are inactive. Although the health benefits of physical exercise are well documented, estimates indicate only 10–20% of the adult population between the ages of 18 and 65 exercise with the intensity and frequency that would lead to positive health outcomes. Many of today's adults and, alarmingly, children lead a sedentary lifestyle.

If being fit and muscular is considered the vogue, then why are so many adults inactive? Interventions that focus on factors that influence physical activity are thought to be more useful in increasing physical activity among populations. An intervention protocol that focuses on self-efficacy, social support, perceived benefits of exercise, and perceived barriers to physical activity may result in behavioral changes (Pender, Murdaugh, & Parsons, 2010). Perhaps many adults believe they were born to be overweight and have no control over their weight. Some may accept weight gain as a normal aging process. Some may lack confidence in their ability to change. Others may think they are too out of shape, are too tired, or do not have time to exercise. The negative consequences associated with exercise, such as exercise taking too much time and causing pain and sore muscles, may be enough to stop some from trying. Also, the results from exercise—lost pounds and inches—are not immediate. Visible results take weeks of consistent effort.

Conceivably, the primary reason many Americans resist change is that they continue to search for a painless, quick fix. A number of people claim to be experts who try to appeal to our desire for immediate results. In fact, dieting and weight control have become big business. Billions of dollars are spent annually in America on weight loss. Indeed, even a quick glance at a typical magazine or book rack will probably reveal an assortment of eye-catching titles like *Weight-Loss: Tips That Work; Lose Fat Faster;* or *Lose Ten Pounds in Ten Days.* Unfortunately, there are no quick and easy fixes. In most cases, these quick fixes actually compound problems.

As might be surmised by now, the causes of obesity are not usually well understood. Some individuals have a genetic predisposition; others have neurological or hormonal disorders that contribute to obesity. Others may live a very sedentary lifestyle or lack responsibility for their health and well-being. Studies suggest that about 25–40% of individual differences in body weight and body fat depends on genetic factors. Evidence also suggests that some people are more susceptible to either weight gain or weight loss than others. Obesity and overweight are not always the result of a lack of adherence to prescribed dietary modifications. Obesity may be related not only to genetic tendencies but also to ethnicity and ethnic disparities (Black & Hawks, 2005). Although genetic tendencies for overweight and obesity are often observed in family units, obesity is more prevalent among certain ethnicities. The reasons for this are not clear, so it is necessary to consider culture in a sensitive manner when developing health-promotion approaches.

CHILDHOOD AND ADOLESCENT OBESITY

Unfortunately, obesity affects more than just adults. Obesity in children is a very serious problem that may cause health and social problems into adulthood. Obesity beginning in early childhood is likely to persist throughout the lifespan. Overweight and obese children are targets for bullying, and the destructive psychological effects can last a lifetime. Teaching healthy behaviors and promoting lifestyle changes in early childhood are important because change always becomes more difficult with age.

It is estimated that about 17.6% of adolescents (ages 12–19) and 17.0% of children (ages 6–11) are obese. Childhood obesity has doubled since 1976 and almost tripled in adolescents (American Heart Association, 2011). This increase in obesity among American youth over the past two decades is dramatic and must be addressed by health care professionals. Overweight and obesity in children is considered to be epidemic and is regarded as the most common prevalent nutritional disorder of U.S. children and adolescents, as well as one of the most common problems seen by pediatricians.

Parents may not recognize the consequences of obesity. Being overweight does not mean that the child is well nourished. Obesity can lead to many complications that are similar to those that occur in obese adults. Figure 17-1 depicts the various complications in relation to a child's body systems. Obesity can increase the risk for hypertension and heart disease. It can also lead to the bowing of legs and pain in the hip joint as a result of the excessive weight. Chances of diabetes mellitus, elevated cholesterol, and gallbladder disease also increase. Physical activity and appropriate nutrition are essential to preventing obesity. A health-promotion approach in children and adolescents should focus on proper nutrition, selection of low-fat foods, increased exercise, and reduction in sedentary activities such as watching television, playing video games, and so forth.

Childhood Obesity Complications

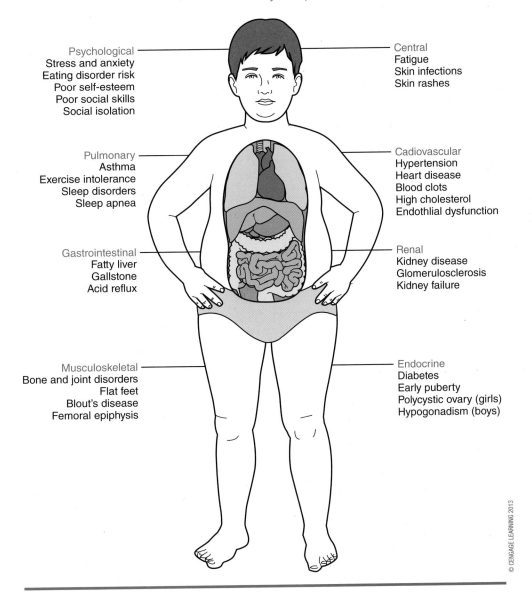

Psychological
Stress and anxiety
Eating disorder risk
Poor self-esteem
Poor social skills
Social isolation

Pulmonary
Asthma
Exercise intolerance
Sleep disorders
Sleep apnea

Gastrointestinal
Fatty liver
Gallstone
Acid reflux

Musculoskeletal
Bone and joint disorders
Flat feet
Blout's disease
Femoral epiphysis

Central
Fatigue
Skin infections
Skin rashes

Cadiovascular
Hypertension
Heart disease
Blood clots
High cholesterol
Endothlial dysfunction

Renal
Kidney disease
Glomerulosclerosis
Kidney failure

Endocrine
Diabetes
Early puberty
Polycystic ovary (girls)
Hypogonadism (boys)

© CENGAGE LEARNING 2013

FIGURE 17-1 Complications of obesity in children.

DOMAINS INFLUENCING OBESITY, WEIGHT CONTROL, AND EATING BEHAVIORS

A number of theories may help explain why some people are prone to excessive accumulation of fat and have difficulty achieving weight control. There is no common agreement, however, among experts on what causes overweight and obesity to be prevalent among some individuals. Understanding factors influencing weight control and obtaining knowledge on how some of the health-promotion domains influence obesity and weight control may help nurses intervene more appropriately. The biological, environmental, psychological, and social domains are primary focus areas when discussing and identifying intervention strategies to prevent overweight and obesity.

BIOLOGICAL DOMAIN

Are some people born to be fat? Many biological factors influence whether an individual becomes obese or remains lean throughout a lifetime. According to the theory of genetics and obesity, genetics influences human body mass and stature. The underlying assumptions of this theory are that people resemble their biological parents and that obesity and fat deposition are largely under genetic control. These assumptions, however, should not be taken to mean that a person will become obese regardless of dietary behaviors. The following are some biological factors influencing whether an individual will become obese.

Theory of Thermogenesis and Weight Control

According to the theory of thermogenesis and weight control, weight control is the result of a balance between caloric intake and energy expenditure. When there is an imbalance, that is, when the calorie (energy) intake exceeds the calories used, the surplus calories are stored as fat (Lutz & Przytulski, 2006). Because adipose tissue is the major energy storage organ, body weight increases as body fat deposits increase. Therefore, obesity results from overeating, a decreased expenditure of energy (inactivity), or a combination of both. Overeating appears to be an important factor in the cause of obesity.

The Five-Hundred Rule states that to lose one lb of body fat per week, a person must eat 500 kcal fewer per day than the body expends for seven days. To gain a pound of body fat per week, a person must eat 500 kcal more per day for 7 days than the body expends. As such, weight control is very influenced by expenditure of energy through activity. Decreased energy expenditure may cause or perpetuate obesity (Lutz & Przytulski, 2006). To maintain a balance between caloric intake and energy expenditure, dietary patterns should be adjusted. Energy expenditure depends on the **basal metabolic rate**, which is the amount of energy required to carry out involuntary activities at rest (e.g., breathing, body temperature, circulation) (Craven & Hirnle, 2007). In other words, if too much food is consumed, a person will gain weight or be in what is referred to as a positive energy balance. **Positive energy balance**, then, occurs when the amount of food consumed exceeds the energy used by the body. Conversely, if a person's energy needs exceed that produced by the food consumed, a **negative energy balance** occurs. For body weight to remain constant, food intake must equal energy needs.

Therefore, to lose weight, a person must burn more calories each day than the calories consumed.

Theory of Equilibrium Set-Point of Weight Control

Body weight usually remains relatively constant. This point is particularly significant when one considers that the amount of calories required to function varies widely from hour to hour or day to day. Some individuals who are more prone to gain weight are thought to require fewer kilocalories to perform normal body functions than do lean individuals. Some experts believe that some obese individuals have a slow metabolism. The **set-point of weight control theory** states that all individuals have a unique, stable, adult body weight that is the result of several biological factors. The obese person is thought to have a higher set-point than does the lean individual (Lutz & Przytulski, 2006). The underlying premise of this theory is analogous to setting a thermostat to maintain a constant room temperature. If you set the thermostat at 76°, an air conditioner will turn on or off to maintain room temperature at 76°. The thermostat is equivalent to the set-point for body weight, whereas the air conditioner is equivalent to either an increase or decrease in metabolic activity required to maintain this body weight (set-point). Each person has an internal set-point that is established by biological or genetic factors and controlled by the hypothalamus. Because of this set-point, starving or overfeeding is followed by a rapid return to the original weight. In other words, during times of famine, the body survives by lowering its set-point or energy requirements (basal metabolic rate).

The set-point of weight control theory may help explain excessive weight gain. When a person diets, the basal metabolic rate is lowered. The body does not know a person is dieting to lose weight on purpose. The body interprets extreme calorie deprivation as starving and tries to compensate. After the dieting has ended, the effects of the lowered metabolic rate continue. Many researchers believe that stringent dieting triggers binge eating. Eating after starving may be as natural as gasping for air after being deprived of oxygen.

Weight cycling is losing and regaining weight, as seen in yo-yo dieting. Yo-yo dieting is the repeated practice of dieting followed by the return to normal eating patterns or in some cases overeating and then dieting again. This practice is not only counterproductive but may have potentially harmful effects. Weight cycling appears to alter the set-point for weight control. When the basal metabolic rate is lowered, as with a diet-only approach, the muscle-to-fat ratio is altered. Muscle is lost and fat is gained. The energy required to sustain life is taken from muscle. Thus, the results of dieting may be a loss of muscle mass and a gain in body fat.

Although the results are inconclusive, diets very low in calories (800 cal/day or less) may lead to a protein-sparing effect. It bears mentioning that dieting results in loss of not only body fat but also of protein because lean body mass is more metabolically active and burns more kilocalories than fat tissue (Lutz & Przytulski, 2006, p. 377). The greater the amount of weight loss, the more organ and muscle mass is lost.

The long-term detrimental effects of weight cycling remain undetermined. However, the health risks associated with obesity are known. Therefore nurses should encourage those who have a history of weight cycling to gain control of their weight through lifestyle changes. Nurses can be instrumental in assisting patients with life-long commitments to better eating and activity patterns.

Theories of Biochemical Influences and Eating Behaviors

Out-of-control eating and obesity may be the consequence of a malfunctioning brain or central nervous system. According to the theory of biochemical influences and eating behaviors, obesity may occur as a result of a malfunction of the mechanisms within the brain that regulate appetite and satiety (Payne & Hahn, 2000). Although the physiology of eating is a poorly understood complex process, the limbic system and the hypothalamus have been identified as the command centers of the brain that control hunger, food intake, and satiety. The hypothalamus, located at the base of the brain, serves as a mediator between the brain and body by regulating the endocrine system (Guyton & Hall, 2006). The ventromedial hypothalamus has been identified as the satiety center, where electrical stimulation (an action potential) of this area reduces appetite. Innervation, or electrical stimulation, of the ventrolateral hypothalamus increases hunger and appears to initiate feeding behavior. Studies with mice have shown that electrical stimulation of the feeding center evokes eating behavior and destruction of the satiety center leads to hyperphasia and hypothalamic obesity (Ganong, 2005).

Many neuroscientists believe that the problem in the brain leading to obesity is a breakdown in neurotransmitter systems. Within the central nervous system, of which the hypothalamus is a part, cells (neurons) communicate with each other through chemicals called neurotransmitters. Molecules seep out of one cell and excite another cell, triggering electrical signals (action potentials). Norepinephrine (also known as noradrenaline) and serotonin are two neurotransmitters that have been implicated as playing an integral role in appetite, eating behaviors, and satiety. The norepinephrine-containing cells originate in the brainstem and ascend in a netlike manner (like electrical wiring) through the midbrain, the hypothalamus, and throughout the cerebral cortex. The serotonergic system also originates in the brainstem and projects to portions of the hypothalamus, the limbic system, the cerebral cortex, and the spinal cord (Ganong, 2005).

Anorectics (antisuppressing drugs) presented for the treatment of obesity are not intended as a cure for obesity, but rather as an adjunct treatment while an individual makes lifestyle changes in eating and activity behaviors. Currently, few appetite-suppressing drugs are being prescribed by health care providers. The question of risk versus benefit has come under great scrutiny with these drugs. After the approval in the 1940s and 1950s of a number of amphetamine and amphetamine-like compounds for the treatment of obesity, the U.S. Food and Drug Administration struggled to define the efficacy and safety of these agents. Labeling restrictions on duration of use and warnings about abuse and addiction ultimately have contributed to the reduced use of anorectics. The reduced use of prescribed anorectics continued until the mid to late 1990s, when the off-label use of fenfluramine plus phentermine (fen-phen) and the approval of dexfenfluramine gave rise to widespread, long-term use of anorectics to treat obesity. The adverse effects that have come to be associated with fenfluramine and dexfenfluramine, leading to their eventual withdrawal from the market, have given pause to regulators, health care providers, patients, and drug companies alike. Phentermine, phendimetrazine, and diethylpropion are appetite-suppressant medications approved by the Federal Drug Administration for promotion of weight loss by decreasing appetite or increasing the feeling of being full. These medications make you feel less hungry by increasing one or more brain chemicals that affect mood and appetite. Phentermine is the most commonly prescribed appetite-suppressant in the United States

(Weight Control Information Network, 2010). Xenical (orlistat) is a lipase inhibitor that has been approved for over-the-counter purchase. It is weight loss drug that reduces the body's ability to absorb dietary fat by about one-third. It does this by blocking the enzyme lipase, which is responsible for breaking down dietary fat. When fat is not broken down, the body cannot absorb it, so it is eliminated and fewer calories are taken in.

✳ NURSING **ALERT**

Anorectics as Treatment for Obesity

Sibutramine (Meridia), once determined to be an effective drug in the treatment of obesity, has been withdrawn from the U.S. market. The recall, issued October 8, 2010, was based on findings that link the drug to an increased risk of cardiac problems including heart attack and stroke.

Health care providers and patient must be aware of the risks involved in pharmacologic treatment of obesity to determine whether the benefits of weight loss are worth the health risks.

Not all theories of biological influences and the development of obesity are widely accepted. According to another theory of biochemical influences and eating behaviors, the hypothalamus does not act alone. It influences and is influenced by other systems. The endocrine system is a group of glands located throughout the body. The hypothalamus communicates with these various glands through substances known as hormones. Hormones are chemical messengers that travel through the bloodstream in order to reach the glands they control. The hypothalamus receives continuous feedback from the organs of the endocrine system, which also produce hormones. It is through this feedback system that the hypothalamus monitors the pituitary (Guyton, 2010). The thyroid has been considered an important gland in the endocrine system contributing to obesity. Thyroid hormones increase metabolic rate and energy expenditure. Conversely, a deficiency of thyroid hormone causes a decrease in metabolic rate. One could conclude that a hypometabolic state produced by deficient quantities of circulating thyroid hormones could cause obesity and that treatment with thyroid hormones would increase the resting metabolic rate and reduce hunger. However, long-term treatment of obesity with thyroid replacement has not proven successful.

ENVIRONMENTAL DOMAIN

Of course, other factors influence whether a person will become obese. The environment, for example, plays an indirect—but powerful—influence. This is good news, because nurses may assist individuals with learning how to modify their environment to promote weight control. The environment is thought to be a major determinant of overweight and obesity. Environmental influences are related to food intake and physical activity behaviors. The overabundance of food in the United States plus the aggressive marketing of foods promote high calorie consumption. It seems that the U.S. environment is intent on perpetuating and promoting overweight and obesity, whereas the U.S. government is intent on controlling overconsumption and obesity.

SPOTLIGHT **ON**

Environmental Influences and Obesity

Parents may unwittingly program their children to overeat by teaching them to associate food with comfort, love, and pleasure. Children may also learn to eat when they are not hungry. For example, Jane, a 36-year-old overweight female, enjoys cooking for her family. She prepares meals the way her mother did for her when she was a child. Her favorite meals include southern fried meats, rich gravies, cream sauces, and plenty of fresh vegetables cooked with butter or pork fat. She complains about being overweight because she can't stop overeating. She says that she not only finishes all the food on her plate but also any food that is left on her children's plates. She says that as a child she was taught to always clean her plate.

Theories of Environmental Influences

Nature versus nurture has been debated for years. As previously stated, there appears to be some genetic component to the development of obesity, but the environment clearly influences whether someone becomes obese. According to cognitive-behavioral theorists, people's early environmental experiences influence behaviors. Eating patterns stem from the home environment. If the home environment encourages overeating, then overeating becomes an ingrained pattern of behavior. In other words, people may be obese because they were taught to eat large meals high in calories and fat.

Moreover, according to cognitive-behavioral theorists, people learn to eat excess amounts of food because of the abundance of foods available to them. In other words, in prosperous environments where foods are plentiful, there is

a parallel rise in obesity. Conversely, in poorly developed environments where foods are less available, the incidence of obesity is far lower.

Recognizing that obesity is probably the result of both genetic and environmental forces interacting with each other, nurses should assist patients in modifying their environments to reduce the risk of developing obesity. Perhaps something as simple as pointing out that grocery shopping on an empty stomach may influence the selection of fat-laden, calorie-rich foods is all the information that a patient needs to modify this behavior. Patients must also recognize that learned unhealthy behaviors may be unlearned.

PSYCHOLOGICAL DOMAIN

The psychological domain influences and is influenced by weight-related lifestyle behaviors. Emotional status is very important to weight control since emotions can affect eating patterns. Some people tend to eat more when they are sad, upset, depressed, anxious, or stressed. This may create a vicious cycle because overeating may lead to overweight that can then have psychological consequences. These psychological consequences can result in overeating, thus continuing the cycle. Research has shown that psychological factors are in part responsible for obesity and overweight. These psychological factors must be addressed if weight loss is the ultimate goal. In addressing health promotion in overweight patients, the nurse must recognize that a person-centered approach that enables understanding of the psychology behind eating behaviors is essential (Annesi & Whitaker, 2009).

Understanding the psychological consequences of being overweight cannot be minimized. Traditional models of obesity treatment and management have sometimes neglected to include the psychological domain. One important psychological consequence of obesity is **body image disturbance** (Lutz

? ASK **YOURSELF**

The Environment and Overeating Habits

The next time you go grocery shopping, notice the vast amounts of foods available. Do you purchase more food than you need for energy purposes? Do most people you see grocery shopping do the same? Do the variety and abundance of foods in the grocery store influence you to buy things that you really don't need? Do you find yourself shopping more on the "outside" aisles, where fresh fruits and vegetables are displayed, or the "inside" aisles, where foods that are processed, packaged, and preserved are found?

✻ NURSING **ALERT**

Theories of Obesity and Nursing Practice

The theories of heredity influences, environmental influences, and biological influences have several important implications for nursing practice. Nurses must remember that:

1. Obesity is not necessarily the result of a person's weakness, gluttony, or lack of pride in appearance.
2. Pharmacologic approaches to the treatment of obesity are based on biological theories and have adverse consequences.
3. Although persons cannot control their genetic predisposition for obesity, people can modify behaviors to alter their set-point metabolic rate.
4. Individuals can alter their health behaviors to reduce the risk of adding pounds and extra fat deposits.

& Przytulski, 2006), which is the distorted image that a person has of himself or herself. This distorted image can lead to eating disorders such as anorexia or bulimia (see Chapter 15). Obese patients may also present with poor self-esteem, self-worth, and self-confidence. There are clear obesity-depression links in the literature, but there is no conclusive evidence as to which comes first (Sharman, 2004).

SOCIOCULTURAL DOMAIN

The sociocultural domain is also integral to a discussion about weight control. Societal expectations include having a lean and trim body. The United States seems, in particular, to be obsessed with leanness. Our society often equates attractiveness with thinness, especially in women. Societal expectations may cause those who are overweight or obese to feel unattractive and ashamed. The assumption is that overweight and obese people are gluttonous, lazy, or both. This, of course, is not true. Obese people face prejudice or discrimination at work, at school, while job hunting, and in social situations every day. Feelings of rejection, shame, or depression are common. Obesity has severe psychological consequences in all age groups. Overweight or obese children also encounter prejudice and discrimination in society. Many children are teased or receive negative comments that they remember throughout life.

Cultural expectations as well as ethnicity also influence weight control. The foods that we eat and the type of activity that we participate in may also be related to acculturation factors. There may be a lack of pressure to lose weight among certain cultures. There are also sociocultural differences in preferences and attitudes about diet, body weight, and body image. A health-promotion approach to weight control in obese and overweight patients must incorporate culturally based food preferences and reinforce healthy food choices.

Economics has also been associated with weight management. Lower-cost foods make up a greater proportion of the diet of low-income individuals in the United States. A study by the Department of Agriculture found that female recipients of food assistance had diets containing more processed foods higher in fat, consumed fewer vegetables and fruit, and were more likely to be obese. Healthy Eating Index scores are inversely associated with body weight and positively associated with education and income (Darmon & Drewnowski, 2008).

ISSUES RELATED TO WEIGHT CONTROL

Many issues are related to weight control. It seems that on a daily basis Americans are bombarded with the latest fad in weight management and control. Fads such as the Sugar Busters, Atkins, Zone, South Beach, Ornish, and Low Glycemic Index diets have been quite prevalent over the last few years. The thinking behind these diets is that some foods are worse than others in impacting weight control. These diets limit sugars and sweets (Sugar Busters), are low in carbohydrates (Atkins), include only the right carbohydrates and the right fats (South Beach), are vegetarian and low-fat (Ornish), and banish foods based on their effect on blood levels (Low Glycemic Index), to name a few. People all over the world are turning to trendy exercise routines, a myriad of fad diets, pills or supplements, and even hypnotism to battle obesity. Even restaurants are now offering weight control in the form of food choices that are part

of a particular fad diet. Lawsuits pitting people who are obese against fast-food restaurants are not unheard of. Admittedly all these efforts have made an impact, but still a number of people have had little or no success using these methods. Bariatric surgery seems to be the answer for those who are severely obese (100 lb or more over ideal weight). Bariatric surgery involves reducing the size of the stomach in order to reduce the amount of food a person consumes. The use of bariatric surgery is considered the only permanent treatment for morbid obesity (100 lb or more over healthy weight). The success rates of various surgical treatment options are as follows:

- Diet and exercise alone achieve an average long-term weight loss of only 10%.
- Gastric bypass surgery averages 60% excess weight loss after 5 years.
- LAP-BAND surgery averages 55% excess weight loss after 5 years.
- Duodenal switch surgery averages 60–80% excess weight loss (Bariatric.us, n.d.).

Obsession with weight management and control can lead people to accept the latest fad diet or bariatric surgery as the answer to weight loss. Among all the choices of fad diets and surgery, research affirms that fad diets do not work on a long-term basis and that bariatric surgery is only long-term for 50% of those undergoing the surgery. Research also reaffirms that weight loss can best be accomplished through a reduction in the number of calories consumed, coupled with an increase in exercise. Those interested in weight control and maintenance should be advised that there are no quick fixes but rather that small changes in eating behaviors will produce desired results. Eating well and exercising regularly can result in a healthier status. A change in lifestyle as opposed to diet deprivation is the best way to ensure that the pounds will stay off. Eating a variety of foods such as lean proteins, low-fat dairy items, legumes, fruit, vegetables, and whole grains is recommended for controlling or maintaining weight or both. Box 17-2 presents suggestions on maintaining or controlling weight or both.

BOX 17-2

WEIGHT CONTROL AND MAINTENANCE SUGGESTIONS

- Eat breakfast daily.
- Eat a low-calorie/low-fat diet.
- Avoid sugar-laden soft drinks.
- Surround yourself with a support system.
- Engage in physical activity.
- Eat a variety of foods from all of the food groups.
- Substitute healthy alternatives for fat-laden favorite foods.
- Avoid fast-food restaurants.
- Don't eat standing up or while watching TV.
- Eat only when you are hungry.
- Measure progress in small increments.
- Maintain a daily food and activity log.

HEALTH PROMOTION THEORY LINK

The Transtheoretical Model of Health Behavior Change and Weight Management

The Transtheoretical Model posits that health behavior change involves progress through six stages of change: precontemplation, contemplation, preparation, action, maintenance, and termination. The six stages, as applied to weight loss, are as follows:

1. *Precontemplation: The "I'm oblivious" stage*—In this stage, others may see the need, but the person is unaware or underaware that he or she has a problem with weight management and has no expressed desire to make a change.

2. *Contemplation: The "I should" stage*—Awareness that there is a problem occurs at this stage, and the person has begun to consider what can be done about it. Shortness of breath or tighter fitting clothing may be part of this awareness, and a connection with health may be realized but no action is planned.

3. *Commitment: The "I will" stage*—Greater awareness occurs at this stage, and the person becomes motivated to take action. Dislike for self and feelings of self-consciousness can be apparent.

4. *Preparation: The "I could" stage*—A decision is made to change, and options to effect the change are evaluated. Thoughts of possibilities range from realistic to unrealistic, such as using savings to pay for a personal trainer, working out for hours every day, or eating only lean frozen dinners. In essence, a battle plan is devised.

5. *Action: The "I am" stage*—In this stage, a person is physically, psychologically, and emotionally ready to make the change(s) to improve life and is committed to the in-place plan. Results toward reaching a weight loss goal are evident. Self-efficacy is increased as well as self-esteem as progress toward the weight loss is seen.

6. *Maintenance: The "I did it" stage*—Better habits have become part of the person's lifestyle. Self-confidence is higher, and the person does not want to return to the old habits that created the weight gain. Going back to them is just not an option.

Adapted from: Prochaska, J. O.., & DiClemente, C. C. The transtheoretical approach. In J. C. Norcross, & M. R. Goldfried (eds.). *Handbook of psychotherapy integration*. 2nd ed. New York: Oxford University Press; 2005. p. 147–171

THE NURSING PROCESS IN WEIGHT CONTROL

Chapter 4 covered the role of the nurse in health promotion and included the use of the nursing process in identifying the health needs of patients and in determining health-promoting strategies. Likewise, the nurse caring for an obese patient utilizes the nursing process in gathering and interpreting data essential to the formulation of a plan that includes weight control strategies. This nursing process focuses primarily on health-promotion planning and utilizes the original steps of assessment, diagnosis, planning, implementation, and evaluation.

ASSESSMENT

Assessment is the foundation for the nursing process. The purpose of doing an assessment is to develop a baseline of information in order to identify problems or potential problems that a patient may have and to plan how to assist a patient in making necessary changes to promote health. Understanding what factors may have contributed to an individual's obese state depends on the nurse's effectiveness in obtaining appropriate information. Critical to this process is the ability of the nurse to communicate with a patient in such a way that promotes a therapeutic relationship.

As described in Chapter 5, effective communication involves an awareness of communication skills and attitudes toward others. This awareness is especially important when dealing with obese patients. By developing some insight or self-awareness about negative thoughts or emotions, it may be possible to avoid acting on them. Only by taking a nonjudgmental approach to patients can nurses build therapeutic relationships. A nonjudgmental approach may best be defined as accepting patients without harsh criticism and encouraging them to express their thoughts and feelings (the individual's point of view).

In performing a nursing assessment, nurses must appreciate the difficulties someone may encounter in making needed lifestyle changes. Conceivably, the greatest obstacles to overcome may be related to some commonly held myths about how to achieve an optimal body composition. In fact, nurses may also believe some of these same myths. To do an accurate assessment and follow through with a health-promotion plan, nurses must be knowledgeable about these commonly held myths. Box 17-3 provides a listing of some commonly held myths.

The first myth listed in Box 17-3 is one of the most difficult to dispel. It is critical that nurses are knowledgeable about the normal aging process and provide appropriate information to patients. If a patient states that she has gained weight after hitting 40, remember that, although gaining weight after turning 40 years old may be common, it is not necessarily a normal process. Overeating and inactivity are more likely to account for the excess weight gain. A decline in overall physical and mental health may be more related to lifestyle than to a natural process of aging.

In the role of a health-promotion educator, the nurse is asked for advice by many people. At some point, patients, primarily female, will approach the nurse for some advice on how to get rid of that special fat called cellulite. Although the news and television media may frequently provide information on so-called fat busters and special lotions and treatment that eliminate cellulite, cellulite is not a special kind of fat. The dimpling effect is nothing more than connective tissue

---

BOX 17-3

COMMON MYTHS RELATED TO WEIGHT CONTROL

1. It is a normal part of aging for people over 40 to gain weight.
2. Cellulite is a special kind of fat.
3. The best way to gain control of weight is by dieting.
4. Gaining control over weight means avoiding certain foods.
5. The terms *low-fat* and *fat-free* mean a product is low in calories.
6. Obese people are weak and lack the willpower to resist overeating.
7. Some people were born to be fat.
8. Gaining control of weight requires large amounts of time exercising.
9. Some people are too out of shape to exercise.
10. Everyone can have a perfect body.

SPOTLIGHT **ON**

Low-Fat or Nonfat Foods and Calories

Even though some foods are labeled low-fat or fat-free, they still contain calories. Most low-fat and fat-free foods have excessive amounts of sugars. Weight control, then, involves learning to eat smaller portions of a variety of foods.

---

surrounding a layer of excess fat beneath the skin. Many advertisers who are in the business of promoting books, diets, or equipment for profit are guilty of misleading the public in that they have given ordinary fat a fancy name. Appealing to a desire to have smooth, tight, and firm thighs, they have attempted to convince the public that this type of fat, cellulite, requires special treatments, such as body wraps, rolling machines, or intense massages. Nurses can educate patients about the best approaches to reducing fat, which include balancing nutrition with physical exercise.

Thinking that dieting is the best way to control weight gain is another very difficult myth to dispel. Dieting may lead to a short-term weight loss, but chances are the weight will be regained. Unfortunately, there are no quick fixes or miracle cures. Attempting to shed pounds by dieting pits the dieter against the body's own physiology. Dieting is a negative word that probably should be deleted from our vocabularies. Nurses working with patients who are trying to control their weight must inform them that learning moderation, eating a variety of foods, and including physical exercise will lead to positive results. Nurses may also assist patients by teaching that the best way to lose weight forever is by eating the same healthy foods in reasonable amounts that they will continue to eat after they have lost weight.

One of the best ways to sabotage a weight-control program is to avoid certain foods. This way of thinking automatically sets one up for failure. For example, Jill, proud of her efforts to change her unhealthy eating habits, ordered broiled fish, dry, no oil, a tossed salad without dressing, steamed vegetables with no butter, and no dessert. Although we have increased public awareness about the importance of reducing fat intake, many like Jill have taken this message to an extreme. The food industry has capitalized on our obsession to avoid fats. No-cholesterol, no-fat, or low-fat products sell quite well. Although overloading on fats can cause weight gain and increased risks for health problems, some fat is essential for life. Fat supports the cell walls within the body. Fat enables the body to absorb, circulate, and store fat-soluble vitamins. Fat provides a layer of insulation that

is needed for the production of hormones and surrounds vital organs for protection and support. Avoiding all fats not only is unhealthy but reduces the chances of making a lifelong change in eating behaviors. The key to success is learning to balance intake with energy expenditure. The message of weight control is that it's okay to have a pizza—just not the extra-large one.

Another one of the most common myths is that low-fat and fat-free foods are also low in calories. This is a common mistake. Many believe that because foods are labeled as low-fat or fat-free, people can consume larger amounts of them. Joe sampled a bite of a low-fat coffeecake and said, "This is great! I bet I could eat the whole thing." He did. Does this sound familiar?

As explained, one of the hardest barriers to overcome is the mistaken belief that obese people are weak people who lack the willpower to resist overeating. This broad generalization is unfair, especially when even experts do not have a full understanding about the causes or physiology involved.

Although some people may be genetically susceptible to obesity, modifying lifestyles by balancing food intake with physical activity can help control weight. Exercising may require no more than 20–30 minutes, three days a week, to improve health and control weight. Generally, people find the time for the things that are important to them, and it is important to make exercise a priority. Not all people can engage in more strenuous exercise (Figure 17-2), but the myth that some individuals are too out of shape to exercise must be debunked. The truth is that people should exercise because they are out of shape. If they wait until

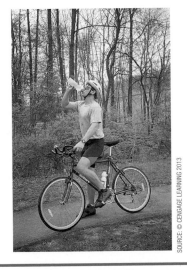

SOURCE: © CENGAGE LEARNING 2013

FIGURE 17-2 Everyone can benefit from exercise.

TABLE 17-1 Nutrition Assessment for Adults and Adolescents

Nutritional screening:

Height _____ Usual weight _____ Actual weight _____

Has your weight changed in the past six months? _____ yes _____ no

If yes, how much? _____ Describe associated events _____

_____

Have you been on a weight-reduction diet? _____ yes _____ no

Have you had any recent change in appetite? _____ yes _____ no

Do you have any food allergies? _____ yes _____ no

If yes, please list _____

Do you take any medication? _____ yes _____ no

If yes, please list prescription

If yes, is your appetite affected? How? _____

Nutritional practices:

Who plans the meals? _____

Who shops for groceries? _____

Who prepares the meals? _____

How many days a week do you eat? _____

A morning meal? _____

A lunch or midday meal? _____

An evening meal? _____

During the evening or night? _____

How many days a week do you have snacks and when do you have them? _____

In midmorning? _____

In midafternoon? _____

In the evening? _____

During the night? _____

Where do you usually eat your meal? _____

Morning_____ Mid-day_____ Evening _____

How many times a week do you usually eat away from home? _____

Describe mealtime (who is present, when, where, and atmosphere?) _____

Would you say your appetite is good? _____ Fair? _____ Poor? _____

Are you on a special diet? _____ If yes, what kind? _____ Who prescribed? _____

Are there foods you don't eat for other reasons? _____

What foods do you particularly like? _____

Dislike? _____

Do you add salt to the food at the table? _____

Do you use canned or packaged foods? _____

© Cengage Learning 2013

they are in shape, it will never happen. Exercising helps individuals get into shape. They should make the effort, begin slowly, and gradually build muscle strength and endurance.

The myth that everyone can have a perfect body is also difficult to discount. Human bodies are genetically coded, and, for some, even faithful adherence to a healthy lifestyle will not result in a perfectly sculptured body. Therefore, all people should focus on reaching an attainable or reasonable weight. A reasonable weight is one that an individual can maintain over time.

Professional nurses make an assessment that includes many facets of a patient's lifestyle, including a review of individual dietary habits. Information obtained about overall food consumption patterns can enhance one's understanding of the nature of the problem, can serve as a way of making a patient aware of individual eating behaviors, and serve as the basis for decisions regarding change. A guideline for gathering information on nutritional practices is offered in Tables 17-1 and 17-2. In addition, a 3- or 7-day food diary kept by a patient may serve

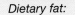

Dietary fat:

How many times per week do you eat the following (at any meals or between meals)?

Red meat, fish, and poultry   0 1 2 3 4 5 6 7 > 7

Specify: _____

Cheese _____   0 1 2 3 4 5 6 7 > 7 What kind?

Cold cuts   0 1 2 3 4 5 6 7 > 7

Eggs   0 1 2 3 4 5 6 7 > 7

Fat in cooking   0 1 2 3 4 5 6 7 > 7

Milk, dairy products   0 1 2 3 4 5 6 7 > 7

Butter or margarine   0 1 2 3 4 5 6 7 > 7

Complex carbohydrate and fiber:

How many times per week do you eat the following?

Fruit   0 1 2 3 4 5 6 7 > 7 (juices, fresh, canned?)

Vegetables   0 1 2 3 4 5 6 7 > 7 (canned, frozen, fresh?)

Bread   0 1 2 3 4 5 6 7 > 7 (whole grain, white?)

Pasta   0 1 2 3 4 5 6 7 > 7

Potatoes   0 1 2 3 4 5 6 7 > 7

Sugar consumption:

Do you use sugar in cooking? Do you buy candy, pastries, sweetened cereal?

Do you eat desserts? _____ If yes, how often? _____

Do you use sugar substitutes in packet form or in drinks? _____

Alcohol consumption:

How often do you use alcohol? _____

Caffeine:

How much coffee, tea, or cola do you drink per day? _____

Water consumption:

Do you drink water? How often during the day? _____

How much each time? _____

Economics:

Do you receive any supplementary income to purchase food items? _____

Source of nutrition information:

School, journals, magazines, friends, family members, health food stores _____

as an assessment tool to evaluate dietary status and related behaviors, as well as a patient's thoughts and feelings about eating.

Before a nurse and patient may continue to develop the next phases of the nursing process, the degree of obesity must be determined. **Optimal body composition** refers to the proper balance among body fat, muscle mass, and bone. Ideal body weight and optimal body composition are not necessarily one and the same. A person may be within an accepted range of ideal weight, as determined by height, weight, and frame charts, but have a high body fat composition. The percentage of body fat for the average male should be 15–19% and for the average female 18–22% (Lutz & Przytulski, 2006). The minimum body fat acceptable for good health is 5% for males and 12% for females. Low body fat may be found in athletes who believe that low body fat is related to athletic performance. Although the body fat percentage is increasing in the United States and Europe, a low body fat percentage is a major health problem (About.com, 2006). Although some of the body's

TABLE 17-2 Physical Activity Questionnaire for Adults and Adolescents

Please place a check by the statement that most accurately describes you.

_____ I currently do not exercise.

_____ I do not exercise but I am thinking about starting.

_____ I exercise some but not regularly.

_____ I exercise regularly.

If you marked a space indicating that you exercise, what sort of activities do you do? _____

_____

If you currently exercise, how much time per session do you spend? _____

How many days per week do you exercise? _____

Do you exercise alone or with someone else? _____

If you are considering starting an exercise program, what sort of exercises would you enjoy? _____

_____

Do you feel confident that you can participate in regular exercise? yes _____ no _____

What are some of your concerns about starting a regular exercise program? _____

_____

What are some of the benefits of regular exercise? _____

_____

What are some of the barriers to exercising? _____

_____

composition is genetic, for most of us the percentage of body fat is directly related to poor eating and exercise behaviors as well as to lifestyle. Box 17-4 demonstrates assessment methods for determining body composition.

Generally accepted and reliable techniques used to determine the ratio of body fat to lean muscle mass are hydrostatic weighing, bioelectrical impedance, densitometry, and skin fold measurements. The drawback with these techniques is that they require special equipment and charts, thus making their use impractical for the general population. Therefore, although a less reliable indicator of body fat percentage, a derivation of the Mahoney Formula may be used to determine ideal body weight (Healthy/Living Radio, 2005). The formula is as follows: For men, multiply the height in inches by 4, then subtract 128; for women, multiply the height in inches by 3.5, then subtract 108. If the skeletal frame is large (wrist size greater than 7 in. for men and 6.5 in. for women), add 10% to the total. If the skeletal frame is small (wrist size less than 7 in. for men and 6.5 in. for women), subtract 10% of the total. For example, a small-boned woman 5 ft, 6 in. tall should weigh 111 lb.

Although the Mahoney Formula has been used to measure ideal body weight for a number of years, other methods can also be used as easy methods of assessing body composition. One method to calculate ideal body weight is to add 5 lb for women and 6 lb for men for each inch over 5 ft of height to a baseline of 100 lb for women and 106 lb for men. Adjustments for frame

BOX 17-4
ASSESSMENT METHODS FOR BODY COMPOSITION

Hydrostatic (underwater) weighing:

1. Weigh patient on land.
2. Seat patient on a scale.
3. Have patient blow out air in lungs.
4. Submerge patient for about 5 seconds.
5. Record registered weight on the scale.
6. Calculate fat percentage according to formula.

Biolectrical impedence:

1. Attach electrodes to patient's right hand and right foot.
2. Record results from portable instrument.

Skinfold method:

1. Use caliper to measure skinfolds:

Female	Male
Triceps	Chest
Iliac crest	Abdomen
Midthigh	Midthigh

2. Measure each skinfold three times and average.
3. Sum the three skinfolds.
4. Calculate fat percentage according to formula.

size are made by adding or subtracting 10% from the obtained weight. For example, a small-framed woman 5 ft 6 in. tall would ideally weigh 117 lb (130 lb minus 13). After the ideal weight is calculated, the current weight divided by the ideal weight multiplied by 100 will provide the percentage of ideal body weight. A percentage of the ideal weight over 110% is considered overweight, over 119% is considered obese, and over 200% is morbidly obese (Dudek, 2006). Anything under 90% is considered malnourished. Taking the same example, if the woman weighs 139 lb, her percentage over ideal body weight is 119%. She is considered to be overweight (139 ÷ 117 × 100 = 118.8%).

Although these formulas for determining ideal body weight are limited in the information they provide, they act as a frame of reference from which to measure outcomes and may also be useful for calculating a baseline daily caloric intake.

The hip-waist circumference ratio and the body mass index (BMI) may be used to determine risks associated with fat and weight distribution (Black & Hawks, 2009). The hip measurement in millimeters (1 mm = 1/16th in.) is divided into the waist measurement in millimeters. Less than 0.90 for men and 0.80 for women is considered low risk. For example, Sue, a 35-year-old female, measured her hips and waist. She had a hip measurement of 35.5 in. (35.5 × 16 = 584 mm) and a waist measurement of 26.5 in. (424 mm). Her hip-waist circumference is 0.73 (424 ÷ 584 = 0.726 or 0.73). Therefore, she is considered low risk for the development of cardiovascular disease.

$$\frac{\text{Abdominal circumference}}{\text{Hip circumference}}$$

The BMI defines the level of fat composition according to the relationship of weight to height, independent of frame size. The BMI is an indicator of optimal weight for health and considers only weight and height. It is an indicator of risk for disease and can be used by health care providers in clinical settings. It is important to note, however, that the BMI may not be accurate in patients who have much muscle mass, such as weightlifters and body builders. A BMI of 20–25 is considered normal for those individuals who do not have large muscles. Anything over 30 is considered obesity, and any BMI over 40 is considered morbid obesity (Lutz & Przytulski, 2006).

To determine the BMI, take the weight in kilograms (weight in pounds divided by 2.2 = weight in kilograms), and divide by the height in meters squared (height in inches multiplied by 0.0254 = height in meters).

$$\frac{\text{Weight (kg)}}{\text{Height (m)}^2}$$

For example, Gloria is 5 ft 6 in. tall and weighs 122 lb. Her BMI is calculated as follows:

$$\frac{122/2.2}{(66 \times .0254)^2}$$

Gloria's BMI is 19.67. According to this value, is Gloria at risk for early death? The answer is no. She has a good fat percentage and should not be at risk for early death from obesity or obesity-related diseases.

NURSING DIAGNOSIS

As described in Chapter 4, the next step of the nursing process is the determination of a nursing diagnosis. This nursing diagnosis is formulated after objectively analyzing all of the patient's data. Since this chapter deals with weight control as a strategy for health promotion, the most likely nursing diagnosis(es) deal with nutrition, although other nursing diagnoses may also be related to weight control. For example, a person's nursing diagnosis of situational low self-esteem may also relate to the need for control of weight. However, whether a patient is trying to reduce weight or gain weight, the most likely nursing diagnosis related to weight control will be risk for imbalanced nutrition: more than body requirements related to excessive intake and sedentary activity level: less than body requirements related to inability to digest food (NANDA, 2009).

The nursing diagnosis may deal with actual identified needs or ones that could develop in the future. With that in mind, then, risk for imbalanced nutrition: more (or less) than body requirements might also be a nursing diagnosis to address.

PLANNING

Once the nursing diagnoses are determined, the plan of care is then formulated and implemented. Some basic knowledge about nutrition and physical exercise is necessary to effectively assist the patient in setting reasonable goals and selecting ways to increase the likelihood that the goals may be accomplished. The goals should be stated as realistically as possible and accomplished within a designated time frame. For example, to set a goal stating that a significantly obese individual will lose 10 lb/month may not be realistic. For that reason, the planning stage is of considerable importance and should be determined in collaboration with the patient. All goals should be stated in measurable terms in order for them to be evaluated.

Dietary guidelines for reducing chronic disease risk are recommended (see Box 17-5). These recommendations include (1) reducing fat intake to 20–35% or less of the total calories consumed daily (saturated fats should not exceed 10% of calories and cholesterol should not exceed 300 mg/day); (2) daily intake should include sufficient servings from all five food groups, as well as green and yellow vegetables and citrus fruits; (3) choosing fiber-rich fruits and vegetables; (4) selecting lean cuts of meat and maintaining protein intake at a moderate level (0.36 g of protein per pound of ideal body weight per day). These guidelines may be incorporated in the planning phase for the patient.

BOX 17-5

DIETARY TIPS TO CONFRONT THE OBESITY EPIDEMIC

- Enjoy your food, but eat less.
- Avoid oversized portions.
- Make half your plate fruits and vegetables.
- Switch to fat-free or low-fat (1%) milk.
- Compare sodium in foods like soup, bread, and frozen meals, and choose the foods with lower numbers.
- Drink water instead of sugary drinks.

Source: U.S. Department of Agriculture and Health and Human Services. (2005)., *New Dietary Guidelines to Help Americans Make Healthier Food Choices and Confront the Obesity Epidemic*, Washington, DC: U.S. Government Printing Office. Released January 31, 2011.

The most realistic nursing approach for obese patients is to encourage them to (1) focus on the total daily consumption of food rather than on individual foods; (2) avoid thinking of foods as either good or bad; and (3) balance food intake with a variety of foods in a moderate amount. Eating a variety of foods is particularly important, because varying foods provides a much greater range of nutrients. In addition, eating a variety of foods increases the probability that a change in eating behaviors can be sustained over time. Eating the same foods, as with many diets, is boring.

The total caloric intake should not be less than 1,200 cal/day for women and 1,500 cal/day for men. In addition, to either lose weight or maintain weight, most of the total caloric intake should occur early in the day. In other words, eat a light supper and avoid snacking before going to sleep.

The best way to achieve weight control is through a lifestyle change that includes balancing proper nutrition and physical exercise. The human body is not designed to be sedentary. Sitting for long periods causes fatigue and sluggishness. When less energy is expended than consumed, an imbalance is created, which results in those added pounds. Physical activity burns calories. Regular physical exercise must be included to achieve and maintain a balance between fat and lean.

Although exercising specific areas, such as doing abdominal crunches, enhances muscle tone, trying to eliminate a flabby midsection cannot be achieved by working that area alone. The body burns calories uniformly. To lose excess adipose deposits, the calories burned must exceed those consumed. Therefore, probably the best way to achieve the optimal body composition is to include a combination of aerobic (calorie burning) and isotonic (muscle toning as shown in Figure 17-3) exercises along with a proper diet (Dudek, 2006).

Nurses should recognize the difficulty most people have in changing long-standing behavioral patterns. Helping patients break goals into smaller, more achievable short-term objectives may increase their confidence that they can make lifestyle changes. Patients should establish reasonable goals to avoid becoming overwhelmed with the tremendous amount of weight they need to lose. Setting a short-term goal for losing 1–2 lb instead of focusing on the entire number of pounds to be lost can build confidence that an overall goal can be accomplished.

IMPLEMENTATION

How can nurses motivate patients to change long-standing behavioral patterns? Despite the considerable efforts directed toward motivating individuals to adopt healthy lifestyles, to date

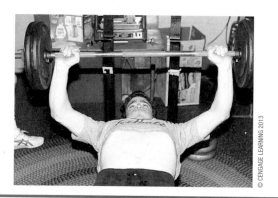

FIGURE 17-3 **Regular physical activity is essential to maintain weight.**

there has been little progress. Although researchers have sought to identify factors relevant to an individual's decision to make significant lifestyle changes, most health treatment plans continue to be determined by the nurse. Even though nurses are taught to include the patient in formulating a treatment plan and recognize the importance of gaining the patient's cooperation for therapies requiring self-care, input from the patient's point of view is seldom encouraged. Individuals are viewed as passive recipients of care. They are given directions in the guise of patient education, and it is assumed that knowledge will lead to behavioral change.

Health intervention strategies for weight control typically include diet instructions and an exercise program. Generally, limited information is given to the patient on the positive effects of weight loss and exercise or the risk associated with obesity and inactivity. Feedback about the patient's intentions to carry out the prescribed plan is often excluded.

? ASK YOURSELF

Discharge Planning

How many times have you witnessed a nurse reciting a long list of discharge plans as the patient is packing to leave the hospital? Usually the importance of social support and individual perceptions regarding the benefits and barriers to adopting a lifestyle change are omitted. How can we expect patients to comply with our treatment plans if they have not been included in devising the plan?

HEALTH-PROMOTION MODEL AND WEIGHT CONTROL

Derived from social learning theory, Pender's Health-Promotion Model may be an alternate, more effective approach because it explores human behavior in terms of a continuous interaction among cognitive, behavioral, and environmental factors (Pender, Murdaugh, & Parsons, 2010). As described in Chapter 3, the Health-Promotion Model may help explain why people adopt health-promotion behaviors when there is no perceived threat. In other words, people do not have to wait until they experience a heart attack to make a behavioral change. According to this model, behaviors may be either health protecting or health promoting. Health-protecting behaviors are aimed at stabilizing, whereas health-promoting behaviors are directed toward developing an increased level of well-being. Within this model, concepts have been categorized into cognitive-perceptual factors (individual perceptions) and modifying factors (variables affecting the probability of action).

For example, Marissa, who has a family history of heart disease, has been primarily sedentary for years. After reading a magazine article about how exercise reduces the risks of heart disease, she joined a fitness center. Even though she initially changed behaviors because of a perceived threat, she continued to attend regular exercise classes because she enjoyed the company of others, felt more energetic, and liked the way she looked.

The importance of knowledge cannot be negated; however, knowledge cannot be considered separate from other factors that have been identified as essential motivational determinants of behavioral change. In conjunction with knowledge, other factors proposed by the Health-Promotion Model as directly affecting the likelihood of behavior change are (1) individual characteristics and experiences such as those related to self-esteem, (2) perceived benefits of action, (3) perceived barriers to change, (4) perceived self-efficacy or the confidence in one's ability to make the change, and (5) interpersonal influences such as family, peers, and social support. In addition, situational factors and behavioral factors, such as previous experience with dieting and exercise, indirectly influence behavioral change (Pender, Murdaugh, & Parsons, 2010).

NURSING **ALERT**

Behavioral Change and Weight Control

Before deciding to initiate a behavioral change, such as weight control, a person must develop self-awareness. According to Bandura (1986), enduring behavioral patterns are sustained because they are cued and reinforced by aspects of the environment. Interventions for enhancing a person's decision to alter diet and to include physical exercise involve the promotion of the individual's awareness of existing and important behaviors, feelings, or attitudes. The nurse's responsibility is to raise patient awareness by asking the patient to engage in self-observation and self-judgment. Ask the patient to list the anticipated gains or losses associated with weight control or to keep a diary recording eating and activity patterns along with associated thoughts and feelings.

BEHAVIOR, ATTITUDE, AND WEIGHT CONTROL

Attending to specific behaviors, attitudes, or feelings associated with weight control enables a participant to become aware of the factors that fostered an unhealthy lifestyle. Understanding what conditions lead to certain behaviors allows for the possibility of modifying things to effect change (Sharman, 2004). For example, if pain or discomfort is associated with exercise, ways to reduce or prevent muscle soreness can be discussed. Also, if a person discovers passing a doughnut shop on the way to the office without stopping is impossible, altering the route may reduce the temptation to indulge. However, record keeping should be considered a short-term (one week) intervention strategy. The goal is not to create people who obsess about food and calories, but to increase their awareness about habits and the conditions that foster those habits, and to get a general idea about total caloric intake. In addition, it is not practical to expect patients to carry calorie counters and diaries around with them forever.

SPOTLIGHT **ON**

Self-Awareness and Implementing Change

Jonelle is very aware that exercise and weight control are important to her health. Jonelle had good intentions when she joined the gym. She dutifully pays for her membership but has made it to the gym only twice since she signed up six months ago. A friend saw her at the grocery store and asked why she had not been going to the gym. Jonelle responded that she has to be at work early each day and that she does not get home until after 6:00 p.m. every evening. How realistic is this excuse? Having knowledge of what is good for a healthy outcome does not always result in lifestyle changes.

Identifying triggers or cues to behavior is an important step toward change. To successfully modify one's habits, environmental changes to support the desired behaviors and to weaken the competing behaviors must be made (Bandura, 1986). Careful scrutiny of current situations may reveal conditions that suppress desired behavior (weight control) and facilitate unwanted behavior (overeating). Sometimes the simplest solution is to modify the environment. For example, if a patient finishes all the food on her plate because that is what she has been taught to do, she can learn either to remove herself or the plate from the dinner table when she is full. Using a smaller plate or serving smaller portions may also modify existing habits.

Another strategy that may be effective in promoting behavioral change is cognitive restructuring, that is, correcting maladaptive thinking. For example, if an individual says that there is no time to exercise, question whether the lack of time is real or artificial; most people seem to find the time for things that are most important to them.

Restructuring thoughts about dieting is also important. Many people think that eliminating one meal per day is a logical way to lose weight. For example, Carol stopped eating breakfast, because she figured she could cut approximately 3,500 cal/week, the amount needed to lose a pound. Her problem was she more than made up for this calorie reduction at supper. In addition, she found that she was feeling sluggish most of the day. She did not lose weight. Grazing or eating small amounts throughout the day is a more effective way to lose weight. Not only is this more nutritionally sound, but it also helps control appetite and increases the basal metabolic rate. Just as a car needs fuel to run, so does the human body.

SHAPING AND GUIDED PRACTICE WEIGHT CONTROL TECHNIQUES

There are no quick and easy fixes. Dieting, appetite suppressants, and surgery do not work for the long term. Shaping

RESEARCH NOTE

The Internet and Weight Management

STUDY PROBLEM/PURPOSE

The internet has become a popular source of weight management interventions, including basic information, assessment tools, and diet plans. Unfortunately, most sites inundate consumers with multitudes of products for purchase with little or no behavioral change support systems available. The purpose of this study was to provide a review of weight management components as a means for developing suggested guidelines for online program development or selection.

METHODS

Forty-two published studies associated with Internet programs focusing on weight loss were reviewed. Studies included online weight management components: tailored feedback, social support, self-monitoring, and interactive components.

FINDINGS

Five key principles are associated with Internet-based weight management programming including those that (1) recreate the human experience, (2) personalize to the individual, (3) create a dynamic experience, (4) provide a supportive environment, and (5) build on sound theory.

IMPLICATIONS

Patients as consumers of health care have a variety of resources available to them. As consultants and educators, nurses need to be aware of e-tools for patients seeking weight reduction including principles that support behavior change in order to offer guidance in the development or selection of online weight management programs.

Source: Bensley, R. J., Brusk J. J., & Rivas, J. (2010). Key principles in internet-based weight management systems. *American Journal of Health Behavior 34*(2), 206–213.

and guided practice may be useful techniques. Rather than prescribing a weight reduction diet and a rigorous exercise program, teaching patients to try putting three-quarters of their usual portions on their plate for the first week and then half of the usual portions thereafter may assist them in altering their eating habits without feeling deprived. In addition, balancing foods to reduce the fat content and increase complex carbohydrates (fruits, vegetables, and grains) and lean proteins is not only nutritionally sound but helps to suppress appetite. Moreover, thinking in terms of making a healthy lifestyle change instead of thinking in terms of dieting is more likely to lead to adherence to the suggested behavioral changes. Altering eating habits, with the goal of losing 1 or 2 lb a week, is a more reasonable approach than undertaking more drastic and potentially harmful measures such as fasting, skipping meals, fad diets, appetite suppressants, laxatives and diuretics, binge eating and purging, or surgical removal of fat. Focusing on the attempts to change rather than reaching an ideal body composition may increase the likelihood of success.

The principle of shaping behavior should also be applied to exercise. If a person has been generally inactive, exercising at the recommended intensity and duration to achieve cardiovascular fitness will be overwhelming and will increase the chance of dropping out. Beginning at a relaxed pace (low intensity) for 10 minutes or less and gradually increasing the time and intensity will increase the chance that the person will change behavioral patterns. Even taking a relaxed walk to the end of the block and back is beneficial because it is an increase over a previous activity level and alters existing behavioral patterns. In addition, patients should be encouraged to choose physical activities that they enjoy. They are much more likely to engage in regular exercise if it is fun. Moreover, patients should be encouraged not to weigh themselves daily. Because changes are not readily apparent, weighing

daily may reinforce returning to the previous, more comfortable sedentary lifestyle.

Developing a positive support system may be the most important factor influencing behavioral change. Social support consists of the social interactions that are perceived as being available and supportive or that actually provide support. Positive social support can be of an emotional nature, can be advisory or informational, can include provision of resources, can lead to personal introspection, or all of these (Pender, Murdaugh, & Parsons, 2010). Patients should be encouraged to get their social support systems such as families or friends involved in their weight control program.

EVALUATION

The last phase of the nursing process is the evaluation phase. During this phase, a nurse uses professional judgment in determining whether the goals determined in the planning phase have been achieved. Any changes that have been observed, whether it is the patient's attitudes and behaviors or in actual weight loss or gain, should be duly noted. Some of the questions that come to mind when evaluating the patient's progress include the following: Have the goals been attained? Do the goals need to be modified? What types of lifestyle changes have taken place? Is the patient watching her nutritional intake? Exercising? Has weight been gained or lost? Does the patient seem to have developed self-awareness regarding appropriate nutrition? These questions are only meant only as a guide. Naturally the important questions in the evaluation phase are those that adequately describe the changes that the patient has exhibited as a result of focusing on weight control as a means to achieve health promotion. Table 17-3 provides an example of how the nursing process may be used in promoting health in the patient requiring weight control. A case study for an individual who has weight control issues is also included at the end of this chapter.

TABLE 17-3 Nursing Process for the Sedentary Overweight Patient

Assessment

A small-framed, 35-year-old female; weight = 150 lb, height = 5 ft, 6 in.; does not engage in any exercise; average daily caloric intake = 1,690; ideal body weight = 117 lb

NURSING DIAGNOSIS(ES)	GOALS/OUTCOMES	INTERVENTIONS
Activity intolerance related to sedentary lifestyle as evidenced by deconditioned status	Will engage in physical activity by ___ (date).	Have patient list anticipated barriers to exercise and ways to overcome them. Encourage patient to keep a diary to record thoughts and feelings. Examine types of exercise to include in program. Utilize behavioral contracting to encourage some exercise commitment.
Imbalanced nutrition: More than body requirements	Will lose 1–2 lbs/week.	Have patient keep diary to record types of foods, eating patterns, thoughts, feelings. Reduce caloric intake to 1,400 cal/day. Schedule time for breakfast, lunch, and dinner. Balance meals with various food groups. Reduce serving portions. Limit weighing to 1–2 times/week. Drink 8–10 glasses of water/day.

© Cengage Learning 2013

SUMMARY

Obesity and obesity-related problems are of concern to the health care community. Consequences are associated with being overweight. A majority of the problems that patients experience are life-threatening and related to obesity states. Health-promoting strategies that focus on weight control and obesity are important to the professional nurse dealing with patients who are in need of education and support. The professional nurse recognizes the obstacles encountered in weight control and utilizes the nursing process in developing a weight control health-promotion plan.

The obese not only suffer the health consequences of their size but also are faced with psychosocial as well as economic consequences. They face public intolerance and have difficulty finding employment. Individuals who have difficulty controlling their weight must also deal with the propaganda in the advertising world that promises miracles. Finally they are often faced with the fact that obesity is generally misunderstood.

Many theories address the reasons for obesity. Some theories are related to genetics, biological, and environmental influences. Not all theories are widely accepted. For that reason, it is easy to see why individuals in need of weight control strategies receive erroneous or misleading information. The nurse's responsibility is to assist the patient with decision making related to fads, drugs, diets, and exercise. The public looks to the professional nurse for advice on how best to control weight.

The nursing process is appropriate for addressing the health needs of a patient and in devising a realistic plan to address these needs. This nursing process utilizes concepts found in the health-promotion model to determine appropriate health-promoting strategies for those in need of weight control. Use of the assessment, planning, implementation, and evaluation phases of the nursing process demonstrates an effective method for patients who need assistance in controlling their weight.

CASE STUDY

Alma Sandoval: Weight Control and Management

OBJECTIVES/GOALS: Through participation in a discussion of this case study, participants will have the opportunity to:

1. Identify appropriate weight ranges for certain individuals.
2. Describe methods that promote weight control in the morbidly obese person.
3. Discuss theories related to weight control and management.

(Continues)

HEALTH-PROMOTION CONCERN, HISTORY AND PHYSICAL, PRESENT HEALTH STATUS, PAST HEALTH STATUS, FAMILY HISTORY, AND SOCIAL HISTORY

Alma Sandoval is a 28-year-old Mexican American female with a long history of being overweight. She is a pharmaceutical representative with a professional degree and lives with a former college roommate, who works for the same pharmaceutical company. Alma is 5 ft, 7 in. tall and weighs 190 lb. Alma is active in her community and church. She enjoys cooking and entertaining friends on weekends. As part of her job, she is expected to take potential clients to dinner three to four times a week. She sees her nurse practitioner every 12 months for her gynecological checkups or more often if she needs to. Alma's parents are both alive, and her family history is negative for any major illnesses. Alma is frustrated with her yo-yo dieting patterns and wants to achieve a normal weight so that she can look better in her clothes. She needs information on what choices she has in terms of managing her weight and what resources are available to her in her community.

REVIEW OF PERTINENT DOMAINS

Biological Domain

Physical exam reveals an obese young woman with no major health complaints. She has not had any major illnesses and no surgeries, but due to her weight she is at risk for diabetes mellitus and hypertension. She denies any problems with alcohol but does enjoy having mixed drinks with her meals and includes alcoholic beverages when she entertains. She exercises only occasionally, and her favorite form of exercise is walking. She does not smoke and finds that she experiences an allergic reaction if she is around a lot of smoke.

GASTROINTESTINAL: Reports no problems in this area. She has occasional constipation due to the fact that she likes to eat highly refined foods such as baked goods and any type of breads. She loves to eat and gets very little fiber from her dietary habits.

GENITOURINARY: Nonremarkable. She reports no problems in this area. She urinates frequently with no discomfort. Urine is clear, straw colored, with no foul odor. Her dietary pattern is varied. She rarely eats breakfast because she is always in a hurry to get to work. She eats lunch and dinner out most of the time. She does not usually frequent any fast-food restaurants because she has an expense account to take her clients to fine dining establishments.

DIAGNOSTIC TESTING: All of Alma's blood tests are normal.

Psychological Domain

COGNITIVE: Cognitively, she is an intelligent individual with a degree in business administration. She is well aware that she is having a problem controlling her weight. She has gained 10 lb in the last year, which coincides with employment with her company. Her source of entertainment is watching movies and television. With the exception of feeling "fat," she seems happy most of the time. She and her roommate have a lot in common and get along very well. She recently broke up with her boyfriend, who would occasionally point out that she needed to lose weight.

Social Domain

Alma is very gregarious. She gets along well with her family and enjoys an active social life.

Environmental Domain

Part of Alma's problem is that her job requires her to entertain her clients socially. She usually takes her clients to the best dining establishments. Alma has very little self-control when it comes to food.

Cultural Domain

Alma is a Mexican American, and her mealtimes are very important, especially if she is socializing with friends and family. She tends to like high-calorie Mexican fried dishes, such as fried stuffed chili peppers and homemade flour tortillas.

Technological Domain

Alma can afford to buy some of the most sophisticated exercise and weight control equipment available. She is very technologically adept at using computerized calorie counters and exercise machines. Using sophisticated equipment does not pose any challenge for her.

QUESTIONS FOR DISCUSSION

1. Because of her long history with weight control issues, Alma is very frustrated and wants to know what her ideal weight should be. What information would you give her?
2. Alma wants to know whether she would be a good candidate for a gastric bypass. What would you tell her?
3. Alma has not been able to lose more than 30 lb every time she attempts to diet. She says that she has been able to lose the weight, but her weight always fluctuates between 160 and 162 lb. She wants you to tell her why.

KEY CONCEPTS

1. Many common health problems are linked to lifestyle.

2. Weight control health-promoting strategies can alleviate many of the health problems associated with sedentary, hedonistic, and technologically enhanced lifestyles.

3. Numerous physiological consequences are associated with obesity such as diabetes mellitus, hypertension, coronary artery disease, some forms of cancer, and lipid disorders.

4. Obesity has important psychosocial and economic consequences, such as discrimination, lowered self-esteem, and poor economic compensation.

5. Inactivity, difficulty with behavioral changes, a lack of personal responsibility, and quick-fix attitudes related are major obstacles to achieving weight control.

6. A number of theories are associated with the excessive accumulation of fat and difficulty achieving weight control. These include hereditary, environmental, and biological theories.

7. The nursing process can be utilized in formulating a plan of care for the obese patient.

8. Effective communication skills, along with recognition of commonly held myths, are essential to the performance of an adequate assessment of the patient.

9. The degree of a patient's obesity can be assessed by means of several techniques: bioelectrical impedance, hydrostatic weighing, skinfold measurements, hip-waist circumference, and body mass index.

10. Pender's Health-Promotion Model can be used effectively in planning approaches to dealing with the patient in need of weight control.

11. Self-awareness regarding specific behaviors, attitudes, or feelings associated with weight control issues enables patients to recognize unhealthy lifestyle behaviors.

CHAPTER REVIEW

Learning Activities

1. Perform and record a nutritional and activity assessment on a patient.
2. Plan a weight control program for someone who has a history of unsuccessful attempts at dieting.
3. Plan an educational program designed to assist a patient in learning the difference between dieting and weight control.

Multiple Choice

1. Central obesity refers to:
   a. an accumulation of body fat in the hips and upper thighs.
   b. a condition of being overweight or of being more than 20% over the ideal body weight.
   c. a pattern of obesity with body of fat localized around the abdomen and upper body.
   d. a plan that centers on whole-person involvement in achieving weight control.

2. Negative energy balance occurs when:

   a. a person's energy needs exceed that produced by the foods consumed.

   b. fatigue results from excess energy output.

   c. more calories are burned each day than calories consumed.

   d. the amount of food consumed exceeds the energy used by the body.

3. The five-year postintervention success rate has been shown to be highest in which one of the following?

   a. Diet and exercise

   b. Duodenal-switch surgery

   c. Gastric bypass surgery

   d. Lap band surgery

4. An overweight female, age 25, wants to lose weight. She has an average frame, is 5 ft., 6 in. tall, and weighs 160 lb. Using the Mahoney Formula, how much weight should she lose?

   a. 27 lb

   b. 37 lb

   c. 47 lb

   d. 57 lb

5. Appetite suppressants are based on which of the following theories?

   a. Biological

   b. Environmental

   c. Genetic

   d. Social learning

6. A patient would like to lose weight. She asks the nurse which diet is recommended. The nurse's best response would be which of the following?

   a. "Eating an assortment of foods in moderate amounts is the best way to lose weight."

   b. "I lost weight on the grapefruit diet. You may want to consider it."

   c. "If you increase your proteins, you will lose weight."

   d. "To lose weight, you should eliminate all fats from your diet."

7. A male patient, age 25, has a BMI of 25. He is concerned that he might be at risk for cardiovascular disease related to obesity. The nurse's best response would be which of the following?

   a. "Body mass index has no relationship to the risk of developing heart disease."

   b. "I think you should discuss your concerns with your doctor."

   c. "If you are concerned, you need to reduce your calories and exercise more."

   d. "Your BMI of 25 indicates that you are at low risk for the development of heart disease."

8. A patient is 30 lb overweight. You plan on including strategies to help your patient lose weight. Of the following, which is your highest priority?

   a. Asking the patient how she feels about making a change

   b. Consulting with a dietician

   c. Performing a history and physical

   d. Providing her with a list of foods to avoid

9. A male patient is 20 lb overweight. You are to assist him with learning how to balance his nutrition. His total caloric intake is 1,600 cal. Approximately what percentage of his total calories should come from protein?

   a. 20%

   b. 30%

   c. 40%

   d. 50%

10. A 62-year-old female patient is 5 ft, 9 in. tall and has an abdomen/waist measurement of 32.5 in. and hips 44 in. Based on these physical facts alone, what is her risk for developing cardiovascular disease?

   a. No risk

   b. High risk

   c. Low risk

   d. Super risk

ORGANIZATIONS AND WEBSITES

American Academy of Sleep Medicine: Involved in advancing sleep medicine and improving health: **http://www.aasmnet.org**

American Sleep Apnea Association: Comprehensive site that addresses problems associated with sleep apnea and offers practical health information related to this disorder: **http://www.sleepapnea.org**

American Obesity Association: Founded to combat a condition affecting more than one-quarter of all adults and one in five children; focuses on changing public policy and perceptions about obesity; the authoritative source for policy makers, media, professionals, and patients about the obesity epidemic: **http://www.obesity.org**

International Food Information Council: Communicates science-based information on food safety and nutrition to health and nutrition professionals, educators, journalists, government officials, and others providing information to consumers; supported primarily by the broad-based food, beverage, and agricultural industries: **http://www.ific.org**

REFERENCES

About.com. (2006). Body composition basics. About.com, a part of the New York Times Company. Retrieved from http://sportsmedicine.about.com

American Heart Association. (AHA). (2011). Overweight in children. Retrieved from http://www.heart.org/HEARTORG/GettingHealthy/Overweight-in-Children_UCM_304054_Article.jsp

American Sleep Apnea Association. (2006). *Enhancing the lives of those with sleep apnea.* Retrieved from http://www.sleepapnea.org

Annesi, J. J., & Whitaker, A. C. (2009). Psychological factors associated with weight loss in obese and severely obese women in a behavioral physical activity intervention. *Health Education Behavior.* DOI: 10.1177/1090198109331671;

Bandura, A. (1986). *Social foundations of thought and action: A social-cognitive theory.* Englewood Cliffs, NJ: Prentice Hall.

Bariatric.us. (n.d.). Bariatric surgery results. Retrieved from http://www.bariatric.us/

Bensley, R. J., Brusk J. J., & Rivas, J. (2010). Key principles in Internet-based weight management systems. *American Journal of Health Behavior, 34* (2), 206–213.

Black, J. M., & Hawks, J. H. (2009). *Medical-surgical nursing: Clinical management for positive outcomes* (7th ed.). St. Louis, MO: Elsevier Saunders.

Centers for Disease Control and Prevention (CDC). (2011a). Childhood overweight and obesity. Retrieved from http://www.cdc.gov/obesity/childhood/

Centers for Disease Control and Prevention (CDC). (2011b). The health effects of overweight and obesity. Retrieved from http://www.cdc.gov/healthyweight/effects/index.html

Childhood Obesity Foundation of Canada. (n.d.a.). *Welcome.* Retrieved from http://childhoodobesityfoundation.ca/

Childhood Obesity Foundation of Canada. (n.d.). *What are the complications of childhood obesity?* Retrieved from http://www.childhoodobesityfoundation.ca/complicationsOfChildhoodObesity

Colman, E. (2005). History of medicine: Anorectics on trial; A half century of federal regulation of prescription appetite suppressants. *Annals of Internal Medicine, 143*(5), 380–385

Craven, R. F., & Hirnle, C. J. (2007). *Fundamentals of nursing: Human health and function* (5th ed.). Philadelphia, PA: Lippincott Williams & Wilkins.

Darmon, N., & Drewnowski, A. (2008). Does social class predict diet quality? *American Journal of Clinical Nutrition, 87*, 1107–1117,

Dudek, S. G. (2006). *Nutrition essentials for nursing practice* (5th ed.). Philadelphia, PA: Lippincott Williams & Wilkins.

Finkelstein, E. A., Trogdon, J. G., Cohen, J. W., & Dietz, W. (2009). Annual medical spending attributable to obesity: Payer- and service-specific estimates. *Health Affairs, 28* (5), w822–w831.

Flegal, K. M., Carroll, M. D., Ogden, C. L., Curtin, L. R. (2010). Prevalence and trends in obesity among US adults, 1999–2008. *Journal of the American Medical Association, 303*(3), 235–241.

Ganong, W. F. (2005). *Review of medical physiology* (22nd ed.). New York: Lange Medical Books/McGraw-Hill.

Guyton, A. C., & Hall, J. (2010). *Textbook of medical physiology* (11th ed.). Philadelphia, PA: W. B. Saunders.

Healthy Living Radio. (2005). http://www.cooperaerobics.com/radio

Lutz, C., & Przytulski, K. (2006). *Nutrition and diet therapy.* Philadelphia: F. A. Davis.

NANDA. (2009). *Nursing diagnoses: Definitions and Classification 2009–2011-.* Indianapolis, IN: Wiley-Blackwell

National Heart, Lung, and Blood Institute, Obesity Education Initiative. (2000). The practical guide: Identification, evaluation, and treatment of overweight and obesity in adults. Retrieved from http://www.nhlbi.nih.gov/guidelines/obesity/prctgd_c.pdf

Parikh, R. M.. Shashank, J. R., Kirti. P. (2009). Index of central obesity is better than waist circumference in defining metabolic syndrome. *Metabolic Syndrome and Related Disorders, 7*(6), 525–528.

Payne, W. A., & Hahn, D. B. (2000). *Understanding your health* (6th ed.). Boston, MA: McGraw-Hill.

Pender, N. J., Murdaugh, C. L., & Parsons, M. A. (2010). *Health promotion in nursing practice* (6th ed.). NJ: Pearson Prentice Hall.

Sharman, K. (2004). From compliance to concordance: A psychological approach to weight management. *Healthcare Counseling and Psychotherapy Journal, 4* (4).

Shields, M., Carroll, M. D., & Ogden, C. L. (2011). *Adult obesity prevalence in Canada and the United States.* National Center for Health Statistics, U.S. Department of Health and Human Services. Retrieved from http://www.cdc.gov/nchs/data/databriefs/db56.pdf

Statistics Canada. (2011). Canadian Health Measures Survey: Adult obesity prevalence in Canada and the United States. Retrieved from http://www.statcan.gc.ca/daily-quotidien/110302/dq110302c-eng.htm

Sturm, R. (2003). Increases in clinically severe obesity in the United States, 1986–2000. *Archives of Internal Medicine, 163* (18), 2146–2148.

U.S. Department of Health and Human Services (USDHHS). (2011). *Healthy people 2020.* U.S. Government Printing Office. Retrieved from http://healthypeople.gov/2020/topicsobjectives2020/objectiveslist.aspx?topicId=29

Weight Control Information Network. (2010). Prescription medications for the treatment of obesity. Retrieved from Weight Control Information Network, 2010, http://win.niddk.nih.gov/publications/prescription.htm

BIBLIOGRAPHY

American Dietetic Association. (2008). Position of the American Dietetic Association: Dietary guidelines for healthy children ages 2 to 11 years. *Journal of the American Dietetic Association, 1038–1047.* DOI: 10.1016lj.jada.2008.04.005.

International Food Information Council Foundation (2003). Calories count: Balancing the energy equation. *Food Insight* (March–April), 1, 6.

National Alliance for Nutrition and Activity (NANA). (2002). *From waistline to wallet: The hidden costs of supersizing.* Retrieved from http://www.cspinet.org/w2w.pdf

U.S. Department of Agriculture Food and Nutrition Information Center. (2009). *Weight management and obesity information list January 2009.* http://www.nal.usda.gov/fnic/pubs/bibs/topics/weight/consumer.pdf

CHAPTER 18
Avoiding Tobacco, Alcohol, and Substance Abuse

DEBRA OTTO, DM, MN, WHNP-BC

KEY TERMS

addiction
comorbidity
cross-tolerance
detoxification
drug abuse
drug misuse
dual diagnosis

environmental tobacco smoke
  (ETS)
half-life
over-the-counter (OTC) drugs
polypharmacy
prescription drugs
primary prevention
protective factors

psychotropic drugs
relapse prevention
risk factors
secondary prevention
tertiary prevention
tolerance
triad diagnosis

OBJECTIVES

Upon completion of this chapter, the reader should be able to:

- Describe the impact of substance use, abuse, and addiction on society.
- Differentiate among prescription, nonprescription, and psychotropic drugs.
- Explain the mechanics of drugs.
- Differentiate among drug misuse, abuse, and addiction.
- Compare the biological and psychosocial bases of addiction.
- Describe the effects of nicotine, alcohol, and psychotropic drugs on the body and the brain.
- Relate patterns of substance abuse to gender, age, and ethnicity.
- Discuss substance abuse among nurses.
- Identify the relationship of comorbidity, mental health, physical health, and spirituality to substance abuse and addiction.
- List health-promotion and preventive strategies related to tobacco, alcohol, and other drugs.
- Describe the role that nurses have in preventing abuse of and addiction to drugs.

INTRODUCTION

Human use, abuse, and addiction to drugs in some form or another has always existed. There is reference to alcohol consumption and drunkenness in the Bible. Over 3,000 years ago, the Aztec and Toltec Indians used the hallucinogenic flowering head of the peyote cactus during sacred rites and for healing. Perhaps the first drug crisis in America happened in the sixteenth century when the Spaniards, desiring to keep the Indians subordinate, deprived the Indians of the peyote cactus because they revered the cactus more than they did the Spaniards (James, 1998). Other drugs, including cocaine and caffeine, have been part of human consumption for centuries.

The use, abuse, and/or addiction to tobacco, alcohol, and other drugs continue to play a major part in the lives of a significant number of individuals in our society, and everyone is susceptible. The short- and long-term effects of tobacco, alcohol, and other drug use and abuse present serious problems for individuals, families, and society. Indeed, 41 areas are targeted in *Healthy People 2020* that focus on the use of tobacco and alcohol and other drugs in adults and adolescence (U.S. Department of Health and Human Services [USDHHS], 2010, n.d.).

Many people, including nurses and other health care professionals, have limited knowledge regarding substance use and abuse. To promote health, nurses must have a fundamental understanding of the concepts and issues involved with substance use and abuse regardless of the practice area. Promoting healthy behavior is essential whether the nurse is involved in wellness programs aimed at enhancing health, primary prevention services that screen clients for health problems, tertiary care for clients with acute and chronic disease, or programs directly targeted to treat clients with use and abuse problems.

Why do people turn to these substances? Why do people abuse drugs and alcohol to the point of addiction? These are age-old questions and questions whose answers continue to be elusive. Finally, once a person is using or abusing or addicted, is there room for health promotion?

This chapter covers the basic health-promotion and disease-prevention strategies related to tobacco, alcohol, and other drugs. A general discussion of drug effects and the bases of addiction is presented. The effects on the body and the brain of the most commonly used substances are addressed. Health-promotion and prevention strategies are arranged according to the extent of substance use. These strategies are further addressed according to use by gender, age, ethnicity, and presence of **comorbidity** (another disability present in addition to the substance use disability). An additional area of emphasis is on nurses, their role in prevention, and their use and abuse of drugs.

SUBSTANCE USE AND ABUSE

The use and abuse of tobacco, alcohol, and other drugs have been and continue to be devastating to people of all ages in our society and in countries around the world. There are over 440,000 smoking-related deaths in the United States each year (Centers for Disease Control and Prevention, 2010). It is estimated that there are an additional 100,000 alcohol-related and 20,000 drug-related deaths each year in the United States as well, and these numbers will continue to rise (Centers for Disease Control and Prevention, 2010).

Death is not the only measure of the devastating effect of drug use and abuse. There are premature infants born with human immunodeficiency virus (HIV) or addiction to cocaine, teenagers with brain cells destroyed by inhalants, adults crippled from drunk drivers, and older adults who suffer liver and kidney damage from unknowingly combining medications. These are just a few examples of the damaging effects of drug use and abuse across the life span. Damages are suffered not only by individuals but also by families, communities, and nations.

GLOBAL HIGHLIGHTS IN HEALTH PROMOTION
Drug Use around the World

The use of illegal drugs is a worldwide phenomenon. Although varying from country to country, the three main substances are cannabis, opiates, and cocaine. Because individual countries have their own drug laws, law enforcement varies greatly from country to country. The enormous economic impact of drug production on source countries makes the elimination of this production nearly impossible. In poor nations, people usually consider the cash opportunities worth the risks. Often, the risks are decreased by corrupt governments that take huge profits from the illicit drug production. Some countries simply lack the resources or manpower to combat illicit drug growing and production. The *World Drug Report 2010* authors state that world patterns of illicit drug consumption are changing. Cocaine consumption in the United States has decreased significantly, while rising sharply in European nations. Cannabis remains the world's most widely produced and consumed illegal substance; however, its use is declining in the United States and some European markets.

Source: United Nations Office on Drugs and Crime. Retrieved from http://www.unodc.org/unodc/en/press/releases/2010/June/unodc-world-drug-report-2010-shows-shift-towards-new-drugs-and-new-markets.html

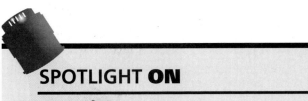

SPOTLIGHT **ON**
Drugs and You

In the broad sense, all chemicals are drugs. Many people fail to realize the extent to which they are exposed to and use drugs. Think about a typical day in your life from the time you get up until the time you go to bed. Try to remember all the products you have used. Think about the air you have breathed. Did you take any medications? How many chemicals have you applied, inhaled, absorbed, ingested, injected, or instilled?

TABLE 18-1 Routes for Drug Administration with Examples

METHOD	EXAMPLE
Inhalation	Bronchodilators, tobacco smoke, pollutants
Instillation	Eye drops, ear drops, nose drops
Oral ingestion	Tablets, capsules, teas, alcohol
Mucous membrane absorption	Mouthwashes, dental pastes/gels, suppositories
Intramuscular injection	Antibiotics, illegal drugs
Intravenous injection	Antibiotics, blood transfusions, illegal drugs
Subcutaneous injection	Insulin, immunizations
Transdermal absorption	Hormones, nicotine, deodorants, hair dye

© Cengage Learning 2013

WHAT ARE DRUGS?

To comprehend and discuss substance abuse, one must have a basic understanding of what drugs are, where they come from, and how they are categorized.

Drugs are any substance that, when taken into a living organism, may modify one or more of its functions (Venes, 2010). More simply, all drugs affect the processes of the mind or the body. They can be taken or administered in many ways, as listed in Table 18-1. Drugs are substances that can have either helpful or harmful effects on the body and may be found in ordinary household products as well as in medicines and herbal supplements.

SOURCES AND CATEGORIES OF DRUGS

Drugs are derived from four basic sources: plants, animals, minerals, and synthetic chemicals. Morphine, which is commonly used to control pain, comes from the opium poppy of the plant kingdom. People with diabetes inject insulin that is manufactured from the pancreas of animals. Aspirin comes from coal tar, a mineral. Human-made drugs, such as oral contraceptives, are produced in laboratories using various scientific techniques.

There are three major categories of drugs pertinent to the discussion of substance use and abuse: prescription, nonprescription, and psychotropic.

PRESCRIPTION DRUGS

Prescription and nonprescription drugs are taken for health problems that have been diagnosed by a physician or nurse practitioner. Taking these drugs is considered to be within social norms. **Prescription drugs** are prescribed for us by a physician or nurse practitioner and contain substances that aid in the prevention of disease, the diagnosis of a condition, or the alleviation of symptoms, or they help in the recovery from a disease or disorder. The Food and Drug Administration regulates approval for the use of these drugs in the United States. Some examples are antibiotics, narcotics, anticoagulants, diuretics, and cardiovascular drugs.

NONPRESCRIPTION DRUGS

Nonprescription drugs, or **over-the-counter (OTC) drugs**, are those that we can purchase from our pharmacy or supermarket for use when our symptoms are of a minor nature. OTC drugs, like prescription drugs, have gone through testing and approval and are regulated by the U.S. Food and Drug Administration. Examples are analgesics, cold medications, decongestants, vitamins, and sleep aids, to name a few.

PSYCHOTROPIC DRUGS

Psychotropic drugs (including alcohol) affect psychic function, behavior, or experience; they modify mental activity and are normally used to treat mental disorders. This third category of drugs consists of substances that are taken outside the social norm or for the purpose of altering feelings. Many drugs can be classified as intentionally psychotropic, but many other drugs also occasionally may produce undesired psychotropic side effects (Thomas & Taber, 2010). Several classes of psychotropic drugs are used legitimately in treatment, including antidepressants and neuroleptics (tranquilizers). Also in this category are stimulants (caffeine, amphetamines, and cocaine), opiates (morphine, heroin, and methadone), and hallucinogens (marijuana, mescaline, LSD, and PCP), which are not used in the treatment of mental disorders.

DRUG MECHANICS: HOW THEY WORK

Think for a moment about putting a key into a lock, turning the key, and opening the door. Drugs and body cells act much like the key and a lock. As shown in Figure 18-1, each cell has receptor sites, like keyholes, that are engaged to act when the appropriate key or transmitter fits into it. An example of a naturally occurring transmitter is the hormone epinephrine, which unites with heart muscle cells to stimulate their action, resulting in increased heart rate and blood pressure when more oxygen is needed. Other neurotransmitters, such as serotonin, can slow the body processes, enabling rest and sleep to occur.

Inside the brain and throughout the nervous system, nerve cells transmit information. Neurotransmitters (chemicals) work to facilitate, modify, or cancel normal transmissions between nerve cells at the synapses between the dendrites (Figure 18-2). Psychotropic drugs act directly on nerve cells and their neurotransmitters to alter brain chemistry and function. Figure 18-3 shows the brain, which is composed of the cerebrum, cerebellum, and brain stem, and the division of the cerebrum into lobes with specialized functions. Psychotropic drugs modify or affect our thoughts and feelings, with resulting

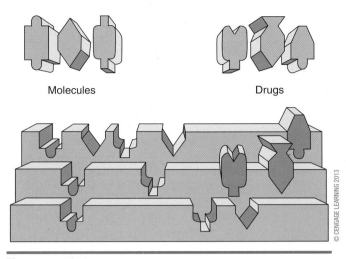

Molecules   Drugs

FIGURE 18-1 Drugs interact with the normal function of the body because they share similar structures with the body's own molecules. As a result, drugs compete for receptor sites on cells.

behaviors, by altering the natural physical processes in the body and brain (National Institute on Drug Abuse Research Report Series, 2010).

DRUG MISUSE, DRUG ABUSE, AND ADDICTION

Prescribed drugs and OTC drugs always have directions for proper use, an explanation or indications for their use, and possible side effects. Drugs are rarely harmful if taken as directed. **Drug misuse**, however, can occur if a drug is used inappropriately. Misuse generally results from a lack of understanding of the directions for use or from polypharmacy. **Polypharmacy** occurs when multiple medications are used without the knowledge of a supervising physician or nurse practitioner. Seeking health care from more than one care provider, or from self-medication with OTC drugs, or from a combination of these can result in polypharmacy.

The result of practicing polypharmacy can be disastrous. For example, decongestants decrease the effectiveness of antihypertensive medications prescribed to prevent strokes in middle-aged and older adult clients.

Drug abuse, or substance abuse, is the use of a drug or drugs inconsistent with social norms, usually to alter feelings or mood, and without relation to medical or health reasons. Drug abuse begins when a person makes a conscious decision to continue the use of the drug or substance for the altered feeling it produces.

Drug abuse leads to the deterioration of health in a biological and psychosocial sense. Biologically, the continued use of the drug eventually causes changes in the brain itself, creating a need to use the drug, not for the original altered feeling it gives but for the drug itself. Psychosocially, the drug abuser creates a perpetuation of drug use because of social rejection and guilt. **Addiction** is a gradual process that occurs when a person has developed both a biological and a psychosocial dependence on the substance of use.

BIOLOGICAL BASIS OF ADDICTION

The National Institutes of Health (2010) studies have revealed that substances tending to be abused act on brain centers to

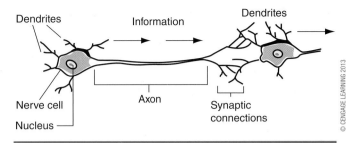

FIGURE 18-2 The transmission of information among nerve cells along the axon, dendrite, and a synapse.

activate pleasure. The more the pleasure centers are turned on, the more an individual wants to use drugs. This is why individuals use and continue to use drugs.

The more the individual uses a drug, the more the brain learns to depend on it to bring about the sensation of pleasure. By activating the pleasure circuits, many addictive drugs make the brain act as though the drug itself was as important for survival as food. The continued use of addictive drugs can actually change the way the brain works. They alter the normal process of chemical neurotransmission. This is the biological basis of addiction.

THE EFFECT OF DRUG WITHDRAWAL

The opposite effects of drugs occur after they are metabolized out of the system. This is known as a withdrawal syndrome (bounce-back effects). Symptoms tend to appear after use is discontinued (e.g., depressant drugs result in anxiety, stimulants result in depression). These negative effects perceived by the individual do not seem to be a major deterrent to use, abuse, or addiction. In fact, use, abuse, or addiction often continues in order to avoid the effects of withdrawal.

Drugs have a **half-life**, or a half-time. The half-life of a drug is half the time it takes for the drug to be metabolized out of the system. Different drugs have different half-lives. For example, the half-life of alcohol is 30 minutes, and cocaine's half-life is less than 90 minutes, whereas the half-life of a typical amphetamine is more than 4 hours, and methadone's half-life is about 15 hours. Basically, during the first part of a drug's half-life, the drug produces its perceived positive effects (altered state of consciousness). In the last half of a drug's half-life, the user perceives the negative (withdrawal) effects.

Detoxification refers to taking a drug user off the drug. Several methods accomplish detoxification. One method is slow withdrawal by using lesser amounts of the same drug. Other drugs that have a **cross-tolerance** (drugs that are similar to each other and produce similar effects on the body and brain) to the drug may be used in a similar fashion. An example is substituting the drug methadone for heroin, thereby eliminating the craving for the narcotic.

PSYCHOSOCIAL BASIS OF ADDICTION

Drugs produce emotional states that are initially perceived as pleasurable. Drugs produce these states on demand. It has been well documented that users expect a drug to produce a perception of well-being (National Institute of Mental Health, 2010). A sense of well-being and the natural highs are more difficult to obtain and happen less frequently without drug inducement. Individuals have difficulty obtaining these states naturally on demand.

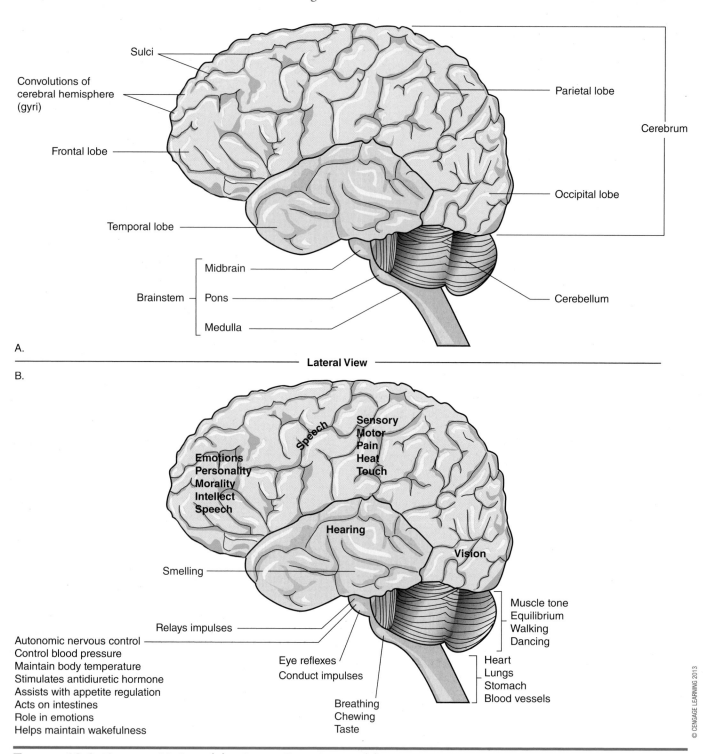

FIGURE 18-3 The parts of the brain (A) and areas of brain function (B).

Drugs of use, abuse, and addiction produce **tolerance** (Mayo Foundation for Medical Education and Research, 2010). Tolerance to a drug occurs when a progressive increase in the amount of a drug is required to obtain the desired effects. Highly tolerant individuals may be prone to more severe withdrawal symptoms. Thus increased frequency and dose of a drug to obtain the desired results produces physical and psychosocial dependence. For example, cocaine appears to produce psychological dependency because it directly stimulates the pleasure centers of the brain responsible for

the reinforcing properties of food, water, and sex (National Institute on Drug Abuse Research Report Series, 2010a).

Drugs also can condition and control behaviors by acting as positive and negative reinforcement. Positive reinforcement occurs when an event (a reinforcer) is experienced as positive (e.g., pleasurable effects of drug use) and increases the likelihood that the behavior will occur again. Negative reinforcement occurs when a negative circumstance is eliminated (e.g., drug use takes away negative feelings), and the removal of the negative circumstance increases the likelihood that the

TABLE 18-2 Psychosocial and Biological Progression of Events Leading to Addiction

PSYCHOSOCIAL PROGRESSION	BIOLOGICAL PROGRESSION
Drug/substance abuse ↓	Drug/substance abuse ↓
Social rejection ↓	Damage to brain cells and neurotransmitters in the central nervous system ↓
Development of guilt and shame ↓	Altered transmission of impulses in brain for normal thought processes ↓
Positive and negative reinforcement leading to increased substance/drug use ↓	Positive and negative reinforcement leading to increased substance/drug use ↓
Reconciliation attempts with family and friends Formation of new peer group associated with drug/substance use ↓	Poor judgment from damaged brain cells and altered neurotransmission ↓
Positive and negative reinforcement leads to increased substance/drug use ↓	Positive and negative reinforcement leads to increased substance/drug use ↓
Social withdrawal from former friends and family Greater acceptance by new peer group of substance users ↓	Physical dependence on drug to avoid effects of withdrawal Development of tolerance leading to increased amount of drug/substance use Development of intensive craving for drug/substance ↓
Psychosocial addiction	Biological addiction

behavior will reoccur. The individual then seeks the drug for reinforcement. Drugs that tend to be abused meet these criteria. This is the psychosocial basis of addiction.

Drugs bring about physical dependence by their very nature. Some produce physical dependence more rapidly than others. For example, heroin produces rapid physical dependence, whereas the physical dependence of alcohol is slower.

Physical dependence, however, is not addiction. Although tolerance and physical dependence may be necessary preconditions, addiction must also include psychosocial dependence on the drug. Individuals who are on pain medication, for example, become physically dependent and develop tolerance, but once the need for the drug is past, they are able to give it up.

Individuals who have physical and psychosocial dependence continue to use and abuse because they rely on the drug for their very psychosocial existence. Thus addiction includes physical and psychosocial dependence. Alcohol and heroin are examples of drugs that have both biological and psychosocial addiction processes. Table 18-2 summarizes the biological and psychosocial consequences of drug abuse that result in addiction. Note that all psychotropic drugs do not fit the same pattern for addiction to occur. Controversy exists, for example, regarding a clearly identifiable pattern of tolerance and withdrawal for cocaine and marijuana to be addictive in the biological sense.

COMMONLY ABUSED PSYCHOTROPIC DRUGS

Substances referred to by such names as ecstasy, yellow sunshine, snow, cotton candy, and rainbow sound exciting, comforting, and inviting. This is exactly what some drugs tend to create for their users. For some people, using these substances appears to make life better. The short- and long-term effects of using these substances, called street-drugs or recreational drugs, pose many dangers.

OPIATES

Opiates include opium, morphine, and codeine (naturally occurring opioids) and derivatives such as heroin (synthetic substances). The brain has natural opiate receptors (the endogenous opioid system) that operate to regulate mood and the sensation of pain. Opiates bind to these natural receptors and replace the natural opioids. Natural opiate receptors are distributed throughout the brain and body (National Institute on Drug Abuse Research Report Series, 2010). This is why opiates are some of the more powerful chemicals that reduce pain and alter mood.

Opiates act to depress the central nervous system while reducing the ability to experience pain. Aftereffects (withdrawals) include a heightened sensitivity to pain, chills, and sweating. Perceived positive feelings include a sense of well-being, relaxation, and feeling at one with the universe. Many individuals in treatment call heroin the cotton candy drug because it reminds them of when they were children enjoying the sweetness and softness of cotton candy. Several individuals who used or abused heroin have said, "If you ever used heroin or any of the opiates, you would not be able to stop because it makes you feel so much in harmony with the world." Signs of opiate use are an appearance of sedation, a decrease in respiratory rate, and a narrowing of the pupils, as well as needle marks and nasal discharge. Addiction to heroin is extremely rapid.

In addition to addiction, the long-term effects of heroin are very serious and life-threatening. Continued use can cause damage to all major body systems. There can be damage to the skin and veins, bacterial infections, and infections of the lining of the heart and heart valves. Arthritis can develop, as well as kidney and liver disease and other infectious diseases, including acquired immunodeficiency syndrome (AIDS) and hepatitis.

HALLUCINOGENS

Examples of the hallucinogens include lysergic acid diethylamide (LSD), cannabis santiva (marijuana), phencyclidine (PCP), mescaline, peyote, and psilacybe mushrooms. Hallucinogens include a wide variety of responses, but the main effect is to produce hallucinations. Some, such as LSD, produce hallucinations in small doses, whereas others require higher doses of the active ingredient (e.g., marijuana that includes the active ingredient of tetrahydrocannabinol).

These agents, in general, tend to produce visual, auditory, and other sensory hallucinations such as time distortion; short-term memory difficulties, mood changes, and performance problems. In addition to producing hallucinations, PCP is also a stimulant and an anesthetic. PCP is unpredictable in its effects from one batch to the next and can result in long-term cognitive deficits (e.g., schizophrenic symptomology). MDMA (also known as ecstasy) is a hallucinogen with stimulant properties. Tetrahydrocannabinol, the active ingredient in marijuana, in high doses produces hallucinations. It also has stimulant and depressant effects.

Signs of hallucinogenic use are agitation; increased heart rate; dilated pupils; and altered perceptions of time, sounds, colors, tastes, textures, and patterns. The short-term effects of hallucinogen use can be deadly because users may attempt dangerous feats and can develop severe anxiety leading to panic. Long-term effects include respiratory disease, cancer, altered reproductive abilities, and depressed immune system.

HOUSEHOLD DRUGS

Household drugs of abuse include agents such as glue, nail polish remover, correction fluid, freon, propellant in spray cans, and some paints and varnishes. Many of these drugs are found in most homes and produce an altered sense of consciousness when inhaled. Signs of household drug abuse include rash around the mouth or nose, red eyes, and headaches.

Household drugs of abuse enter the bloodstream through the lungs and then pass into the brain and nervous system to produce euphoria (Office of National Drug Control Policy, 2008a). The euphoric feeling results because the oxygen in the blood is replaced with the household drug. Parts of the brain then tend to shut down. The resultant physical problems are loss of memory functions and coordination problems.

SPOTLIGHT **ON**

Marijuana and Cancer

Some individuals believe that smoking marijuana is safe. In fact, the use of marijuana for chronic pain relief has gained some support. Studies, however, have indicated that chronic smoking of marijuana can cause cancer. These studies report that marijuana smoke is more dangerous than tobacco smoke and that a person who smokes five marijuana joints a week could be inhaling as many cancer-causing agents as a person who smokes a full pack of cigarettes in one day.

STIMULANTS

In addition to nicotine, other drugs that stimulate the nervous system include cocaine, amphetamines, and caffeine. Caffeine, although it is abused and results in addiction, is not discussed here because it does not produce an altered state of consciousness to such a degree that behavior is altered and comes to the attention of health care providers. There may be physical repercussions, but the effects of caffeine on health are inconclusive.

Stimulants increase perceptions of well-being and alertness and decrease perceptions of anxiety and fatigue. They also decrease hunger and are used to reduce weight gain. In contrast to the positive feelings, stimulants also produce negative feelings such as irritability and anxiety. Essentially they act on the body by increasing cardiac output. High doses may cause paranoia and unpredictable violent behavior. Animals will choose stimulants over sex, food, alcohol, sedatives, hallucinogens, and PCP. Human beings appear to respond the same when

SPOTLIGHT **ON**

Tobacco Addiction

Addiction to tobacco is prevalent among all age groups. Regardless of the tobacco product used, increased health risks are associated with smoking. Risk of cancer, stroke, and heart disease increases as a result of tobacco use. Inhaled tobacco smoke causes lung cancer, sinus disease, and chronic obstructive lung disease. Even pipe smokers who do not inhale the smoke are at increased risk for lung, larynx, throat, esophagus, pancreas, and colon-rectal cancer. There is also an increased risk of coronary artery disease, emphysema, chronic bronchitis, and stroke.

Source: Tobacco facts: Dangers of tobacco. Retrieved from http://www.tobacco-facts.info

given free access to all of these stimulants. Stimulants activate the dopaminergic pathways (dopamine is a neurotransmitter), but the neurochemical mechanisms responsible are not clear (Office of National Drug Control Policy, 2008a).

TOBACCO USE AND ADDICTION

Tobacco is an ancient plant that has created many modern problems. Before Columbus set foot in America, only the American Indians knew tobacco and thought it to be a way to connect with the gods. To these ancient Indians, tobacco was the most precious of possessions. The rest of the world was introduced to tobacco only after the Spanish brought it back to Europe in the fifteenth century. And the detriments of tobacco use have been known or suspected for most of the next 400 years.

Tobacco comes in several forms. The two forms most widely used are those that can be inhaled, such as in cigarettes and cigars, and those that may be chewed, as in snuff and chewing tobacco (spit tobacco). The cigarette industry spends billions of dollars on advertising and promotions every year, especially to young people. Children, referred to by cigarette marketing researchers as "consumers in training," are special targets of marketing (Centers for Disease Control and Prevention, 2010).

Addiction to nicotine in tobacco is, by far, the most prevalent, costly, and deadly of all substance abuse addictions. Death from smoking is the most preventable cause of death and disease in our society. It is estimated that each year more than 443,000 deaths in the United States, or one out of every five, are the result of tobacco use. About half of these deaths occur in smokers between the ages of 35 and 69 (American Cancer Society, 2010; American Cancer Society, 2011a). In addition to the tragedy of death are the numerous diseases and conditions (listed in Box 18-1) that produce untold suffering.

ENVIRONMENTAL TOBACCO SMOKE

Even those who don't use tobacco in any form are at risk for exposure to **environmental tobacco smoke (ETS)**. Also

---

BOX 18-1

CONDITIONS LINKED TO CIGARETTE SMOKING

Lung cancer	Atherosclerotic peripheral vascular disease
Laryngeal cancer	
Oral cancer	Gastric ulcers
Esophageal cancer	Fetal growth retardation
Bladder cancer	
Cervical cancer	Low-birth-weight babies
Stroke	
Coronary heart disease	Sudden infant death syndrome (SIDS) or crib death
Chronic bronchitis	
Chronic obstructive pulmonary disease	Early menopause

Source: Adapted from American Cancer Society. (2011b). Learn about cancer: Cigarette Smoking. Retrieved from http://www.cancer.org/Cancer/CancerCauses/TobaccoCancer/CigaretteSmoking/cigarette-smoking-who-and-how-affects-health

---

BOX 18-2

CHILDREN AND HEALTH RISKS FROM ETS

Conditions that have been linked to exposure of children to ETS:

Pneumonia	Upper respiratory infections
Bronchitis	
Asthma	Sinus infections
Influenza	Pharyngitis
Ear infections	Eye irritation
	SIDS or crib death

---

known as involuntary, sidestream, or secondhand smoke, ETS is known to be detrimental to smokers and nonsmokers of all ages. Each year about 3,400 nonsmoking adults die of lung cancer directly attributed to ETS. In addition, an estimated 46,000 deaths from heart disease are attributed to ETS (American Cancer Society, (2011a, p. 37). Box 18-2 lists the many health risks for children exposed to secondhand smoke.

NICOTINE

The active ingredient in tobacco is nicotine, although the tars, gases, and chemicals contained in the cigarette smoke also cause damage to the body (National Institute on Drug Abuse Research Report Series, 2010). Over 5,000 chemicals have been identified in tobacco smoke, 43 of which are known carcinogens (National Institute on Drug Abuse Research Report Series, 2010). Hundreds of the other chemicals are poisonous and cause mutation or cellular changes in body cells. A partial listing of these chemicals and where they are commonly found other than in tobacco smoke is in Table 18-3. Although most physical problems attributed to tobacco use (e.g., heart attacks, strokes, and emphysema) are diagnosed many years after exposure, even short-term tobacco use may be harmful.

Nicotine, which is both a stimulant and a sedative, reaches the brain in about 8 seconds when inhaled. It activates the area in the brain that initiates a feeling of pleasure. The nicotine in

---

TABLE 18-3 Harmful Chemicals in Tobacco Smoke and Where They Are Commonly Found

CHEMICAL	COMMONLY FOUND IN
Acetone	Nail polish
Acetic acid	Vinegar
Ammonia	Floor/toilet cleaner
Arsenic	Rat poison
Butane	Cigarette lighter fluid
Cadmium	Rechargeable batteries
Formaldehyde	Embalming fluid
Methanol	Rocket fuel
Napthalene	Mothballs
Stearic acid	Candle wax

© Cengage Learning 2013

RESEARCH

NOTE

Harmful Effects of Environmental Tobacco Smoke (ETS)

STUDY PROBLEM/PURPOSE

The effects of maternal cigarette smoking during pregnancy are well documented and include spontaneous abortion, placental abruption, growth restriction, preterm rupture of membranes, preterm birth, miscarriage and stillbirth, resulting in increased perinatal morbidity and mortality. Longer-term adverse effects include higher rates of attention deficit hyperactivity disorder, asthma, adverse effects on the immune system and possibly childhood cancers. The purpose of this study was to evaluate the effects of environmental tobacco smoke (ETS) on perinatal outcomes.

METHODS

In this retrospective cohort study, non smoking women with a singleton gestation who delivered 1 April 2001–31 March 2009 and self-reported exposure to ETS were compared with those who reported no exposure. Univariate analyses and multivariate linear and logistic regression analyses (adjusting for maternal age, parity, partnered status, work status, level of education, body mass index, alcohol use, illicit drug use and gestational age) were performed and odds ratios(OR; or adjusted differences) with 95% confidence intervals were calculated. Main outcome measures included: Birth weight, birth length, head circumference and stillbirth. Secondary outcomes included gestational age at delivery, preterm birth <37 and <34 weeks of gestation, premature rupture of membranes, Apgar score, endotracheal intubation for resuscitation, neonatal intensive care unit admission, congenital anomalies, respiratory distress syndrome, intraventricular hemorrhage, neonatal bacterial sepsis, jaundice and neonatal metabolic abnormalities.

FINDINGS

A total of 11,852 women were included in the study. Of those women: 1202(11.1%) exposed to ETS and 10,650 (89.9%) not exposed. Exposure to ETS was an independent risk factor for lower mean birth weight (−53.7 g, 95% CI −98.4 to −8.9 g), smaller head circumference (−0.24 cm, 95% CI −0.39 to −0.08 cm), shorter birth length (−0.29 cm, 95% CI −0.51 to −0.07 cm), stillbirth (OR 3.35, 95% CI 1.16–9.72, $P = 0.026$), and trends towards preterm birth <34 weeks (OR 1.87, 95% CI 1.00–3.53, $P = 0.05$) and neonatal sepsis (OR 2.96, 95% CI 0.99–8.86).:

IMPLICATIONS

The exposure of nonsmoking pregnant women to ETS is associated with a number of adverse perinatal outcomes including lower birth weight, smaller head circumference and stillbirth, as well as premature rupture of membranes and shorter birth length. This information is important for women who anticipate pregnancy, their families and health care providers. The results of this study reinforce the continued need for increased public policy and education on prevention of exposure to ETS .:

Source: Crane, J,. Keough, M., Murphy, P., Burrage, L., & Hutchens, D. (2011). Effects of environmental tobacco smoke on perinatal outcomes: A retrospective cohort study. *British Journal of Obstetrics and Gynaecology,118*(7), 865–871.).

chewed or inhaled tobacco is an addictive and mood-altering drug. In fact, as Box 18-3 shows, nicotine is as addictive as cocaine and heroin.

Throughout the day, tobacco users maintain a predictable nicotine blood level. They usually have an initial intake of nicotine soon after awakening because the body has depleted its supply of nicotine. Most users of tobacco cannot choose to use one day and not the next.

ALCOHOL USE AND ADDICTION

Alcohol (also known as ethanol) is a well-known depressant drug whose effects have been widely studied. Alcohol is considered to be a legal drug and is readily available to adults, illegally obtained by adolescents, and often left unchecked to be misused by children. In small and moderate amounts, alcohol consumption can be associated with benefits, such as protection against heart disease and maintenance of bone density in postmenopausal women. The results of heavy alcohol use, however, can be devastating.

The problems of alcohol abuse and alcoholism affect millions of people world-wide. The social consequences of alcohol abuse are present every day in the form of accidents, violence,

BOX 18-3

HOW POWERFUL IS NICOTINE ADDICTION?

Addiction is defined as mental and emotional dependence on a substance. Nicotine is the addictive drug in tobacco. Regular use of tobacco products leads to addiction in many users.

Of the 70% of smokers who state they want to quit, 40% try to quit each year with 4–7% succeeding without help. Smokers not only become physically dependant on the nicotine, there is a strong emotional (psychological) dependence as well. This is what leads to relapse after quitting. The smoker may link smoking with social and many other activities. Smokers also may use cigarettes to help manage unpleasant feelings and emotions, which can become a problem for some smokers when they try to quit. All these factors make smoking a hard habit to break.

Source: What Is in Tobacco? (2010). American Cancer Society. Retrieved from http://www.cancer.org

---

BOX 18-4
PHYSICAL EFFECTS OF ALCOHOL ABUSE

Gastritis	Malnutrition
Gastric ulcer	Nerve damage
Gastric hemorrhage	Hepatitis
Cirrhosis of the liver	Cancer
Liver failure	Stroke
Anemia	Delayed puberty
Osteoporosis	Pancreatitis
Heart disease	Esophageal varices

---

crime, and family neglect, just to name a few. Current statistics indicate that almost 14 million Americans, or one in every 13 adults, abuse alcohol or are alcoholic. Sadly, several million more adults and adolescents participate in patterns of drinking alcohol that place them at risk of becoming alcoholics.

The age at onset of drinking appears to correlate with the development of alcoholism in later years. The younger persons are when they begin drinking, the more likely they are to become alcoholic. Studies find that over 40% of respondents who started drinking before the age of 15 were later classified as alcoholic later in their lives (National Institutes of Health, 2010).

The harmful effects of alcohol on the body are extensive and often deadly (Box 18-4). When used during pregnancy, alcohol can be detrimental to a developing fetus, causing low birth weight and a syndrome of developmental, cognitive, and behavioral problems. Withdrawal from alcohol, without medical supervision and treatment, may result in severe psychological trauma and potentially fatal seizures.

SPOTLIGHT **ON**

Alcohol and Osteoporosis

Moderate alcohol consumption may help to increase bone density in postmenopausal women by facilitating two physiologic actions in the body. One of these ways is to stimulate an increase in the amount of estrogens made in the body. Estrogen is a hormone that stimulates bone formation. The second way to increase bone density is to promote the secretion of the hormone calcitonin from the thyroid gland. Calcitonin helps to regulate the amount of calcium in the body by inhibiting the absorption of bone.

Excessive intake of alcohol is toxic to the bone because it destroys bone cells. This can result in a fragile bone disease called osteoporosis. Older women who drink excessively have a double risk of developing osteoporosis because they also lose the bone-enhancing effect of estrogen after menopause.

? ASK **YOURSELF**

Alcohol and You

There are various thoughts and theories on why people become addicted to alcohol. How has alcoholism affected your life? How do you feel about caring for a person who is ill as a result of alcohol use?

WHY PEOPLE DRINK

There are a number of theories to explain why people drink. Many people drink during events of happiness and celebration. Although abuse of alcohol may occur, this type of drinking rarely leads to alcoholism. Individuals with poor self-esteem who drink out of boredom, when they are stressed, when they are depressed, or just out of habit are most likely to become alcoholic.

An issue of debate is whether psychosocial influences or biological makeup predispose one to becoming an alcoholic. Certainly environment has a great effect on an individual's patterns of behavior. What is learned from one's parents, peer pressure in adolescence, and influences from adult social groups all come into play. There is substantial evidence, however, that alcoholism has a biological basis. This basis for this theory is that some individuals inherit a genetic predisposition for addiction.

There are conflicting views on whether alcoholism is a disease in itself or causes disease. Whatever the case, alcohol addiction can ruin personal and social lives. Alcoholism has been identified as a major factor in dysfunctional families, child abuse, spouse abuse, and impaired job performance. Half of all Americans have someone in their family who abuses alcohol. Multiple drug use often includes alcohol.

ALCOHOL AND THE CENTRAL NERVOUS SYSTEM

Even with all of the research on alcohol, its action on the central nervous system is still not clearly understood. It probably alters neuron cell membranes to alter neurotransmission. Certain individuals may be more prone to these neurochemical abnormalities than others. Alcohol tends to stimulate the release of some of the neurotransmitters such as serotonin, dopamine, and noradrenelin in these particular individuals. Minor tranquilizer drugs (e.g., Valium, Librium) and barbiturates (also known as sleeping pills) produce these same kinds of effects. As such, these drugs have a cross-tolerance to alcohol.

Depressant drugs, like alcohol, initially produce perceptions of relaxation, well-being, and a decrease in anxiety and insomnia. After effects include nausea, headache, and agitation. Signs of depressant drug use are slurred speech, lack of coordination, difficulty with recent memory, and dilated pupils.

SUBSTANCE ABUSE PATTERNS

Differences in substance use, abuse, and addiction patterns exist or are purported to exist among groups. Some careers lend themselves to a high level of stress, especially those that require caring for others. Nurses are especially vulnerable to substance use. Some groups are related to gender, age, comorbidity, and ethnicity.

BOX 18-5

A PROFILE OF TOBACCO USERS IN THE UNITED STATES

Current trends of smoking in the United States:

- Between 1965 and 2004, cigarette smoking among adults aged 18 and older declined by half from 42% to 21%. Since 2004, rates have changed little. In 2008, an estimated 21%, or 46 million, Americans continued to smoke.

- Although cigarette smoking peaked higher and earlier in men, the gender gap narrowed in the mid-1980s and has since remained constant. As of 2008, there was a 3% absolute difference in, the prevalence of smoking in non-Hispanic white women versus men, an 8% difference between African American women versus men, a 10% difference in Hispanic white women versus men, and an 11% difference between Asian women versus men.

- Smoking continues to be most common among the least educated. Although the percentage of smokers has decreased in every level since 1983, college graduates had the greatest decline of 13% in 2008. By contrast, those with a high school diploma decreased by 7% in the same time period.

- While cigarette smoking among U.S. high school students increased significantly from 28% in 1991 to 36% in 1997, the rate declined to 20% by 2007.

Source: Cancer Facts and Figures 2010. American Cancer Society. Retrieved from http://www.cancer.org

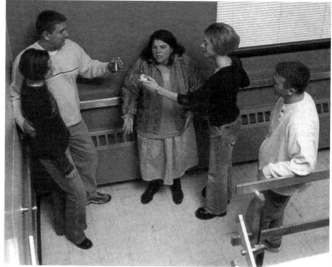

FIGURE 18-4 Smoking typically begins in adolescence from peer pressure and in response to role models, including parents.

GENDER

Males and females differ mostly in consumption patterns rather than in an increase in problem behaviors. Females tend to consume drugs in relation to interpersonal dynamics, and males tend to consume drugs to maintain their sense of manliness. Females are identified less often than males as having problems because of their protected status in society (i.e., they tend to be shielded from others' gaining knowledge about their use or abuse of substances). Females are also less prone to discuss substance use/abuse/addiction patterns in their lives. Many times, it is only at the tertiary prevention stage that a female is identified as having a problem.

Regarding smoking, the group that is reported to have among the lowest smoking rates are white-collar males. Their female counterparts (white-collar female employees), however, have a higher incidence of smoking than do blue-collar female workers. Box 18-5 provides a profile of tobacco users in the United States.

AGE

Substance use, abuse, or addiction or all three occur at any age. There are, however, two age groups that are particularly vulnerable: adolescents and the elderly.

ADOLESCENTS

Many adolescents eventually grow out of their use of drugs. The reasons are not totally clear, but most tend to move into acceptable roles in society. This acceptance then allows drugs to be replaced by other social and personal reinforcers. Those who continue toward addiction tend to struggle with acceptance by society and with self-value. Peer groups for these individuals tend to be those who continue to use and abuse drugs and who engage in antisocial or asocial role modeling. Thus, role identity becomes intricately entwined with drug use and abuse and behaviors that produce conflict.

Tobacco use typically begins prior to the age of 18 primarily in response to peer pressure and to role models, including parents, who use tobacco. There is growing evidence that tobacco use is increasing in the younger age group (Figure 18-4). A recent National Youth Tobacco Survey revealed that the percentage of current cigarette smokers among 12- or 13-year-olds dropped from 2.1% in 2008 to 1.4% in 2009. The percentage of current cigarette smokers remained steady among 14- or 15-year-olds (7.6% in 2008 and 7.5% in 2009) and among 16- or 17-year-olds (16.8% in 2008 and 16.9% in 2009) (Substance Abuse and Mental Health Services Administration, 2009).

ELDERLY

Another age group at risk for substance use and addiction are senior citizens. Substances abused in this age group tend to be alcohol and prescription medications.

The senior citizen tends to be in a dependent role with loss of clear role definition, loss of income, and loss of a support system. In addition to misuse as a result of physical problems (such as loss of vision), cognitive problems (misunderstanding of directions), and polypharmacy, drugs may become an avenue to alter perceived negative emotional states resulting from life changes.

ETHNICITY

Studies abound indicating that ethnicity plays an important role in the development and support of substance use, misuse, abuse, and addiction. Perhaps the basis for future problems with substances is more embedded in devaluation and exclusion rather than in ethnicity itself.

Drug use, abuse, addiction, or all three appear to be more closely related to the age group than to the ethnic group. Children who have behavioral difficulties are at risk regardless of ethnicity (Substance Abuse and Mental Health Services Administration, 2009). Acceptance by the peer culture is critical to preadolescents and adolescents.

The issues of devaluation and exclusion are reflected in the changes in substance use over time. With the exception of tobacco, substance use, misuse, abuse, and/or addiction risk among Whites tends to decrease with age, whereas the risk among African Americans, Hispanics, and Asian Americans tends to increase. In regard to alcohol, however, the Native American tends to have a higher rate of alcohol use and abuse than any other group across age and gender.

Use of tobacco also tends to be higher among Native American adolescents than any other cultural group. African American adolescents have shown lower rates for tobacco use than other ethnic groups except Asian Americans, who have the lowest rates. Smoking rates for White adolescents are usually double the rates found for African American adolescents, yet African American adults have higher prevalence rates than Whites. This suggests that, as White users move into adulthood, they successfully relinquish tobacco use more often than do African Americans.

Adolescent males continue to have the highest prevalence for smokeless tobacco. The prevalence is greatest for White males at 20%, followed by 6% among Hispanics, and 4% among African Americans (U.S. Department of Health & Human Services, 2010).

NURSES

Beginning in the 1970s and 1980s, much attention was focused on drug abuse among nurses. Because of the stress inherent in their occupation and the availability of drugs, nurses were believed to be at risk for substance use, misuse, abuse, and addiction to illicit drugs and narcotics. Some nurses were found to have obtained drugs by withholding medications from clients, forging prescriptions, or stealing the drugs from available supplies.

More current research has indicated, however, that abuse of these substances among nurses is no greater than the general population and may, in fact, be even less. Much of the evidence pointing the finger at nurses as addicts was based on individual accounts, not on scientific research. Exaggeration of illicit drug use among nurses could have been done to amplify the drug problems of society in order to gain funding for rehabilitation (Taylor, 2003; Dunn, 2005).

This is not to say that there is no problem of drug abuse among nurses. Estimates of drug abuse or of chemical impairment among nurses in the profession continue to vary from 3% to 5%. Chemically impaired nurses are at risk of making poor judgments, resulting in varying degrees of harm to those in their care. In recognition of this, prevention programs have been made available through the State Board of Nursing, the regulating body of the profession, in every state to assist nurses having difficulties with personal drug use. These programs are in place to initiate an intervention, monitor progress, and maintain support for chemically impaired nurses. The National Council of Boards of Nurse Examiners offered the premises listed in Box 18-6 to be considered by each State Board of Nurse Examiners when addressing regulatory issues

---

BOX 18-6

PREMISES OF THE NATIONAL COUNCIL OF STATE BOARDS OF NURSING FOR PEER ASSISTANCE PROGRAMS

Each State Board of Nursing should consider the following premises regarding peer assistance programs:

1. Consumers have the right to receive safe and effective care from nurses licensed in their state.
2. To practice, licensed nurses should be physically, mentally, and emotionally capable.
3. Substance abuse or dependency is an illness on the wellness-illness continuum.
4. Because it is an illness, those with substance abuse should be treated rather than punished.
5. Boards of Nursing must be able to reassure the public regarding health, safety, and welfare.
6. State Boards of Nursing have constitutional authority over those they license. To obtain or maintain licensure, nurses must comply with the requirements of their State Board of Nursing.
7. Privacy and confidentiality of nurses involved in peer assistance programs should be evaluated against the State Board of Nursing's responsibility to protect the health, safety, and welfare of the public and to protect the public from receiving unsafe, incompetent care.

Source: Endorsement Issues Related to Peer Assistance/Alternative Programs. (2005). National Council of State Boards of Nursing. Retrieved from http://www.ncsbn.org/files/publications/positions/peerassistance.asp

---

of peer assistance programs and chemically impaired nurses in their state.

Chemically impaired nurses are less likely to approach and counsel others about drug use, abuse, and/or addiction. Because nurses are in key positions to provide support and counsel to others about drug use, they must address and resolve their problems rather than allowing them to progress to the loss or suspension of their licenses because of illegal drug use.

COMORBIDITY

The effects of drugs on the body eventually take their toll. An individual in need of treatment for substance abuse problems is often also in need of treatment for mental, spiritual, and physical health problems. This is called **comorbidity**, when another disability is present in addition to the substance use/abuse/addiction. Treating individuals with a **dual diagnosis** (substance abuse along with mental or physical health concerns) or perhaps a **triad diagnosis** (a mental health issue, a physical health issue, and a substance abuse issue) requires a multidisciplinary team approach. Many substance abuse issues come to light only when the individual enters treatment for a mental or spiritual health issue or a physical complaint.

MENTAL HEALTH ISSUES

Substance abuse issues and mental health issues are better approached as separate syndromes. Because drugs produce feelings, thoughts, and behaviors that mimic mental health problems, confusion may occur as to which is the primary disability. Also, an underlying mental health issue may have preceded and perhaps was exacerbated by substance use.

There are many examples of people with psychological disabilities who may be predisposed to substance use problems. Some of the high-risk groups with mental health problems who are prone to developing substance abuse problems are those with schizophrenia, mood disorders such as depression, anxiety and bipolar disorder, and personality disorders. The three camps of mental health, physical health, and substance abuse issues are divided by philosophy and by physical location. Thus, these individuals are many times bounced from one treatment approach to another without the pooled benefit of the experts most concerned with their well-being.

PHYSICAL HEALTH ISSUES

Physical health issues are related to the detrimental effects of the drugs themselves and to injuries from accidents as a result of using the drug. An individual with a physical disability that occurs during drug use or an individual who already has a physical disability is at risk to continue or develop substance abuse problems. An individual's risk for obtaining a physical disability increases with the use of drugs.

SPIRITUAL HEALTH ISSUES

Drug use, abuse, or addiction or all three create a void in one's spiritual health. It might also be said that poor spiritual health could lead to drug use. It may be debatable to exactly define the human spirit; a number of various perspectives make the human spirit difficult to define. The human spirit, in essence, may be described as the very depth of the soul. It is the quintessence of the being that we call human. The body, mind, and spirit make up a person, but the spirit seems to maintain the body and the mind. Without the spirit, the body and mind

cannot exist. If the spirit is not healthy, the body and the mind may have to struggle to be healthy.

Drug use, abuse, addiction, or all three appear to rob one of one's spirit. After drugs take their toll, the body and mind may be salvaged to the extent of the damage, but the spirit must heal. The healing of the spirit comes, in part, through the acceptance of oneself and others.

STRATEGIES FOR HEALTH PROMOTION

Promoting health in all individuals involves supporting healthy behaviors that entail making healthy choices. Health-promotion strategies, therefore, are to prevent individuals from making unhealthy choices including exposure to tobacco, alcohol, and other substances that may lead to use, abuse, and eventually addiction or irresponsible use or both.

Prevention may be arranged according to the degree of substance use and the approaches used to prevent use, continued use, abuse, or addiction. Primary prevention occurs prior to any use. Secondary prevention may be in the form of treatment, but most often it targets those who are using and possibly abusing;. Tertiary prevention is most often in the form of long-term treatment, the goal of which is to prevent early death and disability.

The evaluation of individuals with substance abuse issues is usually not an easy task because minimization or secretiveness many times surrounds their relationship with drugs. Few nurses are formally educated or trained to recognize substance use, abuse, and/or addiction; to provide appropriate referrals; and to initiate effective prevention strategies. Yet nurses are in positions that lend the opportunity to provide prevention at all levels. Training nurses to evaluate, refer, and treat substance use, abuse, and addiction is essential to overall prevention efforts.

The Agency for Healthcare Research and Quality of the U.S. Department of Health and Human Services has developed guidelines for the health professional to use for smoking cessation (Agency for Healthcare Research and Quality, 2008). Similar guidelines could be helpful for clients with other types of substance abuse as well. The premise behind the development of these guidelines is that health care professionals are in key positions to identify the smokers and to plan interventions for smoking cessation. Four basic strategies are identified to guide the health care professional: ask, advise, assist, and arrange. Primarily aimed for use in clinics and medical offices, these strategies involve asking clients about smoking at every office visit, advising the smoker to quit, assisting the smoker in developing a quit plan, and arranging for follow-up contact. Table 18-4 shows how asking, advising, and assisting could be incorporated into substance abuse prevention at the primary and secondary levels in medical offices and hospitals.

IDENTIFICATION OF RISK AND PROTECTIVE FACTORS

Implementation of health-promotion strategies for individuals who are at risk for substance use and abuse problems requires that the nurse recognize factors that place an individual at risk for substance use and factors that protect an individual from substance abuse. **Risk factors** include situations or conditions or both that increase an individual's vulnerability to substance abuse. **Protective factors** are factors that build resiliency against substance abuse and increase the likelihood that an individual will resist substance abuse. Research has

SPOTLIGHT **ON**

Long-Term Effects of Alcohol Abuse

Harry was a 36-year-old male who appeared to be in his 60s. He had abused alcohol since he was 14 years of age. He was independently wealthy and lived alone. His brother, who made weekly visits, found him unconscious one day. When he was admitted to the hospital, his physical health had deteriorated to the point that his system was no longer able to function. He died shortly thereafter. What do you think could have contributed to his alcoholism? What interventions do you think could have changed this scenario?

TABLE 18-4 Substance Abuse Prevention Guidelines for the Health Professional

STRATEGIES	SUGGESTIONS FOR PRACTICE APPLICATION
Ask Ask the supervisor in your agency about the existence of a method to identify clients with substance use, misuse, abuse, or addiction problems. Establish a system that assesses for substance use at every office visit or hospital admission.	1. Incorporate asking about use of tobacco, alcohol, or other substance use into the confidential data collection form used at each office visit or admission assessment to the hospital. 2. Denote a special area on the record for documenting these data. Include questions about the use of prescription drugs, nonprescription drugs, herbs, vitamins, tobacco, alcohol, marijuana, cocaine, heroin, and other substances.
Advise Provide professional advice appropriate to the client and in accordance with your agency protocol.	1. If no problem exists, encourage the client to continue healthy behavior. 2. If a problem of use, misuse, abuse, or addiction exists, advise the client of the importance of behavior change.
Assist According to your agency protocol, offer resources available to help with the problem.	1. If change is desired, explain options available for assistance. Options will vary according to resources in the community. 2. If change is not desired, offer motivation and offer continued support for change. 3. Offer educational materials that are culturally sensitive and educationally appropriate.

© Cengage Learning 2013

shown that the more risk factors that are present in an individual, the more likely it is that a substance abuse problem will develop. Scientists have found that both risk and protective factors are critical components in preventing substance abuse. Prevention programs must utilize the body of knowledge related to both risk and protection areas of study. Risk and protective factors extend to all areas of a person's life, and multiple interventions in those areas that increase substance use risk can enhance outcomes (Center for Substance Abuse Prevention, 2010).

A number of factors can protect individuals against substance abuse. Some of these relate to internal factors, and some are more externally based. Internal factors that protect individuals from substance abuse include an individual's belief in self and in the ability to accomplish meaningful tasks. Other factors include social confidence, or the degree to which an individual gets along with others and contributes to a social group. How an individual relates to family and peers, such as in grade school, can assist in protecting against the temptations of substance use, especially during the formative and adolescent years. Research indicates that the risk for substance use during adolescence is strongly related to environmental characteristics in which the adolescent lives. Family supervision, school environment, community opportunities, and the quality of life all influence the development of positive or problem behaviors in youth (Center for Substance Abuse Prevention, 2010). Box 18-7 depicts risk and protective factors associated with substance use. Nurses developing and implementing health-promotion strategies for individuals at risk for substance use should familiarize themselves with all of the risk and protective factors associated with substance use and abuse.

PRIMARY PREVENTION

Primary prevention with regard to substance use is defined as prevention for those who have not used tobacco, alcohol, or other drugs. The goal is to prevent exposure to and experimenting with drugs.

Primary prevention has been touted in the schools, particularly in the early grades, as an effective strategy for the prevention of subsequent substance abuse and other high-risk behaviors. Many programs with various approaches have been attempted. There is little scientific evidence to indicate that school-based preventative programs are effective in preventing substance abuse problems either in younger children or in adolescents. Studying the effectiveness of these prevention programs is difficult because the individuals in whom primary prevention may be effective would not be identifiable; they would not progress to secondary or tertiary prevention levels.

Tobacco prevention education programs in schools that provide skill-training approaches appear to be effective in reducing the onset of tobacco use (Centers for Disease Control, 2010). To be effective, these programs need to target youth before they initiate tobacco use. Individuals who develop smoking habits early in life are more likely to become heavy users and to have a greater chance of developing smoking-related diseases due to long-term use.

Are schools expected to replace the family in ethical, moral, and preventive behaviors? Some describe primary prevention as multidimensional with a recommendation that prevention, particularly in the early years, be strategies that promote healthy development (USDHHS, 2010b). Schools can be highly influential in building the motivation and social competence that children need as they engage in behaviors that promote health

BOX 18-7

SELECTED SUBSTANCE USE AND ABUSE RISK AND PROTECTIVE FACTORS

- Youth who believe that drugs and cigarettes are harmful are less likely to smoke or use drugs.
- Sensation-seeking personalities are more likely to smoke and do drugs.
- Inappropriate expressions of anger increase the risk of substance use.
- Aggressive and disruptive classroom behavior may predict substance abuse.
- Youths who have conventional values are less likely to abuse substances.
- Poor parenting practices can predict adolescent substance abuse.
- Parental monitoring and supervision protect against substance abuse.
- Outstanding school performance reduces the likelihood of drug use.
- Peer substance use is among the strongest predictors of substance use.
- Sustained involvement in structured peer activities is linked to a low level of drug use.
- Ready access to tobacco, alcohol, and other drugs increases use of these substances.
- Stress in the workplace may elevate alcohol consumption.

Source: U.S. Department of Health and Human Services, Substance Abuse and Mental Health Services Administration, Center for Substance Abuse Prevention. (n.d.). Preventing drug abuse among children and adolescents: Risk factors and protective factors. Retrieved from http://www.nida.nih.gov/Prevention/risk.html

SPOTLIGHT **ON**

Secondary Prevention for Substance Abuse: Troy's Case

Imagine yourself as a school nurse in a local high school. Troy is 18 and a senior in your school. His grades have recently dropped, and he is losing weight. His friends are concerned that Troy might be using drugs because he is hanging out with individuals known to use cocaine and speed (amphetamines). The recent death of Troy's older brother has had a devastating effect on his entire family. He no longer feels that his family cares about him, and he is feeling isolated and lonely. Drugs, he feels, make him feel more valued as a person. What can you do to promote health for Troy?

and as they are exposed to risky behaviors such as substance abuse.

Primary prevention in adults is aimed primarily at educating them about the unhealthy attributes of drug use and toward responsible use of legal drugs. Prevention programs aimed at increasing self-esteem in adults are probably most effective at the secondary prevention level.

SECONDARY PREVENTION

Secondary prevention includes strategies aimed at preventing substance abuse by those considered at risk to develop problems and those who are using substances. Groups of individuals who are considered at risk for substance abuse problems include (but are not limited to) adolescents, elderly, lesbians/gays, minorities, and people with disabilities. The common thread in these groups is exclusion from and devaluation by society. Other high-risk groups are those in vocations that they perceive to be highly stressful. One of these groups is the health care professional.

Users of substances are considered to be at risk for the development of substance abuse and possible subsequent addiction. By experimenting or using, individuals place themselves at risk for abuse and addiction.

Secondary prevention appears to be a tool to identify individuals who are prone to develop problems or who have moved into substance use and at times abuse. Many times, the potential substance use problems come to light through other avenues during secondary prevention.

TERTIARY PREVENTION

Tertiary prevention in substance use refers to the prevention of death and disability of individuals in long-term treatment. Tertiary prevention is appropriate for two populations: those who are considered in need of treatment but who maintain control over their behavior (substance abuse) and those who are considered in need of treatment but who clearly are not in control of their behavior (substance addiction). Many of these individuals tend to use more than one substance. Many use tobacco but do not consider the use of this drug as a cause for concern.

The primary treatment goal in tertiary prevention is to learn to live life without drugs. This entails a total change in lifestyle. Education on the effects of drugs may be useful to increase an individual's awareness, but the underlying feelings of self-acceptance and acceptance by others appear to be the more crucial variables in adjustment to a life without drugs. Relapse prevention tends to occur in conjunction with tertiary prevention. Relapse is the return to drug use, and **relapse prevention** is the prevention of this behavior. Several relapse prevention programs encompass physical and psychosocial addiction processes.

IN CONTROL

Individuals who are maintaining control over their behavior but are abusing substances are considered to be in control of their use or, perhaps, abuse of drugs. These individuals have intact families, careers, and physical, mental, and spiritual health, although they may be bordering on the loss of any one or all of these. They are usually identified after the loss of one or more of these parts of their lives, or they may at times identify themselves prior to any losses. They tend to have a sense of in-vulnerability to the adverse consequences of their substance use or abuse or both. Many use and abuse drugs to provide them with an altered state of consciousness to gain relief from the inner psychological pain.

OUT OF CONTROL

Individuals who are considered to be out of control of their be-havior are considered to have moved into addiction. They have lost their family, friends (other than those who are using or abus-ing substances), income and career, and their sense of them-selves. Their physical, mental, or spiritual health or all three have been compromised. They are usually identified by their family, friends, employers, by law enforcement and at times by them-selves. Drugs have penetrated their every waking moment and have ceased to provide them with a means to seek relief from the internal physical and psychological turmoil and a sense of well-being. Many have experiences that predispose them to an in-ability to live life without numbing their memories. Drugs have now become a way of life. The intake of drugs takes on a compul-sive nature, and the loss of control is reflected in the frequency, amount, duration, dosage, and behavior of the individual. See the Case Study for an individual with alcohol issues and addiction.

🧍 HEALTH PROMOTION THEORY LINK

Dorothea Orem's Self-Care Theory

Dorothea Orem's Self-Care Theory is based on the assumptions that people should be self-reliant and responsible for their own care. In the application to drug and substance use, Orem's development of the Self-Care Deficit is useful to determine the client's difficulty in developing and maintain-ing optimal self-care. In her theory, Orem states that two main phases of self-care can be applied to drug and substance use: the decision and the action.

Source: Dumas. (1992). The Nursing Process According to Orem. A Concrete Very Simple Example Explains How to Follow this Nursing Process. http://www.ncbi.nlm.nih.gov/pubmed/1600504

SUMMARY

The overall goals of *Healthy People 2020* are designed to in-crease the quality and years of healthy life, eliminate health disparities, create social and physical environments that pro-mote good health for all, as well as healthy behaviors across all life stages (USDHHS, 2010b). As such, strategies aimed at risk-reduction, behavior change, and preventive services are at the core of health promotion of all ages, at varying degrees of health, and in diverse groups.

The prevention of substance use, abuse, and addiction ap-pears complex, but it is no mystery. Whether the underlying rea-son is psychological, social, or physical, individuals' decisions to use substances are based on a desire to alter their perceptions of themselves and the world. An individual who feels good and has a sense of belonging to self and to the world has no need to alter subjective perceptions and feelings. In an ideal world, a child raised with limits and structure among those who love, respect, and trust may have no need to change perceptions of self and the world. In such cases, health is promoted and pri-mary prevention is taking place. Secondary prevention relates to preventing a fall into abuse and/or a way to responsible use. Tertiary prevention essentially is to prevent the destruction of the body, mind, and spirit.

CASE STUDY

Jane Davey: At Risk for Alcohol Abuse and Addiction

OBJECTIVES/GOALS: Through participation in a discussion of this case study, participants will have the oppor-tunity to:

1. Identify factors that can lead to alcohol abuse and addiction.
2. Describe the physical effects of alcohol abuse and addiction.
3. Describe the psychosocial effects of alcohol abuse and addiction.

HEALTH-PROMOTION CONCERN, HISTORY AND PHYSICAL, PRESENT HEALTH STATUS, PAST HEALTH STATUS, FAMILY HISTORY, AND SOCIAL HISTORY

Jane Davey is a 29-year-old Caucasian female who is currently a stay-at-home mom. Her day includes homeschool-ing her three young boys, maintaining the family home, and shopping and cooking for the family. She has a college degree in business and always thought she would someday develop her own company. Jane's husband of 6 years is

(Continues)

CASE STUDY

(Continued)

a successful lawyer who works 14 or more hours a day with hopes of making partner within the next 5 years. He is home less and less due to his demanding career. Jane starts drinking alcohol early in the day to "relax and get through her very long days." Jane thinks she has been able to hide her drinking for several months now.

REVIEW OF PERTINENT DOMAINS

Biological Domain

Physical exam reveals an overweight individual who is 66 in. tall and weighs 205 lb with a previous weight of 230 lb.

GASTROINTESTINAL: Ms. Davey has a history of unexplained weight loss. Her dietary patterns have not changed. She usually tries to eat three well-balanced meals a day but admits to drinking at least one soft drink with her meals and snacking and drinking in the evening. She has been feeling very tired lately.

DIAGNOSTIC TESTING: Glucose and cholesterol readings are significantly above normal.

Psychological Domain

Ms. Davey was diagnosed with postpartum depression shortly after her third birth. She discontinued the prescription treatment against medical advice. Jane feels she has become more isolated since the birth of the children.

Social Domain

Ms. Davey dedicates her entire day to homeschooling the children, as well as to taking care of the home environment. She no longer has social contact with family and friends; however, she does attend her husband's occasional social events with the law firm. She is isolated and has feelings of decreased self-esteem.

Environmental Domain

Ms. Davey finds her environment stressful and nonstimulating intellectually. Although she homeschools her children, she is also responsible for taking care of all the household chores and making dinner daily.

QUESTIONS FOR DISCUSSION

1. What are the signs of depressant drug use such as alcohol?
2. What are the social consequences of alcohol abuse?
3. Develop a plan to help Ms. Davey with her social isolation and reliance on alcohol.

KEY CONCEPTS

1. The misuse, abuse, and addiction to substances such as tobacco, alcohol, and psychotropic drugs affect the well-being of individuals, families, communities, and nations. The effects range from the destruction of personal lives and relationships, to millions of dollars spent in health care and treatment, and to hundreds of thousands of lives lost nationwide.

2. Use of prescription, nonprescription, and psychotropic drugs each can lead to misuse, abuse, and addiction.

3. All drugs are designed for specific actions and interactions with our body cells. Drugs that tend to be abused alter the normal body processes specific to the brain at the level of the neurotransmitters.

4. Individuals can become addicted biologically, psychosocially, or in a combination of both way.

5. Nicotine, alcohol, and psychotropic drugs act on the pleasure centers of the brain, altering mood and, in some instances, perceptions.

6. Diversity exists in patterns of substance use according to gender, age groups, and ethnicity, and according to the particular substance.

7. Comorbidity, mental health, physical health, and spirituality are issues influencing drug use among individuals.

8. Knowledge about drugs and substance abuse is powerful for promoting health and in prevention of use and abuse among those at risk.

9. Nurses are in key positions to ask about substance use, to advise individuals of the health risks of using, and to assist those who are using and desire to quit.

CHAPTER REVIEW

Learning Activities

1. Describe the difference between drug misuse and drug abuse.
2. List at least five ways that drugs may enter the body.
3. How is physical dependence different from psychosocial dependence?
4. Describe the effects of environmental tobacco smoke (ETS).
5. How can nurses be effective in primary and secondary drug abuse prevention efforts?
6. How can nurses get help if they have a problem with substance abuse?

Multiple Choice Questions

1. Which of the following may be an effect of drug use and abuse?
   a. Cerebral palsy
   b. Early puberty onset
   c. Eczema
   d. Prematurity
2. All of the following are basic sources from which drugs are derived *except*:
   a. animals.
   b. minerals.
   c. plants.
   d. soil.
3. Psychotropic drugs do which of the following?
   a. Act by affecting the stomach lining, increasing absorption
   b. Affect respiratory function
   c. Alter mental activity and are used to treat mental disorders
   d. Do not affect thoughts and feelings
4. Bladder cancer is a condition linked to which of the following?
   a. Cigarette smoking
   b. Drug inhalants
   c. Opiate drug use
   d. Psychotropic drug use
5. Which of the following statements is true?
   a. Ethnicity does not play a role in the development of substance abuse.
   b. Drug use and drug abuse in nurses are no greater than in the general population.
   c. Men and women do not differ in drug consumption patterns.
   d. No age groups are particularly vulnerable to drug abuse.
6. The biological basis for addiction is in the alteration of which process of chemical neurotransmission?
   a. Average
   b. Clinical
   c. Normal
   d. Subclinical

ORGANIZATIONS AND WEBSITES

Action on Smoking and Health: Provides information for people concerned about smoking and nonsmokers' rights, smoking statistics, quitting smoking, smoking risks, and other smoking information: **http://www.ash.org**

Centers for Disease Control and Prevention (CDC): One of the 13 major operating components of the U.S. Department of Health and Human Services, which is the principal agency in the U.S. government for protecting the health and safety of all Americans and for providing essential human services, especially for those who are least able to help themselves; committed to achieving true improvements in people's health: **http://www.cdc.gov/**

National Institutes of Health (NIH): A part of the U.S. Department of Health and Human Services and the primary federal agency for conducting and supporting medical research; NIH scientists investigate ways to prevent disease as well as the causes, treatments, and even cures for common and rare diseases: **Health.nih.gov**

National Institute on Drug Abuse (NIDA): Leads the nation in bringing the power of science to bear on drug abuse and addiction; NIDA-supported research addresses the most fundamental and essential questions about drug abuse, ranging from the molecule to managed care and from DNA to community outreach: **www.nida.nih.gov**

Partnership at Drugfree: Provides information on child drug use and keeping children off drugs. Includes intervention and treatment information: **http://www.drugfree.org**

Tobacco Information and Prevention Source, Centers for Disease Control and Prevention: Information on smoking statistics, smoking cessation, and other tobacco-related health problems: **http://www.cdc.gov/tobacco**

United States Food and Drug Administration (FDA): Responsible for protecting the public health by assuring the safety, efficacy, and security of human and veterinary drugs, biological products, medical devices, our nation's food supply, cosmetics, and products that emit radiation; also responsible for advancing the public health by helping to speed innovations that make medicines and foods more effective, safer, and more affordable, and for helping the public get accurate, science-based information about medicines and foods to improve their health: **http://www.fda.com**

REFERENCES

Agency for Healthcare Research and Quality (2008). Treating tobacco use and dependence. Retrieved from http://www.ahrq.gov

American Cancer Society (2010a). Cancer facts and figures. Retrieved from http://www.cancer.org

American Cancer Society. (2010b). What is in tobacco? Retrieved from http://www.cancer.org/Cancer/CancerCauses/TobaccoCancer/CigaretteSmoking/cigarette-smoking-tobacco

American Cancer Society (2010c). Cigarette smoking: Introduction. Retrieved from http://www.cancer.org/Cancer/CancerCauses/TobaccoCancer/CigaretteSmoking/cigarette-smoking-tobacco

American Cancer Society. (2011a). *Cancer facts & figures 2011*. Retrieved from http://www.cancer.org/acs/groups/content/@epidemiologysurveilance/documents/document/acspc-029771.pdf

American Cancer Society. (2011b). Learn about cancer: Cigarette Smoking. Retrieved from http://www.cancer.org/Cancer/CancerCauses/TobaccoCancer/CigaretteSmoking/cigarette-smoking-who-and-how-affects-health

Center for Substance Abuse Prevention (2010). Annual report of science-based prevention programs. U.S. Department of Health and Human Services, Substance Abuse and Mental Health Services Administration.

Center for Substance Abuse Prevention. (2010). *The national cross-site evaluation of high-risk youth programs: Understanding risk, protection, and substance use among high-risk youth*. Monograph Series No. 2. U.S Department of Health and Human Services, Substance Abuse and Mental Health Services Administration. Retrieved, from http://www.samhsa.gov

Centers for Disease Control and Prevention. (2010). *Health effects of cigarette smoking fact sheet*. November 2010. Retrieved, from http://www.medofficeinc.com

Crane, J,. Keough, M., Murphy, P., Burrage, L., & Hutchens, D. (2011). Effects of environmental tobacco smoke on perinatal outcomes: A retrospective cohort study. *British Journal of Obstetrics and Gynaecology,118*(7), 865–871.

Dumas, L. (1992). The nursing process according to Orem. A concrete very simple example explains how to follow this nursing process. Retrieved from http://www.ncbi.nlm.nih.gov/pubmed/1600504

Dunn, D. (2005). Substance abuse among nurses—intercession and intervention. *AORN Journal* (November 2005).

James, J. (1998). *Peyote & mescaline: History & uses of the "divine cactus."* Tempe, AZ: Do It Now Foundation.

Mayo Foundation for Medical Education and Research. (2010). Pain pill-addiction: What's the risk? Retrieved from http://mayoclinic.com/

National Council of State Boards of Nursing. (2005). Endorsement issues related to peer assistance/alternative programs. Retrieved from http://www.ncsbn.org

National Institute of Mental Health. (2010). Medications publication 2010. Retrieved from http://nimh.nih.gov

National Institute on Drug Abuse. (2003). Stress and the brain: Developmental, neurobiological, and clinical implications. Retrieved from http://www.drugabuse.gov/

National Institute on Drug Abuse Research Report Series. (2010). Cocaine abuse and addiction. Retrieved from http://www.drugabuse.gov/ResearchReports/Cocaine/cocaine.html

National Institute on Drug Abuse. (2010). Smoking/nicotine. Retrieved from http://www.drugabuse.gov

National Institutes of Health. (2010). The brain—Lesson 4—Longterm effects of drugs on the brain. Retrieved from http://science.education.nih/

Office of National Drug Control Policy. (2008a). Inhalants. Retrieved from http://www.whitehousedrugpolicy.gov

Office of National Drug Control Policy. (2008b). Drug czar unveils new resource for youth drug prevention. Retrieved from http://www.whitehousedrugpolicy.gov

Substance Abuse and Mental Health Services Administration. (2009). *The 2010 National Survey on Drug Use and Health*. Office of Applied Studies, NSDUH Series H-27, DHHS Publication No. SMA 05-4061. Rockville, MD. Retrieved, from http://oas.samhsa.gov/

Taylor, A. (2003). Support for nurses with addictions often lacking among colleagues. *American Nurse, 35* (September/October 2003), 10–11.

Thomas, C. L., & Taber, C. W. (eds.). (2010). *Taber's cyclopedic medical dictionary*. Philadelphia, PA: F. A. Davis.

United Nations Office on Drugs and Crime (2010). World drug report 2010: Drug use is shifting towards new drugs and new markets. Retrieved from http://www.unodc.org/unodc/en/frontpage/2010/June/drug-use-is-shifting-towards-new-drugs-and-new-markets

U.S. Department of Health and Human Services, Substance Abuse and Mental Health Services Administration, Center for Substance Abuse Prevention. (n.d.) Preventing drug abuse among children and adolescents: Risk factors and protective factors. Retrieved from http://www.nida.nih.gov/Prevention/risk.html

U.S. Department of Health and Human Services (USDHHS). (2010a). Health promotion and disease prevention objectives for 2020. Retrieved from http://www.os.dhhs.gov

U.S. Department of Health and Human Services (USDHHS), National Institutes of Health, National Institute on Drug Abuse. (2010b). Preventing drug abuse among children and adolescents. Retrieved from http://www.drugabuse.gov/prevention/

Venes, D. (ed.). (2010). *Taber's cyclopedic medical dictionary, thumb-indexed version*. Philadelphia: F. A. Davis.

BIBLIOGRAPHY

Boles, S. M., Joshi, V., Grella, C., & Wellisch, J. (2005). Childhood sexual abuse patterns, psychosocial correlates, and treatment outcomes among adults in drug abuse treatment. *Journal of Child Sexual Abuse, 14*(1), 39–55.

Krowchuk, H. V. (2005). Effectiveness of adolescent smoking prevention strategies. *American Journal of Maternal-Child Nursing, 30*(6), 366–372.

Kuper, H. (2002). Tobacco use and cancer causation: Association by tumour type. *Journal of Internal Medicine, 252*, 206–224.

Rea, T. D. (2002). Smoking status and risk for recurrent coronary events after myocardial infarction. *Annals of Internal Medicine, 137*, 494–500.

Usher, K., Jackson, D., & O'Brien, L. (2005). Adolescent drug abuse: Helping families survive. *International Journal of Mental Health Nursing, 14*(3), 209–214.

Williams, C. M. (2002). Using medications appropriately in older adults. *American Family Physician, 66*(10), 1917–1924.

CHAPTER 19
Enhancing Holistic Care

Janice A. Maville, EdD, MSN, RN

KEY TERMS

ayurveda
complementary and alternative
   medicine (CAM)
capacity building
chakras
cognitive restructuring
energy
energy field

heliotherapy
holistic healing
holistic nursing
imagery
learned helplessness
meditation
modeling
nurse healers

phytochemicals
presence
reflexology
Relaxation Response
role modeling
therapeutic touch

OBJECTIVES

Upon completion of this chapter, the reader should be able to:

- Create a personal definition of a healing nurse.
- Discuss how the nurse can help the patient discover and meet health needs.
- Explore the concept of the human energy field and its relevance to nursing.
- List two ways to become conscious of and change unwanted thoughts.
- Discuss how imagery can be used to promote health.
- Practice and teach the Relaxation Response technique.
- List two ways the nurse can use light and sound for health promotion.
- Demonstrate the use of Centering and Grounding as used in Therapeutic Touch and Healing Touch.
- Demonstrate the use of touch therapy by using reflexology or massage to help balance the body for relaxation and healing.
- Choose among methods of nurturing the self and managing stress, and describe how they can be used for health promotion.
- Describe how healing and health can be promoted through human caring and love.

INTRODUCTION

Today, people use a wide variety of methods to help heal themselves, and these and other methods are finding their way into professional health care practice. With the growing concern in the health professions and health care delivery systems about the cost of health care, greater emphasis must be placed on promoting health and finding alternatives to traditional health care.

This chapter discusses what is meant by holistic healing, what a nurse healer is, and how incorporating holistic care can enhance health promotion. The importance of the relationship of nurses with their own inner being, as well as with the patient, is explored. Ways are suggested to help the patient and nurse discover what each needs to allow healing to occur and how to meet those needs. Many holistic healing modalities are introduced, and ways the nurse can incorporate them into nursing practice are discussed. The goal of this chapter is to offer new tools and new points of view that you as a nurse can use in the ongoing quest to help your patients and yourself to be healthy.

WHAT IS HOLISTIC CARE?

Providing nursing care is more than giving medicines, changing dressings, and charting. It is eye contact, smiles, touch, time, and caring. It is considering patients as individuals with unique needs and fears. It is helping them to feel in control by meeting those needs and comforting those fears. At vulnerable moments, it is helping others with private activities of daily living when they cannot help themselves. It is looking at, and interacting with, patients holistically.

Nursing has always been holistic. **Holistic healing** means considering all aspects of a person's internal and external environment that may contribute to health and well-being, as well as being willing to entertain a wide variety of options to help that person heal. Nurses view this total picture when suggesting which modalities patients might use to help correct imbalances in their state of health. **Holistic nursing** is looking at a person as a whole greater than the sum of the parts. Another view of holism is that human beings are holograms, which means that each part reflects the whole (Eliopoulos, 2009).

What are these aspects of the human being? They are both the physical and energetic aspects of the body, the mind or thoughts, the emotions and feelings, and the spirit. Central to the holistic health philosophy are as follows:

- Holism of the person (body, mind, and spirit) is in interaction with the environment.
- Health promotion and disease prevention are the focus rather than treatment of symptoms.
- Disease, illness, or imbalance are opportunities for positive growth.
- Patients are responsible and active participants in their own health.
- Collaborative relationships among patients and practitioners are emphasized.
- Cultural diversity is a highly valued component.
- Complementary and alternative modalities are part of a worldview perspective (Bright, Andrus, & Lunt, 2004).

Holistic nursing considers a person's total environment whether at work, at home, in school, or in the community. A person's environment includes everything. It includes feelings of social support, stressors and how they are handled, the quality of air and water, the food ingested, type and location of home, presence of animals or pets, and habits of daily living such as sleep, exercise, and play. Holistic nursing care means considering the whole person. It looks at all that contributes, or that has contributed in the past, to make patients who they are, and it discovers how all those factors affect health and the disease process. Nurses consider these factors when assessing, planning interventions, and evaluating progress. Nursing is inherently holistic. Very few nurses consider the state of a person merely by the physical body. Because nurses are intuitive and caring, they consider a person's thoughts, feelings, and family life to one degree or another.

People are multifaceted beings with all aspects of their selves and their lives constantly interacting to produce all degrees of health and illness. To help patients discover and achieve their unique desired level of wellness, all these facets must be considered.

WHAT IS HEALING?

A core component to nursing is helping people to heal. What it means to heal is unique to each individual.

The words *healing* and *holy* both come from the root word *hal* (hale), which means to make whole. As people begin to feel the connection between spirit, thoughts, feelings, and bodies, healing happens. Those who are conscious of their total being make changes that create lives that are fun and fulfilling. This is healing.

In the heart of each person, people are and always have been whole and complete. Events in life such as childhoods that were less than supportive, disappointing relationships, anger, and even lack of sleep can cause individuals to forget their inherent state of wholeness. Healing is remembering one's true nature. Nurses use many tools to help people remember, such as prescription drugs, surgery, prayer, massage, exercise, play, and many, many others.

The natural state of the body is to heal itself, to have abundant energy, and to have no pain. Disease or imbalance occurs when people deprive themselves of physical, mental, emotional, or spiritual needs. Symptoms such as constipation, headaches, pain, depression, and low energy are wake-up calls. The individual who makes the necessary changes may prevent both acute and chronic illness. By removing the resistances that are self-inflicted and by providing needed nourishment instead, the mind and immune system can become powerful allies for health maintenance and restoration.

WHAT IS A NURSE HEALER?

Nurses are health professionals who provide services for health promotion, restoration, maintenance, and general well-being. Nurses support, nurture, cherish, and care to enable healthy growth and development throughout the lifespan. Involving patients and their families in decision making for health and well-being is an important part of nursing. Two terms associated with facilitative decision making are *empowerment* and *capacity building*. Empowered patients have control over and confidence in their decision making, which is central to health promotion and healing. However, nurses do not empower patients. Patients become empowered by mobilizing their own strengths, abilities, and resources. This is called **capacity building**, which is a developmental process that results in independence and self-confidence. Nurses facilitate the capacity of patients to empower themselves through trust, support, guidance, and education.

Nurse healers help patients discover what they need to heal and meet those needs. Nurses help patients find their own definition of health and set their own goals for healing. They are empowered to help themselves by helping themselves feel worthwhile and capable, in control of their lives. Furthermore, by learning how to care for themselves, they make positive change in their lives.

Being a nurse healer means many things. It is about **presence,** or being with another in a meaningful way, giving of one's self in the current moment; listening, and providing unconditional acceptance (Potter & Frisch, 2007). These are the most important qualities. Nurses who put presence into their practice help their patients feel cared for and safe and may assist them in listening to their own inner voice to discover what they need to heal.

Nurse healers speak with the patient and/or family about their health goals, needs, and strategies for meeting needs. They may choose to practice and teach holistic healing techniques that they find effective. Some of these may include Therapeutic Touch, massage, Healing Touch, or reflexology. These nurses teach the patient and/or the patient's family about self-care, and may give them information about nutrition, herbs, communication, exercise, meditation, visualization, and prayer.

Finally, nurse healers begin to apply holistic principles in her own life including:

- Examining thoughts and feelings about healing and nursing.
- Being aware of thoughts, tones of voice, and words used when with the patient.
- Incorporating the use of holistic healing techniques into the nurse's own life.

Nurses are much more effective in teaching patients about the benefits of holistic health care when they speak from personal experience. They can choose how and where they want to begin to try some holistic ideas. They need not wait until all of these ideas have been fully incorporated into life to begin sharing them with patients. Nurses can teach as they learn.

HOLISTIC NURSING: PAST, PRESENT, AND FUTURE

Where did this "new" form of healing begin? It may be helpful to look at the history of holistic healing and its place in nursing.

THE PAST

Holistic healing is as old as humankind. Early tribes all over the world believed that all things in the universe were connected. Humankind, the animals, sky, rocks, sun, rain, plants—all had spirits that affected and were intimately related to each other. These cultures had shamans or medicine men and women to help them in the healing process. As described in Chapter 1, the healing practices of the Greeks of 700 BCE–CE 300 centered on the ideals of holism. They believed that the ideal was to have balance in all areas of life with a strong mind, body, and spirit. Many healing temples existed for hundreds of years that incorporated healing techniques including looking at dreams, music, art, massage, rest, laughter, hot baths, herbs, diet, and feelings of love and kindness. The primary belief of Hippocrates, the father of modern medicine, was that the purpose of the healer was to help the body heal itself.

Beginning as early as 2000 BCE and continuing to the present, a very holistic form of medicine has been practiced in India called **ayurveda**. Ayurveda, as a healing modality, recognizes the holistic concept of body, mind, and soul connectedness and covers all aspects of health and wellness in life from birth to death (Qutab, 2005). This form of healing focuses on physical health and spiritual growth, using meditation, sound,

---

🚶 HEALTH PROMOTION THEORY LINK

CAM use in Europe

Complementary therapies have historically been more popular in Europe than in the United States. Herbs are commonly used in CAM. A majority of research on herbs has been conducted in Germany, and herbs are an integral part of German health care. Across the world, CAM therapies are the main mode of health care. One estimation is that 70–90% of persons worldwide use complementary therapies as a routine part of their health care.

In the first Europe-wide study of CAM and cancer patients, members of the European Oncology Nursing Society surveyed 956 patients in clinics in 14 countries. They found that the use of CAM varied from a low of just under 15% of cancer patients in Greece to a high of nearly three-quarters of patients in Italy. Patients' ages ranged from 17 to 91 years, and over 60% were women. In most countries approximately a third used CAM, with only Italy, the Czech Republic, and Switzerland showing high levels of use and Greece showing very low levels. CAM users tended to be female, younger, and more highly educated, and patients with poor prognosis used CAM significantly more often than other patients. A total of 58 different CAM therapies were used with herbs, specific to each country, as the most common treatment. Homeopathy was among the top five therapies used in seven countries, as were medicinal teas, with vitamins or minerals appearing in the top five in nine countries. Spiritual therapies were more strongly reported by Israel, Denmark, Italy, Spain, Greece, and Iceland.

Sources: Snyder, M., & Lindquist, R. (2001). Issues in complementary therapies: How we got to where we are. *The Online Journal of Nursing Issues, 6*(2); retrieved from http://www.nursingworld.org; European Society of Cardiology (2005, February 8). Third of European cancer patients use complementary and alternative therapies. *Science Daily*.; retrieved from http://www.sciencedaily.com/releases/2005/02/050205080531.htm

massage, herbs, the breath, and types of food specific to the individual to help balance the body and its energy field.

Fabiola, considered the patron saint of nursing, established the first free Christian hospital in Rome in CE 390. In approximately CE 800, nursing came to be regarded as the work of God because it was caring for the sick with no expectation of earthly reward. By the 1300s, orders of nursing nuns had begun using caring, nurturing, prayers, songs, and herbs for healing. In the 1700s, the religious hospitals began to close, leaving only city hospitals. The religious hospitals had had gardens, clean water, and lots of room, with nurses who ministered to the spirit of the patients.

At the time when hospitals were places to go to die instead of to get better, Florence Nightingale entered the world of health care. In 1854, at the age of 38, she became the head of the nurses in a hospital during the Crimean War. She and her 39 nurses cleaned the filthy sickrooms, fixed nutritious meals, opened windows, and cared for wounds. Nightingale believed that if the nurse could provide the basics for the mind, body, and spirit, nature could do the healing. Within a 5-year time frame, she reduced the mortality rate from 60% to 1%. She was the first nurse to prove that quality nursing care could affect healing (Joel, 2006).

Until the discovery of sulfa in the 1930s, America was on its way to creating a very holistic health care system. There were homeopathic medical schools in America, physicians in their practices were using reflexology, and light and color were being used in hospitals. With the advent of drugs, these modalities were considered nonscientific.

In the 1940s, Scherrer discovered that experiencing stress affected the endocrine system. In 1956, Hans Selye proposed his General Adaptation Theory. Many nursing theories are built on this theory stating that, if organisms do not cope well with the stressors of life, physical and mental imbalance and disease will result (Selye, 1956). This was the beginning of research into the connections between the thoughts of the mind, the feelings, and the health of the body.

THE PRESENT

Two important nurse theorists made great contributions to holistic healing. In the 1970s, Dr. Martha Rogers, RN, introduced the idea that the nurse, the patient, and everything in their environments are interconnected and constantly interacting. In the mid-1970s, Dr. Dolores Krieger, RN, began doing research on her technique Therapeutic Touch, which uses the hands to help balance the energy field to aid healing.

During the 1970s, holistic healing centers sprang up in many cities in America. The majority of the health care community, including physicians and nurses, did not yet believe that the philosophies and techniques of holistic healing were sound or had much to do with health. At that time, little research had been done in America on the mind-body-spirit health connection or on holistic techniques. Much of the rest of the world was using both traditional holistic techniques and so-called modern medicine.

Some pioneers, however, among physicians, nurses, psychologists, and other health care providers, supported the benefits and practices of holistic healing. They began giving seminars and writing books for the public, providing testimony in favor of holistic techniques. By 1975, reflexology, massage, Therapeutic Touch, polarity, color, sound, music, fasting, herbs, diet, yoga, and meditation were all becoming more popular.

From all walks of life, people were beginning to search for and find answers to how they could understand the body-mind-spirit connection and heal themselves. This popularity was evidenced in 1998, when the National Center for Complementary and Alternative Medicine (NCCAM) became one of the 27 institutes and centers that make up the National Institutes of Health (NIH). NCCAM recently reported on a nationwide government survey conducted in 2007, revealing that 38%, or two in five of U.S. adults age 18 years and older, and 12% of children, or one in nine, use some form of **complementary and alternative medicine (CAM)** (see Figure 19-1).

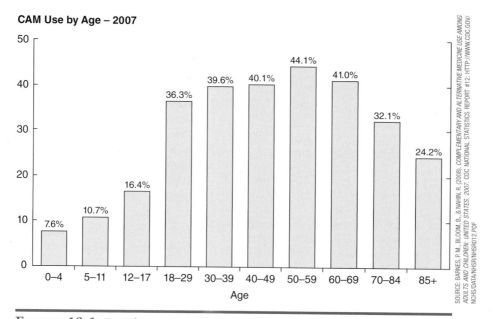

SOURCE: BARNES, P. M. BLOOM, B. & NAHIN, R. (2008). COMPLEMENTARY AND ALTERNATIVE MEDICINE USE AMONG ADULTS AND CHILDREN: UNITED STATES, 2007. CDC NATIONAL STATISTICS REPORT #12: HTTP://WWW.CDC.GOV/NCHS/DATA/NHSR/NHSR012.PDF

FIGURE 19-1 Complementary and Alternative Medicine use among adults and children: United States, 2007.

National Center for Complementary and Alternative Medicine (NCCAM) defines CAM as a group of diverse medical and health care systems, practices, and products that are not currently considered to be conventional medicine or that is practiced by medical doctors or other health professionals, such as physical therapists, psychologists, and registered nurses (NCCAM, 2008). More specifically, complementary modalities are used as an adjunct to conventional medicine, while alternative modalities are used instead of conventional medicine.

Reflective of the growing interest in holistic healing, the American Holistic Nurses Association (AHNA) and the American Holistic Medical Association were established in the early 1980s by Charlotte McGuire, RN, and Norm Shealy, MD (cofounder), respectively. By the late 1980s, membership in AHNA was growing, and the organization was defining itself. Nurse researchers such as Erickson, Parse, Newman, and others were proposing nursing theories that addressed body-mind-spirit environment. Nurses all over the world are now researching, practicing, and teaching Therapeutic Touch, Healing Touch, and Holistic Nursing in hospitals, universities, clinics, private practices, and with families and friends. It is now possible to become a Certified Holistic Nurse. The AHNA endorses certificate programs in aromatherapy, guided imagery and visualization, and holistic nursing.

THE FUTURE

Nurses have always been holistic healers in theory and practice. What makes nurses unique, with regard to other health care professionals, is that they have always looked at the patient's total inner and outer environment, and its relationship to body, mind, and spirit. Martha Rogers brought the study of energy fields to nursing before they were part of popular conversation.

Now many health professionals are realizing that people are not happy and healthy if only the body or only the mind or only the environments are taken into consideration. Nurses have been doing this all along. Holistic care fits well within the nursing model of practice that emphasizes disease prevention and health promotion, health restoration, and health maintenance.

In the future, nurses will be primary consultants, teachers, and practitioners of holistic healing in the hospital, home health, private practice, and educational settings. Nurses are already leading practitioners of holistic modalities. The potential exists for holistic healing clinics in every state with nurses as directors and practitioners. It is time for nurses to take leadership roles in the research, teaching, and practice of holistic healing as a unique role in the emerging new paradigm of health care.

THE NURSE-PATIENT RELATIONSHIP

Attitudes about healing that allow individuals their own unique views of health and to explore all avenues toward that health create an open mind and heart where many possibilities can emerge. Individual nurses' attitude about healing and about themselves influences the type and quality of the nurse-patient relationship. Because holistic nursing involves the entire world of the patient, nurses become part of that world. The way nurses view themselves, their personal thoughts and feelings, and how perceptions about patients when providing care for them all play a part in the quality of the healing relationship.

THE NURSE'S ATTITUDE ABOUT HEALING

Healing does not always mean a perfectly functioning body, a totally clear mind, or being completely happy. As nurses begin working with patients, it is helpful to examine their personal definition of healing. This definition greatly affect how one interacts with patients. If the word *heal* comes from the word *hal* which means whole, what does *wholeness* mean? Nurses can ask what is needed to feel whole or to heal. Wholeness or health is a balance of body, mind, emotions, and spirit that is unique to each individual. Often healing requires making change of some kind. Nurses' attitude about what healing colors all interactions with patients and can enhance or hinder their healing.

THE NURSE'S ATTITUDE ABOUT SELF

A characteristic of a great nurse is the presence with which the nurse moves through all aspects of life, especially when with patients. To contemplate presence, or being, the nurse can look within and explore the inner self.

For nurses to fully practice holistic healing, they must be willing to look at themselves: their comfort in body, feelings, thoughts, and world; discovering where they are happy and where they are not. In the areas where they are not happy, they must begin to choose changes in thoughts, feelings, and actions. To be the most effective healer possible, nurses must be able to choose their responses to the unpleasant as well as to the pleasant circumstances in life.

Everyone is in a constant state of Becoming. The healing work is creating the balance between Being and Becoming. As people are more conscious or awake in each moment, they realize that healing is the balance between Being present in the moment (just observing) and Becoming, which is learning, changing, and growing. When people are still, they feel their feelings, discover their needs, listen to others, and create an open space for intuition to arise. When people are Becoming, they are open to pursuing opportunities that come their way for growth, learning, and service. These opportunities are constantly leading all people along their own unique healing journey. Whichever area is focused on most eventually leads to the balance of both. The path is different for each one. Some begin with great personal awareness and few techniques to share with patients. Others know many techniques but have not yet become comfortable with themselves.

Nurses who desire to enhance their healing abilities must become conscious in the moment. All people are responsible for the thoughts and tones of voice they choose to have and the words they choose to speak. Positive thoughts or affirmations increase confidence, energy, and hope, whereas those that are negative result in the tightening of the body as well as increases in blood pressure, breathing, and heart rate (Dossey & Keegan, 2005). Assessing and analyzing our thoughts enhances our ability to clarify our goals, examine our options, and gain control of situations we encounter.

Negative emotions experienced by the nurse, including such feelings as inferiority, frustration, sadness, or anger, should be recognized as a red flag to stop and reflect. The nurse's environment away from work affects the type of person the nurse is with patients. If events of life are stressful, the nurse may use many techniques to create an outer world that is healing.

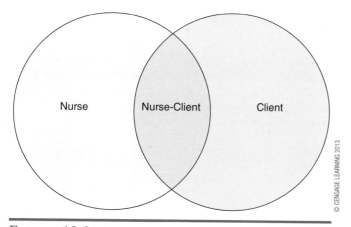

© CENGAGE LEARNING 2013

FIGURE 19-2 The nurse-client relationship.

INTERACTION BETWEEN NURSE AND PATIENT

There are three parts to the nurse-patient relationship, as depicted in Figure 19-2. Given their role, nurses cannot directly change the patient. Only the patient can do that. What nurses may do is look at the interaction between themselves and the patient. As health care professionals, the nurse should be able to be more conscious in the interactions between the self and the world, as well as discover that transforming relationships can occur—helping to get both the nurse's and the patient's needs met. So all parties benefit.

Being conscious in the moment, or choosing responses to others, may be more difficult than it sounds. As a nurse enters a patient's room with every intention of being kind and caring, the patient may react negatively because the call light was not answered fast enough or the pillow is not in the right place. Such reactions may create a negative feeling in the nurse, but the nurse who is conscious in the moment will recognize the emotion, analyze why it is being felt, and choose a caring response.

Certain questions often cut through the exterior gruffness and get to the heart of the connection: "What can I do for you?" "What do you need?" If a nurse views all people and patients as precious beings, then the actions selected help everyone heal.

Words, tone of voice, and body language help to create a feeling of trust and caring. Behaviors that help people feel safe are eye contact; soft, low tones of voice; sitting close to patients; touching or holding their hand; really listening to what is being said and not being said; and smiling. The nurse must use judgment to decide which of these is most effective with different patients.

When a person feels safe, it is easier to open up and explore what is needed to heal. This varies with each individual. The nurse must ask each patient what he thinks he needs to heal. One patient who is an athlete with a broken leg may want to be able to run again, a patient with emphysema may want to breath without having to think about it, and another may want to make it through a day without grieving for her deceased child. When needs are met, healing is facilitated. Table 19-1 provides tips for the nurse to help patients discover and meet their needs. The questions and statements in the table are related to five major areas in which the nurse can determine the needs of patients and involve them in a plan for meeting those needs. These tips are applicable to patients or clients as

TABLE 19-1 Tips for Helping Patients Discover Their Needs	
1. Description	Describe what is happening to you. What do you think it this is related to? What do you think caused this to happen?
2. Needs	Has this happened to you in the past? What has helped you feel better in the past? What will help you feel better now? You know best what you need to heal.
3. Expectations	What do you think is going to happen? What would you like to have happen?
4. Resources	How can you help yourself? How can I help you to help yourself? Who else can help you?
5. Goal	When do you think you will feel better? What would it take to have that happen?

© Cengage Learning 2013

⊕ HEALTH PROMOTION THEORY LINK

Erickson's Theory of Modeling and Role Modeling

Dr. Helen Erickson, RN, developed the Theory of Modeling and Role Modeling, which says that, for people to heal, their needs must be met. Sometimes nurses or family members can meet those needs for the patient. Sometimes the nurse helps patients discover their needs and how to meet them. To meet those needs, patients must look at the stressors in their lives and resources for coping with those stressors. Nurses can be most facilitative when they have made the effort to acknowledge and understand patients as individuals and to see situations through the world of the patient (**modeling**)—a world reflective of life's experiences, values, culture, knowledge, and so forth. In **role modeling**, the nurse plans interventions that facilitate growth, development, and healing at the patient's own pace based on the unique model of the patient's world.

Sources: Erickson, M. E. (2002). Modeling and role-modeling. In A. M. Tomey & M. R. Alligood. *Nursing theorists and their work* (5th ed.). St. Louis: Mosby, pp. 443–464; Frisch, N. C., & Bowman, S. S. (2002). The modeling and role-modeling theory. In J. B. George, *Nursing theories: The base for professional nursing practice* (5th ed.). Upper Saddle River, NJ: Prentice Hall, pp. 463–487.

SPOTLIGHT **ON**

Being Conscious in the Moment

Sara is a staff nurse caring for 10 patients on a busy medical-surgical unit. It's been a very hectic day, but her shift is nearly over. Mr. R's call light is on. She hurries to answer it after being stopped for a moment by the charge nurse asking Sara to work an extra 4 hours. As she arrives in Mr. R's room, he shouts angrily, "Where've you been? Why doesn't anyone give me attention?" He continues to complain about his bed, the room temperature, and lack of service. Sara takes a deep breath, pulls a chair close to his bed, makes direct eye contact, and says, "I'm here now. How can I help you to feel better?"

? ASK **YOURSELF**

Using a Framework to Meet Needs

Do you encourage yourself and others to evaluate situations, discover needs, identify expectations, review resources, and define goals? Have you used this framework for decision making? How did it make you feel? How do you think it would make a patient feel?

individuals, families, groups, or communities. Inherent is the interaction between the nurse and patient whereby the nurse creates a safe, comfortable, and caring space allowing the discovery of the patient's needs, strengths, and resources needed to create goals and plan interventions that promote health and well-being.

HOLISTIC TECHNIQUES FOR HEALTH PROMOTION

Having explored the importance of the nurse's relationship with healing, and the patient, it is important to briefly discuss several holistic healing modalities or tools that may be incorporated into nursing practice. The focus of these tools is to establish and maintain health and well-being rather than to treat a specific illness. These tools may be used by a nurse for personal growth and healing, and they can be shared with family and friends. The nurse can choose those that are appropriate in the practice setting or taught to patients and their families for self-care and health promotion at home. Nurses may teach these techniques to students, other nurses, and health care providers

to use in their practices. This chapter is intended to provide an introduction to these tools and some simple ways to use them in nursing practice.

Very often it is an imbalance or illness that inspires a person to seek any kind of health care, including holistic care. Holistic modalities may be used when there is illness to help restore balance and health to the system. Just as importantly, however, they may maintain health so that disease or illness occurs much less frequently. That is the goal.

As discussed earlier in this chapter, many people incorporate complementary and alternative medicine (CAM) into their lives for health and healing. NCCAM (2008) has noted that the list of what is considered CAM is in constant change as evidence grows regarding the safety and effectiveness of tested therapies and as new approaches to health care are adopted. Table 19-2 identifies major categories of CAM recognized by NCCAM and examples of modalities associated with each.

THE TEACHING AND LEARNING OF HEALING TECHNIQUES

Because many of these techniques or modalities involve teaching in one way or another, it is necessary to examine teaching for a moment. First, there has to be a learner; that is, patients must want the information, connect with how it will meet their needs, and fit with their view of health. Nurses often project onto people their own definition of health and their own health goals. If they are not the same as the learner's, even the best teaching is ineffective.

By listening carefully, the nurse hears exactly what patients need and how best to proceed with teaching.

People are ready for different levels of learning at different times. If many new things are going on in life at the same time, positive or negative, only a small amount of information may be absorbed. Sometimes the nurse must teach in short increments for the patient to learn effectively. Sometimes only one thing can be changed at a time.

When patients learn that they can control their health, they become empowered. How can nurses assist in empowering patients? They can teach them tools to use for health promotion. How can nurses encourage patients to use those tools? Briefly, they can share the benefits of the tools and the results that other people have gotten using these modalities. Nurses must help them realize that the body and mind are designed to feel good most of the time. Pain and emotional upset are warning signals to change something. Nurses can remind patients that they deserve to feel good. Sometimes people have learned from childhood not to expect good health or that individuals have no control over their health. Sometimes people have learned that they are not capable and cannot learn new things or that they do not deserve to be happy and healthy. These are issues of self-esteem. Cognitive learning theories from educational psychology present effective methods for teaching people new information.

To learn and to change, people must feel they are in control of their environment or have the ability to choose and affect their environment. If individuals feel safe and are asked, they know best what they need to create health and happiness in their lives or at least to take a first step. The nurse can ask these questions, help the patient explore choices, and become a key figure in the empowerment of patients.

TABLE 19-2 CAM Categories of Practice and Examples of Associated Modalities

CAM CATEGORY AND DESCRIPTOR	ASSOCIATED MODALITIES EXAMPLES	
Natural products include natural substances, special diets, or vitamins (in doses outside those used in conventional medicine).	Herbal medicine (unrefined plant-based products) Phytotherapy (plant derivatives) Botanical medicine (herbs and plants) Orthomolecular medicine (other nutritional supplements) Probiotics (live organisms such as in yogurt)	
Movement therapies include those from Eastern and Western cultures that promote physical, mental, emotional, and spiritual well-being	Feldenrais method Alexander Techniques Pilates Rolfing Structural Integration Trager Psychophysical Integration	
Traditional healers are also considered a form of CAM.	Traditional healers, such as American Indians, use methods based on indigenous theories, beliefs, and experiences handed down from generation to generation.	
Energy medicine based on energy fields (magnetic or biofields) subcategorized as veritable, which can be measured and putative, which have yet to be measured.	Reiki and Johrei (Japanese) Qi Gong (pronounced "chee-GUNG") (Chinese) Healing Touch Therapeutic Touch	Huna (Hawaiian) Bioelectromagnetics Intercessory prayer (prayer on behalf of another)
Manipulative and body-based practices are based on the manipulation or movement of one or more body parts.	Chiropractic manipulation Craniosacral therapy (skull massage) Feldenrais method (movement) Massage therapy (pressure and movement) Reflexology (foot and hand massage)	Rolfing (deep tissue massage) Trager bodywork (slight rhythmic rocking and shaking of the body) Tui Na (pressure on acupoints) Pilates exercise
Mind-body medicine uses techniques for enhancing the mind's ability to affect bodily functions and symptoms.	Relaxation hypnosis Visual imagery Meditation Yoga Biofeedback Tai Chi	Qi Gong Cognitive-behavioral therapies Group support Autogenic training Spirituality
Whole medical systems based on complete theory and practice developed apart from conventional Western medical practice.	Traditional Chinese medicine (TCM) Ayurvedic medicine (India) Homeopathy Naturopathy	Other systems from various cultures (Native American, African, Middle Eastern, Tibetan, and Central and South American)

Source: National Center for Complementary and Alternative Medicine (NCCAM). (2008). The use of complementary and alternative medicine in the United States; retrieved from nccam.nih.gov; Catalano, J. T. (2006). *Nursing now! Today's issues, tomorrow's trends*. Philadelphia: F. A. Davis.

USING ENERGY AS A HEALING TOOL

What is energy? **Energy** is a dynamic quality or power with the capacity for doing work. The concept of the energy field in nursing is not a new one. Martha Rogers, considered to be one of the first nurse theorists, proposed her theory, the Science of Unitary Human Beings, in 1970. This theory suggests that all living things are continually interacting energy fields and that these fields are infinite in space and time connecting all things, even at great distances. Some say the **energy field** is a field of energy composed of constantly changing vibrational frequencies that surrounds and connects all matter. According to Dr. Rogers, people and all living things are energy fields that affect and are affected by all other forms of energy, creating health and disease. Rogers based much of her theory on Albert Einstein's work in physics. He found that all matter is energy in motion. Therefore, the nurse, patient, family, and the total environment of all of them are continually affecting each other.

Dr. Dolores Krieger, RN, used Martha Rogers's theory as the foundation of her work on therapeutic touch (TT) (Krieger, 2002). In **therapeutic touch**, the caregiver uses the hands to facilitate the balance of the energy field in order to enhance relaxation and healing. TT is used by thousands of nurses worldwide in all types of nursing scenarios.

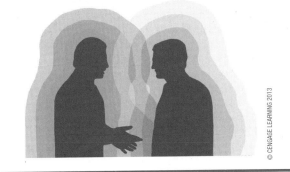

FIGURE 19-4 Interaction of human energy fields.

SPOTLIGHT **ON**

Roots of Biofield Therapeutics

The biofield is the energy field around the body. Biofield therapeutics, often called energy healing or the laying on of hands, is one of the oldest forms of healing known to humans. The earliest Eastern references are from China dating nearly 4,000 years ago. Hieroglyphics depict biofield healings in ancient Egypt. Hippocrates, in ancient Greece, is credited with coining the term *biofield* as "the force which flows from many people's hands." Over 25 terms for biofield have been identified from various cultures the world over.

body being the most dense area of the field. She reports that the human field extends 2–3 ft around the body. It is composed of layers of different vibrational frequencies, colors, and patterns that respond very quickly to thoughts and feelings, especially those held over long periods of time. Figure 19-3 depicts the four major layers of the human energy field, and Figure 19-4 shows how human energy fields can interact.

Human energy fields are not separate from but are part of, or connected with, the universal field, or Higher Power, as understood by the individual. Within the energy field layers are **chakras**, which are spinning wheels of energy that help move healing energy from the universal field through the layers of the individual field (spiritual, mental, emotional, etheric) to the human body. This is visualized in Figure 19-5. The body uses this energy to maintain health.

Dora Kunz, the co-originator of TT, was born with the ability to see energy fields of living objects and used her perceptions as a guide for the hands-on healing of TT (Eliopoulos, 2009). The energy field contains several layers of varying frequencies of vibration: one corresponding to the body, one to thoughts, one to feelings, and one to spirit, with the physical

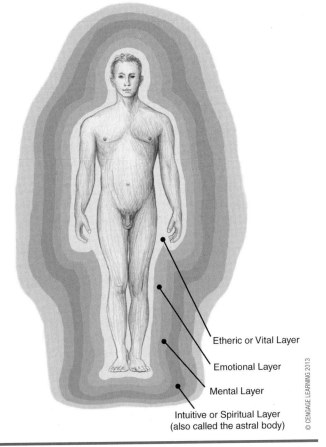

Etheric or Vital Layer

Emotional Layer

Mental Layer

Intuitive or Spiritual Layer
(also called the astral body)

FIGURE 19-3 Layers of the human energy field extending beyond the physical boundaries.

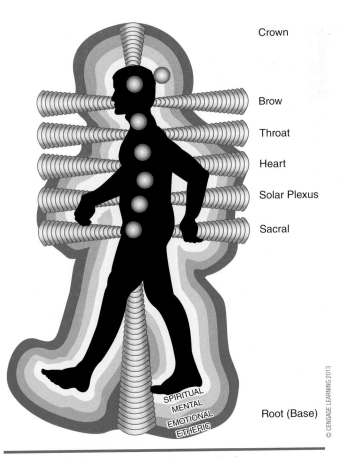

Crown

Brow

Throat

Heart

Solar Plexus

Sacral

SPIRITUAL
MENTAL
EMOTIONAL
ETHERIC

Root (Base)

FIGURE 19-5 The chakras in relation to the human energy fields.

Many researchers have studied and continue to study the characteristics of the energy field around living things, how it changes in health and disease, and what can be done to promote health (Jobst et al., 2009; Hover-Kramer, 2009; Krieger, 2002; Kreitzer & Snyder, 2002; Leigh, 2004).

The energy field, including the functions of the chakras, have been part of ayurvedic medicine for hundreds of years. The fields and chakras have specific connections to feelings, thoughts, endocrine glands, and nerve plexus. Balancing the chakras and energy field can aid the healing and maintain balance in areas of the body that correspond to the chakra areas (Hover-Kramer, 2009; Krieger, 2002). For example, the second chakra, sacral, is below the navel, and balancing it aids in the function of the intestines.

The energy field is constantly vibrating because it is constantly moving when the person is healthy and in balance. An imbalance in the mind, body, or spirit is reflected in the energy field and can be perceived through the hands as an area in the field that is not moving, as it should. The Law of Resonance in physics says anything that vibrates is affected by all other vibrations. When nurses look at what may help to balance the energy field, they consider light, color, sound, music, and thought because all of these are forms of energy waves or vibrations. The energy coming from the hands is also a form of vibration affecting the field.

Considered controversial by some, the North American Nursing Diagnosis Association (NANDA, 2008) has included "Disturbed Energy Field-00050" as a diagnostic domain. NANDA addresses the definition of this diagnostic domain as well as the following areas: related factors, defining characteristics, desired outcomes/evaluation criteria, actions/interventions, and documentation focus. Nursing interventions such as Therapeutic Touch and Healing Touch address this diagnosis.

THE POWER OF THOUGHTS AND FEELINGS

Thoughts and feelings are forms of energy with vibrations that affect personal energy fields and those of others near and far. Only in the last 25 years have people begun to realize that what is thought and felt is a strong determinant of health or illness. Prior to this time, thoughts and feelings were considered unimportant to health, perhaps because they seem to have no material substance, are fleeting, and are "only in the mind."

Almost 20 years ago, the formalized study of the body-mind connection called psychoneuroimmunology (PNI) was born. PNI, discussed in detail in Chapter 8, is the study of how thoughts and feelings affect the body. Much research has been done to discover the effects of different thoughts and feelings on the health of the body. Emotional states such as anger, fear, depression, learned helplessness, joy, and perceived control have been examined to determine their effects on different aspects of physiology, such as the immune, cardiovascular, digestive, and endocrine systems.

One very important example of PNI is **learned helplessness** (Abramson, Seligman, & Teasdale, 1978), which holds that, if one believes one has no control over one's experience (whether positive or negative) or that what one does cannot get a positive outcome, one learns to become helpless. Some characteristics of learned helplessness are decreased immune function, lack of motivation and creativity, and depression. It affects health, as well as success in school, job, and relationships.

Learned helplessness may be reversed when persons learn that they can affect their world.

Thoughts and feelings cause chemicals to be released from the brain and the organs of the immune and endocrine systems. These chemicals travel through the bloodstream and enhance or depress the functions of all the others. What people habitually think and feel, or worry about, causes physiologic change in the body.

Knowing about PNI is important for nurses who may feel out of control, angry, frustrated, or depressed in the work setting. These feelings can lead to stress and the burnout syndrome. If the nurse feels out of control at work, this may often be balanced by incorporating even one regularly practiced stress management technique into work or home life.

Patients often feel helpless when they are in a health care setting. Realizing the deleterious effects on health that these feelings can create, the nurse can find ways to help patients feel more in control of their experiences. Some of these ways might be choosing what they want to eat and when, what they wear, when visitors come, when activities are scheduled, and any other choices they can possibly make. The nurse may also encourage patients to focus on being hopeful and appreciative because both have positive effects on the body.

Thoughts are also very powerful in the area of stress. It is not what happens, but how events are perceived, that creates a physiological stress response. Patterns of faulty thinking lead to cognitive distortion that has a negative effect on our thoughts, behaviors, and experience with stress. A situation occurs and a reaction results before the situation is fully assessed. This reaction is often anger, fear, resentment, guilt, or another negative emotion. Such feelings and words set the stress response in motion with all of its physiologic, mental, and emotional outcomes. In communication with others, words often happen so fast that they may go from being kind and friendly in one moment to being curt and angry in the next.

How can one learn to be aware of thoughts and therefore be selective among responses? **Cognitive restructuring**, also known as cognitive reframing, is a process of recognizing, challenging, and changing cognitive distortions and negative thought patterns (Scott, 2007). With cognitive restructuring, individuals can learn to control those thoughts in a positive and realistic way. When people are able to change their thinking, they can approach their daily lives and problems with more energy, control, and confidence.

Box 19-1 describes cognitive restructuring tips for recognizing and changing thoughts. Nurses may use these suggestions for themselves and teach their patients as part of their self-care, which fosters empowerment.

People's perceptions of and responses to stress are considered to contribute to the majority of all disease. Nurses can therefore no longer dismiss symptoms as, "Oh, it's just stress." They must address the causes of stress.

The problem is never only one event for a short time. When many stressful events continue for prolonged periods, health problems result. Nurses can help patients look at all of the factors in their lives that are stressful over a long period and help them see how and where they can make changes.

THE BREATH

The breath is a powerful tool for balancing the body for healing and promoting health. It is the one part of the autonomic nervous system that may easily be controlled. The autonomic

---

BOX 19-1

COGNITIVE RESTRUCTURING TIPS FOR RECOGNIZING AND CHANGING THOUGHTS

Cognitive restructuring begins by evaluating your thoughts and fears, as well as whether they are rational or irrational. Crating an awareness of thoughts, recognizing the power to change, avoiding negativity, focusing on the positive, and staying in the present are key to restructuring thoughts. Questions to ask yourself are:

- What the is ultimately worst possible outcome of this situation?
- Is this truly harmful to me or my family?
- Am I viewing this situation correctly? What proof is there for my fears?
- Can I really manage this situation even though I have doubts about myself?
- What steps can I take to change this situation?

Source: Adapted from Rodriguez, D. (2011). Cognitive restructuring: Change your thoughts, change your attitude. *Everyday Health*. Retrieved from http://www.everydayhealth.com/emotional-health/ understanding/cognitive-restructuring.aspx

---

BOX 19-2

BREATHING EXERCISE FOR WELL-BEING

1. Find a quiet place.
2. Sit comfortably, extremities uncrossed, and rest your arms in your lap.
3. Focus on how you feel in the moment (mentally, physically, emotionally).
4. Exhale deeply, and contract your stomach muscles at the same time.
5. Inhale slowly, and think about your abdomen expanding.
6. Inhale further, more deeply, expanding your chest and raising your shoulders up toward your ears.
7. Hold the inhaled breath for a few seconds.
8. Slowly exhale, reversing the process: relaxing the shoulders, relaxing the chest, and contracting the stomach muscles until all air is exhaled and your body feels limp.
9. Repeat the process two or three times with increasing ease.
10. Reexamine how you feel in the moment.

---

nervous system affects all automatic functions, such as the immune system for healing, digestion and assimilation, heart rate, and the like. The breath usually occurs automatically, but it may be consciously changed, either the rate or the depth. The rate of breath affects heart rate and brainwaves. Slowing the breath creates relaxation, and speeding it up is stimulating.

Slow, deep, continual breathing has its physical, mental, and emotional benefits. In the stress response, the body shifts to chest breathing. Chest breathing is shallow and quick. Chronic chest breathing can recreate feelings of stress in the body. Slow breaths can create feelings of relaxation and clarity. The lungs can hold 2 pt of air, but the average breath is less than 1 pt. Adequate oxygen is crucial for combining with food to produce heat and energy for the body. Deep breathing can enhance the oxidation of lactic acid in sore muscles, increase physical energy levels, and lead to more efficient metabolism. Slow, diaphragmatic breathing allows the abdomen to expand with the inhale and contract with the exhale. This movement allows the greatest filling of the lungs and is the most relaxing breath. It is generally accepted that slow, diaphragmatic breathing can help to decrease anxiety, release negative emotions, and diminish the stress response. There are many variations of diaphragmatic breathing exercise. Try the breathing exercise suggested in Box 19-2.

Changes in feelings are reflected by changes in breathing. Anger, fear, and sorrow have specific patterns of breathing. Often, unpleasant emotions create a constriction of energy and a holding of the breath. Unconscious reactive decisions and actions often follow. Consciously changing breathing patterns changes the emotion being felt. Full breaths relax the mind and allow a flow of energy to occur that fosters greater choice of word and deed. Deep, slow continual breaths can bring conscious awareness to the present moment, and they offer an opportunity to examine and choose thoughts and feelings.

The spirit and breath have much in common. In fact, the word *breath* is a derivative of the Latin word *spiritus,* which comes from the verb *spirare,* which means to breathe. The breath is our vehicle to consciously still the thoughts of the mind, allowing an experience of our spirit and a connection with a Higher Power.

When nurses have been very busy for the entire shift, "out of breath" and stressed, they can immediately become more still and calm—and reduce stress levels—by taking a few deep breaths. Before entering a patient's room, taking a few deep breaths allows the nurse to bring about an awareness to the present and be better able to choose the feelings and words with which to interact with the patient. Taking 5 minutes at lunch to sit and breathe lets confusion and mental tension drift away and invites a sense of calm and peacefulness.

Learning about the power of the breath for relaxation and the ease with which breathing patterns may be changed is a valuable tool for patients. They may use this tool at any moment to help reduce muscle tension, pain, the anxiety, fear, and depression that often accompany illness.

For health promotion, in the absence of illness, continued deep breathing is energizing, stress reducing, and calming for the ever restless mind and emotions. Focusing on the breath is a beginning step to practicing meditation and imagery because it quiets the mind and brings the person's awareness to the present moment.

IMAGERY

Imagery is another method by which a person may consciously use thoughts and feelings to create a variety of desired physiologic conditions such as relaxation, increased sports performance, or decreased blood pressure. One can focus on the desired outcome and/or the steps that need to be taken to achieve that outcome. **Imagery** focuses on thoughts and feelings and then uses them to create images that are desired to make changes in life. When an image is held in the mind, the body begins responding to it to try to make it happen. Imagery is a communication mechanism between perception, emotion, and bodily change.

The most effective images for creating physical change are those that use all five senses plus movement and emotion. Imagery gives the subconscious mind a plan for constructing reality.

NURSING **ALERT**

Breathe for Relaxation

- At least once every hour remember to take five or six deep, slow, continuous breaths, like long sighs.
- In times of emotional or mental stress, noticing and changing the breathing pattern to a slower, deeper pattern changes the emotional or mental outlook.

Thoughts can also be used to scan the body from head to toe. By focusing in an area, a person can note if the area is holding tension. By directing a breath or two to each area, the tension can melt away with each exhale. Nurses can teach patients and families to use imagery for specific health improvements and for relaxation.

To enhance the effects of imagery, relax first. Progressive relaxation is a very effective technique for becoming aware of

---

SPOTLIGHT **ON**

A Case Study for Imagery

A nurse named Lou was preparing her patient, Mr. B, for surgery. Mr. B was very afraid and did not want to go. Lou asked him to think about his favorite place, a place where he felt safe and comfortable. He told Lou about the flowers, the trees, the weather, the road, the location, and the breeze near the lake he was imagining. Lou handed him a pencil and said, "Take this to surgery. When you feel afraid, hold it, and think of this moment." Mr. B came through surgery just fine. Later, he found Lou and told her that the pencil helped him remember his safe place and that he wasn't afraid. He still comes to see her, a year later.

---

and releasing tension. Tighten and relax each muscle group from feet to head, one at a time. This method can be practiced before imagery or by itself to relax tight areas.

MEDITATION

There are many forms of meditation: Transcendental Meditation, Siddha Yoga, Mindfulness Meditation, and many others. What most have in common is bringing awareness of the everyday, rampant thoughts of the mind. When not focused on hectic or troubling thoughts, the body relaxes, and the stress response ceases. People have the opportunity to experience greater peace and creativity, and they may get in touch with a Higher Power.

Meditation may be done with the body in a stationary position or with movement. Examples of both types are discussed here.

Herbert Benson, MD (1975, 1996), studied many forms of meditation and noticed two steps that most of them have in common. When people practice these steps, which he calls the **Relaxation Response**, they notice a sense of relaxation that interrupts the stress response. Benson has been researching the Relaxation Response since 1975. Box 19-3 describes the two steps in the practice of this technique. The benefits of using the Relaxation Response technique include decreased blood pressure, heart rate, muscle tension, and cardiac dysrhythmias, along with increased alpha brain waves (produced during relaxation and creativity), concentration, ability to cope with stressors, and stimulation of the immune system. It is recommended to practice this 10 minutes, twice a day. If that is impractical, try 5 minutes once a day. It is an easy technique that may be taught to patients, can be practiced anywhere, and can have many physiologic benefits.

T'ai Chi, Qi Gong, and Yoga are three forms of moving meditations. They have been practiced for hundreds of years in China and India for relaxation, balance, and healing of the body, mind, emotions, and spirit. They focus on the breath and

---

NURSING **ALERT**

Using Meditation

Meditation is taking a moment to become conscious of who one is. One simple way for anyone to do this is to set a timer for 5 minutes and sit down, be still, and focus on happy times or thoughts.

---

slow precise movements designed to connect and balance all areas of the physical body, energy field, and the life force or chi (chee) or prana.

As the life force begins to flow freely through the body, the benefits include:

- Stress reduction
- Deeper respirations
- Relaxation of spine and muscles
- Increased energy to the nervous system
- Stimulation of internal organs

These techniques may be learned by watching videotapes, but it is recommended to take classes from teachers

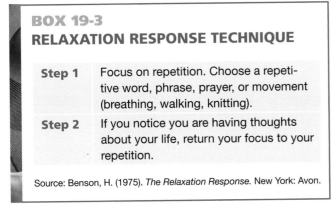

BOX 19-3
RELAXATION RESPONSE TECHNIQUE

| Step 1 | Focus on repetition. Choose a repetitive word, phrase, prayer, or movement (breathing, walking, knitting). |
| Step 2 | If you notice you are having thoughts about your life, return your focus to your repetition. |

Source: Benson, H. (1975). *The Relaxation Response*. New York: Avon.

SPOTLIGHT ON

Using Prayer for Patient Health

Choose a specific patient in your practice to pray for. In three or four 30-second intervals over 2–3 days, offer prayers for that person or send positive thoughts and feelings, wishing the best possible outcome. Assess changes in body, mind, and/or spirit that occur.

who have practiced and taught these techniques for some time. There are classes for all levels of expertise, physical condition, and age.

THE POWER OF PRAYER

Religions the world over believe in the power of prayer. Since humankind began, prayer has been viewed as a way to communicate with a Higher Power and to aid one's self and others. The reports of healing with prayer became so numerous that scientists finally became interested. Spiritual practices such as prayer have been found to positively affect many kinds of living entities such as enzymes, red blood cells, plants, cancer cells, and bacteria (The proof that prayer works, n.d.). Epidemiological and medical literature documents hundreds of studies in which spiritual and religious practices have been statistically associated with positive health outcomes. Opposing views also exist on the merits of prayer on effecting positive health outcomes. The recognition of prayer as a separate complementary or alternative medicine (CAM) modality has become questionable in that there is no conventional understanding of the what prayer is and there is lack of distinction among various forms of spiritual healing used by practitioners (Tippens, Marsman, & Zwickey, 2009). It has been recognized that including prayer in evaluating the use of CAM inflates and distorts statistics; therefore, the most recent assessment of CAM use in the United States does not include prayer. Nonetheless, the role of religious involvement in the promotion of health and well-being is receiving increasing attention from researchers and is integral to providing holistic nursing care.

Prayer has been found to have an effect on one's self as well as on others who are nearby or at great distances. Studies indicate that it does not seem to matter what religion or type of prayer is used. Each person may be inspired to pray in different ways at different times for different reasons: by speaking, singing, chanting, or in silence; individually or in groups; in public or in private; for forgiveness, direction, thanks, concern for others. In fact, prayer has been categorized into four distinct types: (1) adoration (worship and praise for God), (2) confession (faults, misdeeds, sins acknowledged), (3) supplication (requests for divine intervention in a life event), and (4) reception (awaiting divine wisdom, understanding, or guidance) (Laird et al., 2004). Some people include techniques such as visualization, guided imagery, or relaxation, and movement such as walking, dancing, or drumming (Burkhardt & Nagai-Jacobson, 2005).

Dr. Larry Dossey (1994), physician and cochair of the Panel on Mind-Body Interventions of the Office of Alternative Medicine at the National Institutes of Health in Washington, D.C., reported on over 100 studies on the effects of prayer/visualization in his 1994 book, *Healing Words*. More than half showed an effect on everything from seed germination to wound healing and positive effects on hypertension, heart attacks, headaches, and anxiety. Dr. Dossey summarized that the results occurred not only when people prayed for explicit outcomes but also when they prayed for nothing specific.

There are varied reports on the mechanism by which prayer works. Although studies show that people receive images or physical sensations at great distances that others are imaging, there is no energy in the classical physical sense recorded as being sent or received. Quantum physics has discovered through research that a field of energy connects all things in the universe. In this field, nonlocal connections are events that happen between subatomic particles. Nonlocal connections happen instantaneously, where the activity of one particle affects the activity of another even at great distances.

A Higher Power and all things in the universe may be connected by this pervasive field with prayer as a vibrational frequency that helps to amplify the vibrations of health and balance in self and others. Prayer may be letting the mind or daily thoughts go while connecting with, and lending support to, the Universal Whole that connects all things.

The nurse, if so inclined, may pray for and with patients, holding them in thought, and wishing them the best possible outcome. The nurse may educate the patients on the power of prayer as a tool for self-healing.

LIGHT AND COLOR

Light and color have been used for promoting health since ancient times. Around 500 BCE, the Greeks used **heliotherapy**, the use of sunlight for healing. In the early 1900s, hospitals used ultraviolet (UV) light with patients to kill bacteria up to 8 ft away at a strength that would not create redness even on fair skin. UV light has been used as a treatment for tuberculosis, streptococcal infections, viral pneumonia, mumps, the flu virus, and fungal infection of the skin.

Light is energy that is constantly moving in vibrating waves. Colors are the different frequencies (some fast, some slow) of light. Sunlight contains the full visible spectrum of the rainbow plus UV light and many other frequencies.

Sunlight, or full-spectrum light, is nourishing to the human body. Until recent times, humankind lived outside bathed by sunlight. Everyone needs exposure to full-spectrum

BOX 19-4
HEALING EFFECTS OF CONSISTENT NORMAL EXPOSURE TO SUNLIGHT

ENHANCES:	DECREASES:
Tolerance to stress	Lactic acid in the blood following exercise
Energy, strength, and endurance	Blood pressure
Ability of the blood to carry oxygen	Respiratory rate
Ability of the blood to absorb oxygen	Blood sugar
Mood	Resting heart rate

SPOTLIGHT **ON**
Sunlight

In our daily lives, in all seasons, most of us are outside very little. We wear sunglasses and sunscreen when we do go outside. We spend much of our time inside, often in rooms with limited or no outside light. Many of our inside environments have fluorescent lights or incandescent lightbulbs. Could we be creating our own seasonal affective disorder (SAD)?

light every day. The healing effects of sunlight in Box 19-4 can be obtained with as little as 5 minutes a day without UV protection on the eyes or skin. More is not better, however. In homes or hospitals, patients may greatly benefit by sitting by windows or in sunrooms, by going out on porches to look at sunlight, or having sun shine on them for short periods of time.

Dr. John Ott, a pioneer in light research, studied the health effects of full-spectrum light and suggested that malillumination, or lack of adequate full-spectrum light, may be the cause of many physical health problems (Ott, 1973). Today, we know that seasonal affective disorder (SAD) is a type of depression that occurs more commonly in winter when exposure to full-spectrum light is decreased.

Researchers have connected the development of SAD to the regulation of serotonin (wakefulness) and melatonin (sleep-inducing), two hormones regulated by the pineal gland in the brain (Miller, 2005). It is suggested that melatonin contributes to the development of SAD in individuals deprived of sunlight. Sunlight, as shown in Figure 19-6, has a direct neurological pathway via the retina (optic nerve) to the pineal gland. Stimulation by sunlight prevents the pineal gland from converting serotonin to melatonin. When possible, using full-spectrum fluorescent bulbs can create a healthier environment, especially for people who cannot go outside and for nurses working inside. Box 19-5 provides further suggestions for enhancing the healthful benefits from natural light.

Just as people need a wide variety of foods, they also need a wide variety of colors. The ancient Egyptians were the first to have temples of light in which color was used for

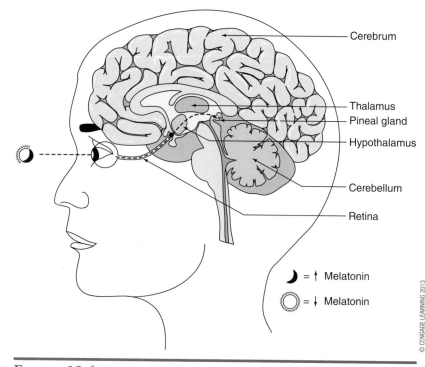

© CENGAGE LEARNING 2013

FIGURE 19-6 The neurological connection between sunlight and melatonin.

BOX 19-5

TIPS TO ENHANCE HEALTHFUL BENEFITS FROM LIGHT

1. Go outside, and allow the sun to shine on your body for at least 5 minutes a day without sunscreen.

2. While outside, avoid using sunglasses, regular glasses, or contact lenses coated to shield UV rays, for 5 minutes a day.

3. Avoid exposure to harmful UV rays, highest between the hours of 10 a.m. and 2 p.m.

4. Trim bushes and trees to allow more natural sunlight through windows.

5. Sleep and work in rooms facing the east.

6. Replace regular fluorescent lightbulbs with full-spectrum fluorescent lighting.

SPOTLIGHT **ON**

Using Color in Practice

- Incorporate all colors into your life for balance.
- Use blue for relaxation and for aiding pain relief.
- Imagine yourself or your patient surrounded by a wash of color that corresponds to the need.

NURSING **ALERT**

Using Care with the Color Red

The color red is stimulating in small amounts but can be energetically overwhelming in large amounts. Red is known to stimulate heart rate, blood pressure, and appetite. Many restaurants use red tablecloths for appetite stimulation. If you are trying to limit food intake, a dark blue or black tablecloth or placemat is a better color choice.

---

healing. Physicians, nurses, optometrists, and chemists have researched the specific effects of the individual colors on the body and mind (Harvard Medical School, 2008). Many health practitioners throughout the twentieth century have used color as therapy, alone and in combination with other therapies.

It has been observed that different colors may also aid the healing of different parts of the body and the mind. Nurses can use the principles of light and color to help themselves, their patients, and patients' families. Table 19-3 lists the general effects of the color spectrum for promoting health. The warm colors are used to stimulate the body, including the function of the liver, pancreas, sinuses, and intestines for digestion, assimilation, and elimination. They can help to loosen chronic congestion. Green can aid the healing of muscles and tissue and balance physical conditions. Magenta (a combination of red and violet) is effective in balancing emotions and physical and emotional heartache. The cool colors are relaxing and used to calm acute conditions. They are effective for anxiety, pain relief, insomnia, boosting immune function, fevers, and skin conditions, and to enhance meditation.

Color can be added to the nursing environment in many creative ways. Pieces of cloth can be put in patients' field of vision, or they can wear colored clothing. Nurses can wear colored uniforms or jackets or pins. Flowers, curtains, and pictures can add color. Visualizing a particular area of the body filled with a color or seeing one's entire person surrounded by a color is also an effective way to use color to promote health. Color may be projected onto the body using colored light bulbs, and plastic or cloth can be put on a window or lamp.

SOUND

Many cultures and religions believe that the world was created by sound. Some American Indian tribes believe that the spoken word "Inyan" was the creative word. In the ayurvedic tradition of India, "om" is a primordial sound believed to be the first breath of creation. The Christian tradition says that in the beginning was the Word. Hans Jenny, MD, and Peter Manners, MD, performed experiments showing that sound creates three-dimensional form. Using sounds from the voice, musical instruments, and other tones, particles of various types of inert matter (such as iron filings suspended in water and oil) formed different three-dimensional shapes and patterns in response to different sounds. These shapes and patterns were very similar to many patterns found in nature. Mandala patterns formed by the sound "om" resemble patterns in snowflakes. Certain sounds produce shapes that resemble the spinal column. Spiral patterns like those seen in sea shells, human fingerprints, the human red blood cell, and many other places are created by certain sounds. Cymatics, the study of patterns of shapes evoked by sound, has shown how sound affects shapes and influences change in shapes (Volk, 2002).

TABLE 19-3 Colors and Associated Energies and Positive Emotions

Red	Survival, security
Orange	Nurturance, creativity, passion
Yellow	Personal power, goals, intellect
Green	Healing, emotions, confidence, compassion
Blue	Calming, communication, mental creativity
Indigo	Intuition, insight
Violet	Spiritual energy, connection to a higher power, healing

Source: Eliopoulos, C. (2009). *Invitation to holistic health: A guide to living a balanced life.* Sudbury, MA: Jones & Bartlett.

TABLE 19-4 Qi Gong Healing Sounds for the Body

Practiced daily, the following sounds benefit certain parts of the body by enhancing the flow of chi, or energy.

ssss	Lungs
haw	Heart
wooo	Kidneys
shhhh	Liver
whoo	Spleen
heee	Body relaxation

Source: Chia, M. (2009). *The six healing sounds: Taoist techniques for balancing chi*. Rochester, VT: Destiny Books.

Using one's voice is the most effective way to use sound to balance one's own energy field. The voice may also be used to help balance the energy field of others. Toning is one way to use the voice for healing. When toning, people get comfortable, take a breath, and let sounds come spontaneously. The body knows what sound vibrations it needs to balance or heal itself. Sounds can be made quietly if in a public place. At home, let the sound come out in whatever tone or volume it emerges. Spending 1–60 minutes per day toning can be relaxing, rejuvenating, and healing, and the practice can aid in pain relief.

The vagus nerve is one way that the effects of sound are carried throughout the body. The vibrations of sound are also transmitted through the bones of the skeleton.

The tones of words can greatly affect the listener and the tension level of muscles. Sound activates memory and feeling. Primordial sounds that are used in ayurvedic medicine are thought to vibrate certain areas of the body, bringing them into balance. Table 19-4 offers some healing sounds for specific body areas used in Qi Gong, which is a component of traditional Chinese medicine that combines movement, meditation, breathing, and sound to enhance the flow of qi, or vital energy, in the body to improve blood circulation and enhance immune function.

Environmental sounds, those within and those beyond people's control, can create states of relaxation or tension. Sounds of nature such as running water, rain, the ocean, birds, and frogs can create relaxation. Sounds like motorcycles, lawn mowers, airplanes, traffic, and machines can cause the body and mind to feel tense.

MUSIC

Sound in the form of music has been a part of healing rituals as revealed in some of the oldest accounts of medical practices. Its effect on health can be explained by modern physics.

According to physics, all vibrations are rhythm, or repeated patterns. Vibrations are waveforms. In passive resonance, a waveform triggers a vibration in a resting source. Active resonance or entrainment happens when one vibrating source changes the vibration of another vibrating object. Music consists of vibrations with rhythm or repeated patterns. Music with 60 beats/minute, such as some Mozart largos, have been found to entrain the heartbeat, lowering it from 72–68, and to entrain brain waves, lowering them to alpha frequencies of 3–7 cycles/second. Alpha frequencies are those of meditation, relaxation,

SPOTLIGHT ON

Using Sound and Music in Nursing Practice

Here are some suggestions for using music for yourself and for your patients.

1. For stress relief, start with music that matches your current feelings. If you are stressed, pick something with a fast rhythm. After 5 minutes, switch to something slower and more relaxing.

2. Be mindful of your tone of voice when speaking to patients. A lower-pitched voice at a slower pace can be very calming.

3. Teach patients and families about toning techniques for the release and balancing of feelings and tension in the body.

4. Encourage the family to bring a recording of the patient's favorite music. If they do not know what the patient likes, you can suggest some of the following for balancing the entire body:
   a. Nature sounds—frogs, waves
   b. Indian ragas—tabla and sitar, Ravi Shankar, for example
   c. Gregorian chants—medieval church music
   d. Largos—a type of classical music such as in Mozart largos

5. Take 5 minutes of silence and stillness each day, even if you must use earplugs.

and creativity. Lullabies played in neonatal intensive care nurseries have been found to entrain the breathing rhythms of babies to the rhythm of the music, resulting in a decrease in the amount of time needed for the discharge of premature babies.

Many studies have been done on the beneficial effects of music to promote the health of the body. Some of the effects range from decreasing blood pressure, respirations, blood levels of ACTH, pulse, and heart rate, to increasing beta endorphins that promote feelings of well-being. These beneficial results are most often found when the music is of the patient's choosing (Dunn, 2004).

ENERGY-BASED THERAPIES: THERAPEUTIC TOUCH AND HEALING TOUCH

Energy as a healing tool was discussed earlier in this chapter. Two specific modalities originated by nurses that use energy as a healing tool are Therapeutic Touch (TT) and Healing Touch (HT). With these modalities, the hands are used to perceive and help to balance the energy field that exists around all living things. TT focuses on balancing the entire field with attention to areas in the field where the energy is not moving. HT

RESEARCH NOTE

Music Therapy for Anxiety Reduction in Women with Cancer Receiving Chemotherapy Treatment in Italy

STUDY PROBLEM/PURPOSE

To investigate the effect of musical therapy on anxiety in a population of breast cancer patients receiving conventional chemotherapy medical treatment. This study was the first of its kind to be done in Italy.

METHODS

Using a clinical experimental design, a sample of 60 female patients with stage I–II breast cancer receiving postsurgical chemotherapy treatment were randomized into two groups: the control group receiving standard assistance with no music therapy prior to receiving chemotherapy and an experimental group that was able to choose and listen to pretaped musical themes with Walkman and earphones for 15 minutes prior to receiving chemotherapy. Speilberg's State-Trait Anxiety Inventory–Italian version (STAI-Y) was used to assess self-reported state of anxiety and traits of anxiety before and after receiving chemotherapy.

FINDINGS

The experimental group showed a significant reduction in state anxiety. Comparison of scores on the STAI-Y confirmed the positive effects that music has on cancer patients. Data analyzed suggested that the anxiety levels in both groups were moderate, chemotherapy is an unpleasant and stressful event, and anxiety is problematic for breast cancer patients awaiting chemotherapy.

IMPLICATIONS

On a short-term basis, musical interventions can be useful in nursing practice to reduce anxiety. It is not costly, is noninvasive, and gives the sense of empowerment when the patient is involved in the choice of music. The limitations of this study are that it was a small sample size, which limits generalizability, and it investigated only the short-term effects of music therapy.

Source: Bulfone, T., Quattrin, R., Zanotti, R., Regattin, L., & Brusaferro, S. (2009). Effectiveness of music therapy for anxiety reduction in women with breast cancer in chemotherapy treatment. *Holisti Nursing Practice, 23*(4), 238–242.

it helped them gain weight. Studies have been done indicating that TT aids in pain relief after surgery, is helpful for headaches, and for wound healing. TT has also been shown to decrease respiratory and heart rates, pain, anxiety, nausea, and shortness of breath. It has been shown to increase warmth in extremities and to enhance immune function in both the practitioner and the recipient. TT may be done in 3–20 minutes, is very effective, and is easy to learn and teach to patients and their families.

Healing Touch was founded in 1989 by Janet Mentgen, RN. HT incorporates several energy-based healing techniques including TT, and many of Janet Mentgen's original techniques. HT techniques include balancing the entire field, working with specific techniques for chakra balancing, and working with specific pain problems such as in the spine and migraines.

Energy-based therapies do not require many classes. Legitimacy of the practitioner, however, is provided through certification for some therapies. For example, Healing Touch certification is achieved through completion of a sequence of five courses in addition to documented evidence of practice and mentorship. Almost anyone can learn to feel the energy field and its disturbance with the hands with practice. Practicing the techniques sensitizes the hands and allows the brain to better interpret the signals the hands receive. The brain is not familiar with interpreting non-three-dimensional stimuli. Also in a short time one can learn to help balance the field using TT and HT. For these reasons, both techniques are ideal for teaching to patients and their families for relaxation, pain relief, and wound healing. The Krieger-Kunz method of TT includes four basic phases: (1) centering and grounding; (2) assessment; (3) unruffling; and (4) directing and modulating energy (Bright, 2004).

? ASK YOURSELF

The Energy Field and Nursing

Have you ever walked into a room with people and noticed a particular feeling about the room? If we are connected to others through the interconnections of energy fields, how might our thoughts affect our own and another's field?

TOUCH THERAPIES: REFLEXOLOGY, MASSAGE, AND ACUPRESSURE

One of the most healing things a nurse can ever do for patients is to touch them. Touch conveys more than words ever may. A touch on the arm can say, "I understand, I'm here, I care." Of course, the nurse must use her professional judgment to determine whether a patient is receptive to being touched.

Some nurses may be uncomfortable with simply sitting and holding a patient's hand. Many types of touch can be therapeutic. All nurses should be aware of the importance and use of touch as a therapy. Some techniques, however, require special training, licensure, or certification. With any touch therapy, nurses must observe the following general guidelines:

1. Examine personal feelings about touch.
2. Understand the patient's culture in relation to touch.

addresses the entire field with attention to these areas and the chakras. Nurses may use both techniques on themselves as well as on patients.

Kunz and Krieger began teaching TT to nurses in the early 1970s. Dr. Krieger's early study of TT indicated that it could raise hemoglobin levels. This became the foundation for the research that has followed. Nurses have studied the effects of TT and found it to be beneficial with premature and full-term infants in the neonatal nursery who had respiratory distress, and

3. Obtain the patient's permission to use touch therapy.
4. Respect the patient's privacy.
5. Offer explanations before and during the session.
6. Move slowly.
7. Exercise extra care and gentleness with the frail, elderly, and critically ill, and with infants.
8. Inform the patient when the session is over, allowing time for reorientation.
9. Obtain feedback from the patient.

ASK YOURSELF

Touching a Patient

Have you experienced touch as being especially comforting? How do you feel about touching a patient in a caring way? What does it mean to you to touch a patient in a caring way? How would you feel about sitting down on the bed and holding a patient's hand?

REFLEXOLOGY

Reflexology is an ancient healing technique based on the belief that the entire body is reflected in the ears, eyes, palms of the hands, and soles of the feet. When the pad of the thumb is used to apply pressure to specific points in these areas, it increases circulation and relaxation of the corresponding areas of the body. The right hand and foot correspond to the right side of the body. Applying the reflexology technique to the entire foot, even if the exact points are missed, can provide a feeling of relaxation and well-being for patients. At this time, there is no certification required, so reflexology may be practiced by anyone who feels competent.

There are many anecdotal accounts of the benefits of reflexology. Although there are few scientific studies on this practice in the United States, extensive research has been done in China and Denmark. Pressing a reflexology point is thought to increase circulation to the corresponding areas, bringing nutrients and oxygen and carrying off waste, increasing nerve flow, and removing blockages in the energy field, helping to restore balance to the body. This balance enhances the healing process.

Hieroglyphs in the Physician's Tomb in Egypt from 4,000 years ago show physicians pressing on the feet of patients. Around 1900, William Fitzgerald, MD, used pressure point therapy for anesthesia in his medical practice. In 1925, Joe Riley, MD, wrote a reflexology book for physicians based on Fitzgerald's findings. Eunice Ingham worked in Riley's office and began using these points on the feet and hands of all Dr. Riley's patients. She coined the term *reflexology* and is considered the originator of modern-day practice. After 17 years of mapping the feet and hands and coordinating points with patients' experiences, she wrote *Stories the Feet Can Tell* (Ingham, 1959) and *Stories the Feet Have Told* (Ingham, 1963). Reflexology is practiced and taught globally, with other people adding their own flavor and changing the name somewhat. It should be noted that reflexology is not for diagnosing, but only for helping the body rebalance itself for healing.

BOX 19-6
REFLEXOLOGY TECHNIQUE

The technique for reflexology involves three basic actions. With the pad of the thumb, press on the area of the foot desired and perform one or more of the following:
1. Hold steady firm pressure.
2. Make small clockwise circles.
3. Inch the tip of the thumb along the foot by bending and straightening the first thumb joint.

Reflexology is an excellent tool for nurses because usually, no matter how restricted a person is, the nurse can always get to the feet or hands. Having the feet touched feels wonderful and relaxes the whole body. Much benefit can be gained with just 1–2 minutes of work, making it perfect for nurses. The basic technique is described in Box 19-6.

Reflexology can be used for overall relaxation by working on the entire foot. If someone has pain or a particular health problem, focus on the part of the foot or hand corresponding to that part of the body in addition to the entire foot.

Some advantages of knowing reflexology are that it may be used to help people with conditions that cannot be touched, like burns, broken bones, internal organs, the immune system, skin rashes, and the eyes and ears.

Reflexology may be used on most people with most conditions. It can be done with socks or on bare feet. If someone is ticklish, just hold the foot for a moment before beginning. This can be taught to patients to do on themselves or to families to do for the patient and each other.

MASSAGE

Massage is another ancient healing art. As early as 1800 BCE, mention of rubbing is found in the healing practices of China and in ayurvedic medicine in India. Hippocrates, the father of modern medicine, said that massage and exercise were crucial parts of medicine. In the 1800s, the word *massage* was first used by the French for rubbing the body. In the early 1800s, Ling and Mesger of Sweden created Swedish massage and named the specific strokes of that form of massage. They founded the first massage schools. In 1871, George Taylor, MD, wrote a book on massage and its effects on the physiology of the body.

SPOTLIGHT ON

Reflexology in Nursing Practice

To help someone sleep, work on all points of both feet, very slowly. If someone has back pain, find the bone that goes from the heel along the arch on the inside of the foot to the bunion joint. Rub along the entire bone on both feet.

Currently, every state in the United States has its own massage laws. In some states, to be called a massage therapist, one must graduate from a massage school licensed by the Department of Health. Nurses can do massage within the scope of their practice, whether in the hospital or in private practice under their nursing license, but cannot use the term *massage therapist*. Nurses must find out what the regulations are in their state.

Massage has been part of nursing care since the beginning of nursing. It was taught in nursing schools and was a standard part of evening care until the late 1960s. Nurses who do massage for patients find the patient needs less medication for sleep and for pain. Patients report feeling happier and cared for after receiving a massage.

Massage can enhance circulation, lymph flow, digestion, and elimination. It can help reduce swelling of joints, speed healing of fractures, and improve the quality of the skin. Massage is not just for relaxation, although in today's world, the reduction of the stress response may be its most useful characteristic. There is nothing better at relieving muscular tension and pain than a massage. Often tight muscles press on the nerves, creating pain and numbness. Tight muscles can cause headache and neck pain. When the back muscles are tight, they interfere with nerve and blood flow from the spine to the rest of the body. Dr. Tiffany Field, of the Touch Research Institutes, is currently one of the leading researchers of the physical and emotional benefits of massage. She has found that massage greatly benefits preterm and full-term infants, reduces pain of arthritis, headaches, and lower back, and enhances immune function. It also alleviates depression and anxiety (Touch Research Institute, 2011).

Massage interrupts the stress response, which is covered in detail in Chapter 8. In brief, it is understood that, when people perceive something as a stressor over a long period of time, the immune system and endocrine system are compromised. By affecting the stress response, massage aids healing on the physical as well as mental and emotional levels.

The healing effects of massage benefit all areas of nursing including maternity, pediatrics, gerontology, cardiovascular, rehabilitation, orthopedic, and home health. Nurses can teach these techniques to families to use on each other. Nurses can also treat each other to a shoulder rub to promote health in the workplace.

Massage may be done in a chair, on a bed, or on a massage table. Massage may be with or without lotion, and it may cover just the back, feet, head, or the entire body. It can last

SPOTLIGHT **ON**

Simple Massage for Relaxation

1. Massage for the back with lotion:
   a. Apply *warmed* lotion to the back, slowly, from the base of the neck to the tailbone using long smooth strokes with your palm.
   b. Press with the heel of your palm starting in the sacrum area (below the waist by the tailbone) along the side of the spine (*not on it*) from the sacrum to the top of the shoulder.
   c. Repeat slowly several times to both sides of the spine.
2. Massage without lotion for headaches and neckaches:
   a. Make slow circular movements with your fingers and thumb.
   b. Press up under the occipital ridge (where the neck connects to the skull) starting behind the ears and rub with the fingers and thumb, simultaneously, in toward the spine.
   c. If the person is sitting, hold the forehead in the palm of one of your hands for support.
   d. Rub the entire scalp with the pads of the fingers, using fast or slow motions according to the patient's preference.

for 1 hour or be very beneficial in just 3–4 minutes. It is easily adapted to a nurse's schedule. Figure 19-7 shows a therapeutic back massage.

ACUPRESSURE

Acupressure is a touch therapy that may be very useful to nurses and easy to teach patients. The technique of acupressure involves firm pressure that is applied with the pad of the thumb,

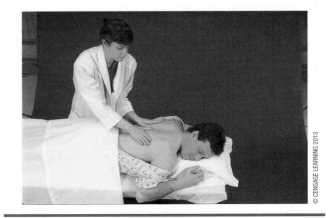

FIGURE 19-7 **A therapeutic back massage.**

© CENGAGE LEARNING 2013

in most cases, to specific points to help balance the body and stimulate healing.

In the ancient Chinese healing system of acupuncture, needles are put into the points that are located along meridians, or lines of energy, that flow from the head to toe. Each meridian corresponds to a different organ of the body. In acupressure, pressing on these points also helps the energy to flow through these meridians, energizing and balancing the corresponding organ. When the energy is properly flowing through all meridians, the body is in balance and able to maintain health.

Much detail may be learned and practiced for working with complex situations. However, the nurse can begin to use certain techniques. The complete system of acupressure is best learned from an experienced practitioner and teacher.

The nurse must also recognize that any therapy has its liabilities. Box 19-7 identifies areas of legal risks to consider for integrative therapies.

🌼 NURSING **ALERT**

Using Acupressure in Nursing Practice

The following method of acupressure has been used to enhance immune function and to help relieve headaches, constipation, vertigo, allergies, sinus problems, toothache, and menstrual cramps.

1. Using the pad of the thumb and first finger, apply pressure to both sides of the web between the thumb and forefinger of one hand of your patient.
2. Hold the pressure steady or rub gently in a circle.
3. Continue for 1–5 minutes or until the pain subsides.

NURSES AND SELF-CARE

This section briefly mentions areas that are covered in greater depth elsewhere in the book. These areas are mentioned here because no discussion of holistic healing and promotion of health would be complete without mentioning the importance of caring for the self. With a focus on caring for others, nurses often are remiss in caring for themselves in a nurturing way that enhances personal well-being and fosters the ability to perform at an optimum level.

ENVIRONMENT

The environment is often taken for granted. Noise levels, the cleanliness of the air, water, chemicals emitted from central air ducts, carpets, paint, perfumes—all affect the health of the body. When only one exists, and only occasionally, the immune system can cope. When the immune system has to handle an environment with multiple toxins, plus stress, plus viruses and bacteria, it often becomes overloaded and cannot perform its function of keeping the body healthy. Allergies, asthma, fatigue, rheumatoid arthritis, infections, colds, skin eruptions, and other diseases may occur or become exacerbated by the environment.

BOX 19-7
INTEGRATIVE THERAPY AND LEGAL RISKS

Nonvitamin, nonmineral natural products, deep breathing, exercises, meditation, chiropractic therapy, massage, and yoga are among the most reported uses of CAM. Therapeutic touch, massage, and acupressure are among many modalities in integrative health care. Nurses who choose to practice any of these need to know about the following.

1. *Standards and scope of practice*—Do the standards and scope of nursing practice in your state allow for the inclusion of the integrative therapy on and off duty?
2. *State laws regulating integrative therapy*—Is a license required?
3. *Employer policies and job description*—Does the scope of employment include the use of the integrative therapy?
4. *Financial risk*—Are your actions covered by your employer's insurance? Does your own liability insurance cover the integrative therapy you choose to practice?
5. *Informed consent*—Did you obtain verbal permission from the patient for the integrative therapy to be used, such as therapeutic touch, massage, or acupressure?
6. *Documentation*—If you practice an integrative therapy, have you properly documented the date, permission granted from the patient, any teaching provided, the nature of the treatment, and the patient's response?

Source: Cady, R. F. (2009). Legal issues related to complementary and alternative medicine. *JONA's Healthcare Law, Ethics, and Regulation, 11*(2), 46–51.

What can nurses do themselves and suggest to clients? Box 19-8 lists suggestions for coping with environmental stressors.

SLEEP

Sleep is often the first thing to go when persons' lives become hectic. When a person is feeling confused, irritable, depressed, sleep is often a good first step. All of these are symptoms of sleep deprivation. While we sleep, the body repairs itself. The immune system is repaired at night, memories are processed and preserved, and internal pacemakers are set that regulate the circadian rhythms of the body—like the release of hormones and the sleep-wake cycle. The room should be as dark as possible for proper secretion of the hormone melatonin, which aids sleep. Often 8 hours of sleep for 3 days in a row improves one's outlook.

EXERCISE

Exercise is often a dreaded word. For some patients exercise may be holding a can of peas in each hand and raising and

TIPS TO COPE WITH ENVIRONMENTAL STRESSORS

1. Wear earplugs if noise is inevitable.
2. Create time for silence.
3. Use water filters for tap water you drink, and frequently change air filters.
4. Spend time with nature and bring natural colors inside.
5. Minimize exposure to perfumes and chemicals.
6. Minimize exposure to electromagnetic fields such as microwaves, electric blankets, and alarm clocks.
7. Don't try to control what is out of your control.

lowering their arms. Walking is considered to be a form of exercise that is the most beneficial with few side effects. Whatever the exercise, doing 20 minutes of it 2–3 times a week is recommended. The body was made to move. When we do not move it or do repetitive tasks, the muscles, nerves, circulation, and lymph system do not function in the most healthy way.

COMMUNICATION

Communicating in relationships is one of the most challenging and potentially stressful and difficult things we humans do. If you watch other animals like dogs, cats, horses, insects, and fish, they all have very clear signals and methods of conveying their needs, wants, and ideas. In childhood, people learn the meaning of tone of voice and facial expressions. Because all childhoods were different, people attach different meanings to these cues.

Most people were never taught to communicate their needs, wants, and ideas clearly, especially in situations with high levels of emotion. Assuming that another person knows how one feels often causes big trouble. To help patients heal, nurses must ask, "What do you need right now?" For more detailed information on communication, refer to Chapter 5.

NUTRITION

Nutrition is vital to enhancing holistic care. There are more opinions on how people should eat, and books written on it, than can even begin to be cited. Opinions vary from pure vegetarianism, to vegetarian with dairy and eggs, to high protein including meat.

Different diets are needed because people are unique. Humans require nutrients from the six food groupings, but how these nutrients are consumed is open to debate. Two things that can benefit all people are to drink at least 1 qt of water a day and to enjoy the food eaten. The main thing is to choose foods that help one feel healthy, relaxed, have plenty of energy and maintain a comfortable weight. See Chapter 15 for more information on nutrition.

HERBS

The use of **phytochemicals** from herbs or plants to promote and maintain health and cure disease is an ancient art. Every traditional culture has had a medicine man or woman who knew which plants to pick, when to pick them, what part of the plant had which effects, and how to prepare the herbs. For some situations, the entire plant is used, and in others, just the flower, leaf, root, or berry. Herbs may be grown at home, bought in health food stores, and even ordered by mail. They can be ingested as a tea, capsule, or liquid tincture (herb extracted in alcohol). Salves and creams containing herbs can be rubbed on the body. Many of our drugs today are made from plants. A growing concern over the loss of the rainforests is that plants that could be cures for disease and enhancers of health may be lost.

The study and practice of herbology is enjoying renewed popularity. A few simple herbs can be part of any medicine cabinet, or the study can become complex with combinations of herbs to address all health situations. These situations include enhancing the immune system, helping women cope with menopause, aiding in prevention of colds and flu, aiding sinus and allergy conditions, decreasing blood pressure, and enhancing the digestive and eliminative functions. There are stimulating, calming, nutritive, and cleansing herbs. In fact, the number and combinations of herbs are so extensive that almost all health situations can be addressed through the proper use of herbology. For example, aloe vera is extremely effective for healing minor burns. Peppermint in any form is excellent for promoting calmness and digestion and easing an upset stomach. Arnica oil is beneficial when rubbed into muscles and tissues affected by sprains, strains, and tension. Black cohosh is used for menstrual cramps and menopausal symptoms.

The most popular legal herbal products purchased and used are ginkgo biloba, St. John's wort, ginseng, garlic, echinacea, saw palmetto, and kava (Sand-Jecklin & Badzek, 2004). The benefits and risks of these are described in Table 19-5. Herbal supplements are not regulated by the U.S. Food and Drug Administration, and the strengths and dosages are not standardized. Studies on the benefits, risks, and dosages of herbal therapies are inconclusive, and, therefore, they must be used with knowledge by the consumer. Although millions of people use herbal therapies for health-related reasons, many of these individuals, along with physicians and nurses, lack knowledge about their benefits and risks (Sand-Jecklin & Badzek, 2003, 2004; Sohn & Loveland-Cook, 2002). Health care professionals need to become educated on herbal therapies in order to promote, protect, and preserve the health of their clientele. Workshops are available for both the beginner and the advanced practitioner.

NURSING **ALERT**

Use Caution with Herbal Supplements

Even when a product is labeled "natural," it can harmful. Interaction with other medications must be considered. Dosages for children should be reduced. Pregnant women and infants should not take or be given herbal supplements. Consultation with a health care practitioner knowledgeable in the use of herbs is important.

TABLE 19-5 Benefits, Risks, and Cautions for Seven Commonly Used Herbs

HERB	MAJOR BENEFITS	IDENTIFIED RISKS
Echinacea	Enhances immune system, anti-inflammatory, antibacterial, prevents/reduces colds, flu	Rare: Can cause flare-ups in some autoimmune diseases such as lupus, some forms of arthritis, and AIDS
Garlic	Improves circulation, enhances cholesterol levels and blood pressure, thins blood	Odor, indigestion; interacts with vitamin E and other medications used for blood thinning
Ginkgo biloba	Improves memory in dementia, reduces ringing in the ears, reduces blood clots	Inhibits clotting (like aspirin), interacts with other medications used for blood thinning
Ginseng	Sold as energy booster or aphrodisiac (studies inconclusive)	Interacts with other medications used for blood thinning, may cause breast tenderness in women, increases blood pressure
Kava	Reduces anxiety	Toxic to liver, interacts with alcohol, damage to central nervous system
Saw palmetto	Reduces enlarged prostate, also used in the treatment of upper respiratory infections, ovarian pain and cysts, and infertility	None known
St. John's Wort	Reduces anxiety and depression, menopausal symptoms, gastrointestinal inflammation, and peptic ulcers	Sensitivity to light, interacts with other drugs such as blood thinners and oral contraceptives

Source: National Center for Complementary and Alternative Medicine (NCCAM). (2011). Herbs at a Glance. Retrieved from http://nccam.nih.gov/health/herbsataglance.htm

AROMATHERAPY

Aromatherapy is the use of the essential oils from plants for beneficial effects on body, mind, emotions, and spirit. The essential oils are steam distilled from plants and flowers. Oils are 75–100% more potent than the plants from which they are distilled. The term *aromatherapy* implies that a scent is inhaled; however, it also includes the application of essential oils in massage and in bathing (Buckle, 2003).

Whether used in a bath, massage, or inhaled as a scent, aromatic oils have long been known for their therapeutic effects. Babylonian clay tablets and Egyptian tombs indicate that as long as 7,000 years ago oils and scents were used for healing. The term *aromatherapy* was coined in 1928 by a French chemist named Gatefosse. He badly burned his arm and plunged it into a vat of lavender. The pain was immediately reduced, and there was minimal scarring (Buckle, 2003). Jane Buckle, RN, is currently a leader in the teaching of aromatherapy for nurses and other health care professionals.

Our brain recognizes approximately 10,000 scents. When one inhales a scent, tiny molecules of the substance travel from the nose to the olfactory part of the brain, which is directly connected with the limbic area of the brain. The limbic area affects memory, emotions, and learning and is connected to the hypothalamus, which controls the autonomic nervous system. People react immediately and involuntarily to scent.

These oils have healing properties such as being calming, analgesic, stimulating, antibacterial, deodorizing, and antiviral (Buckle, 2003; Thomas, 2002). Combinations of oils may increase the circulation of endorphins, which aid in pain reduction; enkephalins, which can cause us to feel happy; serotonin, which helps to reduce insomnia; and noradrenalin, which can be stimulating.

Because essential oils can be very effective and some are not advised with certain conditions, the advice of an experienced practitioner is recommended. However, the beginner can use some. For example, French lavender is very safe, calming, sleep inducing, healing, and antibacterial, and peppermint aids in digestion.

Because essential oils can be so powerful, they should not be applied directly to the skin. One or two drops on a pillow (not pillowcase), cottonball, or handkerchief can be inhaled. The essential oil can be poured into a porous clay pot, and it will diffuse into the room. Diffusers use a heat source. Essential oils can also be absorbed through the skin and travel via the blood to the organ on which they have an effect. There are about 150 essential oils (Thomas, 2002). Table 19-6 provides a sample of some of these and their reported effects.

LOVE AND HEALING

This world is much more than meets the eye. People are not just three-dimensional conglomerates of matter that operate *only* according to all the physical laws accepted in science up to this moment. Humans are on the brink of new discoveries of how the universe works and what it is to be human.

There is evidence suggesting that humans and all animals, plants, and all matter in the universe are beings of energy, vibrating at different frequencies. All other forms of vibrating energy, such as sound, light, thoughts, and feelings, affect these bodies of energy. A field of energy connects us all. There is no separation.

Many researchers in the arts and sciences are now studying exactly how all this is connected. Human beings, animals, and plants heal and thrive in the presence of caring and loving. Many healers say that love is the power that allows

TABLE 19-6 Some Essential Oils and Their Effects

ESSENTIAL OIL	EFFECTS
Basil	Refreshing, clarifying, concentration enhancing
Chamomile	Refreshing, relaxing, calming
Frankincense	Relaxing, rejuvenating, rids fears
Jasmine	Relaxing, confidence-building
Lavender	Refreshing, relaxing, calming
Lemon	Stimulating, motivating
Lemongrass	Toning, fortifying
Marjoram	Warming, sedating
Myrrh	Toning, strengthening, rejuvenating
Orange	Refreshing, relaxing
Peppermint	Cooling, refreshing, head clearing
Thyme	Antiseptic, immune strengthening

© Cengage Learning 2013

healing to happen at a distance. For so long in nursing it was recommended not to touch patients except to do necessary procedures and not to get "emotionally involved" with patients. Hundreds of studies on social support and touch are now telling us what common sense has always known. Humans need to be touched, physically and emotionally. They need each other to be healthy and happy. Social support can be a friend who listens, a pet, a church group, family, a feeling of connection to a Higher Power, plants people care for, a social group, or wherever one feels loved and accepted.

The literature abounds with studies on social support and the positive effects it can have. Among those effects are increased feelings of self-esteem, self-identity, and control over one's environment (which tends to result in enhanced immune function), higher life expectancy, low incidence of heart disease, faster recovery from surgery, decreased blood pressure, and decreased anxiety levels.

SPOTLIGHT ON

Love and Caring in Nursing Practice

Take a moment with a patient who perhaps seems difficult for you to work with. Take a breath. Feel love, appreciation, or caring for the patient or for someone or something in your life. Imagine the two of you being surrounded by a warm light. Come back to your patient. Notice whether you feel differently about her. View her as a precious thing, someone that may feel very vulnerable and afraid. How would you feel in her shoes?

A lack of social support has been linked to general mortality rate, the onset and progression of disease, decreased ability to learn and remember information, increased asthma, pregnancy complications, arthritis, hypertension, depression, coronary disease, cancer, autoimmune disease, and infectious disease.

Love is a very powerful force. Research studies and anecdotal accounts indicate that love and caring create connection over time and great distances, affecting physical change (Watson, 2002a, 2002b, 2005, 2008). If one doesn't have love, one continually seeks it. Yet no one can say exactly what love is or how to get it or how it is lost. Love is an energy that promotes health and facilitates healing.

What does this imply for nurses? Love, caring, and empathy are energies that create healing in ways not fully understood at this time. Nurses need to create ways to support each other. Patients need their loved ones around them to facilitate healing. When a loved one cannot be present, a picture or object can help the patient feel loved and supported. Sometimes the nurse is the only person in a patient's experience to help her feel loved and cared for. No words are needed. Sitting down for a moment or holding a hand can create a heart connection that opens a space for the mystery of healing.

SUMMARY

Each nurse has a personal definition for healing and what it means to be a nurse. For most nurses some part of the decision to be a nurse had to do with wanting to help people feel better. The days are gone when people believed that the health of the body is separate from the health of the mind and the fullness of the spirit. For human beings to realize their full potential, it is necessary to consider their whole nature as body, mind, feelings, spirit, and energy field, and how all of these aspects interact with each other and with all other living things in this universe.

Enhancing health promotion by incorporating holistic principles and modalities into nursing practice gives nurses new tools for embracing the entire human nature and helping patients do the same to achieve maximum desired individual health goals. Holding patients and ourselves as nurses as the most precious of beings helps the heart to open, promotes health, and allows for healing to happen.

CASE STUDY

Charles Fowler: Living with Painful Arthritis

OBJECTIVES/GOALS: Through participation in a discussion of this case study, participants will have the opportunity to:

1. Discuss the effect of the nurse's attitude toward healing on patient outcomes.
2. Describe a holistic approach to healing.

HEALTH-PROMOTION CONCERN, HISTORY AND PHYSICAL, PRESENT HEALTH STATUS, PAST HEALTH STATUS, FAMILY HISTORY, AND SOCIAL HISTORY

Charles (Charlie) Fowler is a 75-year-old white non-Hispanic male with painful arthritis in both knees. He is a retired farmer, has been married 48 years to his wife Helen, and has four adult sons. Two years ago, he sold his farm when the pain in his knees was so great that he could no longer physically perform the work required. He and Helen recently moved into a small home in a nearby town. He is 5 ft, 9 in. tall and weighs 164 lb. As prescribed, he is currently taking acetaminophen 650 mg q 4 hr and capsaicin cream 0.025% applied twice daily to both knees. He is emphatic about avoiding knee replacement surgery. He would like to know what nonmedical methods or treatments are available for help in easing his knee pain. He has also asked about using saw palmetto, which he read was good for prostate problems.

REVIEW OF PERTINENT DOMAINS

Biological Domain

Physical exam reveals an elderly male of appropriate weight for body stature who is experiencing moderate pain to both knees. There is varus (turned inward) deformity of both knees as well as moderate inflammation. His vital signs were: B/P 132/62, pulse 78 and regular, respirations 12, and temperature 98.2°.

GASTROINTESTINAL: Reports no problems in this area. He has regular bowel movements. His diet is well balanced with fruits and vegetables, and he rarely eats at fast-food restaurants.

GENITOURINARY: He reports having "spells" within the past year of frequent urge to urinate with sometimes only a small stream of urine produced. There is no history of urinary tract or reproductive problems, but he thinks it is his prostate that is "getting old, like me."

MUSCULOSKELETAL: Complains of pain in the joints of both knees and knee joint stiffness when sitting too long and upon rising in the morning.

Psychological Domain

Charlie graduated from high school and says he enjoys reading science and agriculture magazines. He also reports reading more and taking a greater interest in personal wellness to "keep away" from taking medication. Charlie states he has lived a fulfilled life and feels blessed with the love of his wife and children. He says he has tried to be a "good" person and feels rewarded that his farming has made a difference in the lives of many. He has a great sense of humor and enjoys telling jokes and stories to make his wife laugh.

Social Domain

Charlie plays shuffleboard at the local senior citizen center when his knees aren't "acting up." He also enjoys sitting with his retiree friends, just "gabbing" about life. He and Helen have taken many trips to visit their four children, who live 50 to 750 miles away, but driving has become a painful experience because of his knees.

Environmental Domain

Charlie lives in a one-story home with five steps leading up to the front door. He says that using steps is painful at times. He loves to attend to the small garden in the back yard.

Spiritual Domain

Charlie is a member of the local Presbyterian church and attends services weekly. He believes in a "higher power" and says he prays for good health for his family first and then himself. He says his great-great-grandfather was a Cherokee Indian and feels that his "Indian blood" is why he feels a connection with nature.

Technological Domain

Charlie's younger son purchased a computer and software for Charlie and Helen and gave them basic instructions on how to access the Internet and use email. Charlie says he gets a "kick" out of "surfing the Web without ever getting wet."

QUESTIONS FOR DISCUSSION

1. How can the nurse's attitude toward healing affect Charlie's desire for alternative or complementary health care or both?
2. How can the nurse help Charlie discover what his needs are and develop a plan to meet them?
3. Identify two areas of caution for Charlie and how the nurse should address them.

KEY CONCEPTS

1. What it means to be a healing nurse is unique to each individual. To help discover a personal definition, nurses can consider what healing means to them, what their goals for self-healing are, and what their role is in helping patients heal.

2. When people's needs are met, the body, mind, and spirit can heal. Nurses can help patients discover needs and create strategies to meet them by asking them to describe their health now, what they think they need to heal, what they expect to happen, how they or others can help them, and what their goals are and what has to happen to reach those goals.

3. Energy fields are part of and surround all living things. Balance in the field affects the health of the body. The nurse can use energy-based therapies such as TT, HT, light, color, sound and music, and thought to help create balance in the field.

4. The thoughts people think affect their physiology and their energy fields. By consciously choosing their thoughts, people can affect health and relationships. Cognitive restructuring can be used to recognize distorted thoughts and replace them with realistic ones to enhance relationships, reduce fears, and increase self-confidence,

5. Imaging is creating a picture in the mind that incorporates the five senses. The picture is what a person wants to occur in the body or events in life. Imagery is used for relaxation, stress reduction, and enhancing healing of the body.

6. The Relaxation Response relaxes the autonomic nervous system, counterbalancing the stress response. The technique utilizes principles from various types of meditation.

7. The nurse can teach patients to visualize a blue color to enhance relaxation and pain relief. Other colors have different effects on humans. Music of the patient's choosing has been shown to increase immune function and decrease the stress response.

8. Centering and grounding are techniques to use before working with patients in any way, especially energy-based therapies like HT and TT. Centering encourages the nurse to clear the mind, bringing her attention to the present. Grounding connects the nurse to the Earth as a steady source of energy and to the universal source of healing energy.

9. Reflexology points on the feet can be pressed to help relieve pain and encourage relaxation in corresponding parts of the body. Simple massage to the head, neck, and shoulders can relieve pain and promote sleep and a feeling of being cared for.

10. Techniques for nurturing the self can be used by nurses and taught to patients. There are many to choose from, and they are effective primarily because they reduce stress and increase feelings of health and happiness. Among them are communication, sleep, nutrition, and love.

11. Because of people's energy nature, all are connected in very real ways. The unique role of the nurse is to help to promote health and to heal by appreciating each patient, providing direction and support, and by helping when patients cannot help themselves in the most vulnerable of times.

CHAPTER REVIEW

Learning Activities

1. What qualities do you have, or want to learn, that would make you feel that you are a nurse healer?

2. A patient tells you he is having headaches and pain in his neck, shoulders, and back, is unusually irritated, is having diarrhea, and is not sleeping well. Using your knowledge of holistic principles, you believe he is experiencing more stress than he can handle. Discuss how you would help him discover the causes of his stress and what he might do about it using the Modeling and Role Modeling techniques presented in this chapter.

3. A patient has had a mild heart attack and wants to create a health-promotion plan to prevent future health problems. She has heard of holistic healing and wants you to help her incorporate it into her plan. Use the holistic modalities presented in this chapter and create a plan for this patient.

Multiple Choice Questions

1. Which of the following is central to the holistic philosophy?
   a. Cultural diversity is more important than any other component.
   b. Disease, illness, and imbalance are opportunities for positive growth.
   c. Environment is separate and distinct from the person.
   d. The treatment of symptoms is the focus of health promotion and disease prevention.

2. A recent survey of adults in the United States found the use of complementary and alternative medicine, excluding prayer, to be prevalent in:
   a. 1 of 10 adults.
   b. 1 of 20 adults.
   c. 2 of 3 adults.
   d. 3 of 5 adults.

3. The National Center for Complementary and Alternative Medicine (CAM) has reported that highest use of CAM in adults is in which one of the following age groups?
   a. 17–29
   b. 30–39
   c. 50–59
   d. 70–84

4. Reiki, Healing Touch, and Therapeutic Touch are examples of which one of the following categories of complementary and alternative medicine identified by the National Center for Complementary and Alternative Medicine?
   a. Biologically based practices
   b. Energy medicine
   c. Manipulative and body-based practices
   d. Mind-body medicine

5. Which one of the following colors can be overwhelming in large amounts and is known to stimulate heart rate, blood pressure, and appetite?
   a. Blue
   b. Green
   c. Red
   d. Yellow

6. Which of the following Qi gong sounds can benefit the heart?
   a. Haw
   b. Sss
   c. Shhhh
   d. Woo

7. Which of the following terms is a developmental process that results in independence and self-confidence of the patient for health promotion?
   a. Capacity building
   b. Empowerment
   c. Grounding
   d. Heliotherapy

8. Recognizing, challenging, and changing cognitive distortions and negative thought patterns is a type of therapy known as cognitive:
   a. learning.
   b. grounding.
   c. reorganization.
   d. restructuring.

9. A nurse plans interventions that facilitate growth, development, and healing at the patient's own pace based on the unique model of the patient's world. This is an example of which one of the following nursing theories?
   a. General Adaptation Theory
   b. Science of Unitary Beings
   c. Theory of Modeling and Role Modeling
   d. Theory of Transpersonal Nursing

10. The term *biofield* was first described by which of the following persons?
    a. Albert Einstein
    b. Dolores Kreiger
    c. Hippocrates
    d. Janet Mentgen

11. As a nurse, which of the following is an important general guideline for you to observe with a patient for any touch therapy?
    a. Communicate when the session is over to allow for reorientation.
    b. Discuss your personal feelings about touch therapy before the session.
    c. Make movements quickly and quietly for greater efficiency.
    d. Permission includes the signature of the patient for legal purposes.

ORGANIZATIONS AND WEBSITES

Alternative Medicine Foundation: Nonprofit organization providing consumers and professionals with responsible, evidence-based information on the integration of alternative and conventional medicine; resource guides on a variety of alternative treatment modalities and health issues and a primer on medical research studies are provided: **http://www.amfoundation.org**

Ayurvedic Institute: A recognized school and ayurveda health spa, established in 1984 to teach and provide the traditional ayurvedic medicine of India, including herbs, nutrition, panchakarma, cleansing, acupressure massage, yoga, Sanskrit, and Jyotish (Vedic astrology): **http://www.ayurveda.com**

Center for the Study of Complementary and Alternative Therapies (CSCAT): Located at the University of Virginia and established in 1995 as one of the original NIH-funded centers for research, collaboration, and information about complementary and alternative medicine (CAM): **http://www.Healthsystem.virginia.edu**

Healing Touch International Inc.: A nonprofit membership and educational corporation established in 1996 to administer the certification process and facilitate healing through the practice, teaching, and research of Healing Touch: **http://www.healingtouchinternational.org**

Healthy.net: Offers a general overview of mind/body medicine, including articles on introduction to mind/body medicine, mind/body therapies, and mind/body approaches to health disorders; includes links to interviews with Larry Dossey, MD, Deepak Chopra, MD, and James Gordon, MD: **http://www.healthy.net**

Herb Research Foundation: Considered a reliable source of accurate, science-based information on the health benefits and safety of herbs, and expertise in sustainable botanical resource development: **http://www.herbs.org**

International Center for Reiki Training: Offers a wealth of information about Reiki practice and teaching; a free download for articles, including free Reiki practice and teaching materials; streaming audio files, a slide show, and a free online newsletter are also available as well as the opportunity to purchase materials: **http://www.reiki.org**

National Center for Complementary and Alternative Medicine (NCCAM): One of the 27 institutes and centers that make up the National Institutes of Health (NIH). The NIH is one of eight agencies under the Public Health Service (PHS) in the Department of Health and Human Services (DHHS). NCCAM exists to explore complementary and alternative healing practices in the context of rigorous science, train complementary and alternative medicine (CAM) researchers, and disseminate authoritative information to the public and professionals: **http://www.nccam.nih.gov**

National Institute for Clinical Applications of Behavioral Medicine: Offers continuing education on mind-body topics for health care practitioners; offers training for mind-body practices and techniques for health practitioners: **http://www.nicabm.com/**

REFERENCES

Abramson, L. Y., Seligman, M. E. P., & Teasdale, J. D. (1978). Learned helplessness in humans: Critique and reformulation. *Journal of Abnormal Psychology, 87*, 49–74.

Barnes, P. M., Bloom, B., & Nahin, R. (2008). *Complementary and alternative medicine use among adults and children: United States, 2007.* CDC National Statistics Report #12: http://www.cdc.gov/nchs/data/nhsr/nhsr012.pdf

Benson, H. (1975). *The relaxation response.* New York, NY: Avon.

Benson, H. (1996). *Timeless healing.* New York, NY: Simon & Schuster.

Bright, M. A. (2004). Therapeutic touch. In M. A. Bright (ed.), *Holistic health and healing.* Philadelphia, PA: F. A. Davis, pp. 171–179.

Bright, M. A., Andrus, V., & Lunt, Y. (2004). Health, healing, and holistic nursing. In M. A. Bright (ed.), *Holistic health and healing.* Philadelphia: F. A. Davis, pp. 31–46.

Buckle, J. (2003). *Clinical aromatherapy: Essential oils in practice.* New York, NY: Churchill-Livingstone.

Bulfone, T., Quattrin, R., Zanotti, R., Regattin, L., & Brusaferro, S. (2009). Effectiveness of music therapy for anxiety reduction in women with breast cancer in chemotherapy treatment. *Holisti Nursing Practice, 23*(4), 238–242.

Burkhardt, M. A., & Nagai-Jacobson, M. G. (2005). Spirituality and health. In B. M. Dossey, L. Keegan, & C. E. Guzzetta (eds.), *Holistic nursing: A handbook for practice* (4th ed.). Sudbury, MA: Jones & Bartlett, pp. 137–172.

Cady, R. F. (2009). Legal issues related to complementary and alternative medicine. *JONA's Healthcare Law, Ethics, and Regulation, 11*(2), 46–51.

Catalano, J. T. (2006). *Nursing now! Today's issues, tomorrow's trends.* Philadelphia, PA: F. A. Davis.

Chia, M. (2009). *The six healing sounds: Taoist techniques for balancing chi.* Rochester, VT: Destiny Books.

Childre, D. (1998). *Freeze frame: One minute stress management.* Boulder Creek, CA: Planetary Publications.

Dossey, B. M., & Keegan, L. (2005). Self-assessments: Facilitating healing in self and others. In B. M. Dossey, L. Keegan, & C. E. Guzzetta (eds.), *Holistic nursing: A handbook for practice* (4th ed.). Sudbury, MA: Jones & Bartlett, pp. 379–393.

Dossey, L. (1994). *Healing words.* San Francisco, CA: HarperCollins.

Dunn, K. (2004). Music and the reduction of post-operative pain. *Nursing Standard, 18*(36), 33–39.

Eliopoulos, C. (2009). *Invitation to holistic health: A guide to living a balanced life.* Sudbury, MA: Jones & Bartlett.

European Society of Cardiology (2005, February 8). Third of European cancer patients use complementary and alternative therapies. *ScienceDaily.* Retrieved from http://www.sciencedaily.com/releases/2005/02/050205080531.htm

Harvard Medical School. (2008). *Complementary and alternative medicine: Color therapy.* Retrieved from http://www.intelihealth.com/IH/ihtIH/WSIHW000/8513/34968/358753.html?d=dmtContent

Hover-Kramer, D. (2009). *Healing touch guidebook: Practicing the art and science of human caring.* Clifton Park, NY: Delmar Cengage Learning

Ingham, E. (1959). *Stories the feet can tell.* Rochester, NY: Ingham Publishing.

Ingham, E. (1963). *Stories the feet have told.* St. Petersburg, FL: Ingham Publishing.

Jobst, K. A., Niemtzow, R. C., Curtis, B. D., & Curtis, M. L. (2004). Special issue on science and healing: From bioelectromagnetics to the medicine of light. *Journal of Alternative and Complementary Medicine, 10,* 1–222.

Joel, L. A. (2006). *The nursing experience: Trends, challenges, and transitions* (5th ed.). New York, NY: McGraw-Hill.

Krieger, D. (2002). *Therapeutic touch as transpersonal healing.* New York, NY: Lantern Books.

Laird, S. P., Snyder, C. R., Rapoff, M. A., & Green, S. (2004). Measuring private prayer: Development, validation, and clinical application of the multidimensional prayer inventory. *International Journal for the Psychology of Religion, 14*(4), 251–272.

Leigh, B. K. (2004). Incorporating human energy fields into studies of family communication. *Journal of Family Communication, 4*(3/4), 319–335.

McKivergin, M. (2005). The nurse as an instrument of healing. In B. M. Dossey, L. Keegan, & C. E. Guzzetta (eds.), *Holistic nursing: A handbook for practice* (4th ed.). Sudbury, MA: Jones & Bartlett, pp. 233–254.

Miller, A. L. (2005). Epidemiology, etiology, and natural treatment of seasonal affective disorder. *Alternative Medicine Review, 10*(1), 5–13.

National Center for Complementary and Alternative Medicine (NCCAM). (2011). Herbs at a glance. Retrieved from http://nccam.nih.gov/health/herbsataglance.htm

National Center for Complementary and Alternative Medicine (NCCAM). (2008). The use of complementary and alternative medicine in the United States. Retrieved from http://www.nccam.nih.gov

North American Nursing Diagnosis Association (NANDA). (2008). *Nursing diagnoses: Definitions and classification 2009–2011.* Indianapolis, IN: Wiley-Blackwell.

Ott, J. N. (1973). *Health and light: The effects of natural and artificial light on man and other living things.* Old Greenwich, CT: Devin-Adair.

Potter, P. J., & Frisch, N. (2007). Holistic assessment and care: presence in the process. *Nursing Clinics of North America, 42*(2), 213–228.

The proof that prayer works. (n.d.). Retrieved, from http://www.1stholistic.com/Prayer/hol_prayer_proof.htm

Qutab, A. (2005). Ayurveda. In B. M. Dossey, L. Keegan, & C. E. Guzzetta (eds.), *Holistic nursing: A handbook for practice* (4th ed.). Sudbury, MA: Jones & Bartlett, pp. 273–283.

Rodriguez, D. (2011). Cognitive restructuring: Change your thoughts, change your attitude *Everyday Health.* Retrieved from http://www.everydayhealth.com/emotional-health/understanding/cognitive-restructuring.aspx

Sand-Jecklin, K., & Badzek, L. (2003). Nurses and nutraceuticals: Knowledge and use. *Holistic Nursing Practice, 21*(4), 384–397.

Sand-Jecklin, K., & Badzek, L. (2004). Know the benefits and risks of using common herbal therapies. *Holistic Nursing Practice, 18*(4), 192–198.

Scott, E. (2007). Cognitive restructuring for stress relief. *About.com Guide.* Retrieved from http://stress.about.com/od/professionalhelp/a/Restructuring.htm

Selye, H. (1956). *The stress of life.* New York, NY: McGraw-Hill.

Snyder, M., & Lindquist, R. (2001). Issues in complementary therapies: How we got to where we are. *The Online Journal of Nursing Issues, 6* (2). Retrieved from http://www.nursingworld.org

Sohn, P. M., & Loveland-Cook, C. A. (2002). Nurse practitioner knowledge of complementary health care: Foundation for practice. *Journal of Advanced Nursing, 39*(1), 9–16.

Thomas, D. V. (2002). Aromatherapy: Mythical, magical or medicinal? *Holistic Nursing Practice, 17*(1), 8–16.

Tippens, K., Marsman, K., & Zwickey, H. (2009). Is prayer CAM? *Journal of Alternative and Complemenary Medicine, 16*(7), 435–438.

Touch Research Institute. (2011). *Touch research institute research.* Retrieved from http://www6.miami.edu/touch-research/About.html

Volk, J. (2002). Sound insights. *Kindred Spirit, 60,* 14–17.

Watson, J. (2002a). *Instruments for assessing and measuring caring in nursing and health sciences.* New York: Springer.

Watson, J. (2002b). Intentionality and caring-healing consciousness: A theory of transpersonal nursing. *Holistic Nursing Practice, 16*(4), 12–19.

Watson, J. (2005). *Caring science as sacred science.* Philadelphia: F. A. Davis.

Watson, J. (2008). *Nursing: The philosophy and science of caring.* Boulder, CO: University Press of Colorado.

BIBLIOGRAPHY

Dossey, B. M., & Keegan, L. (eds.). (2009). *Holistic nursing: A handbook for practice.* Sudbury, MA: Jones & Bartlett Publishers

Downey, M. (2007). Effects of holistic nursing course: A paradigm shift for holistic health practice. *Journal of Holistic Nursing, 25*(2), 119–125.

Faass, N. (2001). *Integrating complementary medicine into health systems.* Gaithersburg, MD: Aspen.

Fontaine, K. L. (2000). *Healing practices: Alternative therapies for nursing.* Upper Saddle River, NJ: Prentice Hall.

Freeman L. (2004). *Mosby's Complementary and Alternative Medicine: A research-based approach.* St. Louis, MO: Mosby;

Halberstein, R., de Santis, L., Sirkin, A., Padron-Fajardo, V., & Ojeda-Vaz, M. (2007). Healing with bach flower essences: Testing a complementary therapy complementary health practice. *Journal of Complementary and Evidence-Based Medicine, 12,* 3–14.

Jonas, W., & Crawford, C. (2003). *Healing, intention, and energy medicine.* London: Churchill-Livingstone.

Keegan, L. (2001). *Healing with complementary and alternative therapies.* Clifton Park, NY: Delmar Cengage Learning.

Peters, D., Chaitow, L., Harris, G., & Morrison, S. (2002). *Integrating complementary therapies in primary care: A practical guide for healthcare professionals.* Edinburgh, UK: Harcourt Publishers.

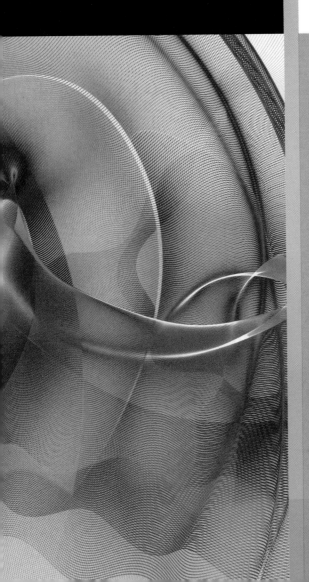

Section V

Health-Promotion Concerns

CHAPTER 20
Concerns of the Health Professional

CAROLINA G. HUERTA, EdD, MSN, RN

KEY TERMS

burnout
electronic health record (EHR)
ergonomics

genogram
hardiness
health behavior patterns

occupational stress
spirituality
stressors

OBJECTIVES

Upon completion of this chapter, the reader should be able to:

- Identify current health-promotion issues that have an impact on nurses and health care professionals.
- Recognize specific factors that affect the nursing profession.
- Discuss health behavior patterns and their implications for the health professional.
- Describe how a health care professional's health-promotion practices influence the biological, psychological, spiritual, sociocultural, environmental, and technological domains.
- Identify strategies for positive health promotion for health professionals.
- Utilize the steps of the nursing process to develop a health-promotion plan for the health care professional.

INTRODUCTION

Nursing as a career choice is extremely rewarding. There is much satisfaction in caring for people and knowing that you are making a difference in people's lives. There are many specialty areas to choose from as well as opportunities for career progression. However, nurses and health care professionals are so invested in helping others maintain or return to a state of health that they sometimes overlook their own health. Busy health care professionals concentrate all of their energies on their responsibilities to help the sick, often ignoring basic health-promotion principles essential for achieving their own maximum wellness. Although researchers from a variety of professions study health care professionals, primarily in relation to issues affecting job performance, the outcomes of such studies have had little impact in alleviating these problems. Master's theses and doctoral dissertations have produced a number of scholarly papers on this topic; however, there is no evidence that the issues affecting the health of health care professionals have been adequately addressed and/or resolved (Missouri State Board of Nursing, 2010; Hunter, Branson, & Davenport, 2010). At a time when radical changes in health care services are taking place, it is important to focus on those **stressors**, or stress-provoking factors, that can impact the health of those who provide health care to others.

Nursing, for example, has become increasingly concerned about the health-related stressors affecting the profession. The *American Nurse Today*, the official journal of the American Nurses Association, dedicates a section in each issue of the monthly journal to the Environment, Health, and Safety. This section focuses on issues that impact the nursing workplace and nurses' personal health. The journal section provides nursing students and nursing professionals with the reality of the nursing profession. To some, it appears that, at times, the health care professions seem obsessed with the negative consequences of the work and seem to blame the individual professions. These findings need to be looked at with objectivity and cool detachment. How different is nursing, for example, from other helping professions such as social work or teaching? Although health care professionals are well paid and usually have job flexibility and career opportunities, they are exposed to a great amount of stress dealing with human frailty and life-and-death situations.

Classroom teachers and social workers, however, may argue that they too are exposed to major stressors in their workplace environment. In all instances, factors in the ever-changing workplace environment, no doubt, contribute to professionals' neglect of their own health-promotion needs. Previous chapters have focused on the concept of health promotion from the point of view of the professional health care giver providing care for the patient. This chapter focuses on the health-promotion needs of health care professionals, specifically nurses, who often ignore these needs and consequently may suffer deleterious effects. Issues impacting nurses and the health care professional as well as strategies that enhance health are also discussed.

CHANGE AND ITS IMPACT ON THE HEALTH PROFESSIONAL

Change sometimes seems to be the one constant in this high-tech information age. In the frenzy to fit into the current and future forms of health care, health care professionals many

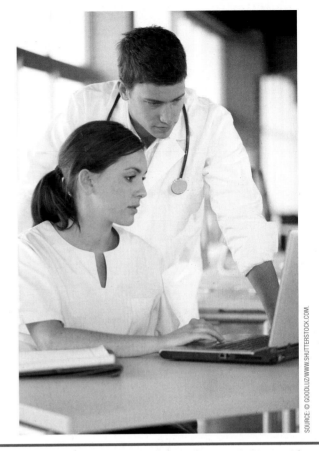

FIGURE 20-1 Becoming technologically competent can also be stressful.

SOURCE: © GOODLUZ/WWW.SHUTTERSTOCK.COM.

times find themselves returning to academic settings for additional education, seeking continuing education in relation to health information technology (HIT) requirements, or moving from acute care settings to community or home-health environments where the pace of the workplace and technological requirements might be slower. Health care professionals who choose to exit the workforce to spend time raising a family or caring for an elderly relative may find numerous technological and pharmacological advances upon reentering the profession (see Figure 20-1). A refresher course or courses may be required to become current.

For example, data collection and recording options have changed frequently in the past 5 years. Today's nurse is expected to collect patient information in a digital format that is then shared across different health care settings. This process automates access to information via an **electronic health record (EHR)**. An EHR is an electronic version of a patient's medical history that may include key clinical data relevant to the person's care, demographics, progress notes, problems, medications, vital signs, past medical history, immunizations, and laboratory and radiology reports (U.S. Department of Health and Human Services, 2010). EHRs allow streamlining of workflow in health care settings with the ultimate goal of increasing patient safety and improving delivery of care efficiency. In this day of specialty focused care, time is also spent learning new things, adapting to changes, hurrying to meet deadlines, and fulfilling responsibilities to others who depend on nurses. No wonder today's caregivers perceive that they have little time to relax, exercise, or play. When inexperienced workers enter the profession, they do so with enthusiasm and gusto. As core workers, they are expected to work hard for a period of time, experience **burnout,** and be replaced by other more energetic core workers. Burnout is a personal coping outcome that results in a state of physical and emotional exhaustion and that occurs when health care givers deplete their adaptive energy sources. Burnout results in feelings of personal ineffectiveness that are then demonstrated as decreased commitment and dedication to the health care professional's job (Lernihan & Sweeney, 2010). Unfortunately, physical and emotional exhaustion can occur among health care professionals who are trying to provide quality patient care while adapting to the technological and social changes in a fast-paced world. Burnout in nursing depletes the professional workforce and its resources. (See Technological Domain at the end of the chapter.)

? ASK **YOURSELF**

Reacting to Change

How have you reacted to change? Do you find yourself running to buy the latest gadget on the market? Have you had to learn multiple computer programs just to progress in college? Do you stress out if you cannot immediately figure out how to use digital electronics? Do you become physically and emotionally depleted, or do you take everything in stride and cope well? What do you do to maintain your health and outlook in your work or classroom environment?

ISSUES IMPACTING THE HEALTH CARE PROFESSIONAL

Health care professionals differ from other types of workers. They are faced with illness and death on a daily basis and are prone to experience **occupational stress,** or job-related stress, which leads to increased physical and mental health risks and decreased work ability and quality of life (Hui et al., 2010). They are expected to find out what the patients' needs are as well as provide comfort and support for all who are in their care. They come face-to-face with human suffering and emotional turmoil on a daily basis and are expected to respond to stress and suffering with compassion and control (Peery, 2010). Health care professionals are given an enormous amount of responsibility and, with the exception of physicians, very little autonomy. Additionally, the population that they serve is ever changing. A mobile society with an increasing aging population presents new challenges to primary, secondary, and tertiary health care providers. These challenges are tremendous and impact the professional caregiver's ability to experience job satisfaction and provide optimum care (Delp et al., 2010).

Several research studies have been done on the stressful issues experienced by physicians, nurses, and other health care workers (Buck, Curley, & Strasser, 2010; Delp, Wallace, Geiger-Brown, & Muntaner, 2010). As a result of the stresses encountered in the health care environment, nurses, physicians, and other health care workers are at high risk for chronic stress and its effects. The consequences of prolonged stress are numerous and devastating. These may include physical as well as psychological problems that can lead to inappropriate coping behaviors, such as excessive drinking of alcohol and/or substance abuse (Epstein, Burns, & Conlon, 2010). (Chapter 18 provides an in-depth overview of the health risks associated with alcohol.) Study results indicate that nursing professionals may experience increasing levels of stress and physical and emotional exhaustion. They experience stress in relation to time pressure, fatigue, role ambiguity and conflict, lack of social support and exposure to environmental hazards (Hughes, 2011).

Nursing literature has also identified issues affecting nurses in their work. This literature reports that nurses are leaving the nursing profession because of workplace issues such as the hospital environment, organizational leadership, quantitative demands such as excessive workloads, and the lack of support for maintaining the quality and safety of patient care (Simon, Müller, & Hasselhorn, 2010). Leiter & Maslach (2009), for example, in their study on why nurses resign from their jobs found that nurses described burnout, values conflict, lack of rewards, and lack of organizational justice and respect as prevalent reasons for their intent to leave a job. Buerhaus, Staiger, & Auerbach (2009), on the other hand, report that nurses who said that they were very satisfied with being a nurse increased from 35% in 2002 to 55% in 2006. This increase in satisfaction is attributed to health care employers' giving nurses more opportunities to influence decisions regarding patient care, recognizing nursing accomplishments, and overall improvement in the nurses' physical health. Additionally, in contrast to previous years, 80% of registered nurses indicated that they would advise a career in nursing (Buerhaus et al., 2007).

New nursing graduates also face stresses associated with their new position. The first few months have the potential to be the most stressful and challenging for the newly graduated nurse. Role stress in new nursing graduates has been found to be relevant to nursing education and practice. The first 6 months, in particular, have been shown to be the most apprehensive period of adjustment for the registered nurse (Benner, Tanner, & Chesla, 2009). Role ambiguity, lack of clarity in terms of the behavior expected, unrealistic expectations, and anxiety have been found to produce stress in the new graduate. For example, anxiety is generated in novice nurses when they attend to immediate patient needs rather than getting their work done on schedule (Benner, Tanner, Chesla, 2009). Interestingly, nursing students are not immune to some of the same stressors experienced by the professional health care employee. Findings from research studies suggest that students experience stress in their clinical practice and in their nursing education program (Jimenez, Navia-Osorio, & Diaz, 2010). These stresses, of course, can also have negative effects on students' health and can impact academic outcomes. In addition to the stresses experienced by students in general, nursing students are faced with the demands of clinical contact with patients and the urgency to master clinical competencies (Burnard et al., 2008). See Box 20-1 for a summary of the issues impacting the health care professional that might also impact the student nurse.

BOX 20-1

ISSUES AFFECTING THE HEALTH CARE PROFESSIONAL

- Aging population
- Aging workforce
- Job security
- Heavy workload
- Human suffering
- Nurse faculty shortage
- Managed care
- Outcomes measurement
- Role conflict
- Role ambiguity
- Stress
- Technological change

SPOTLIGHT ON

Issues Impacting a Nursing Student

Marta, a 32-year-old Mexican American mother of a 6-year-old and a 4-year-old, has decided to return to college after being out of school for 6 years. She has already completed all her prerequisite courses and is now ready to enter the registered nurse program. Her mother and mother-in-law both believe in the traditional role of the mother staying home to care for her young children. They have both been very verbal about that. Although this is stressful to Marta, she is intent on being the first in her family to complete college. She finds herself in conflict sometimes with her parents and her in-laws over her lifestyle choices. Marta becomes preoccupied with her current situation and worries that her husband, who dropped out of high school to provide for his family, will resent her for returning to school. She is aware that she will have little time for family events due to the demands of school and her mothering responsibilities.

FACTORS AFFECTING THE NURSING PROFESSION

The face of nursing is changing rapidly, both for students and for practitioners. The myriad responsibilities that professional nurses assume in the workplace have the potential for affecting their personal and professional functioning. Though a nursing career can be very satisfying and have job-related longevity, these responsibilities may cause individuals to seek other career options or to drop out of the health care arena totally. Although it appears that the nursing shortage of 2006–2011 has eased as a result of the downturn in the United States economy, a joint statement from the Tri-Council for Nursing raises concerns about slowing down the production of registered nurses in the United States (American Association of Colleges of Nursing [AACN], 2010). Some of the data on supply and demand of nurses seems

GLOBAL HIGHLIGHTS IN HEALTH PROMOTION

Nursing Stress Experienced Globally

Nursing stress is not unique to the United States. There is evidence to indicate stress and burnout are universal concerns for nurses in all parts of the world. For example, one study compared Polish and Dutch nurses in relation to stress and burnout. Although the study pointed out that Polish nurses experienced significantly more stress than Dutch nurses, the study concluded that job-related variables produced stress and burnout for both the Polish and Dutch nurses.

Source: Burnout among nurses: A Polish-Dutch comparison. *Sage Journals Online*. Retrieved from http:/jcc.sagepub.com

to give the impression that there is an over-abundance of nurses at present. However, American Association of Colleges of Nursing counters that impression by indicating that the data does not take into consideration that many of the nurses counted in a supply and demand model are not new to the profession of nursing and that many are also not registered nurses (AACN, 2011). Because the U.S. economy is in such a flux, it is not possible to accurately predict when the previous nursing workforce patterns will re-emerge. It is known that the baby boomers are entering retirement years and that this population will increase the demands for health care professionals. In addition, the current health care reform has created the need for nurses with advanced education to serve in faculty, administrator, scientist, primary care providers, and specialist roles. Registered nursing has been identified as the top profession through 2018. Even as the nursing shortage is thought to be abating, registered nurses still identify understaffing, nursing staff turnover, patient acuity, and patient volume increases as the most likely reasons for exiting the profession. These issues may be complicated by the health reform changes that are occurring. Unless these issues are adequately examined by the profession itself, nurses will continue to experience stress and poor health, potentially leading to nurse exit from the profession. Until these issues are resolved through strategies that encourage chief nurse officers to work with nurses, strategies for improving the quality of patient care will not be accomplished. As noted, factors affecting the nursing profession are many and include the current nursing student characteristics, the supply of professional nurses, and the impact of health care reform and managed care.

NURSING STUDENT CHARACTERISTICS

Nursing students are a large group and comprise more than half of all health profession students. These students bring a variety of assets and experiences with them as they prepare for their nursing career. Statistics published by the National Sample Survey of Registered Nurses (U.S. Department of Health and Human Services [USDHHS], 2010) indicate that the average age for the associate degree nursing program graduate is 33.1 years and that the average age for the baccalaureate degree nursing program graduate is 27.5 years. A large percentage of all

RESEARCH NOTE

Stress and Health of Nursing Students

STUDY PROBLEM/PURPOSE

Nursing students are under considerable stress during their clinical practice, putting their education and health at risk. There are potential differences in reports of stress among novice and experienced nursing students.

METHODS

The sample consisted of 357 students from all 3 years of a nursing diploma program in a Spanish college. A cross-sectional research methodology using standard information gathering tools was used. Data was collected over an 8-month period.

FINDINGS

Three types of stressors and two categories of symptoms linked to clinical practice were identified. The stressors related to clinical, academic, and external factors. The two categories of symptoms were physiological and psychological symptoms. Factor analysis identified 6 major sources of stress and 6 important symptoms. Clinical stressors were perceived more intensely than academic or external stressors and showed more psychological than physiological symptoms. All levels of nursing students perceived moderate stress. Experienced students perceived more academic stressors than novices. Second-year students were more vulnerable to somatic and psychic anxiety and common symptoms.

IMPLICATIONS

Nursing students are prone to experience stress while enrolled in a nursing program. Students should be informed about possible stressors associated with their profession and introduced to interventions that support coping.

Source: Jimenez, C., Navia-Osorio, P. M., & Diaz, C. V. (2010). Stress and health in novice and experienced nursing students. *Journal of Advanced Nursing, 66*(2), 442–455.

The preceding statistics are significant in that the wider age ranges as well as previous careers indicate that today's nursing student may be involved in more diverse life tasks such as caring for aging parents and raising children while juggling other multiple roles. Students may also be spouses, parents, single or married, and employed part-time or full-time while in school. Juggling multiple roles presents life challenges that are overwhelming at times and may lead to neglecting personal health practices and needs. In addition, the age at which a student graduates from nursing school is of concern since older graduates become older nurses in the workforce. Older nurses usually have a shorter career life expectancy. The fact that many of today's nursing students are enrolled in technical programs impacts the health care delivery system and the nursing profession as well. An inadequate health care system and fewer years of academic preparation may provoke stress and its consequences in those delivering care.

NURSING STUDENT STRESS

Many students in nursing are described as overachievers who have difficulty setting priorities that include play and having fun. These students are faced with a demanding scientific curriculum that dictates the establishment of new priorities and alterations in lifestyle. Nursing students are faced with many of the same problems encountered by nurses in the profession. They must adjust to shift changes, heavy workloads, and death and dying situations. For these students, anything less than the highest grade signifies failure and may lead to demoralization and stress. This is of concern; high levels of stress can have a major impact on academic outcomes because it has been found to lower academic achievement and increase attrition rates (Huerta, 1990).

? ASK YOURSELF

Learning to Say No!

Are you the type of person who has difficulty saying no? Do you take on too many projects because you are asked to do so? As a student, are you the one who takes the class notes and shares them with others? Do you sometimes feel that the other students do not reciprocate? Do you feel used? Can you say no and mean it?

nursing students have worked in other areas of health care before entering nursing school. Many of these students also have other academic degrees prior to enrolling in nursing courses. In the recent past, the majority of nursing students did not enroll in programs that led to an academic degree; however, current statistics indicate that the trend is slowly advancing to attainment of a 4-year academic degree. It has been reported that 45.4% of all registered nurses have an associate degree as their highest level of education and that 36.8% have a baccalaureate degree as the highest degree (United States Department of Health and Human Services & Health Resources and Services Administration [USDHHS&HRSA], 2010).

Students need to recognize that good grades are important, but not at the cost they often demand. Perfectionism is an unrealistic goal with a big price tag attached. No goal justifies the loss of physical or emotional health. Being the class hero may be a reenactment of being the family hero attempting to meet all the needs of the family growing up or to gain personal recognition in order to feel significant. All this is also true of other health care students who are pursuing an education in a highly competitive field. Sadly, many of the health care professions, including nursing, reinforce these behaviors. These professionals are taught to nurture, comfort, and "fix" those who come to them for help. Unfortunately, students are not taught how to "fix" themselves as well.

PROFESSIONAL NURSING SUPPLY

The demand for professional nurses is very market driven, and shortages have occurred periodically over the years. Nursing shortages were evident in the late 1980s, early 1990s, and in the current decade. As recently as recently as 2011, the nursing shortage in the United States was thought to be quite severe. At present, the nursing shortage has abated; however, the profession should not become complacent about the current employment statistics because the nursing shortage is predicted to become even more severe in the future. According to AACN (2011), once the current economy is stabilized, more registered nurses will be retiring, and the need for nurses will increase as the baby boomers age and the need for health care grows. In fact, the Bureau of Labor Statistics has stated that the need for health care workers is on the rise, with 283,000 jobs added in the health care sector this year (AACN, 2011). The anticipated nursing shortage is expected to be much more acute than in years past. According to AACN (2011), labor statistics indicate that more than 581,500 new registered nurse positions will be created by 2018, increasing the size of the current nursing workforce by 22%. Employment of RNs is expected to increase at a much faster rate than any other health care profession. According to Buerhaus, Staiger, and Auerbach (2009), the shortage of nurses may exceed 500,000 by 2028. Nursing shortages have a negative impact on nursing professionals who are attempting to provide quality patient care.

Lack of the necessary manpower to provide this care will result in workload-related stress; poor health practices such as skipping meals, overeating, or excessive drinking of alcohol; working long hours; and possibly physical and mental exhaustion or profession dropout. To adequately understand the demands placed on nurses and the impact these demands have on nurses' own health care needs, we look at the make-up of professional nurses today in terms of gender, age, ethnicity, and educational diversity.

GENDER

Gender inequities certainly exist in the nursing profession. Between 90% and 94% of all nursing students are female (USDHHS& HRSA, 2010). This lack of diversity is, of course, then reflected in the general nursing population. Trends, however, are showing that more males (see Figure 20-2) are entering the nursing profession than previously. Men enter nursing for a variety of reasons which, of course, include caring for others, but it seems that, according to the literature, their primary motivations are job security and career opportunities. The majority of the men in nursing are concentrated in certain types of jobs such as hospital administration and areas of specialty such as emergency room, psychiatric, and intensive care nursing.

Although current trends may indicate that the male registered nurse population is increasing, these statistics are still of concern to the profession because the majority of registered nurses are female, married, and have children who still live at home. Traditionally, women have been charged with the additional responsibilities of child rearing and making sure that the family life runs smoothly. Fortunately, nursing is a profession that can be exited and reentered based on personal and family needs. This too may sometimes be viewed as a limit in career development. But because nursing is primarily a female workforce, the inherent strengths of women predominate. The skills that males and females bring to the nursing workforce are vital for shaping the changing health care environment of

SPOTLIGHT **ON**

Nursing as a Career Choice for Men

Matthew is a 32-year-old male who has a degree in English literature and has taught at the high school level for 10 years. He has recently decided to make a career change and major in nursing. Matthew chose nursing as his second career because he wants a career that can allow him to express his caring nature and that will improve his economic status. He likes the career flexibility, mobility, and possibilities that nursing offers.

the future. A gender-diverse profession has all the benefits of balance within the profession (Christman, 1998).

AGE

Registered nurses in the United States number close to 3.1 million, with approximately 62% of them employed in direct patient care. Nurses comprise the largest single component of hospital staff employees (USDHHS&HRSA, 2010). The majority of health care services today involves caring for the growing population of older adults and usually includes some form of care by nurses (AACN, 2011). These statistics are frightening in view of the fact that nurses are growing older along with the general population. An aging workforce can result in negative health outcomes both for the patient and for the nurse providing the care.

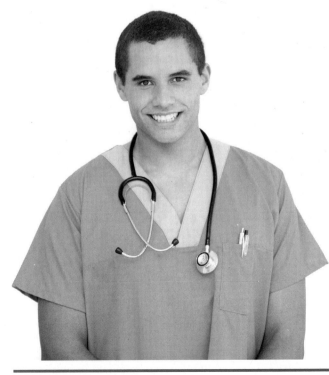

FIGURE 20-2 Men are a growing presence in nursing.

SPOTLIGHT **ON**

Delivering Culturally Competent Care

Mi-Ling, a 27-year-old Asian American, newly graduated BSN-prepared nurse, has been hired in an obstetrics floor in an institution that cares for a predominantly Hispanic population. A new mother tells Mi-Ling that she plans to care for her baby's umbilical cord so that it may dry quickly and fall off. In her conversation, she tells Mi-Ling that it is traditional in her ethnic group to bury the baby's dried umbilical cord. Mi-Ling has never encountered this practice. She is feeling stressed out by the number of things that she still needs to learn about her patient population. She determines that she needs to increase her awareness of different cultural practices associated with childbirth by going to the library and reading about the different cultural groups that she will care for. She has a strong desire to deliver culturally competent care.

The average age of the registered nurse in this country is 47 years, up from 46.8 years in 2004. It is estimated that 45% of all registered nurses are older than 50 and will leave the workforce within the next 10 years. In 1980, 25% of all nurses were under the age of 30. Current statistics, however, show that these numbers have actually gotten worse, with approximately 11% of all nurses being under the age of 30 (USHHS & HRSA, 2010). Nursing schools have tried to increase the number of younger RNs and have responded to the state and national pressure to increase enrollments in schools of nursing. In particular, nursing schools have attempted to increase the number of students admitted to bachelor's nursing programs, having a student population that is younger than the population in other initial registered nurse programs.

Obviously, an aging registered nurse workforce will be less mobile and more resistant to change and may be unable to adequately care for the acutely ill patients who receive nursing services today. This is especially true if the nurse caregiver is dealing with personal health problems related to aging. Issues such as health care insurance, retirement prospects, workloads, and career benefits will surely impact the nursing supply, especially when considering the aging of the nursing population. Excessive workloads, increasing stress in providing patient care, and the demands of ever changing technology can all have an impact on the health-promoting behaviors and health status of the professional caregiver.

ETHNICITY

The professional nursing supply definitely lacks ethnic diversity. Although Blacks, Hispanics, and American Indians make up 25% of the United States population, only 9% of the nation's nurses, 6% of the nation's physicians, and 5% of the nation's dentists are ethnic minorities (Health Care Workers Council, 2007). There is obviously an imbalance in the makeup of the nation's health care workforce. Nurses of ethnic minority represent only 16.8% of the total registered nurse population in the United States. These statistics are expected to change in the future because there are more minority nursing students in the education pipeline. Many barriers have been identified as deterrents to enrolling and succeeding in the nursing and health care professions. This lack of ethnic diversity among nurses and other health care workers contributes to the gap in health status and a lack of access to health care for many in our population (USDHHS & HRSA, 2010). Although the enrollment of minorities in nursing has shown a slight increase, the number of nurses from minorities has failed to keep up with the growth of the minority population. The data indicates that the number of minority nurses is substantially less than the number of minorities in the United States.

The numbers of minority populations are increasing rapidly in the United States. Many of these minority populations are first-generation Americans who may be living in poverty, lack access to health care, and be undereducated. Nurses are called upon daily to deliver nursing care to these minority populations with their complex health care needs. Nurses who are predominantly White and not from an ethnic minority may not understand a patient's culture, values, and beliefs but are still expected to provide culturally sensitive care. There is the expectation that professional nurses must provide culturally congruent care. This added responsibility may provoke stress in the nurse and may eventually lead to job frustration and dropping out of the nursing profession.

EDUCATION

Although the number of registered nurses with baccalaureate degrees (BSN) has increased, a large percentage of registered nurses are still educated at the technical level, such as the associate degree. Diploma program graduates are still considered as having degrees at the technical level, though very few diploma programs currently exist in the United States. Associate-, diploma-, and baccalaureate-prepared nurses all take the same licensing exam but are prepared to function at different levels. Baccalaureate graduates are prepared to practice in all health care settings because their education includes a broad spectrum of courses in the sciences and humanities, as well as courses in critical thinking, community health, and leadership (AACN, 2010). Unfortunately, only 36.8% of all nurses hold a baccalaureate degree in nursing as their highest degree, while 50% of all nurses are prepared at the associate or diploma level. Also, fewer than 10% of all registered nurses have graduate nursing degrees (USDHHS & HRSA, 2010).

Although the preceding statistics may not sound alarming, the lack of educational preparation may be reflected in the quality of care received by patients. It is also reflected in the amount of responsibility placed on the nurse, especially one who possesses a baccalaureate degree and is responsible for supervising patient care. Associate degree and diploma nurses provide the majority of the patient care, with the vast majority of nurses with a university degree working in management settings. Managing a poorly prepared workforce, assuming excessive responsibility when inadequately educated, and dealing with the multitude of issues associated with today's nursing environment may lead to unhealthy behavior patterns in the nursing workforce.

IMPACT OF HEALTH CARE REFORM AND MANAGED CARE ON NURSING

In 2010, Congress passed a law signed by the president that provides comprehensive health care legislation and that is now referred to collectively as the Affordable Care Act. The purpose of this legislation is to transform the health care system to provide higher-quality, safer, and accessible health care. These laws demonstrate a future where health care is responsive to individual needs through the delivery of quality, patient-centered care (Institute of Medicine of the National Academies [IOM], 2010). With the passing of the Affordable Care Act, the Institute of Medicine, along with the Robert Wood Johnson Foundation, formed a partnership to assess and respond to the need to transform the nursing profession. This partnership resulted in a report titled *The Future of Nursing: Leading Change, Advancing Health* (IOM, 2010). This report contained four key recommendations related to nursing's future: Nurses should (1) practice to the full extent of their education and training, (2) achieve higher levels of education and training, (3) be full partners with physicians and other health care professionals, and (4) be involved in planning and policy making to improve information collection and infrastructure. These recommendations impact the nursing profession and may be a source of concern for all nurses providing health care. Approaches to the use of health services, including managed care, is a major focus of this report.

Traditionally, health care was delivered by the health care provider only when people sought care for an illness. This lack of emphasis on prevention has been replaced by current health models that focus mainly on levels of prevention. Managed care, however, is a different approach to the use of health services. This model of health care delivery looks at providing services from a cost-containment perspective. Common features that characterize managed care include prenegotiated payment rates, mandatory patient precertification, utilization review, limited choice of providers, and fixed-price reimbursement (Smeltzer et al., 2010). The real concern of managed care seems to relate to reimbursement from insurance companies and Medicare for services rendered. Reimbursement for health care services can have an effect on patient care and an indirect effect on nurses.

Although there are acknowledged benefits to health care reform and managed care, primarily in terms of access to health care, cost containment, and the emphasis on disease prevention, health care reform and managed care models can also become a source of stress and discontent for the professional workforce. Criticism of managed care revolves around the issue of short-term cost containment with little emphasis on quality patient care. The discipline of nursing is centered on core values such as caring, empathy, and preservation of integrity. Taking the time to treat patients holistically is also central to the profession.

Critics of health care reform and the Affordable Care Act are concerned with the issue of who will pay for the services that constitute quality, accessible health care to all citizens. Other criticism revolves around the concept of managed care and its promotion of cost containment at the physical expense of the patient. Patients are admitted to health care institutions in a sicker state and dismissed earlier than ever before. In the effort to reduce expenses, institutions that function under managed care have had to cut back on professional nursing personnel and increase the number of unlicensed health care personnel. These actions only add to the workload stress experienced by nurses working for these institutions. Nurses working under any adverse conditions may also develop unhealthy ways to cope with the stressful environment and suffer dire health-related consequences. Chapter 21 discusses more information on economic and quality concerns associated with managed care.

HEALTH BEHAVIOR PATTERNS

People face important decisions about healthy eating, alcohol use, sexual practices, and exercise patterns. Eating disorders run rampant in our society, which appears fixated on a perfect, thin body. As students enrolled in health care courses learn about disease and health in others, opportunities will arise to evaluate and perhaps change their own health patterns. One way for students to learn about their propensity for future health concerns is to draw their family health **genogram** and observe their family members' age, their health patterns, and their causes of death, or, if living, their current health status (Smeltzer et al., 2010). A genogram is a useful tool that diagrams and depicts family relationships over a period of several generations. See Figure 20-3 for an example of how to construct a genogram.

Most health care professionals have established **health behavior patterns** by the time they become college students. These are health habits that may relate to physical functioning, such as exercise, food, and routine maintenance, or to the person's psychological, spiritual, and/or professional life. The choices made in the early adult years about diet and exercise have a lasting effect. A person who continues to eat junk food and plans to start exercising "tomorrow" may wake up 30 years later still planning to do something about personal health. Health care professionals who ignore their psychological well-being, physical and spiritual needs, and professional health needs lose both individually and collectively.

Health care professionals are very aware of the fact that people's needs change with each life stage and that they, as health care providers, are not immune to these changes. Many times, however, they are more in tune with their patients' changing needs than their own and forget to apply special health care knowledge and principles to themselves. These professionals have a rich source of information about health and health behavior patterns that can improve their general health. This information is gleaned from years of study, professional journals, and personal experiences. For example, nursing and medical professionals know that mortality increases with increased body weight and that being substantially over the recommended body weight increases the chance of death from cardiovascular disease and even from cancer. Yet many of these individuals choose to overlook these facts rather than make the necessary health-promotion changes.

Nurses, of course, are no exception. There is a rich source of information about nurses' health in the Nurses' Health Study, a major longitudinal research study conducted by the Harvard School of Public Health. There are 238,000 nurse participants in this study, which is close to 40 years old. The study has produced landmark data on cardiovascular disease and diabetes that has resulted in studies that have found an increased risk of coronary disease with 6 or more years of rotating shift work. There are also complex findings in the study regarding alcohol, indicating that light to moderate alcohol intake is associated with a lower rate of coronary heart disease but that these same levels are associated with increased risk for breast cancer. Most important, studies based on the data collected

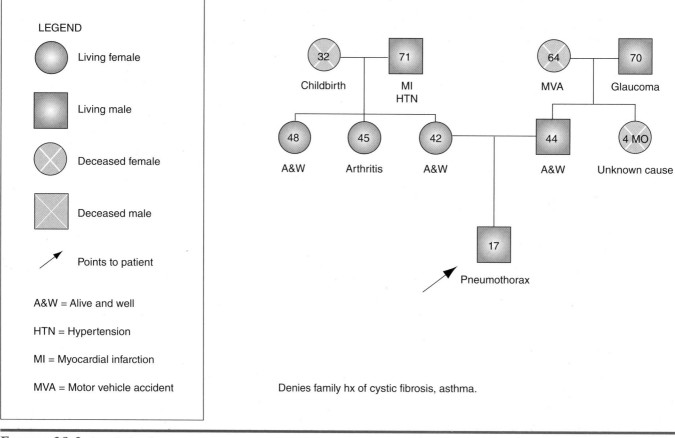

LEGEND

⬤ Living female

◼ Living male

⊗ Deceased female

⊠ Deceased male

↗ Points to patient

A&W = Alive and well

HTN = Hypertension

MI = Myocardial infarction

MVA = Motor vehicle accident

Denies family hx of cystic fibrosis, asthma.

FIGURE 20-3 Sample family genogram.

have demonstrated that diet, physical activity, and lifestyle factors can promote better health (Nurses' Health Study, 2011). These findings and many others related to general health, diet, exercise, family planning, and various risk factors are readily available to nurses, yet many choose to continue with their unhealthy behaviors. Nurses and other members of the health care professional workforce should adopt behaviors that are health promoting so that they may have a long and satisfying life and career. Failure to do so may result in dropout from the profession.

HEALTH PROMOTION THEORY LINK

Planning Health-Promoting Behaviors

Aizen's Theory of Planned Behavior (1991) identifies the variable of perceived behavioral control (PBC) as important in making a personal change in health behavior. PBC is a person's expectations that the performance of a behavior (or the nonperformance of a behavior) is within a person's control. One example of a behavior control expectation is a person's belief that he can quit drinking alcohol though he drinks on a daily basis. The person might initially think, "How likely is it that I won't drink today if I hang around with my nursing student peers and we drink daily after class to relax?" This thinking is followed up by the thought, "If I don't go to the pub with my peers today, how likely is it that I won't go tomorrow?"

HEALTH-PROMOTION PRACTICES BY DOMAIN

Of all occupations, nursing and professional health care rank as the second-highest professions prone to occupational injury and illness in the United States. Many major concerns must be addressed to ensure a healthy and productive nursing population. These concerns include needlestick and back injuries, workplace violence, and exposure to neoplastic agents, among others (Meeks-Sjostrom, Lopuszinski, & Bairan, 2010; Polovich & Giesker, 2011; Howerton-Child & Mentes, 2010). It is vital for nurses and health care professionals to be aware of their physical, emotional, spiritual, and professional health in order to experience a long and satisfying career. The first step is assessing overall health and then determining future goals. The domains provide a framework for assessing overall health in the health professional and for planning strategies to improve health status. Not only do these domains highlight areas that need addressing, they also provide a system for performing a personal evaluation in a holistic manner. When any domain is neglected, ill or unwanted effects may result.

The domains that are of concern are the same as those previously discussed: the biological, psychological, spiritual, sociocultural, environmental, and technological domains.

Change in one domain causes change in the others. This idea is similar to that of different ingredients being mixed in a punch bowl, in which a variety of flavors intermingle and saturate each other to produce a single taste. One-sided growth or deterioration in part of the system is dangerous at any period of life. The demands of working in a high-pressure profession can cause imbalance that may result in serious health concerns.

BIOLOGICAL DOMAIN

In thinking about ways to prevent illnesses that affect the physical or biological domain, obviously, nurses and other health care professionals can do many simple things for themselves to promote their own physical health. For example, they can follow established guidelines on routine immunizations such as tetanus, diphtheria, pertusss, and hepatitis B, which may be overlooked after schooldays are over. Seasonal influenza shots should also become a part of the regular immunizations received by nurses. Regular dental care impacts the future health of teeth and gums. Poor dental health and inflamed gums have been associated with serious health conditions such as cardiovascular disease.

Also, other work-related factors can seriously affect the biological domain and can have lifelong health-related consequences. All health care providers, for instance, who are actually providing bedside care are prone to injuries from lifting and moving patients. Major injuries are well documented in health care workers. Nurses may be on their feet all day, moving their hands and keeping their arms busy doing procedures. These activities may result in many musculoskeletal aches and pains that could eventually force them to drop out of the nursing profession. Of all of the occupation-related injuries suffered by nurses, the largest majority are caused by overexertion to the back or trunk. It is estimated that back injuries affect up to 48% of all nurses and that nursing absenteeism is largely due to back injuries (Missouri State Board of Nursing, 2010). Although patient handling and manually lifting objects are factors that place nurses and other health care professionals at risk, the majority of these injuries are attributed to the act of lifting patients. The American Nurses Association (ANA) is so concerned about musculoskeletal injuries in the workplace that it has published a position statement on the elimination of manual patient handling and advocacy of assistive devices for nurses. ANA has devoted a lot of resources to establishing safe patient handling policies that seek to eliminate the manual lifting of patients. The organization's position is that the nursing

profession can no longer afford to lose nursing professionals because of musculoskeletal injuries (ANA, 2011). Effective and safe patient handling programs using assistive devices greatly reduce back injury risks. Use of safe equipment also offers a more secure, comfortable, and dignified way to handle patients.

Health care disciplines have shown a lot of interest in the field of ergonomics and its application to the workforce. **Ergonomics** involves the study and analysis of human work, particularly as it relates to an individual's anatomy and other human characteristics. The term refers to assessing the work-related factors that may pose a risk of musculoskeletal disorders and recommendations to alleviate them (U.S. Department of Labor, Occupational Safety and Health Administration, 2011). Following appropriate ergonomic principles and pushing for ergonomic standards are strategies that can decrease the risk of injury. Discovering what lifting devices are commercially available and working only in institutions that use these are also strategies that might be helpful in decreasing this type of work-related injury.

Another area of concern affecting the biological domain is risk for chemical hazards. Serious chemical exposure can result from the use of sterilizing agents and chemotherapeutic agents. Reactive airway symptoms and skin problems can occur. Nurses frequently care for patients with cancer who are receiving anticancer drugs. These drugs represent a significant hazard for nurses (Polovich & Geisker, 2011).

Other conditions are not necessarily work-related but warrant periodic screening to prevent development of disease process. These include, but are not limited to, such conditions as hypertension, hyperlipidemia, colon cancer, breast cancer, cervical cancer, prostate cancer, and testicular cancer. In those with risk factors, a regular screening by a dermatologist for mole changes or skin lesions is prudent. Some health-promotion issues are more age specific, such as birth control or the need to check vision for glaucoma and cataracts. Birth control methods include the regular use of condoms, which protects from pregnancy and many sexually transmitted diseases, including acquired immunodeficiency syndrome (AIDS).

Despite the fact that smoking has a well documented negative impact on health, the use of nicotine continues in younger populations, particularly young White females. This is

SPOTLIGHT **ON**

Nurses Caring for Themselves

Nurses provide quality care to their patients but may ignore their own health care needs. Nurses have one of the highest rates of workplace injury among all occupations. Nurses must focus on taking care of themselves so that they may continue to provide quality care to their patients.

? ASK **YOURSELF**

Role Modeling Behavior

How many times have you seen a nurse who is grossly overweight? Who smells of cigarette smoke? Is it the nurse's responsibility to follow a healthy lifestyle? Professionals in health care fields do not always practice what they preach when making personal choices that may affect their health. These professionals, like everyone else, must assume responsibility for their own health. They must interpret research information, contemplate possible lifestyle and health habit changes, and apply what has been learned to themselves.

of concern to the nursing profession whose workforce consists largely of White females. Recognizing that smoking is an unhealthy behavior can often be the first step in seeking help to stop, the next step. Alcohol and other drug abuse also have serious health consequences that need expert treatment. Perhaps, because of the stresses encountered in their work, health care professionals have been noted to have a propensity for drinking excessively and for abusing drugs. Professionals who are aware of this predisposition to alcoholism and drug addiction prevent the associated physical consequences or seek professional care early. Chapter 18 provides a more in-depth discussion on the alcohol use and addiction.

Unfortunately, many of the choices made in youth, such as whether to exercise, take drugs, use alcohol, diet, or smoke, have lifelong physiological effects. The immediate results of such choices on a young person's health may not be seen, and this in itself can create a false sense of security and a continuation of the detrimental behaviors. Good nutrition and regular exercise increasingly show up in research as being essential to good health. Knowledgeable health care professionals have the responsibility to make healthy choices, particularly in view of their potential to serve as possible role models.

ASK **YOURSELF**

Developing Healthy Habits

Andrea, a 22-year-old junior nursing student, has been learning about the different types of cancer in her adult health class. She rarely goes to the doctor and knows very little about cancer and cancer prevention. When Andrea does a genogram as part of her class assignment, she notices that her mother's sister and her grandmother have both been diagnosed with and survived breast cancer. She also notices that depression and alcoholism run in her father's family. In completing her assignment, Andrea notes that she is in a vulnerable group.

- What can Andrea do to prevent or detect breast cancer or both?
- Are there any lifestyle changes that Andrea needs to adopt to ensure that she does not become a victim of alcoholism or drug abuse?
- What would you do in a similar situation?

PSYCHOLOGICAL DOMAIN

Values and expectations impact emotional health. The ways in which people cope with stress impacts everyone. **Hardiness**, or resilience to stress, and perceptions are significant influences on psychological well-being. Burnout can be the natural consequence of not caring, resulting from an extended period of stress, of which there are many sources in the workplace. For example, one significant source is nurse/supervisor conflict and staff/physician conflict. Of course, other areas can cause turmoil and psychological stress in the work area. Stress and turmoil in the nursing workplace is not unique to U.S. nurses

but is a phenomenon reported in other parts of the world (Menzani & Bianchi, 2009). Excessive stress may be related to an inadequate fit between the employee's assigned job and the institution's work policies. A restrictive work environment or one that stifles autonomy has a devastating effect on employee well-being. Stress and burnout can occur in the nursing profession. Leiter and Maslach (2009) found that nurses expressed symptoms of stress and burnout as reasons for their intention to exit the profession. They also found that the workplace is oppressive and creates work cynicism and dissatisfaction among nurses. In assessing stress in the health care professional and in determining strategies that promote psychological health, it is wiser to look beyond individual responses to the broader picture of the work setting and work team.

Physical and mental exhaustion among nurses is associated with anxiety, frequency of illness, and negative job attitudes, as well as with lack of collegial support (Van Bogaert et al., 2009). A positive collegial and supportive network is also associated with feelings of job satisfaction. Strategies that facilitate positive peer relationships increase positive job attitudes and perhaps even job satisfaction. Professionals who seek out or create positive work settings enjoy better psychological health and experience fewer episodes of psychological crisis.

Congruence between personal values and the values held by the employing institution also plays an important role in increasing job satisfaction, decreasing job turnover, and improving the psychological health of the employed professional. Individuals who experience personal conflict between their values and those of their employer are at risk for experiencing low self-esteem and a uncaring attitude. Feelings of autonomy and of control are also important to preventing psychological distress. Buerhaus, Staiger, and Auergach (2009) found that RNs who reported that their organization emphasized quality patient care, recognized the importance of their personal lives, and had positive relationships with colleagues were more satisfied with their chosen profession. Decreases in job satisfaction were predicted in those feeling stress related to too many non-nursing tasks.

The individuals most susceptible to physical and emotional exhaustion are usually bright, perfectionists, hardworking, and idealistic. Hardiness is related to four Cs: control, communication, challenge, and commitment. Four behaviors drain a health care professional's energy: perfectionism, complaining, resisting reality, and judging others. Many positive strategies reduce stress and decrease the energy drain, including seeking

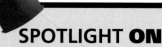

SPOTLIGHT **ON**

Student Stress

Students have unique areas of stress. Grades can be a demonstration of pushing for perfection. When only As are acceptable, anything less can produce anxiety and discontent. Some students argue for hours over a grade of 98% versus one of 96%. Procrastination, on the other hand, is another student-related demon that can cause major psychological distress.

TABLE 20-1 Coping Practices		
Add your scores for each column according to the scale in the table. Do you score higher on healthy or unhealthy coping practices? How can you minimize unhealthy coping?		
HEALTHY COPING PRACTICES		**UNHEALTHY COPING PRACTICES**
Listen to music		Avoid social contact
Express emotions: cry, talk		Drink or use drugs
Exercise: walk, jog, bike, swim	*1 = Often*	Smoke or overeat
Pray, meditate, read	*2 = Sometimes*	Blame others for your problems
Go outdoors, enjoy nature		Yell or curse at others
Practice deep breathing	*3 = Rarely*	Drive fast or recklessly
Attend concerts, plays, events	*4 = Never*	Anticipate worst possible outcome
See a counselor or minister		Ignore the problem
Total Points		Total Points

Cengage Learning 2013

support from psychologically positive individuals, exercising, eating right, and resting when needed. Adopting healthy coping practices is also essential to prevent psychological distress. Table 20-1 illustrates one way to evaluate individual coping strategies.

SPIRITUAL DOMAIN

A spiritual life is a large part of what makes us different from other species. It is a defining characteristic of human nature (Maslow, 1970). **Spirituality** has been identified as an integral component of nursing practice (Pesut et al., 2009). The concept has been defined in many ways, but most definitions include concepts related to religion and states of awareness. Spirituality is concerned with the whole personality and emotional sharing. The word *spirituality* is derived from the Latin *spiritus*, meaning breath and also relates to the Greek word *pneuma*, also meaning breath or the vital spirit of the soul (Dossey & Keegan, 2009). A belief in the sacredness of every person and of every living thing can be included in the definition of spirituality.

The concept of wellness is multidimensional and includes the spiritual domain in addition to all of the other domains. A spiritually well person seeks a harmony between that which lies within the individual and the forces that come from outside the individual. A health-promotion approach to care, whether for the patient or the health care professional, incorporates spirituality. Spirituality can provide personal comfort and is a source of major support for patients. What is not always as obvious is that the spiritual dimension can also be a resource for the health care professional.

Nurses and other health care professionals come into contact with the spiritual dimension of life in their everyday practice. They must have some understanding of this spiritual dimension, not only for themselves but also for assessment of others. Professionals, such as the nurses who provide for the most intimate care of an individual, must be comfortable in recognizing the spiritual needs of patients and providing spiritual care. Most important, they must recognize that spirituality can be a personal strength for themselves in the role of caregiver (Hussey, 2009).

The research literature reveals studies describing measurable indicators of spirituality. Nurses, in particular, are expected to be familiar with these indicators in order to make accurate nursing diagnoses. The North American Nursing Diagnosis Association has identified risk for spiritual distress as a patient diagnosis that refers to the impaired ability to experience and integrate meaning and purpose in life through a person's connectedness with self, other persons, art, music, literature, nature, and a power greater than oneself (Sparks-Ralph & Taylor, 2011). Some specific indicators of spiritual distress include anger at God, depression, lack of hope, loss of meaning and purpose in life, and a refusal to interact with others. Although the spiritual distress diagnosis was developed for patients, the risk for spiritual distress can also be a possibility for all nurses and health care professionals. When understanding how these apply to patients, especially to those who are enduring a physical or mental illness, professional nurses recognize that issues affecting spirituality may really be quite relevant for themselves. For example, patients who have no belief in God or a Higher Power may feel they are completely on their own to combat the fear and anxiety of a poor health state or acute health problem. These individuals may believe that no outside power is available to help support or direct them in their current crisis. Isolation and a lack of significant relationships in one's life may be indicators of poor self-esteem, an inability to give or receive love, and subsequent behavior patterns based on the belief that one must earn another's love and respect by being perfect. These issues can be experienced by the nurse as well and are no different for the nurse caring for the patient. Nurses and health care professionals can experience personal spiritual distress that needs to be addressed. In fact, the nursing process can be applied to nurses as well in order to develop a plan to address their own spiritual distress.

Just as there are instances of risk for spiritual distress, there are also instances when a positive nursing diagnosis of readiness for enhanced spiritual well-being is observed. This diagnosis refers to the ability to experience and integrate meaning and purpose in life through connectedness with self, others, music, literature, nature, and a power greater than oneself (Sparks-Ralph & Taylor, 2011). In assessing a patient, nurses should be ready to do a personal spiritual inventory to determine their

SPOTLIGHT ON

Neglecting Spiritual Health

Spirituality takes many forms. It is not simply a matter of going to church on holidays or special occasions. In fact, spirituality can exist devoid of any church affiliation. People frequently think about their spiritual connection when they are faced with a crisis. Health care professionals may be called upon to resolve issues that relate to crisis and to the spiritual concerns of unfinished business.

own readiness to address personal spiritual concerns. Although health care professionals are aware of the importance of the spiritual dimension from the patient's point of view, most do not stop to assess their own spirituality. Tending to their own spiritual needs can be a source of comfort that adds focus to life and provides a sense of fulfillment. Frankl (1978) describes lack of purpose in life as existential vacuum, a sense of emptiness and boredom that leads to a state of unhappiness with one's life. Often this spiritual boredom is compounded by the stresses that occur in the professional workplace. People have a tendency to make their work their life's priority and do not take time to renew their spiritual life. Many caregivers are uncomfortable with their own spiritual dimension and choose to ignore this aspect of life until they are faced with a crisis. By performing a personal spiritual assessment, knowing themselves spiritually, and taking the time to renew their spirituality, nurses and health care professionals become more comfortable with the spiritual care that they are expected to provide. For a more thorough description of the spiritual domain, refer to Chapter 4.

Box 20-2 provides a spiritual assessment guide for the health care professional.

BOX 20-2
SPIRITUAL ASSESSMENT GUIDE

1. What gives your life meaning?
2. Do you have a sense of purpose in your life?
3. What is the most important or powerful force in your life?
4. What brings you joy and peace in your life?
5. What are your personal beliefs?
6. Do you pray?
7. How do you show love to yourself?
8. Who are the significant people in your life?
9. Do you have close friends or family you can call on for help when you need it?
10. Is it easy for you to forgive yourself and others?

SOCIOCULTURAL DOMAIN

Working as a health care professional in today's society is a major challenge that takes special skills. The changes impacting society today also have an impact on health care. Social issues, such as the ethnic minority population influx, economic challenges, workforce supply and demand, and technological changes, have the potential to overburden nurses and other health care workers. Nurses and health care professionals who make personal health-related changes in response to the stresses experienced at work will enjoy life and express satisfaction in their chosen career.

Many nurses and other providers of health care would prefer to not view health care as a business, but it is. The more that they know about the business end, the more effective they can be. In this business, the patient and often the family are the customers. Maintaining positive interactions with patients and their families can indirectly impact the economics of the employing institution. Also, the nurse's documentation, for example, can directly lead to the bottom line and to the viability of the organization and therefore to the nurse's job. What nurses do and know affects their salaries and the economics of the employing institution. Nurses and health care professionals are power brokers who often form partnerships and important bonds with their patients. It is not unusual for patients to follow their nurses or other health care practitioners to their new jobs, such as in home health or nurse practitioner-run clinic. This patient preference for a specific practitioner is common in other professions but is sometimes viewed with skepticism in health care disciplines other than medicine.

Agencies and hospitals want the nurse to be loyal or to be independent as it suits the employer, whose preferences are usually related to patient census or other bottom lines of economics. But nurses, like other professionals employed in the health care fields, must assume responsibility for themselves. Communicating in clear and respectful ways and being well informed on the economics associated with health care, for example insurance and reimbursement changes, help nurse employees be equal partners in health care. Using effective communication skills, taking ownership for solving problems, and cultivating positive work relationships go a long way in furthering a career. Taking risks, letting go, and embracing change are powerful attitudes for the health care professional to cultivate.

ENVIRONMENTAL DOMAIN

Another significant area of possible stress is the physical environment of the workplace. An unsafe work environment can impact the nurses' personal health and job longevity. The workplace environment can have adverse effects on the recruitment and retention of nurses, as well as on patient safety. It is critically important that nurses develop an awareness of how to maintain their own health and safety in a workplace environment that is not always conducive to personal health (Handleman, 2010). A crowded, noisy area impacts job satisfaction and self-care. If there is little control over the environment, stress and dissatisfaction increase. The elimination of negative factors in the environment is essential to the achievement of the health care employee's job satisfaction.

Nursing can enhance its environment through increased personal control, contact with nature, and the creation of aesthetically pleasing spaces. Surrounding themselves with positive people rather than those who whine or complain is important. Being around complainers drains energy and can decrease morale and productivity.

Many environmental issues are potentially serious for the health care professional. Workplace violence, for instance, has been recognized as a peril for health care workers. Workplace violence is one of the most complex and dangerous hazards facing nurses who work in health care environments. Dangers arise from the exposure to violent individuals and from the fact that violence prevention programs and protective regulations are sorely lacking (Chapman et al., 2010). It is not uncommon to hear about a nurse who was punched in the eye or slammed to the floor. Agitated patients in health care facilities and the emergency room as well as patients with dementia or a history of assault can pose a great risk to the nurse caring for them. Demanding the right to a safe environment is one step in curbing violence in the workplace. The next is becoming aware of the employing institution's policies on violence and how incidents have been dealt with in the past.

Other environmental issues most frequently identified are needlestick injuries, latex allergy, and exposure to physical hazards such as radiation. Needlestick injuries can transmit hepatitis B and C viruses if the injected patient is infected. The hepatitis viruses and human immunodeficiency virus (HIV) affect thousands of health care workers annually, usually by means of needlestick injury (Hospital Employee Health, 2010). Obviously, this is a real environmental hazard in our profession of which nurses must become aware.

Latex allergies are also a source of concern to the health care profession (Bemis & Mullet, 2009). Allergy to the latex in gloves and other medical products occurs in workers in health care institutions. Latex sensitization is most commonly caused by using powdered latex gloves, which allows the latex to become airborne and gain access to the respiratory system. This allergic response can cause minor symptoms such as skin irritation or flushing, but unfortunately it can also cause shock, laryngeal spasms, and cardiac arrest.

> ## ✿ NURSING **ALERT**
>
> ### Health-Promotion Strategies
>
> - Use the energy in anger to make changes and then get over it.
> - Remember life is not a race; pace yourself.
> - Exercise, relax, play, and take time alone. These are essential for well-being.
> - Protect personal time from school or work time.
> - Be clear and responsible in communicating. Ask for what is needed.
> - Appreciate personal humanness and celebrate that with others.

Physical hazards are all around the health care worker's environment. The health care professional must recognize the risks in the environment and formulate a plan that addresses them. It is also essential that the professional become cognizant of the roles of the employee health and risk management departments. Appropriate protection from potentially damaging environmental hazards is a priority.

TECHNOLOGICAL DOMAIN

Technology has transformed the traditional health care industry as well as the delivery of patient care. Although technology has brought better and more advanced care to our patient populations, it has also been a source of stress for nurses and health care workers who recognize the need to update their skills in order to remain competent in the health care setting. Registered nurses (RNs) are the primary information managers in clinical settings. They collect data, transform data to usable digital formats, integrate information from many diverse sources, analyze information, make data-based nursing care decisions, and communicate information to others as appropriate. The skills employed and the technology-related activities undertaken by RNs make them the consummate knowledge workers of today. Nurses are expected to upload and monitor complex data, such as data from computerized monitors and medical records. Along with the cognitive nursing skills needed for such critical thinking activities, nurses are expected to use information technologies to arrive at critical decision making. They must be able to manipulate sophisticated equipment and also deal with various complexities that require the application of technology in the clinical setting. Some clinical areas such as intensive care units, that are probably already stressful to the nurse because of the gravity of a patient's situation, have many electronic monitors, pumps, and other assessment gadgets—all requiring immediate attention when the machines beep. The constant beeping and the need to focus on computerized equipment can be overwhelming and stressful to nurses working in those areas.

Some recent technological developments that have been a source of assistance as well as stress for today's nurses are computerized automated medication delivery systems, bedside charting, electronic health records, and other equipment. Nurses must be able to keep up with the latest technologies and, through the Internet, have the ability to find information from all over the world quickly and without difficulty. The Internet has provided opportunities for nurses to learn about interventions and programs that other countries have established to provide better care. Technological advances, such as the small and portable tablet computers, can also assist nurses in assessing their own health and wellness. Digital technology provides nurses with information at their fingertips such as data on their own blood pressure readings, glucose monitoring, fat analysis, and so forth. This information can be used to make wise lifestyle choices.

NURSING PROCESS AND HEALTH-PROMOTION PLANNING

Previous chapters have established that the nursing process is a problem-solving method useful in gathering and interpreting data in order to formulate a plan of care. This same process can be applied in determining a plan of action to address actual or potential health-promotion problems affecting nurses and other health care professionals. The domains covered throughout the text are useful as the organizing structure for assessing problems and planning interventions for the health care professional who is at risk. For example, an assessment of the biological domain may reveal physical problems such as gastritis and high blood pressure. Further assessment may also reveal that the professional has been experiencing major work-related stress, exhibits angry behavior, and is having difficulty

TABLE 20-2 Nursing Process Plan for the Health Professional

Assessment: Patricia is a 49-year-old African American nurse working on an oncology floor. She is constantly stressed due to the heavy patient load and the gravity of their prognosis. Most days, she is responsible for caring for eight seriously ill patients. She is overweight and is always complaining of fatigue and backache. She acknowledges that she needs to lose weight and has decided to join a weight reduction program. She states that joining will make her feel as if she is "at least in control of that aspect" of her health.

NURSING DIAGNOSIS(ES)	GOALS/OUTCOMES	INTERVENTIONS
Ineffective coping related to inability to manage work-related stress	Will identify three social support networks	Identify social support networks such as friends, colleagues, organizations. Increase awareness of personal coping skills through use of assessment tools. List alternate ways of coping.
	Will learn how to manage time effectively	Invest in time management course. Engage in exercise. Establish work, play, sleep schedules.
Readiness for enhanced nutrition	Will verbalize present understanding of factors that enable and/or hinder enhanced nutritional status	Identify times when she is most likely to overeat.
	Will express positive feelings about herself	Maintain journal on thoughts and behavior. Use positive self-talk.
	Will identify stressors that increase eating behavior	Examine personal coping skills. Maintain food diary. Reward self for positive outcomes. Increase activity. Use friends for support in weight loss. Attend weight reduction support group meetings. Analyze eating patterns. Do not rationalize. Read food labels; use food guides such as the healthy plate guidelines
Readiness to learn regarding risk for work-related back injury	Will verbalize physical risks associated with caring for patients	Read materials on how to prevent back injuries. Become aware of equipment that is ergonomically appropriate for use in lifting patients.
	Will demonstrate appropriate patient handling and transfer techniques	Become aware of physical risks in moving heavy patients. Maintain proper positioning and good posture. Minimize back sprain.

Cengage Learning 2013

communicating with coworkers. The nursing process action plan can then address healthy coping skills, anger management, and communication skills.

The nursing process is useful in assessing personal needs and values, helping in the making of decisions that affect long-term career planning. Career planning is not an accident. Having an idea of what is happening on a personal level and in the health care arena is necessary in planning for the future. The identification of strategies that are useful in preventing career-related health problems is essential in promoting healthy behaviors among the health professional workforce. Table 20-2 provides an example of a nursing process plan addressing areas that affect health promotion by a nurse or health care professional.

SUMMARY

Nurses and health care professionals are faced with many issues that impact their professional lives. In addition to being confronted with life-and-death issues in their daily work, they must adapt to a phenomenal amount of technological change. Health care professionals are impacted by heavy workloads, health care reform laws, managed care, and an increasing focus on cost containment and outcomes measurement. Some health care disciplines seem to have bigger demands than other disciplines. The nursing profession, for example, might have to deal with nursing shortages in some areas of the country in addition to all the issues confronting health care professionals today. Unless plans are made to focus on personal health promotion, occupational stress, frustration, emotional exhaustion, and job turnover are the consequences that health care professionals face.

A positive professional life begins in school. Students can take advantage of the many opportunities that will help them have a more satisfying professional future. Being proactive and in charge of one's career is vital. Health care professionals should know the risks involved in their line of work. Education should include information on work-related risks that affect personal health promotion, finances, retirement benefits, and health insurance. Being professionally healthy means that the nurse is taking responsibility for personal health, staying open to new opportunities, and seeking these out. Key strategies include having positive relationships and networking with others. The investment on a personal level, as well as in terms of career planning, is worthwhile. Individuals engaging in careers in the health care professions should know that these careers are both rigorous and demanding. Those who choose these careers have countless opportunities to meet the needs of patients. As they respond to the call of those whom they serve, health care professionals must remember to put themselves as the priority. Modeling health and wholeness to others requires personal health-promotion skills.

CASE STUDY

David Bordeaux: Sleep Deprivation; Ineffective Health Maintenance; At Risk for Latex Allergy Response; Imbalanced Nutrition: More Than Body Requirements

OBJECTIVES/GOALS: Through participation in a discussion of this case study, participants will have the opportunity to:

1. Identify specific factors or issues or both that may affect a nursing student.
2. Describe how a nursing student's health-promotion practices influence curricular activities and outcomes.
3. Identify strategies for positive health promotion.

HEALTH-PROMOTION CONCERN, HISTORY AND PHYSICAL, PRESENT HEALTH STATUS, PAST HEALTH STATUS, FAMILY HISTORY, AND SOCIAL HISTORY

David Bordeaux is a 40-year-old male from Haiti returning to school for a second career. He is married and has three children, ages 12, 14, and 16. He has a degree in business but is returning to attain a BSN and eventually an MSN so that he can assume an administrative role in a health care institution. David is employed at United Parcel Service (UPS) and works evenings, full-time, Monday through Thursday. He is also attending school on all days of the week. On days that he has clinical lab, he spends 8 hours there and then hurries to his evening job. On the other days, he leaves school at 2:00 p.m. and clocks in to work at 4:00 p.m. He returns home at 12:00 midnight and studies until 2:00 every morning. He sleeps approximately 5.5 hours each night. David is overweight, skips meals frequently, and overindulges later, usually late at night. His health history is nonremarkable.

REVIEW OF PERTINENT DOMAINS

Biological Domain

Physical exam reveals a 5 ft., 8 in. male who weighs 200 lb.

GASTROINTESTINAL: He drinks at least four cola drinks and eats a fast lunch every day. Because his job has "down times" when it is not very busy, he consumes cola and snacks on corn chips. He dislikes vegetables but will eat fruit occasionally. He eats supper whenever he gets home, usually very late at night.

GENITOURINARY: David reports no problems in this area. He has regular bowel movements and urinates with no discomfort.

INTEGUMENTARY: David has been experiencing a rash on his hands, which seems to be getting worse. He is allergic to bananas and some tropical fruits and has a history of a skin reaction to balloons.

(Continues)

Psychological Domain

David is a very intelligent person, but he is making average grades because of his tight schedule, which allows limited time for study. David appears to be exhausted most of the time. His wife reports that he has been slightly depressed. David has trouble staying awake during lectures. He drinks alcohol only during the weekends and not to excess.

Social Domain

David has not been getting along with his family. He becomes very exasperated anytime that he is asked to join in social activities. In addition, even though David is working, he is making considerably less money than he did at his previous job, and he is having problems making ends meet. His wife is having difficulty supporting David emotionally because she is not sure that he should be pursuing a BSN. She has said to him that he must be having so much fun surrounded by "all those young female students."

Environmental Domain

David has been experiencing a rash on his hands that causes redness and swelling. He thinks that his rash is getting worse. He did not have this problem when he was at his job. David thinks that his rash may be stress related.

QUESTIONS FOR DISCUSSION

1. Describe specific factors that might affect David's school performance.
2. Identify three of David's health behavior patterns that are affecting his health status.
3. Identify strategies that David can use to achieve positive health promotion.

KEY CONCEPTS

1. Many stress-provoking factors impact the health of those who provide health care to others.
2. Technological change is forcing many health care professionals to return to the academic setting for additional preparation.
3. Job-related stress, emotional exhaustion, and job turnover are consequences of the enormous responsibility assumed by health care professionals.
4. Students enrolled in health career courses are not immune to some of the same work-related stresses experienced by the health care professional.
5. Nursing supply and demand factors impact professional nursing delivery.
6. Health care professionals are not immune to health problems and must apply their special knowledge and principles to themselves.
7. Back injuries, psychological stress, spiritual distress, needle-stick injuries, and latex allergies are health risks associated with the health care disciplines.
8. The nursing process can address health-promotion problems and risks affecting health care professionals and provide strategies to enhance health.
9. Technological changes can affect stress levels in nurses but can also be used to assess negative lifestyle behaviors.

CHAPTER REVIEW

Learning Activities

1. What are some specific factors that impact nursing students?
2. Describe the difference between occupational stress and burnout. Are these two synonymous?
3. List two health risks that confront health care professionals according to domain.
4. Draw your family genogram. Include age, causes of death, any cancer, cardiac conditions, hypertension, overweight, substance abuse, mental illness, chronic illnesses, and other pertinent findings. Refer to Figure 20-2 as a reference. Ask your family for information. There may be issues that your family members may not want to discuss.

5. After completing the genogram, consider the following:
   a. What health changes might be personally necessary?
   b. What new information did you learn?
   c. Did you discover any risk factors for diseases?
6. Read a current professional nursing journal. Identify technological advances in nursing.

Multiple Choice Questions

1. All of the following are factors affecting nursing students and the profession *except*:
   a. age.
   b. ethnic representation.
   c. genetic environment.
   d. stress.

2. Hardy individuals are more successful in the nursing profession. Hardiness refers to:
   a. susceptibility to burnout.
   b. resilience to stress.
   c. perfectionist behaviors.
   d. physical fitness.

3. Major issues impacting health care professionals include:
   a. an aging population.
   b. supply and demand.
   c. technological advances.
   d. all of the above.

4. Burnout is defined as a state of:
   a. physical fatigue and ergonomic injuries.
   b. hardiness and coping.
   c. established health and emotional behavior patterns that cannot be changed.
   d. depleted adaptive energy resources leading to physical and mental exhaustion.

5. Environmental hazards for nurses in the workplace include:
   a. ergonomics.
   b. dementia.
   c. musculoskeletal injury.
   d. autonomy.

6. Which of the following is an issue affecting all health care professionals?
   a. oversupply of health care workers.
   b. younger nursing professionals.
   c. specific nursing roles.
   d. technological changes.

7. Of the following health conditions, which of the following is the most common among practicing nurses?
   a. Back injuries
   b. Blood-borne infections
   c. Depression
   d. Hepatitis

ORGANIZATIONS AND WEBSITES

American Nurses Association: Represents American's registered nurses and promotes quality nursing care: **http://www.nursingworld.org**

ANA Nursing World: Provides information on preventing needlestick injury in practice; provides a guide to the types of work-related injuries that occur in the workplace: **http://www.nursingworld.org**

Nursing Society: Provides information on all international honor society activities and provides information from disaster preparedness to implementing evidence-based nursing practice: **http://www.nursingsociety.org**

Sigma Theta Tau International Honor Society of Nursing: The only international honor society of nursing; represents the global community of nurse leaders. Members lead in using knowledge, scholarship, service, and learning to improve the health of the world's people: **http://www.nursingsociety.org**

REFERENCES

Aizen, I. (1991). The theory of planned behavior. *Organizational Behavior and Human Decision Processes,* 50, 179–211.

American Association of Colleges of Nursing (AACN). (2010). Your nursing career: A look at the facts. Retrieved from http://www.aacn.nche.edu

American Association of Colleges of Nursing (AACN). (2011). Nursing shortage. Retrieved from http://www.aacn.nche.edu.

American Nurses Association. (2011). Safe patient handling. Retrieved from http://www.anasafepatienthandling.org.

Bemis, P.A., & Mullett, S. (2009). Disabled nurses discover new career paths. *RN, 72* (6), 28–31.

Benner, P., Tanner, C., & Chesla, C. (2009). *Expertise in nursing practice: Caring, clinical judgment, and ethics.* New York, NY: Springer.

Buck, D. F., Curley, A. L., & Strasser, P. B. (2010). Developing and implementing a survey to determine employer satisfaction with care provided to injured workers. *AAOHN Journal, 58*(2), 69–77.

Buerhaus, P., Donelan, K., Ulrich, B., DesRoches, C., & Dittus, R. (2007). Trends in the experiences of hospital employed registered nurses: Results from three national studies. *Nursing Economics, 25*(2), 69–79.

Buerhaus, P., Staiger, D., & Auerbach, D. (2009). *The future of the nursing workforce in the United States: Data, trends, and implications.* Boston, MA: Jones & Bartlett.

Burnard, P., Edwards, D., Bennett, K., Thaibah, H., Tothoba, V., Baldacchino, D., Bara, P. & Mitevelli, J. (2008). A comparative, longitudinal study of stress in student nurses in five countries: Albania, Brunei, the Czech Republic, Malta, and Wales. *Nurse Education Today, 28*(2), 134–145.

Chapman, R., Styles, I., Perry, L., & Combs, S. (2010). Nurses' experience of adjusting to workplace violence: A theory of adaptation. *International Journal of Mental* Health, *19*(3), 186–191.

Christman, L. (1998). Who is a nurse? *Image: The Journal of Nursing Scholarship,* 30(3), 211–214.

Delp, L., Wallace, S. P., Geiger-Brown, J., & Muntaner, C. (2010). Job stress and job satisfaction: Home care workers in a consumer directed model of care. *Health Services Research, 45*(4), 922–940.

Dossey, B., & Keegan, L. (2009). *Holistic nursing: A handbook for practice* (5th ed.),. Sudbury, MA: Jones & Bartlet.

Epstein, P., Burns, C., & Cohen, H. (2010). Substance abuse among registered nurses, *AAOHN, 58* (12), 513–516.

Frankl, V. (1978). *Man's search for meaning.* New York: Beacon Press.

Handleman, E. (2010). Top occupational and environmental tips for healthy nurses. *Maryland Nurse, 10*(2), 1.3.

Health Care Workers Council. (2007). Health care employees cites scarcity of minorities in health professions, identifies solutions. United Steel Workers. Retrieved from http://legacy/USW.org

Hospital Employee health. (2010). Needlestick risks remain but safety goal fades away. *Hospital Employee Health, 25*(12), 137–140. Retrieved from http://www.ebscohost.com

Howerton-Childs, R. J., & Mentes, J. C. (2010). Violence against women: The phenomenon of workplace violence against nurses. *Journal of Mental Health Nursing, 31*(2), 89–95.

Huerta, C. (1990). The relationship between life change events and academic achievement in registered nursing education students. Unpublished doctoral dissertation, Texas A&M University.

Hughes, N. (2011). Environmental health & safety: Confronting job stress. *American Nurse Today, 6*(5), p. 48.

Hui, W., Tie-Shuang, C., Li, C., Lie, W., & Ya-Ping, J. (2010). Occupational stress among hospital nurses: Cross sectional survey. *Journal of Advanced nursing, 66*(3), 627–634.

Hunter, B., Branson, M., & Davenport, D. (2010). Saving costs, saving health care provider's backs and creating a safe patient environment. *Nursing Economics$, 28*(2), 130–134.

Hussey, T. (2009). Nursing and spirituality. *Nursing Philosophy, 10*(2), 71–80.

Institute of Medicine of the National Academies (IOM). (2010). *The future of nursing: Leading change, advancing health.* Washington, DC: The National Academies of Health.

Jimenez, C., Navia-Osorio, P. M., & Diaz, C. V. (2010). Stress and health in novice and experienced nursing students. *Journal of Advanced Nursing, 66*(2), 442–455.

Leiter, M. P., & Maslach, C. (2009). Nurse turnover: The mediating role of burnout. *Journal of Nursing Management, 17*(3), 331–339.

Lernihan, E., & Sweeny, J. (2010). Measuring levels of burnout among care workers. *Learning Disability Practice, 13*(8), 27–33.

Maslow, A. (1970). *Motivation and personality.* New York, NY: Harper & Row.

Meeks-Sjostrom, D., Lopuszinski, S., & Bairan, A. (2010). The wisdom of retaining experienced nurses at the bedside: A pilot study examining a minimal lift program and its impact on reducing patient-movement related injuries of bedside nurses. *MEDSURG Nursing, 19*(4), 233–236.

Menzanie, G., & Bianchi, E. (2009). Stress among Brazilian nurses working in emergency rooms. *Revista electronic de Enfermagen, 11*(20), 327–333. Retrieved from http://www.ebscohost.com

Missouri State Board of Nursing. (2010). The elephant in the room: Huge rates of nursing and health care worker injury. *MBON Newsletter, 12*(2), 15–17. Retrieved from http://ebscohost.com

Nurses' Health Study. (2011). Retrieved from http://www.channing.harvard.edu/nhs/

Peery, A. (2010). Caring and burnout in nursing: What's the connection? *International Journal of Human Caring, 14*(2), 53–60.

Pesut, D., Fowler, M., Reimer-Kirkham, S., Taylor, E., & Swatzky, R. (2009). Particularizing spirituality in points of tension: Enriching the discourse. *Nursing Inquiry, 16*(4), 337–346.

Polovich, M., & Geisker, K. (2011). Occupational hazardous drug exposure among non-oncology nurses. *MEDSURG Nursing, 20*(2), 79–97.

Simon, M., Müller, B., & Hasselhorn, M. (2010). Leaving the organization or the profession: A multi level analysis of nurses' intentions. *Journal of Advanced Nursing, 66*(3), 616–626.

Smeltzer, S., Bare, B., Hinkle, J., & Cheever, K. (2010). *Brunner & Suddarth's textbook of medical-surgical nursing.* Philadelphia, PA: Wolters Kluwer/Lippincott Williams & Wilkins.

Sparks-Ralph, S., & Taylor, C. (2011). *Spark's and Taylor's nursing diagnosis reference manual.* Philadelphia, PA: Wolters Kluwer/ Lippincott Williams & Wilkins.

U.S. Department of Health and Human Services and Health Resources and Services Administration (USDHHS & HRSA). (2010). *The Registered Nurse population: Findings from the 2008 national sample survey of registered nurses.* Retrieved from http:// thefutureofnursing.org.

U.S. Department of Labor Occupational Safety and Health Administration (OSHA). (2011). Ergonomics, safety and health topics. Retrieved from http://www.osha.gov

Van Bogaert, P., Muelemans, H., Clarke, S., Vermeyan, K., & Van de Heyning, P. (2009). Hospital nurse practice environment, burnout, job outcomes, and quality of care: Test of a structural equation model. *Journal of Advanced Nursing, 65*(10), 2175–2185.

BIBLIOGRAPHY

Blais, K. K., & Hayes, J. S. (2011). *Professional nursing practice: Concepts and perspectives* (6th ed.). Boston, MA: Pearson.

Gallager, R., & Gromley, D. K. (2009). *Journal of Oncology Nursing, 13*(6), 681–685.

Hood, L. (2010). *Leddy & Pepper's conceptual bases of professional nursing.* Philadelphia, PA: Wolters Kluwer Health/Lippincott Williams & Wilkins.

Institute of Medicine. (2004). Crossing the quality chasm: A new health system for the 21st century. Retrieved from http://iom.edu

Jenkins, R., & Elliott, P. (2004). Stressors, burnout, and social support: Nurses in acute mental health settings. *Journal of Advanced Nursing, 48*(6), 622–631.

Lee, J., & Akhtar, S. (2011). Effect of the workplace social context and job content on nurse burnout. *Human Resource Management, 50*(2), 227–245.

Magnavita, N., & Heponiemi, T. (2011). Workplace violence against nursing students and nurses: An Italian experience. *Journal of Nursing Scholarship, 43*(2), 203–210.

Van den Tooren, M., & de Jonge, J. (2008). *Journal of Advanced Nursing, 63*(1), 75–84.

CHAPTER 21
Economic and Quality Concerns

DEBRA OTTO, DM, MN, WHNP-BC
DIANE FRAZOR, EdD, MSN, RN

KEY TERMS

capitation
diagnosis-related groups (DRGs)
exclusive provider organization
  (EPO)

health maintenance organization
  (HMO)
managed care
managed care organization

preferred provider organization
  (PPO)
primary care providers
prospective payment system (PPS)

OBJECTIVES

Upon completion of this chapter, the reader should be able to:

- Describe the changes that affect the cost and quality of health care today.
- Describe the factors influencing increases in health care costs.
- Describe efforts made by health care–conscious organizations, the government, and consumers to control health care costs.
- Define managed care.
- Define the different types of managed care organizations.
- Discuss the nurse's role in managed care.
- Identify measures indicative of a quality managed care organization.
- Describe some of the functions of the National Committee for Quality Assurance.
- Describe how national standards and nursing quality issues are affected by managed care.
- Describe how the concept of health promotion relates to managed care and health care costs.

INTRODUCTION

Late in the first decade of the millennium, the health care system in the United States has seen dramatic changes in how the delivery of services is reimbursed. "Reforms under the Affordable Care Act have brought to an end some of the worst abuses of the insurance industry" (USDHHS, 2010a, para 1.) In the past, health care costs were reimbursed to providers as fee for service through the patient's Medicare or Medicaid service, indemnity insurance plan, or other payment options, as arranged by the patient and provider. Traditional fee-for-service health care has gradually become less prevalent as cost-saving health care options such as managed care have become the norm. Managed care health insurance has become the most common type of health insurance coverage in the United States. With health care costs almost constantly on the rise, managed care health insurance has offered a more affordable option to traditional fee-for-service plans (Health Insurance In-Depth, 2011).

Chapters 1 and 3 defined and described the concept of health promotion. This chapter focuses on how health-promotion and health care costs relate to economic as well as quality issues. Factors that have driven health care costs upward are also described. Managed care is introduced as a method to curtail health care costs.

FACTORS DRIVING COSTS UP

Many factors contribute to an increase in health care costs. Box 21-1 presents an overview of factors affecting health care costs. Of the greatest factors contributing to the rise in costs, technology, and prescription drugs top the list.

Second, the availability of the latest technological services and new drug therapies feed the spending on health care because of developmental costs recouped by industry plus a more intense consumer demand for the latest and greatest in treatments even if they are not cost-effective (Kaiser Foundation, 2011).

Third, the changing economic conditions continue to contribute to the rise in health care costs. Softened labor markets and increasing unemployment rates spur employers to control their company's rising health insurance premium expenses through insurance buy-down programs that reduce employee benefits and increase employee cost sharing.

Fourth, over the past century, the nature of health care in the United States has changed considerably. Individuals living longer with chronic disease have placed tremendous strain on the health care system. The prolonged treatment of chronic disease states and extended care services such as nursing homes account for 75% of the overall national health spending (Kaiser Foundation, 2011).

Fifth, the general aging of the population poses yet another health care demand. The oldest members of the baby boomer generation began qualifying for Medicare benefits starting in 2011. Because health care expenses tend to rise with age, there is much concern as many of the costs are shifted to the public sector (Kaiser Foundation, 2011).

Sixth, administrative costs make up at least 7% of health care costs. Some continue to argue that a mix of public and private health systems self-creates overhead costs and uncontrolled profits that fuel additional health care spending (Kaiser Foundation, 2011).

The seventh factor escalating health care costs is the medical care provided to the uninsured. The number of uninsured people exceeds 50.7 million, according to the latest U.S. Census Bureau statistics. That is the equivalent of one out of every 6 U.S. residents (Wolf, 2010). As in 2003 and years prior, "Insuring the uninsured is again a major policy issue" (Hadley & Holahan, 2003, p. 1). One reason for the large increase in the uninsured is that many workers have lost their jobs during the current recession. According to Wolf (2010), workers pay 47% more for family health coverage than they did in 2005, and employers pay 20% more as well. Funding sources such as Medicare and Medicaid make a substantial contribution to support hospitals that treat poor and uninsured patient. Medicaid alone spent $339 billion in 2008, and costs are expected to reach $674 billion by 2017 (USDHHS, 2008). "Absent reform, there is general agreement that health costs are likely to continue to rise in the foreseeable future. Many analysts cite controlling health care costs as key for broader economic stability. President Obama has made cost control a focus of health reform" (Kaiser Foundation, 2011, para. 2).

? ASK **YOURSELF**

Consumer Utilization of Health Care Benefits

How many people do you know who, because they carry health care insurance, go see their health care provider for a minor ailment that requires no treatment? Do you have health care insurance? Do you see your provider for minor ailments too? Does overutilization of health care impact health care cost?

The last factor is the increase in lawsuits, which has had a dramatic effect on the cost as well as the accessibility of health care. Every time health care professionals are sued, their liability insurance rates increase, which, in turn, requires them to charge higher rates for their services to cover the cost. Some physicians actually eliminate services for high-risk conditions, such as obstetrics or emergency care, to avoid being sued and having to pay higher insurance premiums or, even worse, losing their medical licenses. Any time an insurance company has to

BOX 21-1

FACTORS AFFECTING OVERALL HEALTH CARE SPENDING

- Technology and prescription drugs
- Living longer with chronic disease
- Aging of the population
- Hidden administrative costs and profit
- Individuals who are uninsured
- Lawsuits
- Changing economic conditions

Source: Kaiser Foundation. (2010). U.S. Health Care Costs: Background. kaiseredu.org

pay to defend a patient, whether the patient wins or loses, the company passes the cost on to the patient (physician) in the form of increased insurance premiums.

EFFORTS TO CONTROL COSTS

Several attempts to help control costs for health care have been implemented. The following sections describe the effects of the Medicare/Medicaid programs and the prospective payment system on health care costs. Efforts by consumers of health care services and by nurses are addressed as well.

MEDICARE AND MEDICAID

As described in Chapter 1, the U.S. government created the Medicare and Medicaid programs in an effort to assist in the payment of health care costs for the elderly, the chronically ill, children, and the poor. The effects of the Medicaid and Medicare programs on health care costs and health care reforms, and their subsequent effects on the advancement of health promotion, are profound. Terry (2010) states that health care spending in the United States rose an estimated 5.7% to $2.5 trillion in 2009—in the middle of the most severe economic downturn in 80 years. Even more alarming, the percentage of the gross domestic product (GDP) spent on health care jumped to 17.3% from 16.2% in 2008. This translates to the largest one-year increase since 1960. At this rate of accelerated growth, health care costs are predicted to double to $4.5 trillion by 2019. At that point, health care spending will account for 19.3%, or almost a fifth of our GDP.

Over the entire projection period, national health spending growth is still expected to outpace economic growth Table 21-1 presents an overview of Medicare and Medicaid programs with a look at expenditures over the past 38 years. As can be seen in the table, the participant costs and state and federal costs continue to rise.

ACCESS TO HEALTH CARE

Although the Medicare and Medicaid programs were created by the U.S. government to assist children, the chronically ill, the poor, and the elderly with health care costs, there have been reductions in benefits, and this, coupled with the escalating costs of health care, has exacerbated the difficulties faced by the vulnerable populations in accessing care. The elderly, for example, have seen some of their health care benefits sharply reduced. Medicare, the nation's largest health insurer, does not cover all prescription drugs. The elderly frequently face problems with drug access due to affordability. Many elderly live on limited incomes, which may impact their health care. To assist the elderly with prescription costs, Medicare initiated a new outpatient prescription drug benefit in January 2006. The goal of the prescription drug benefit was to assist the elderly in affording their prescription drugs. Studies show that a consistent 8% of the elderly population continued to skip filling at least one prescription drug because of cost (Reschovsky & Felland, 2009). The results of a recent study show that the average price of dozens of brand-name prescription drugs used by the elderly has risen more than twice as fast as general inflation. A study funded by the Kaiser Family Foundation and the Commonwealth Fund found that 25% of the elderly who responded to a survey stated that they were forgoing taking any medications because of cost (http://www.therubins.com). Health care cost must obviously be taken into consideration when determining a health-promotion plan for the elderly.

Children, however, have fared better when it comes to accessing adequate health care. Legislation passed by Congress in 1997 builds on the Medicaid program that started covering

TABLE 21-1 Overview of Medicare and Medicaid

	MEDICARE	MEDICAID
Provisions	Hospital (Part A) and medical insurance (Part B)	Shared federal and state funding to assist states in paying for health care services for the needy
Funded by	Federal government	Federal and state governments
Administered by	Federal government	State government
Eligibility	Over age 65, disabled receiving Social Security benefits, end stage renal disease patients	Poor, medically needy, aged, disabled, and their dependent children and families
1967 participant costs	Part A—$40 deductible Part B—$50/year, $3/month	None
2006 participant costs	Part A—$39.95/month, $952 deductible Part B—$88.50/month, $124 deductible Part D—$32/month, $250 deductible + payment schedule	Minimal to none depending on state
1967 state and federal costs	$5 billion	$2.3 billion
2006 baseline projections for Medicare/Medicaid		
2008 $361 billion		
2010 $419 billion		

Source: Center for Medicaid and Medicare Services. (2010). U.S. Department of Health and Human Services. Retrieved from http://www.cms.hhs.gov

children over four decades ago. The Child Health Insurance Program (CHIP) is a Medicaid program designed to cover health care costs of children living in poverty. Under federal law, all states must cover children up to the age of 6 if their family earns up to 133% of the federal poverty level (FPL), as well as children 6 and older born after September 30, 1983, with family incomes at or under 100% of FPL (U.S. Department of Health and Human Services, 2010c). Although the federal government has recently attempted to cut CHIPs, every state in the nation now has a health insurance program for infants, children, and teens. Even individuals with a variety of immigration statuses are eligible. For little or no cost, the CHIP pays for doctor visits, prescription drugs, and hospitalizations. Most states also cover the cost of dental care, eye care, and medical equipment (USDHHS, 2010c).

PROSPECTIVE PAYMENT SYSTEM

In the early 1980s, health care costs were spiraling out of control despite past containment efforts. As a result, Congress responded with a Social Security Amendment that, beginning in October 1983, changed Medicare's cost-based, or retrospective, method of paying for hospital health care to a **prospective payment system (PPS)**.

The PPS was a method of payment to hospitals based on the concept that similar medical diagnoses result in the same hospitalization costs. Consequently, a fixed predetermined payment was allowed according to the classification of the patient's diagnosis (American Hospital Directory, 2010). The diagnosis classification system used with the PPS was identified as **diagnosis-related groups (DRGs)** and contained 468 diagnoses. Hospitals were forced to control patient costs in order to remain within the reimbursement allowance according to DRGs. Reimbursement to physicians was, in turn, affected as hospital administrators scrambled to curb costs at every angle, including human resources, procedures, equipment, supplies, and construction.

The PPS helped somewhat to contain health care costs for the Medicare patient because administrators began to cut costs by decreasing the length of time a patient stayed in the hospital so that they would not exceed their reimbursement according

to the prospective payment. Many private-pay insurers followed in the government's footsteps and began by reimbursing care providers more on the diagnosis of the patient, thus developing a standard reimbursement for different types of health care services.

Even with these changes in reimbursement, health care costs continue to rise. For this very reason, the United States has seen some remarkable changes in the health care system. On March 23, 2010, the Affordable Care Act became law. The Affordable Care Act has given Americans more freedom and control over their health care choices (USDHHS, 2010b). The development of health maintenance and managed care organizations has also contributed to the changes in health care in the United States and will be discussed in the chapter.

CONSUMER EFFORTS IN COST CONTAINMENT

Because the rising cost of health care has created a major problem that affects many major facets of our society, consumers, as well as health care professionals, must become involved in efforts to contain cost. Solutions to the rising costs of health care are not easy, but consumers can control several factors. One of these is to investigate or shop around for quality health care at the lowest cost. Health care providers are involved in the business of making people well, and, like any other major business, competition exists among the providers. For example, eye examination cost varies depending on whether the eye care provider is self-employed or works for a major discount store. The difference in cost may be significant.

Frivolous lawsuits drive up the costs of health care because even unmerited lawsuits require that the health care provider employ a defense team. The defense costs are passed on to the consumers through increased health care costs and insurance premiums. After all, someone has to pay for the time and effort required to settle the lawsuit. Thus consumers must become educated about frivolous lawsuits.

SPOTLIGHT ON

Cost Containment with the Prospective Payment System

With the PPS, a patient is admitted to the hospital and treated for a diagnosis of pneumonia. According to the PPS, the hospital is reimbursed for that patient based on a preset fee for that diagnosis, regardless of how much money the hospital spent on the patient. If the hospital spends more than the reimbursement amount, then the hospital loses that money. How could this have been avoided? What role does the nurse have in controlling costs in the hospital? If this were a recurrent problem, how do you think the hospital would respond to it?

ASK YOURSELF

Nurses and the Consumer

Do you think that nurses should play an active role in encouraging health care consumers to investigate the costs of different health care services prior to choosing them? Or is it not our place to interfere with consumer health care unless it directly involves the delivery of nursing care? Do you as a consumer of health care "shop around" for your health care plan?

Although the concepts of health promotion and disease prevention are not new and certainly have been discussed in this textbook, health-promotion efforts are often overlooked as potential solutions to decreasing the cost of health care. Health-promoting behaviors must be encouraged in order for individuals to avoid entry into the health care delivery system where treatment of a disease or illness can become costly.

GLOBAL HIGHLIGHTS IN HEALTH PROMOTION
Global Economic and Quality Concerns

Infectious diseases and starvation continue around the world. However, urbanization has reshaped population health problems, particularly among the urban poor, toward noncommunicable diseases and injuries, alcohol and substance abuse, and impact from ecological disaster. Obesity is one of the most alarming concerns, not just healthwise but economically, to have arisen in the past couple of decades. It is a pressing problem, particularly among socially disadvantaged groups in many cities throughout the world. The shift in population levels of weight toward obesity is related to the "nutrition transition"—the increasing consumption of fats, sweeteners, energy-dense foods, and highly processed foods. This, together with marked reductions in physical activity, contributes to the global obesity epidemic. This is due to a variety of factors, including the greater availability, accessibility, and acceptability of processed foods, bulk purchases, convenience foods, supersized portions, and non-nutritional food additives such as high-fructose corn syrup.

Source: Commission on Social Determinants of Health, World Health Organization. (CSDH, 2008, August 28). Closing the gap in a generation: Health equity through action on the social determinants of health, p. 60: http://www.kaiseredu.org

MANAGED CARE

In 1973, the Health Maintenance Organization Act was passed, providing federal funding for health maintenance organizations (HMOs) that followed the federal regulations, which were stricter than the state regulations. The HMO Act also required large organizations to provide an HMO for their employees as a health care option. The establishment of HMOs led to the development of the concept of **managed care**, which is a method of delivering health care that integrates and coordinates the delivery of health care with the costs of that service (USDHHS, 2010d). A **managed care organization** is a health plan that provides consumers access to quality health care at what is considered a reasonable cost by determined health care cost standards. These types of health plans usually rely on **primary care providers**, who are health care providers that the patient sees first for health care services. Primary care providers are physicians, predominantly family practice physicians. The primary care provider acts as a gatekeeper for the consumer's health care and prevents the use of unnecessary or inappropriate health care services, thus resulting in less expensive treatments or interventions (Health Insurance In-Depth, 2011).

Managed care is a prepaid medical plan that is comprehensive in that the plan offers health and medical options, including preventative, specialty, primary, and ancillary health services (Department of Social and Health Services [DSHS], 2011). By encouraging participants in the health plan to participate in health-promotion and disease prevention activities, the organization saves monies that would have been spent to treat preventable illnesses. An example is encouraging patients to exercise regularly because they decrease their weight and cholesterol level and therefore decrease their chances of developing heart disease later in life. This, in turn, saves the consumer's health plan from spending large amounts of money treating its patient who has developed heart disease.

Several types of organizations deliver managed care. The major ones are the health maintenance organization, the preferred provider organization, and the exclusive provider organization. These types of managed care organizations are described in Table 21-2 and are briefly discussed in the following sections.

HEALTH MAINTENANCE ORGANIZATION

A **health maintenance organization (HMO)** is one type of managed care service that provides health care to members

TABLE 21-2 Types of Managed Care Organizations			
HEALTH MAINTENANCE ORGANIZATION (HMO)	**PREFERRED PROVIDER ORGANIZATION (PPO)**	**EXCLUSIVE PROVIDER ORGANIZATION (EPO)**	**CAPITATION**
Has a fixed, usually monthly payment	Members may only use providers within the network.	Members must get all services within the network.	Fixed payment to provide all reasonable and necessary medical services required by plan members
Can be for profit or nonprofit	Providers are paid discounted fees.	Participants must choose a primary care physician.	Fixed payment per member per month charged to employer or insurance carrier
Active in the prevention side of health care	Usually does not have a primary care physician as a gatekeeper.	Primary care physician may refer to other physicians in the network.	Health care organization must maintain some control of physician-generated utilization.
Promotes wellness		Only care allowed outside the network is emergency care.	Primary care provider is gatekeeper.

for a fixed, usually monthly, payment (Health Insurance In-Depth, 2011). HMO organizations can be either nonprofit or for profit. They have a fixed monthly payment that may or may not be part of a benefit package offered by employers. HMOs are very active on the prevention side of medicine. Because of their emphasis on disease prevention, disease risk reduction, and self-care by the patient, HMOs fit in nicely with the concept of health promotion.

PREFERRED PROVIDER ORGANIZATION

Another type of managed care service is the **preferred provider organization (PPO)**, which uses provider networks to deliver health care to its members (Health Insurance In-Depth, 2011). A PPO plan includes preferred health care institutions such as hospitals, preferred provider physicians, insurers, and employers. Individuals enrolled in a PPO may use providers only within the network. PPOs do not require going through a primary care physician as a gatekeeper to obtain services from specialists or other caregivers. The health care providers who meet the qualifications of the PPO are paid discounted fees for being part of that PPO. Charges to the consumer cannot exceed those set by the PPO (Health Insurance In-Depth, 2011).

EXCLUSIVE PROVIDER ORGANIZATION

The **exclusive provider organization (EPO)** is a plan that requires its members to get their services only within that particular network (Health Insurance In-Depth, 2011). The participants usually must select a primary care physician and a hospital that they use exclusively. The primary incentive is that little or no copayment is required when the exclusive provider network is used (Health Insurance In-Depth, 2011). The primary care physician may refer to other physicians in the network if deemed necessary. The only care allowed outside the network is emergency care.

CAPITATION

Capitation is another, and relatively new, type of health care plan that is becoming popular. With capitation, the employer or insurer pays a provider a set fee for all the medical expenses

necessary for each member covered under that plan. This provider may be a hospital that provides all the health care services to the insured. To be profitable, the hospital needs to provide care for less than the set fee. Otherwise, the hospital loses money (Health Insurance In-Depth, 2011).

The hospital and health care providers must work cooperatively to keep health care costs down, or the capitation plan does not work. This requires less hospitalization for the plan members. The hospital's goal is no longer to fill beds, but to keep them empty. The hospital must also develop practice guidelines for the physician to follow so that the physicians maintain controlled utilization. Again, the primary care physician operates as a gatekeeper in keeping these costs down and ensuring that the care given is quality care. Capitation hospitals succeed more often if the physicians profit by cutting costs. This may involve having the physician be a partner in the capitation plan.

NURSING'S ROLE IN MANAGED CARE

Nursing as a profession has embraced the challenge of an ever changing health care environment. Nursing's philosophy makes the profession especially qualified to make the changes needed to move managed care organizations from a paradigm of medicine to a paradigm of health. The managed care nurse functions in many different settings and roles. "In contrast to the traditional role of the nurse to provide direct patient care at the bedside, the managed care nurse's role is to advocate for all patients enrolled in healthcare delivery systems, to administer benefits within the confines of the healthcare delivery system and to provide customer service for all of the nurse's encounters with members of the healthcare delivery system" (American Board of Managed Care Nursing [ABMCN], 2010). As illustrated in Figure 21-1, health care

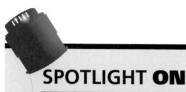

SPOTLIGHT **ON**

Increased Use of Managed Care

Under managed care contracts, the pressure is on hospitals and physicians to use resources more efficiently and effectively and to keep patients out of hospitals as much as possible. Physicians must therefore use more ambulatory care settings to intervene for their patients. Because nurses are the caregivers even in managed care, should they have a role in determining how care can be delivered efficiently and effectively?

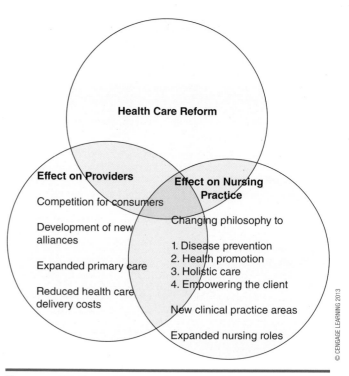

FIGURE 21-1 Health care reform will affect providers and nurses.

reform measures to control costs and meet the health care needs of the nation have implications for both consumers and the profession of nursing.

Because these measures affect the health care provider's financial gains, there is considerable competition for consumers. Consumers, in most cases the employers of the consumers, are thus in a better position to choose the managed care plan that is most reasonable costwise but provides the assurance of quality health care. Expanded primary care services reduce health care costs and increase quality of care.

The effects of managed care and health care reforms affect nursing practice in a very fundamental manner. The nursing profession's philosophy has changed over time in response to some of the health care reform measures. For example, nursing has evolved from a profession focused on treating illness to one that emphasizes disease prevention, holistic care, and health promotion through patient empowerment.

QUALITY MEASURES AND MANAGED CARE

The National Committee for Quality Assurance (NCQA) is a private, not-for-profit organization dedicated to assessing and reporting on the quality of managed care plans. The NCQA provides information to purchasers and consumers of managed health care that enables them to distinguish among plans based on quality, thereby allowing them to make more informed health care purchasing decisions. Accreditation by the NCQA is required by most businesses and organizations that purchase managed care plans (National Committee for Quality Assurance, 2011).

Some of the areas evaluated by the NCQA include quality improvement programs, clinical practice guidelines, clinical measurement activities, and intervention and follow-up for clinical issues. Data is collected through a set of standardized performance indicators led by the Health Plan Employer Data and Information Set and also through employer and business mandates (National Committee for Quality Assurance, 2011).

THE JOINT COMMISSION

The Joint Commission (JC) is an independent, not-for-profit organization, established more than 50 years ago. The JC is governed by a board that includes physicians, nurses, and consumers. The JC sets the standards by which health care quality is measured in America and around the world. The JC

evaluates the quality and safety of care for more than 15,000 health care organizations. To earn and maintain accreditation, organizations must have an extensive on-site review by a team of JC health care professionals at least once every 3 years. The purpose of the review is to evaluate the organization's performance in areas that affect patient care. Accreditation may then be awarded based on how well the organization meets JC standards. During the evaluation phase, the JC is measuring the organization's improvement in areas such as the rights and responsibilities of patient's, continuum of care, education, communication, health promotion and disease prevention, leadership and management, management of information, and improving network performance (Joint Commission, 2011).

NATIONAL STANDARDS AND MANAGED CARE

In the past, consumer groups and HMOs have requested that the federal government develop national standards to guide managed care plans. Ideally, these standards would replace the individual states' regulations, which have not provided the structure desired by the American health care consumer. Rather than incur the cost and time constraints required in developing national standards, not-for-profit organizations such as the NCQA have been encouraged to develop nationally recognized standards called the Health Plan Employer Data and Information Set (HEDIS). HEDIS is a set of standardized performance measures designed to ensure that purchasers and consumers have the information they need to reliably compare the performance of managed health care plans. The performance measures in HEDIS are related to many significant public health issues, such as cancer, heart disease, smoking, asthma, and diabetes. HEDIS also includes a standardized survey of consumers' experiences that evaluates plan performance in areas such as customer service, access to care, and claims processing (National Committee for Quality Assurance, 2011).

NURSING QUALITY ISSUES

The nursing profession continues to express concern over the state of health care reform and quality of care. The American Nurses Association's (ANA) Health Care Agenda 2005 and its subsequent 2009 revised health systems reform agenda (ANA, 2009) state that the U.S. health care system remains in a state of crisis. At this time, the number of uninsured continues to increase, the cost of care continues to rise, and the safety and quality of care continue to be questioned. The ANA remains committed to the following five basic principles:

1. Health care is a basic right, and universal access should be assured to a standard package of health care services for all citizens and residents.
2. The ANA believes the development and implementation of health policies that reflect safe and effective, patient-centered, timely, efficient, and equitable service that is based on outcomes research will ultimately save health care dollars.
3. The current health care system must be redirected away from the overuse of expensive acute hospital-based services to one in which a balance is achieved between high-cost treatments and community-based preventive services.

SPOTLIGHT **ON**

Ensuring Quality in Managed Care

Many states have hired managed care organizations to deliver health care to their Medicaid and Medicare patients. How are they going to ensure that quality care is being given to these patients through these plans?

RESEARCH NOTE

Changes in Access to Health Care among Older Adult Immigrants

STUDY PROBLEM/PURPOSE
The purpose of this longitudinal study was to examine the role of health insurance in access to health care among older immigrants.

METHODS
Using data from the Second Longitudinal Study of Aging, the longitudinal trajectories of having a usual source of care were compared among 3 groups (all 70+ years): (1) late-life immigrants with fewer than 15 years of residence in the United States ("recent immigrants"; $n = 133$), (2) "earlier immigrants" (15 years or longer in the United States, $n = 672$), and (3) U.S. born ($n = 8,642$). A series of hierarchical generalized linear models were run to test the mediating relationship of health insurance between immigrant status and having a usual source of care.

FINDINGS
The probabilities of having a usual source of care increased over time across all three groups. However, recent immigrants were less likely to have Medicare and private insurance over time; this in turn was related to lower probabilities of having a usual source of care (indirect relationship). No direct relationship was found between immigrant status and having a usual source of care.

IMPLICATIONS
To prevent the use of more expensive forms of care in the long run, health care policy efforts should expand elderly immigrants' health insurance coverage by increasing affordable health insurance options.

Source: Choi, S. (2011). Longitudinal changes in access to health care by immigrant status among older adults: The importance of health insurance as a mediator. *The Gerontologist, 51*(2): 156–169.

4. The ANA supports a single-payer model as the most desirable option to reform health care at this time.

5. For health care delivery to be safe, effective, fair, and affordable, there must be an adequate supply of well educated, well distributed, and well utilized registered nurses (American Nurses Association, 2005).

HEALTH PROMOTION THEORY LINK

Marilyn Ann Ray's Theory of Bureaucratic Caring

Marilyn Ann Ray's Theory of Bureaucratic Caring moves away from centered patient care to the broader economic justification of nursing and health care systems. The theory prompts professionals to seek a fuller understanding of how to preserve health care within business or corporate culture.

Source: Marilyn Ann Ray's Theory of Bureaucratic Caring. *Nursing Administration Quarterly* (Winter 1998). Retrieved from http://journals.lww.com/naqjournal/Citation/1989/01320/The_theory_of_bureaucratic_caring_for_nursing.7.aspx

ASK **YOURSELF**

Who Should Monitor Managed Care Organizations?

Knowing that many states are hiring managed care organizations to deliver health care to their Medicaid and Medicare patients, who should regulate these organizations? Should the state government or the federal government be responsible?

HEALTH PROMOTION, HEALTH CARE COST, AND MANAGED CARE

Because the U.S. health care system continues to be in such a state of crisis, the overwhelming problems require significant attention on the part of health professionals, policy makers, and the public (American Nurses Association, 2011). Nurses hold the pivotal role of health care advocate for individuals and families. They are on the forefront of health care with their ability to help patients learn health promotion and disease prevention through education, leadership, and example. By utilizing health-promotion concepts, nurses empower their patients to adopt healthier lifestyles that may also focus on cost containment from the patient's point of view.

SUMMARY

This chapter has focused on how the delivery of health care is in a constant and rapid state of change. These changes can positively affect our rising health care costs in the United States. Many factors are contributing to an increase in health care costs: the rise in hospital spending, changing economic conditions, unprecedented health insurance industry profits, managed care's inability to constrain payment rates for hospital-based care, the role of the consumer, and individuals who are uninsured. These factors continue to drain limited health care resource dollars.

Efforts to control escalating costs have evolved to the current concept of managed care by managed care organizations. Some types of managed care systems, such as health maintenance organizations, emphasize health promotion and wellness in an effort to contain costs. Health promotion and disease prevention are very important measures that consumers of health care can use to affect rising costs. Even those individuals who already have illnesses can learn how to promote the optimal health attainable for them and prevent disease progression or the development of related illnesses.

The nursing profession has experienced many changes with the implementation of managed care systems. Nurses have expressed dissatisfaction with the current system of patient care. The nursing profession's responsibility is to ensure quality patient care. One way is for nurses to empower patients to take control of their own care and to adopt health-promoting behaviors. Learning health-promotion concepts and principles through nursing education is as important to patients as any other skill.

KEY CONCEPTS

1. Health care costs in the United States have continued to spiral and changes are occurring to stop this trend.

2. Factors that contribute to the increases in health care costs are the rise in hospital spending, changing economic conditions, unprecedented health insurance industry profits, managed care's inability to constrain payment rates for hospital-based care, the role of the consumer, and individuals who are uninsured.

3. Managed care is a method of delivering health care that integrates and coordinates the delivery of service and the costs to the consumer.

4. HMOs, PPOs, and EPOs are types of managed care organizations.

5. The regulatory agencies responsible for measuring quality in managed care organizations are the NCQA and the JC.

6. Some of the areas evaluated by the NCQA include quality improvement programs, clinical practice guidelines, clinical measurement activities, and intervention and follow-up for clinical issues.

7. The five basic principles of the 2005 ANA Health Care Agenda are (1) health care is a basic right, (2) the development and implementation of health policies that reflect safe and effective patient-centered care will ultimately save health care dollars, (3) a balance must be achieved between high-cost treatments and community-based preventive services, (4) a single-payer model is desirable for current health care reform, and (5) for health care delivery to be safe, effective, fair, and affordable, there must be an adequate supply of well educated, well distributed, and well utilized registered nurses.

8. By empowering patients to adopt health-promotion lifestyles, nurses can focus on cost containment from the patient's perspective.

CHAPTER REVIEW

Learning Activities

1. List the factors that contribute to the increase in health care costs.

2. Define the three types of managed care organizations: HMOs, PPOs, and EPOs.

3. List the five basic principles of the 2005 ANA Health Care Agenda.

Multiple Choice

1. Factors affecting health care costs include all of the following *except*:
   a. changing economic conditions.
   b. increased number of insured individuals.
   c. increased hospital expenditures.
   d. lawsuits.

2. A managed care organization:
   a. emphasizes treatment, not prevention.
   b. increases health care costs by the consumer.
   c. is maintained through federal funding.
   d. provides consumers with access to quality care.

3. The Joint Commission is an independent, not-for-profit organization that:
   a. evaluates the quality of care provided by all public health agencies in the United States and the world.
   b. exclusively focuses on the rights and responsibilities of health care professionals.
   c. provides leadership training for professionals in the health care arena.
   d. sets standards by which health care quality is measured.

4. The prospective payment system is a:
   a. diagnosis classification system.
   b. fixed predetermined payment system.
   c. payment based on the fact that similar diagnoses result in same hospitalization costs.
   d. reimbursement to physicians according to patient diagnosis classification.

5. Factors affecting increases in health care costs include:
   a. increase in job availability.
   b. increase in lawsuits.
   c. lower insurance premiums.
   d. more insured patients.

6. A PPO plan:
   a. allows consumers to decide on their health care provider.
   b. focuses on disease protection at a set fee.
   c. includes preferred health care institutions such as hospitals.
   d. provides health care to its members at a fixed price.

7. The Joint Commission is an independent, not-for-profit organization that sets the standards by which:
   a. health-promotion and disease-prevention strategies are measured.
   b. health care quality is measured.
   c. nursing personnel are evaluated.
   d. nursing programs are measured.

ORGANIZATIONS AND WEBSITES

Administration on Aging (AOA): Agency in the U.S. Department of Health and Human Services that is one of the nation's largest providers of home- and community-based care for older persons and their caregivers; mission is to develop a comprehensive, coordinated, and cost-effective system of long-term care that helps elderly individuals to maintain their dignity in their homes and communities: **http://www.aoa.gov**

Interfaith Center on Corporate Responsibility: Information on access to health and wellness for all: **http://www.iccr.org/**

Joint Commission: Mission is to continuously improve the safety and quality of care provided to the public through the provision of health care accreditation and related services that support performance improvement in health care organizations. **http://www.jointcommission.org/**

National League for Nursing: Provides information that prepares the nursing workforce to meet the needs of diverse populations in an ever changing health care environment: **http://www.nln.org**

Universal Health Care Action Network: Information on the national campaign for affordable health care for all: **http://www.uhcan.org/**

U.S. Department of Health and Human Services: The principal government agency for protecting the health of all Americans and for providing essential human services, especially for those least able to help themselves; includes more than 300 programs, covering a wide spectrum of activities. **http://www.hhs.gov/**

REFERENCES

American Board of Managed Care Nursing (ABMCN). (2010). The value of certification. Retrieved from http://www.abmcn.org/

American Hospital Directory. (2010). Medicare prospective payment system. Retrieved from http://www.ahd.com

American Nurses Association. (ANA). (2009). ANA board adopts revised health system reform agenda and strategic plan. Retrieved from http://www.nursingworld.org/

American Nurses Association (ANA). (2011). ANA's health care agenda (2005). Retrieved from http://www.nursingworld.org/

Choi, S. (2011). Longitudinal changes in access to health care by immigrant status among older adults: The importance of health insurance as a mediator. *The Gerontologist, 51*(2), 156–169.

CSDH. (2008). Closing the gap in a generation: Health equity through action on the social determinants of health. Final report of the Commission on Social Determinants of Health. Geneva:World Health Organization.

Department of Social and Health Services (DSHS), (2011). Managed care medical programs (Washington). Retrieved from http://hrsa.dshs.wa.gov/healthyoptions/

Hadley, J., & Holahan, J. (2003). How much medical care do the uninsured use, and who pays for it? *Health Affairs Web Exclusive,* 66–81.

Health Insurance In-Depth. (2011). Is a managed care network the right choice for you? Retrieved from http://www.healthinsuranceindepth.com

Joint Commission. (2011). Facts about the Joint Commission. Retrieved from http://www.jointcommission.org

Kaiser Foundation. (2010). U.S. health care costs: Background. Retrieved from http://www.kaiseredu.org

Kaiser Foundation. (2011). Health policy explained. Retrieved from http://www.kaiseredu.org/Issue-Modules/US-Health-Care-Costs/

National Committee for Quality Assurance (NCQA). (2011). Measuring quality: Improving health care. Retrieved from http://www.ncqa.org

Ray, M. A. (1998). Marilyn Ann Ray's Theory of Bureaucratic Caring. *Nursing Administration Quarterly* (Winter). Retrieved from http://journals.lww.com/naqjournal/Citation/1989/01320/The_theory_of_bureaucratic_caring_for_nursing.7.aspx

Reschovsky, J. D., & Felland, L. E., (2009). Access to prescription drugs for Medicare beneficiaries. Retrieved from http://hschange.org/CONTENT/1044/#ib1

Terry, K., (2010). Health spending hits 17.3% of GDP in largest annual jump. Retrieved from http://www.bnet.com/blog/healthcare-business/health-spending-hits-173-percent-of-gdp-in-largest-annual-jump/1117

U.S. Department of Health and Human Services (USDHHS). (2008). Medicaid spending projected to rise much faster than the economy. Retrieved from http://www.hhs.gov/news/

U.S. Department of Health and Human Services (USDHHS). (2010a). Understanding the affordable care act: Introduction. Retrieved from http://www.healthcare.gov/law/introduction/index.html

U.S. Department of Health and Human Services (USDHHS). (2010b). The affordable care act at one year. Retrieved from http://www.healthcare.gov/foryou/betterbenefitsbetterhealth/index.html

U.S. Department of Health and Human Services (USDHHS). (2010c). Center for Medicaid and Medicare services. Retrieved from http://www.cms.hhs.gov/

U.S. Department of Health and Human Services (USDHHS). (2010d.). Managed care. Retrieved from http://www.nlm.nih.gov/medlineplus/managedcare.html

Wolf, R. (2010, September 17). Number of uninsured Americans rises to 50.7 million. *USA Today*. Retrieved from http://www.usa.com.,

World Health Organization Commission on Social Determinants of Health. (2008). Closing the gap in a generation: Health equity through action on the social determinants of health. Retrieved from http://www.globalissues.org/article/588/global-health-overview#GlobalHealthInitiatives

BIBLIOGRAPHY

Chapman, S. A., Wides, C. D., & Spetz, J. (2010). Payment regulations for advanced practice nurses: Implications for primary care. *Policy, politics, and nursing practice. 11*(2), 89–98.

Gresenz, C. R., Rogowski, J., & Escarce, J. (2006). Health Leaders-Inter Study. Total managed care plans data. 2008. Retrieved from http://www.managedcareonline.com/factshts/

Klimmek, R., Snow, D., & Wenzel, J. (2011). Insurance-related and financial challenges reported by managed care enrollees with breast cancer. *Clinical Journal of Oncology Nursing,14*(5), 598–606.

Paterson, B. L, Duffet-Legere, L., Cruttenden, K. (2009). Contextual factors influencing the evolution of nurses' roles in a primary health care clinic. *Public Health Nursing, 26*(5), 421–429.

Wellstood, K., Wilson, K., & Eyeles, J. (2006). "Reasonable access" to primary care: Assessing the role of individual and system characteristics. *Health and Place, 12*(2),

CHAPTER 22
Ethical, Legal, and Political Concerns

Carolina G. Huerta, EdD, MSN, RN
Janice A. Maville, EdD, MSN, RN

KEY TERMS

accreditation
advance directives
assault
autonomy
battery
beneficence
breach of duty
certification
credentialing
crime
deontology

equal protection
ethical principles
ethics
fidelity
informed consent
introspection
justice
law
multistate licensure
negligence
nonmaleficence

paternalism
registration
respect for others
standard of best interest
teleology
tort
values
values clarification
veracity

OBJECTIVES

Upon completion of this chapter, the reader should be able to:

- Recognize ethical, legal, and political issues that can influence the health-promotion goals of professional nursing.
- Identify basic principles of ethics.
- Discuss values clarification.
- Describe legal concerns affecting the delivery of health care.
- Explain the concepts of licensure and professional standards of care and their impact on the delivery of nursing care.
- Describe how nurses can apply ethical-legal concepts in decision making for health promotion.

INTRODUCTION

Complex personal, interpersonal, professional, institutional, and social issues constantly challenge nurses. These issues are rarely confined to caring for the patient in the health care institution. Because nursing's goals are health promotion and the provision of holistic patient care, these constant challenges must be addressed. Responses depend on such variables as contextual factors, patient and family values, relationships, moral development, religious beliefs, spiritual perspectives, cultural orientation, and legal constraints. Historically, nursing has been involved in most aspects of health care delivery and in all aspects of health promotion. Such intimate involvement in the delivery of care has provided nurses with the opportunity to witness countless situations that pose ethical as well as legal dilemmas. To provide quality patient care, nurses must develop an awareness of the ethical and legal considerations pertaining to nursing practice.

Ethical and legal dilemmas are common in the nursing profession. Nurses are frequently called upon to treat patients who may be considered a detriment to society and who are expected to treat them as they would any other patient. For example, a nurse might be called to treat a prison inmate who has been convicted of committing a heinous crime. The attending nurse may be tempted to provide substandard care because of personal feelings toward the patient. This, of course, creates both an ethical and a legal dilemma because, under the **equal protection** clause in the Fourteenth Amendment to the U.S. Constitution, all similarly situated individuals are entitled to be treated similarly (Guido, 2010). Substandard care to this prison inmate involves such basic issues as determining who has the right to receive care and determining what constitutes legal equality in relation to health care. Nurses are called upon daily in their practice to make decisions affecting the patient's care. Frequently, these decisions may pertain to what is right or wrong, and no clear answers are evident. Decisions, however, should be made on sound ethical principles and on professional and legal standards.

The previous chapter discussed health care cost, health care financing, and quality issues associated with the delivery of care. This chapter also focuses on issues related to health care cost, access to health care, and the government's involvement in the delivery of health care but from the standpoint of ethical and legal concerns affecting the delivery of quality nursing care. Issues regarding a patient's choice of treatment and rationing of health care as they relate to health-promotion efforts are also explored. For the reader to fully understand the effect of ethical and legal issues on a patient's health-promotion status, basic principles of ethics and legal concerns are described.

ETHICAL AND LEGAL ISSUES INFLUENCING NURSING CARE

Nurses are expected to provide quality care to all their patients. In providing this quality care, the nurse assumes the role of a patient advocate who speaks up about poor, inadequate, or incompetent care. Because of nursing's advocacy role and because nurses provide the majority of direct patient care, they are frequently expected to make ethical or legal decisions. When nurses make decisions involving ethical or legal issues, these decisions must always be rooted in the professional standards as set forth in the American Nurses Association's (ANA) *Code of Ethics for Nurses with Interpretive Statements* (2001), *Scope and Standards of Practice* (2004), and *Standards of*

Clinical Nursing Practice (1998). (See Chapter 2 for related information.) Nursing decisions must also always be made with an awareness of the patient's rights to receive care. These rights entitle the patient to receive safe and effective care at all times regardless of where the health care is delivered. In fact, several health care organizations have established a bill of rights for patients. The American Hospital Association (AHA) is one of the primary organizations that have established a bill of rights for patients (AHA, 1992). In 2010, President Barack Obama announced new regulations with the Affordable Care Act that included a set of protections that apply to health coverage in the private health insurance market that is intended to put Americans in charge of their own health (U.S. Department of Health and Human Services [DHHS], 2010). These regulations are designed to help children and eventually all Americans with preexisting conditions to gain coverage and keep it, protect all Americans' choice of doctors, and end lifetime limits on the care consumers may receive.

Other entities, such as the U.S. Advisory Commission on Consumer Protection and Quality in the Health Care Industry, have adopted their own bills of rights for patients. Many health plans have adopted these principles, which include the right to information disclosure, choice of provider and plans, access to emergency services, participation in treatment decisions, respect and nondiscrimination, and confidentiality as well as the right to complain about a health plan, a hospital, health care personnel, or a doctor. A patient is also given the right to appeal a decision related to health care plans (American Cancer Society, 2009). The federal government recognizes the need for a patient's bill of rights and has introduced legislation to facilitate patient access to care.

In addition to the professional standards, decisions regarding patient care must abide by legal statutes. The state legislative body sets forth legal rules governing licensure of nursing practice. The provisions that govern nursing can be found in the rules and regulations mandated by the administrative agencies where legislative authority is vested. These regulations are compiled and published by the state board of nursing as the Nursing Practice Act.

ETHICAL ISSUES

Ethical issues have arisen over time as a result of technological and scientific advances. Ethical dilemmas are perplexing to nurses and other health care workers because most of the time there are no clearly right or wrong courses of action (Guido, 2010). Occasionally professional decisions are clear and all the health care providers agree with the course of action (Guido, 2010). This, unfortunately, happens quite infrequently. Interspersed with the dilemmas of ethics are concerns dealing with legalities and concerns of cost and access to health care for all, young or old, rich or poor. The concept of health as a goal of society as described by health-promotion models is both an ethical and legal issue because it questions whether health-promotion behaviors can be imposed on society.

Ethics is the branch of philosophy that is related to moral values and actions. It deals with the rules or principles that distinguish right from wrong or good behavior from bad behavior. Ethical individuals make decisions based on acceptable standards of conduct and moral judgment. Ethical nurses conduct themselves according to fundamental ethical principles and moral reasoning. Nurses therefore need to study ethics in order to fully care for their patients and to provide quality care.

Nurses care for critically ill people and face more difficult and immediate ethical conflicts than do people in other jobs. The patients are ill and less able to fend for themselves, and they need nurses who can make ethical decisions regarding their care and provide them with the information they need to make decisions, frequently involving life and death. Ethical theories and basic principles of ethics are helpful to the nurse involved in an ethical dilemma.

ETHICAL THEORIES

Several theories are important to a discussion of ethical issues. Ethical theories guide by providing the context in which a situation should be viewed. They also provide an integrated view of what values, like pieces in a puzzle, logically fit in and should be considered when dealing with ethical issues. Although there may be more theories related to ethics, teleology and deontology are the familiar ones.

Teleology is an ethical theory that justifies actions based on the results attained by those actions. This theory can easily be summarized by the old adage: The end justifies the means. For example, consider the near-fatal side effects of certain potentially life-saving experimental treatments or the wholesale slaughter of animals for research. This theory lends itself to the judgment that the greatest good is for the greatest number of people. Consequently, if teleology theory is used in decision making in the preceding example, it is logical to have some patients become ill when undergoing experimental treatment or to kill many animals if a cure for diabetes or cancer is found. The problem associated with using teleology to rectify or resolve ethical dilemmas is that there are no rules to determine the rightness or wrongness of an action (Guido, 2010).

Deontology is a theory of moral or professional obligation. The morality of the ethical decision is completely separate from its consequences. For example, health care providers could universally limit organ transplant on the basis of age or gender, with the hypothetical assumption that because there are more female donors, there would be more female recipients. Another example is the belief that alcoholism is a

---

SPOTLIGHT **ON**

Ethical Theories and Decision Making

Effective dietary strategies are very important in the health promotion of communities with a large population of obese individuals at risk for diabetes and obesity-related health problems. The federal government can impose dietary plans in community schools that limit the amount of fats, carbohydrates, and protein served in school cafeterias. These dietary plans may be imposed without regard for dietary cultural differences among ethnic groups. The ethical theory used in this scenario is teleology. Do you think that the result, appropriate nutrition and fewer cases of diabetes, which is in concert with health-promotion concepts, justifies this action?

(♿) HEALTH PROMOTION THEORY LINK

Caring, Clinical Wisdom, and Ethics

Patricia Benner has stated that "[t]he nurse-patient relationship is not a uniform, professionalized blueprint but rather a kaleidoscope of intimacy and distance in some of the most dramatic, poignant, and mundane moments of life" (as cited in Alligood & Tomey, 2010, p. 137). As such, judgments and decisions regarding patient care are integral to nursing practice, sometimes within the context of challenging ethical issues. According to Benner, clinical and ethical judgments cannot be separated and require guidance by being with and understanding human concerns and possibilities. Benner is known for her theoretical model *From Novice to Expert* whereby nurses move through four stages (novice, advanced beginner, competent, and proficient) until attaining the fifth stage of expert. A major concept in her model is ethical comportment that relates good conduct with a sense of belonging to the profession and that comes from being embedded in practices and ways of being and responding to clinical situations that promote the well-being of the patient. The nurse moves progressively through the stages while developing qualities of caring, competence, and wisdom for ethical decision-making.

Alligood, M. R., & Tomey, A. M. (2010). *Nursing theorists and their work* (7th ed.). St. Louis, MO: Mosby Elsevier.

---

self-inflicted disease with increased chances of progression to liver failure. Thus available organs for transplant should be allocated to those recipients deemed more worthy and without a history of self-inflicted disease. These examples are mixed with justice and veracity, two ethical principles to be discussed later in this chapter. Deontology's strength is in its emphasis on the dignity of human beings (Guido, 2006).

BASIC PRINCIPLES OF ETHICS

Ethical decision making involves an understanding of the basic principles of ethics. **Ethical principles** are basic concepts and rules to guide and give direction to nursing practice. If ethical principles are not used, a decision will rest solely on personal emotions and values (Guido, 2010). Table 22-1 lists nine basic principles of ethics.

PRINCIPLE OF AUTONOMY

Nurses are expected to understand the concept of autonomy and be advocates for all patients. **Autonomy** involves independence and freedom and is based on the right to self-determination. The root of the word is *auto*, meaning self, and *nomy*, which refers to control (Ellis & Hartley, 2008). Autonomy is the right to choose what happens to one's own person and gives the patient the right to determine personal care and who gives it. Situations

TABLE 22-1 Basic Principles of Ethics

PRINCIPLE	MEANING
Autonomy	Freedom to make choices
Beneficence	Promote good
Nonmaleficence	Invokes obligation not to harm others
Veracity	Practice of telling the truth
Confidentiality	An individual's right to privacy
Justice	Fair, equitable, and appropriate treatment
Fidelity	Faithfulness to another's cause
Standard of best interest	Assists patient in making decisions about own health care
Respect for others	Acknowledges right of person to make decisions and live or die by those decisions

© Cengage Learning 2013

that involve consideration of this principle include those related to a patient's right to die, receive treatment, or refuse treatment. Informed consent to allow a surgeon to do a procedure on an individual is a legal doctrine reflecting autonomy. However, autonomy does not give the patient absolute rights. Restrictions may be placed on the rights of the patient if these rights interfere with another's safety. For example, a person with a communicable disease may be quarantined, even if he or she does not want to be, if not doing so will expose others to the danger of the communicable disease (Guido, 2010). Occasionally, a patient's capacity for autonomy is brought into question, and a legal opinion must be sought. The courts may then assume the role of surrogate decision maker regarding situations involving the principle of autonomy. Situations that may require legal intervention when patient autonomy is in question frequently involve religious tenets prohibiting treatment or refusal of treatment due to mental illness.

SPOTLIGHT ON

Advance Directives and Autonomy

In 1990, the Patient Self-Determination Act was passed by Congress. This act requires that all health care institutions inform patients of their rights to advance directives, which are written instructions regarding specific procedures to be followed if the patient becomes incapacitated. Because an advance directive provides patients with the right to self-determination and a measure of independence, it upholds the ethical principle of autonomy and is congruent with the concept of empowerment in health promotion.

ASK YOURSELF

Utilizing Beneficence Principle in Determining Risks and Benefits

Newborn twins cojoined at the skull are being considered for a risky surgical separation. Though the beneficence principle indicates that the procedure is necessary for long-term survival, one baby or both babies could die. Can you explain the risks and benefits involved with this procedure to the parents? Are you comfortable with the possible outcomes of the procedure?

PRINCIPLE OF BENEFICENCE

Beneficence is a principle that requires nurses to act in ways that benefit patients. Beneficence provides the groundwork for the trust that society and individuals place in nurses. The primary goal of beneficence is to do good for patients under the care of a health care worker. This principle indicates that in caring for patients, the nurse should always take action to promote good, or what is best for the patient. This principle also maintains that nurses must prevent harm or evil. Although this principle seems very simplistic, the problem with it is determining what constitutes good (Guido, 2010). The *Code of Ethics for Nurses with Interpretive Statements* (ANA, 2001; Fowler, 2008) is quite clear in addressing the nurse's role in promoting the principle of beneficence. The code stresses that the nurse has an obligation to the patient and that this obligation includes protection of the patient from incompetent, unethical, or illegal practice (ANA, 2001). Situations that involve the nurse and the principle of beneficence may include decisions regarding the benefits and risks of certain treatments or procedures that determine who will live and who will die when only one individual can be saved. Nurses in their practice must always function with knowledge of the beneficence principle and will often

ASK YOURSELF

Sharing the Truth with Patients

Sometimes patients ask nurses questions related to their diagnosis and treatment of specific life-threatening diseases such as cancer. Is sharing with the patient details of the condition and prognosis always the right thing to do? What if the physician in charge of the patient's case does not want the patient to know? Will family members' unwillingness to share the truth with the affected family member influence your decision to answer the patient's questions? Does sharing the truth empower the patient and promote psychological health?

encounter situations in which opposing values play against one another (Ellis & Hartley, 2008).

PRINCIPLE OF NONMALEFICENCE

Nonmaleficence requires nurses to act in such a way as to avoid causing harm to patients. The nonmaleficence and beneficence principles are very similar. The primary difference lies in the fact that the beneficence principle strives to achieve what is good while the nonmaleficence principle seeks to do no harm in situations requiring nursing actions. Included in the nonmaleficence principle are actions that produce deliberate harm, risk of harm, or even harm that occurs during the performance of beneficial acts. Prohibited by this principle are procedures performed for monetary gain or experimental research that assumes negative outcomes for the participants. Individual state nursing practice acts address issues related to the nurse's responsibility to do no harm. For example, the Texas Nursing Practice Act specifically addresses a nurse's responsibility in promoting a safe environment for patients and others. It is the nurse's responsibility to report unsafe nursing practice by another RN if there is reasonable cause to suspect unnecessary exposure of a patient to risk of harm as a result of failure to conform to the minimum standards of care (Willman, 2009).

PRINCIPLE OF VERACITY

The principle of **veracity** is simply the practice of telling the truth. It is a universally accepted virtue, and most of us were taught as children to always tell the truth. Telling the truth is promoted in all professional codes of ethics and can certainly be found in nursing's code of ethics. Veracity engenders respect, open communication, trust, and shared responsibility. Not telling the truth is deception, and nurses are not supposed to conceal the truth from patients. Violation of the veracity principle in dealing with patients has serious consequences for nurses. Everyone who knows the truth will remember the deception and be inclined to believe that health professionals cannot be relied on (Ellis & Hartley, 2008). The intimate dealings with patients and their family members usually place the nurse in a position of trust. Questions are asked of the nurse that may deal with delicate issues or that are related to the patient's condition. Although the nurse is taught to uphold the principle of veracity, at times telling the truth may result in awkward or confusing situations because family members have kept important information from the patient. The physician or primary health care giver is expected to share with the patient the truth about the diagnosed illness. This may not always be the case, so it may be incumbent on the nurse to provide the patient with the truth.

PRINCIPLE OF CONFIDENTIALITY

Although most textbooks do not list confidentiality as a principle of ethics, it is not possible to care for patients appropriately without recognizing that all people have a right to privacy. Nurses are privy to information that cannot be made public knowledge without a state or federal court ruling. Again, the *Code of Ethics for Nurses with Interpretive Statements* (ANA, 2001) has a very clear position on the issue of confidentiality. The code asserts that it is the nurse's responsibility to safeguard a patient's right to privacy by protecting information of a confidential nature. A major area of concern related to confidentiality involves the issue of who might have access to

medical records. The Federal Health Insurance Portability and Accountability Act of 1996 (HIPAA) was passed to establish a national framework for security standards and protection of confidentiality with regard to health care data and information. Nurses are expected to comply with HIPAA regulations in protecting the patient's confidentiality regarding health or personal matters. The implications of this federal regulation on the health care community are considerable. For example, some health care institutions are no longer placing a patient's name on the hospital room door so that the patient's name is not visible to others. Although this may ensure a patient's right to confidentiality, this policy may also cause more hospital-related safety infractions.

Confidentiality may be broken only at certain times and only if the nurse knows that the patient is a danger to self or others. Then it is the nurse's legal duty to warn significant others of the impending danger. For example, this is clearly evident in any case involving violent behavior.

PRINCIPLE OF JUSTICE

Justice is the fair, equitable, and appropriate treatment according to what is due or owed to persons, with the understanding that giving to some will deny receipt to others who might otherwise have received those things. In this great nation, excellent health care is available but not to all for various reasons. Nurses are well aware that need is sometimes not the basic factor involved in determining who receives care and who does not. The concept of justice is often expanded to include what is called distributive justice, which states that all people are entitled to be treated equally regardless of gender, marital status, medical diagnosis, social standing, economic level, or religious beliefs (Catalano, 2008). Distributive justice thus includes the idea that all people should have access to health care. Unfortunately, what is not described through this principle is who incurs the costs. For that reason, the principle of justice, specifically distributive justice, is often challenged in health care.

> ### ✳ NURSING ALERT
> #### Institutional Ethics Committees
> Most health care institutions have an active ethics committee to deal with patient ethical issues. Whenever a nursing situation occurs that involves ethics and requires decision making, the nurse should refer the case to the ethics committee.

PRINCIPLE OF FIDELITY

Fidelity is often related to the concept of faithfulness and the practice of keeping promises. Nurses have been granted the right to practice nursing by licensure and certification. As described in ANA's *Code of Ethics for Nurses* (2001), it is the nurse's responsibility to provide services to patients and safeguard their rights to health care. This is considered fundamental to quality nursing practice and addresses the principle of fidelity. The promise to care for the patient is primary. Nurses fulfill that promise in many ways—verbally, mutually contracting or interacting, and a host of other ways. Fidelity relates closely to the concept of accountability.

STANDARD OF BEST INTEREST

The **standard of best interest** is one that allows individuals to share in decision making. This principle is used to assist patients in making choices regarding health care. In using this principle, nurses can assist patients in decision making when they lack the expertise or knowledge and data to make decisions. If the entire decision is taken away from the patient, this principle is obviously avoided (Guido, 2010). The nurse who does not take the patient's wishes into consideration in determining a plan of nursing care is using the concept of **paternalism**. Paternalism encourages individuals to make decisions for others. Obviously, paternalism is an undesirable principle.

PRINCIPLE OF RESPECT FOR OTHERS

Respect for others is seen as the highest ethical principle. It incorporates the concepts found in all the other principles. Respect for others acknowledges that individuals are capable of making decisions for themselves in all areas of their lives, including decisions relating to life or death (Guido, 2010). Nurses are crucial in upholding this principle because they can positively reinforce this principle on a daily basis in their actions with peers, patients, the health care team, and family members. Utilization by nurses of the principle of respect for others includes recognition of the patient's culture, gender issues, religion, ethnicity, and race.

NURSING AND ETHICS

Nurses providing patient care need to be constantly cognizant of the nine ethical principles. They must recognize that there are rarely any black-or-white answers to dilemmas dealing with the variability in human nature. For this reason, each nurse should develop a philosophically consistent framework on which to base contemplation, decision, and action. Ethical and moral principles provide the background for the development of a rational decision-making framework.

ETHICAL DECISION MAKING AND PERSONAL VALUES

In determining solutions for ethical dilemmas, the values with which the nurse was brought up, the values the nurse holds dear, or both of these provide needed direction. Clarification of these values is essential if the nurse is to assist patients in decision making. An awareness of personal values empowers both the nurse and the patient and fosters the achievement of their mutual goal, which is to promote the patient's personal health status. **Values** make up a set of personal beliefs and attitudes about such things as truth, beauty, justice, and the worth of any thought, object, or behavior. In developing values, a person acquires direction and gives meaning to life. Values reflect how people live or have been brought up and are derived from personal life experiences. They affect the disposition one has toward a person, object, or idea. Values are usually not isolated but are interwoven with each other and with specific life events. In addition, values influence each other and are always changing. In sorting through decisions that need to be made,

individuals use their own process for clarifying personal values. This **values clarification** is the process of becoming more conscious of and naming what one values or considers worthy. This process sheds light on a person's personal perspectives.

STEPS IN VALUES CLARIFICATION

Several steps are identified in the values clarification process. These steps provide a systematic approach to obtaining a more comprehensive understanding of how a value is acquired. Although the steps identified in the literature are not always identical, the same concepts are included and considered inherent to the process. By using the steps involved in values clarification, nurses as well as nursing students can understand their own value system as well as that of their patients. Box 22-1 lists several steps that are helpful in clarifying personal values.

The steps involved in values clarification are useful in gaining perspective on personal values. The first step in the process is essential if the nurse wants to deal appropriately with ethical dilemmas. This step involves the mental activity called **introspection**, which is the ability to look inside oneself and examine thoughts and personal meaning for identified values. Without this activity it is almost impossible to determine whether certain situations are wrong or whether they are in conflict with personal values. The act of clarifying values also necessitates recognition that personal freedom does not allow any one value to be dictated and that everyone makes decisions regarding values based on personal meaning and individual situations. The final steps in values clarification are also essential. These require a commitment to the chosen values and demand congruence between value choices and personal actions and behaviors.

BOX 22-1
STEPS IN VALUES CLARIFICATION

1. Engage in personal introspection.
2. Recognize individual freedom to choose personal values.
3. Evaluate personal meaning of value choices.
4. Understand that there are many other individual values.
5. Develop commitment to values.
6. Determine the congruence of actions with values choices.

Values can either be tangible or intangible and are often measured by behavior. Therefore, values are considered to be internal controls for behavior. Many issues facing the practice of nursing today are emotionally charged; if they were not, they would not be considered important. Only by considering all aspects of an issue can a nurse hope to seek understanding of the issue and move into decision making that is beneficial for everyone.

VALUE CONFLICTS

At times, personal values are at odds with the values of the patient or of the institution. This can create friction between the nurse and the employing institution as well as result in poor quality of patient care. The negative outcomes in such a situation can be prevented by becoming more aware of personal values and what actions are acceptable or not acceptable. Values conflict must be dealt with in an effective way, acquiring a conscious awareness of one's own values as well as the perceived values of others. Differences in values arise, and a choice can be made to respond to the other's viewpoint by seeking understanding and common ground.

LEGAL ISSUES

Nursing decisions should reflect adherence to standards of nursing practice and recognition of the associated legal implications as well as ethical ones. In many instances, the clinical practice nurse may be faced with a legal situation. Clinical practice, for instance, can involve legal situations such as disconnection of patients from life support, restraint or medicating of patients against their will, and omission or lack of care, to name a few. Legal issues may also arise when **informed consent** (see Figure 22-1), or a clear explanation of procedures along with associated risks and benefits, is not provided to the patient. Legal situations may also arise when the nurse or a health care professional is thought to have provided inadequate or incompetent care. Patients may then take legal action and attempt to highlight incompetence through the legal system. Nurses must therefore know that the profession is held to the same legal standards as the average citizen as well as to those relating to nursing. Also, as the nursing profession's

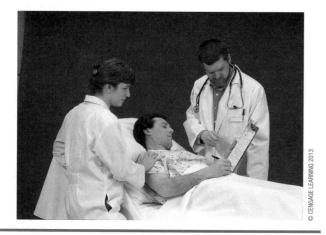

FIGURE 22-1 **The nurse is ethically and legally accountable when engaging in clinical practice. The witnessing of informed consent is one of many nursing responsibilities making the nurse ethically and legally responsible.**

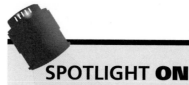

SPOTLIGHT ON

Values Incongruence

Value conflicts occur when two or more values are incongruent. Society is beset with conflicting values. Take, for example, a mother who expresses no concern for her 5-year-old daughter who weighs 82 lb. She refuses to follow nursing advice regarding the need to restrict the child's caloric intake and increase her physical activity. The mother believes she is doing what is best for her child. What would be your response to this? Would the mother's decision conflict with your values?

scope of practice increases, the laws applicable to nursing will continue to evolve.

LAW AND NURSING PRACTICE

Law has been defined in a variety of ways. Law, very simply, can be defined as the sum total of rules and regulations by which a society is governed. Law includes rules and regulations established and enforced by a given community, state, or nation. Laws are created by people and are used to regulate behavior in all persons (Guido, 2010). Laws provide society with rules or standards of conduct that have been determined through legislative bodies and then tested in courts. The ultimate goal of law is to protect and safeguard the public. Likewise, nursing's ultimate goal is to protect the public by providing safe, quality patient care.

Nurses are not exempt from state or constitutional law and must adhere to all civil and criminal statutes. They must adhere to all aspects of the Nursing Practice Act (NPA) and are legally accountable for all actions in their nursing practice, including those that have been delegated to others. This accountability arises from the fact that nurses are licensed to practice through a legal regulatory mechanism (Fowler, 2008). The NPA regulates the practice of nursing in both the United States and Canada. At the same time, each state in the United States and each province in Canada has its own nursing practice act, enacted by individual state or province law.

Nurses in their role as promoters of health act as patient advocates. As patient advocates, nurses are expected to protect patients from unsafe procedures and see that their legal rights to safe and equitable health care are not violated. The standards of nursing practice also guarantee that patients receive quality nursing care and assure that all patients are provided with the information needed to make decisions about health promotion, maintenance, and restoration (ANA, 2004). These standards are used as measurable expectations in a court of law, and nurses are expected to adhere to the standards of practice as well as to the NPA. The registered nurse must also practice within the rules of the Board of Nurse Examiners (BNE) for the state where the nurse is practicing, and within laws relating to the specific practice setting. The rules provided by the BNE provide more detailed guidance to the registered nurse than does the NPA.

HEALTH PROMOTION
THEORY LINK

Competency, Scope and Standards of Practice, and Globalization of Continuing Education

Continuing education is required for nurses to maintain their license to practice and is imperative to maintaining and increasing professional competency. The American Nurses Association has copublished the *Nursing Professional Development: Scope and Standards of Practice* with the National Nursing Staff Development Organization. This document has clearly embraced the fact that the continuing education target audience is now worldwide. Within the continuing education and academic domains, technology has changed the learning environment and the potential target audiences. Once locally or regionally defined, the target audience is now global. Thinking about education has changed to include a globalization concept and how education needs can be assessed across the world. Simulation and virtual reality will become routine as they are incorporated into teaching modalities.

Source: NANA's newly revised scope & standards for nursing professional development reflects 10 years of evolution since last edition. (2010). *NurseZone.* Retrieved from http://www.nursezone.com/Nursing-News-Events/more-news/ANA's-Newly-Revised-Scope-amp-Standards-for-Nursing-Professional-Development-Reflects-10-Years-of-Evolution-Since-Last-Edition_34762.aspx

COMPETENCY INDICATORS

Although it may seem unusual to describe competency indicators as being important to the nurse's role as a promoter of health, the truth is that these competency indicators are essential to the practice role of the professional nurse. These indicators demonstrate that standards of nursing practice are being maintained and that safe, competent care is being delivered. Several measures can be used as indicators of nursing competency and accountability. Table 22-2 lists several indicators of nursing accountability along with their meaning.

LICENSURE

A nurse must attain licensure to practice professional nursing in the United States. This licensure is mandatory and provides a measure of accountability to the general public indicating that the nurse meets minimal competency to provide safe nursing care. Once licensure is attained, the nurse becomes a registered nurse. **Registration** is the listing of an individual's name and other information on the official roster of a governmental or nongovernmental agency. Nurses who are registered are permitted to use the title "registered nurse" or "RN." To be registered, the nurse must complete a basic course of nursing studies in an approved, accredited program and pass the national qualifying examination with an acceptable grade.

Individual states in the United States have their own licensure policies. For example, in the state of Texas, applicants may take the licensing examination every 45 days and within 4 years of completion of graduation requirements. If the exam is not passed within 4 years, applicants must complete a board-approved nursing program (Board of Nurse Examiners for the State of Texas, 2011). This is not true of all states. New graduates of accredited nursing programs in the United States and Canada who are applying for initial licensure are issued a temporary permit after they have been determined eligible. States may vary in these procedures.

Temporary permits differ from temporary licenses. A holder of a temporary license has the same authority to practice professional nursing as does a permanent license holder. This is considered licensure by endorsement without examination and is only for nurses who are licensed as registered nurses in a territory or possession of the United States or foreign country and who demonstrate the same degree of fitness required by the state to which they apply. Licensure by endorsement also applies to nurses who are licensed to practice professional nursing in other states. These are licenses issued after meeting requirements as set forth by each state board.

MULTISTATE LICENSURE

The concept of licensure may soon be a thing of the past. As a result of increased nursing mobility between states, the United States is moving toward the concept of multistate licensure. **Multistate licensure** is the recognition of a single license allowing registered nurses to practice throughout the country. Although not all states in the United States have adopted this type of licensure, compact legislation has been enacted among several states recognizing a single nursing license. This multistate licensure compact provides a process through which states agree to mutually recognize each other's licensees and

TABLE 22-2 Accountability Indicators	
INDICATOR	**MEANING**
Licensure	Indication of the minimum degree of competency to practice safely
Credentialing	Recognition of competence through specialty knowledge, education, registration, certification, licensure, and accreditation
Certification	Judgment of competency by practicing nurses in specialty practice
Accreditation	Recognition of demonstrated compliance with established criteria, usually a symbol of excellence
Standards of care	Guideposts ensuring competent practice

thus discontinues the process of requiring duplicate licenses. The compact requires that nurses be licensed in their home states and comply with the state practice laws of the state in which they practice (Philipsen & Haynes, 2007).

CREDENTIALING

The nursing profession is becoming increasingly more accountable as the general public is becoming more knowledgeable about its right to receive safe and competent care. Like other professions, nursing uses the credentialing process as an indicator of competency and demonstrated accountability. **Credentialing** is a process that recognizes professional achievements such as specialty practice knowledge, educational accomplishments, certification, licensure, and accreditation. The credentialing process is one way in which the nursing profession maintains standards of practice and demonstrates accountability for the educational preparation of its members. The credentialing process is also a means of recognizing technical competence in areas requiring special-level expertise (Ellis & Hartley, 2008). The most highly visible nursing credentialing board is the American Nurses Credentialing Center, which is an independent agency of the ANA and offers various advance practice nursing certifications.

CERTIFICATION

Certification is the process by which an individual registered nurse who has met certain established criteria or qualifications is granted recognition for competency. These criteria may include a judgment of competence by nurses who are themselves practicing in the area of specialization and the completion of certain educational courses and clinical practice. A crucial component of certification is successful completion of an examination that tests knowledge in the specialty area (Fowler, 2008). In many instances, certification is required for entrance into specialty practice such as nurse practitioners, nurse midwives, or certified registered nurse anesthetists.

? ASK **YOURSELF**

Benefits of Multistate Licensure

What benefits does mutual recognition of nursing licensure among states provide? Is multistate licensure of interest to you in your future career goals? What legal implications are there in being licensed in your home state and practicing in another state?

ACCREDITATION

Accreditation is a form of certification or licensure that recognizes demonstrated compliance with established criteria. This certification or licensure is given to agencies or institutions rather than to individuals. Universities, schools of nursing, and hospitals seek accreditation according to the type of business they conduct or service that they provide. For example, the Joint Commission (JC), formerly the Joint Commission on the Accreditation of Healthcare Organizations (JCAHO), is an accrediting body that is very important to health care organizations. The JC's mission is to evaluate a health care institution's performance in all areas that affect health care, with specific focus on the quality and safety of care. To earn and maintain accreditation, an extensive on-site review by a team of Joint Commission health care professionals is conducted at least once every 3 years. Accreditation is awarded based on how well the organization meets the Joint Commission standards (Joint Commission, 2011). Organizations such as hospitals must seek the accreditation process and demonstrate compliance with specific, published criteria. Schools of nursing must meet accreditation standards set by the Board of Nurse Examiners for the state. They may also choose to be recognized as an accredited school by the National League for Nursing (NLN) or the Commission on Collegiate Nursing Education (CCNE), which accredits baccalaureate and graduate nursing education programs. Entry into the armed forces as a commissioned officer requires evidence of having graduated from an NLN- or a CCNE-accredited nursing program. Admission into graduate school usually requires the same evidence.

STANDARDS OF CARE

This chapter multiple references to standards of nursing care. These standards ensure safe practice to the public and serve as guidelines established by the profession for nursing practice. They also serve as parameters and reminders to nurses regarding the boundaries of practice. Standards of care have been referred to as safety checklists. The ANA has established general standards of care as well as standards for such specialty areas as acute care, college health, oncology, pediatric clinical, maternal-child, medical-surgical, geriatric, and surgical nursing. Box 22-2 provides a list of some of the standards of practice developed by the ANA.

A nurse is expected to provide safe and competent care, abide by clinical principles and legal statutes, and do no harm. Within this environment, the nurse contracts with the patient either in an expressed or implied manner. As soon as the patient-nurse relationship is established, the nurse has a legal and binding duty to the patient. The *Lunsford v. Board of Nurse Examiners* (1983) case made it very clear that duty is owed to a patient when a patient-nurse relationship is established.

BOX 22-2
SELECTED ANA STANDARDS OF PRACTICE

Scope and standards of practice in:

- Addictions nursing
- College health nursing
- Diabetes nursing
- Gerontological nursing
- Home health nursing
- Hospice and palliative care nursing
- Neonatal nursing
- Neuroscience nursing
- Nursing administration

- Nursing informatics
- Nursing professional development
- Pain management nursing
- Pediatric nursing
- Pediatric oncology
- Plastic surgery nursing
- Psychiatric mental health nursing
- Public health nursing
- School nursing
- Vascular nursing

By virtue of licensure, this relationship automatically exists whenever a patient seeks care and is met by a nurse (Guido, 2010). The nursing care plan, which is developed by the nurse and the patient or family or both collaboratively, also serves as a contract of an explicit or expressed nature. The responsibility for nursing actions rests solely with the nurse. If the nurse believes an action will be harmful to the patient, the nurse must refuse to carry it out. The validity of the action, as well as the potential consequences, of the action must be documented. In the event that a questionable action has been performed that might be harmful to the patient, it is always best to inform the supervising nurse, document the action succinctly in writing, and keep a personal copy of the report.

TORTS, NEGLIGENCE, AND BREACHES IN LEGAL DUTY

A **tort**, which is a legal wrong committed against a person or property, is settled in civil court and involves some type of compensation, usually money. A tort differs from a **crime**, which is also a legal wrong committed against a person or property. A crime, however, involves a wide range of malfeasance from minor citations to murder and is punishable by the government at the county, state, or federal level (Ellis & Hartley, 2004). Torts may result from a breach of a legal duty and may be intentional, quasi-intentional, or nonintentional acts, and the courts provide a remedy in the form of an action for damages.

Negligence torts are the most frequent basis for liability of nurses, physicians, and hospitals. **Negligence** involves failure to provide the care that a reasonable person would provide in similar circumstances and is considered a civil or personal wrong, to distinguish it from criminal conduct. It denotes conduct lacking in due care and equates with carelessness. Negligence can also include doing something that a reasonably prudent person would *not* do. According to this definition, anyone can be liable for negligence (Guido, 2010). Negligence alone is not enough to establish liability; there must also be an injury caused by the negligence. Four elements must be present in order to establish liability negligence. Table 22-3 lists these elements along with the concepts necessary to understand their meaning.

TABLE 22-3 Elements in Liability Negligence

ELEMENT	CONCEPT
Duty	Duty is owed to a patient.
	Nurse fails to meet standard of care.
	Scope of duty is within professional nursing boundaries.
Breach of duty	Deviation from standard of care is established.
Injury	Financial, physical, emotional harm is established.
Causation	Direct cause for failure to meet standard of care clearly established.

© Cengage Learning 2013

SPOTLIGHT **ON**

Negligence and Causation

An ambulatory elderly patient falls while hospitalized for an unrelated condition and is discharged in a nonambulatory state. He develops pneumonia at home and dies less than 10 days after the fall. Because of the time that passed, the patient's family may be unable to prove causation.

The first element that must be proven in any action for negligence to occur relates to duty. There are two aspects of duty. It must first be proved that a duty was owed to the person harmed, and second it must be affirmed that the scope of that duty is within the boundaries of the profession, usually called the standards of care. The second element refers to the idea that a **breach of duty** has occurred. In other words, there must be a deviation in some manner from the standard of care, which is established on showing that the nurse did something that should not have been done or did no do something that should have been done. Proof of this hinges on showing that the care of the patient was substandard. The third element that must be proven is the establishment of actual injury. Some type of physical, financial, or emotional injury or any combination must be incurred. The actual injury must be demonstrated for negligence to be established. The last element is causation. This final element is probably the most important in establishing negligence. To prove that negligence has occurred as a result of breach of duty, it is essential to establish that the breach of duty without a doubt caused the injury.

RIGHT TO REFUSE TREATMENT

At the core of health promotion is the concept that the patient is the expert in his or her own treatment and care. Thus, in utilizing a health-promotion framework in planning for the patient's care, the nurse must be cognizant of the patient's right to refuse treatment. The law also recognizes that a person has the right to refuse treatment. Additionally, it recognizes that a patient possesses the right to be free from aggression and the threats of actual aggression. If the patient refuses treatment and a nurse provides treatment anyway, charges of assault or battery or both may be filed by the patient. **Battery** involves actually physically touching the person and is considered a physical violation. **Assault** is an infringement on the mental security or tranquility or both of another. Assault is an attempt or threat to touch another person. If a patient refuses a procedure or has certain procedures done without consent, these actions can lead to a civil claim of assault or battery or both (Zerwekh & Claborn, 2009).

Patients cannot be restrained unless they are in danger. Restraints, especially for an extended period, require the order of a physician. Restraining a patient may result in charges of assault, battery, or false imprisonment being filed against the nurse, physician, and the medical establishment. Liability for restraints usually intended to avoid a patient fall or escape

? ASK **YOURSELF**

Student Nurse Liability

When teaching a mother how to take her baby's temperature rectally during her community health rotation, a student nurse gives erroneous information that may result in harm to the baby. If injury to the baby occurs as a result of this information, should the student be held liable? Who else should be held accountable?

that might cause injury to self or others. Courts are more critical when they believe the nurse left the patient unattended in order to do something less important. Failure to provide a restrained patient with a signaling device, failure to restrain a patient properly, and failure to provide attendance when the restraints are removed from a patient are all reasons that the courts can find the nurse liable.

STUDENT NURSE LIABILITY

Student nurses are held liable for their own acts of negligence committed in the course of clinical experiences. If students are performing duties that are within the scope of professional nursing, they will be held to the same standard of skill and competence as a registered professional nurse. A lower standard of care is not applied to the action of nursing students. To fulfill their patient responsibilities and to minimize exposure to liability, nursing students should make sure that they are prepared to care properly for assigned patients and should ask for additional help or supervision if they feel inadequately prepared for an assignment (Guido, 2006). Student nurses are expected to carry personal liability insurance.

ETHICAL, LEGAL, AND POLITICAL CONCERNS RELATED TO HEALTH CARE COST AND ACCESS

Many changes in the last few decades have affected the delivery of care, impacted the finances of health care institutions, escalated health care costs, and made health care literally inaccessible for hundreds of thousands of people nationwide. Although a national health policy was hinted at when the Colonies were first established as far back as the seventeenth century, a national health policy that provides care for all people has not become reality. It is a sad testimony that a nation as rich as the United States still has citizens who are unable to access health care.

Although the nursing profession expects health promotion, restoration, support, and maintenance to be integral components of the nurse's responsibility, ethical and legal concerns still arise over questions of who can receive health care delivery services, who can afford health care services, and who has the right to access health care. Nurses, in their attempt to address these questions, have established that, in addition to health

care access, health-promotion strategies and preventive health care programs should be accessible to all citizens.

HEALTH CARE DELIVERY AND HEALTH CARE COSTS

Rapidly rising health care costs along with unsuccessful attempts to deal with them in the context of the increasingly worrisome federal deficit have had the greatest influence in shaping today's health care system. The high cost of health care has given rise to managed care plans, combining insurance and provider functions, horizontal integration of health care facilities into larger organizations, and hospital expansion into ambulatory surgery, home care, and other centers such as substance abuse treatment centers. The result of all of these measures is that the current health care delivery system is fragmented, delivers poor-quality services, and at times provides inadequate care.

A major restructuring of the hospital workforce has emerged, along with an implementation of cost-cutting diagnostic-related systems that dictate reimbursement rates. All kinds of institutional and alternative delivery systems have been established over the last decade. These have grown as an incentive to provide care at a lower cost. Physicians, for example, are moving toward group practice, and the greatest growth in physician group practice is expected to be in either individual practice associations or preferred provider organizations (PPOs), associated with a health maintenance organization (HMO) or primary case management model. The origination of PPOs and IPAs helps a group of providers negotiate fee schedules with hospitals and third-party reimbursers. The financial shift has gone from the health plans to the physicians. Today, HMOs view themselves as managed care organizations that offer an array of managed care plans. It is important to ask who is responsible for charges for health care services. The availability of private insurance, Medicaid, Medicare, or private pay does not constitute a solution to the delivery of health care in an ethical and cost-effective manner. Sufficient funds must be available to pay for any of these so-called solutions.

? ASK **YOURSELF**

The Right to Health Care: An Ethical or a Legal Concern?

Do you think health care is a right or a privilege? Should all people have access to the same health care services regardless of ability to pay? How should ability to pay influence access to health care services? If you believe health care is a right, how much health care is each person entitled to? As a taxpayer, are you willing to fund taxes that provide health care to all?

HEALTH CARE ACCESS

The decline in access to health care is the most evident in the very young, the very old, and the poor and in minority populations. This decline in accessibility can only be partially

RESEARCH NOTE

Themes of Ethical Conflicts of Nurses and Physicians

STUDY PROBLEM/PURPOSE

Research on clinical ethical conflict has centered on the health care professional in a specialty area of patient care or to a particular segment of the health care professional population. The purpose of this study was to identifies themes of Canadian hospital nurses' and physicians' clinical ethical conflicts across the spectrum of clinical specialty areas and to compare the themes identified by nurses with those identified by physicians.

METHODS

A qualitative descriptive design was used whereby 34 clinical nurses, 10 nurse managers, and 31 physicians working at four different Canadian hospitals and serving on ethics committees formed a convenience sample. They were asked if they ever experienced an ethical conflict and, if so, to describe it and then think of any other examples. Other questions related to ethical conflicts in the organization and barriers in serving on ethics committees.

FINDINGS

From content analysis, nine themes of clinical ethical conflict are common to both hospital nurses and physicians: disagreement about care options; lack of respect for patient wishes; no respect for quality end-of-life care; patient or family behavior; no informed consent; not knowing the correct thing to do; problems with system or organization; conflicting values with patient; and competency of the practitioner. Three physician-specific themes were related to lack of agreement with national clinical practice guidelines, the dilemma of survival versus futility of treatment, and balancing survival over disability in an infant or child.

IMPLICATIONS

This study highlighted that physicians and nurses often face the same ethical dilemmas and also recognized the complexities of intercollaboration across disciplines in ethical situations. It was suggested that these themes could be used to structure basic continuing education across disciplines that could also foster interprofessional understanding, respect, collaboration, communication, and behavior in ethically challenged situations.

Source: Gaudine. A., LeFort, S. M., Lamb, M., & Thorne, L. (2011). Clinical ethical conflicts of nurses and physicians. *Nursing Ethics, 18* (1), 9–19.

not access either preventive or treatment health services is by exploring the sociological and cultural domains.

SOCIOLOGICAL DOMAIN

People do not access care or preventive services or both for many sociological reasons. One overwhelming reason is a lack of resources, which may be material such as a lack of money or living in poverty. The poor and the elderly are very vulnerable to problems with access to care (Allender & Spradley, 2009). Coupled with a lack of financial resources may be fear due to an illegal immigrant status. For example, many undocumented illegal immigrants live in California, New York, and Texas, and they may not seek health care for fear of being deported to their country of origin.

Lack of resources in accessing health care is a major problem related to the cycle of poverty. Many U.S. residents are without access to health care because they are poor and without health services coverage (Allender & Spradley, 2009). This cycle of poverty extends to poor intellectual ability and even to ignorance of where to seek assistance. Inability to communicate in English or the language identified as the predominant language may also pose a sociological barrier to accessing to health care.

CULTURAL DOMAIN

The value that an individual gives to activities involving health care access and health promotion activities frequently reflects cultural or religious beliefs or both. For example, many people may not access modern health care services; they see folk healers or traditional culturally sensitive healers when they are ill. Members of the various ethnic and cultural groups manifest beliefs concerning health, disease prevention, and health promotion. These beliefs play a major part in terms of which health delivery services are sought. Nursing professionals should be sensitive to the fact that certain ethnic groups may first seek help outside the modern health care system. Nursing's code of ethics specifies that nurses are to provide services that recognize human dignity and the uniqueness of the patient. If nurses do not recognize human diversity and the beliefs that are important in accessing care, they are unethical in their nursing performance and are probably guilty of a legal infraction as well.

ETHICAL-LEGAL CONCEPTS AND HEALTH PROMOTION

According to the *Scope and Standards of Practice* (ANA, 2004) and *Nursing's Social Policy Statement* (Fowler, 2008), professional nurses are expected to provide for patient participation in all aspects of health promotion. The nurse is to keep the patient and family informed regarding patient status, collaborate with them in developing a nursing care plan, and provide them with the information needed to make decisions and choices regarding care.

In assuming the responsibility for patient participation in health-promotion activities, the nurse is also expected to abide by the profession's code of ethics and the NPA. These documents spell out nursing's commitment to the caring and nurturing of patients and nursing's clear responsibility to advocate for the patient, communicate with the patient, family, and members of the health care team, and support health actions that restore health.

attributed to a lack of insurance. Actually, lack of health insurance at most explains only a small percentage. Researchers have identified many barriers that delay or prevent access to care, but no one specific factor prevents health care access. One of the better ways, perhaps, to investigate why individuals do

TABLE 22-4 Nurse Roles, Practice Conflicts, and Ethical-Legal Implications

NURSE ROLE	POTENTIAL PRACTICE CONFLICT EXAMPLES	ETHICAL (E) AND LEGAL (L) IMPLICATIONS
Nurturer	A nurse providing home care to a mother suspects child abuse after observing the mother's reaction to her child. The nurse must decide whether to report the situation to authorities and risk having the child placed in foster care.	E Nursing is committed to caring for and nurturing patients. In this example, the nurse must decide who the patient is and how the concept of nurturing applies to the child. L The nurse must find out if reporting the abuse is within the scope of professional nursing. State laws governing reporting abuse must be determined.
Patient advocate	A homeless person without any insurance is being provided substandard care by the medical team.	E Nursing's code indicates that the nurse must act to safeguard the patient at all times. As a patient advocate, the nurse must assist the patient in receiving the care deserved. L The NPA requires that the nurse advocate on the patient's behalf and report unsafe care.
Health-promotion agent	A nurse provides unsolicited dietary counseling to an extremely obese patient being treated for a minor injury.	E The nurse must decide whether nursing professionals have the right to regulate a person's eating habits, even when such advice is unsolicited. L Legally, the nurse owes a duty directly to the patient. A patient has the right to refuse counseling.
Communicator	A community health nurse is informed by a patient that he has been diagnosed with diabetes and requests that no information regarding his illness be shared with his wife.	E Nursing's code of ethics asserts that a patient's right to privacy should be maintained through the protection of confidential information. L The nurse should know that the practice act protects patient confidentiality and that a patient's family or significant other does not automatically have a right to confidential information.
Restorer and supporter of health	A patient who is paralyzed is considering physician-assisted suicide and asks the nurse for help in locating a physician.	E The nurse must review personal feelings about nursing's multiple roles as patient advocate and restorer and supporter of health. L The nurse must investigate whether physician-assisted suicide is legal in the state where he or she is practicing. The NPA should be reviewed to determine whether a nurse can help in physician-assisted suicide.

Many ethical and legal issues arise in nursing practice and in the activities associated with health promotion. Nurses may be expected to participate in decision making surrounding some of these issues. As a member of the profession, the nurse is held ethically and legally accountable. Table 22-4 illustrates examples of potential nurse role/practice conflicts that may be encountered and their ethical and legal implications.

As health-promotion agents, nurses have a duty to advocate quality health care for patients not only at the bedside but also in the community and at the licensing board level (Creasia & Parker, 2006). The profession's accountability and ethical standards thus bind the nurse in the role of health care promoter. However, several ethical and legal questions concerning health-promotion remain. For example, does nursing have the right to determine what constitutes health? If so, does the profession set health agendas for people and decide on uniform health-promotion strategies applicable to everyone?

NURSING AND HEALTH PROMOTION

In responding to the issue of whether nursing has the right to determine what health is and what health-promoting strategies must be espoused by nurses to achieve their patients' health, differentiation of health promotion from disease prevention becomes important. Integral to the concept of health promotion is concern for the problems that compromise health and well-being. Early development of positive health habits can result in a decrease of social problems (Pender, Murdaugh, & Parsons, 2010). Although nursing is concerned with the concept of illness and disease prevention, nursing also focuses on activities that promote social well-being. Accordingly, nursing promotes practices that foster positive health through healthy living and personal as well as family development. Nursing does not prescribe or dictate health-promotion strategies or set health agendas. Nursing, instead, clarifies patient goals and encourages their achievement. People choose to do what they please. Nurses can only empower their patients; they cannot mandate behavior that promotes health.

From an ethical viewpoint, nursing must view health and health promotion from the perspective of supporting self-defined goals, whether of individual patients, their families, or the community in which they reside. Through the support of their patients' self-defined goals, nurses empower them. Ethically, patients are empowered by being allowed to make choices that determine their physical well-being. Nurses support health promotion by providing education regarding choices that can be made and serving as a professional resource.

Legally, nursing is bound by the profession's standards of care and the NPA, both of which demand professional accountability. Health promotion is addressed in these documents in terms of advocating for patients in their pursuit of health and in assuring that a safe environment exists for them. Although nursing's goal is the achievement of positive health and well-being for all, from a legal standpoint a mentally competent patient can refuse all nursing interventions. If there is a possibility of harm to self or others, nursing can intervene through the legal court system, thus indirectly determining health-promotion strategies for patients.

SUMMARY

Nurses are called upon regularly to make decisions that critically affect their patients' lives and well-being. Ethical and legal concerns are closely related and usually interwoven into the decision-making process. When nurses make decisions that have ethical and legal implications, these decisions must be rooted in the professional standards as set forth by the ANA. Decisions related to patient care must also be made with an awareness of legal statutes, particularly those that relate to licensure laws and nursing practice. Ethical theories and principles guide nursing decision making by providing the context in which individual situations should be viewed. A process called values clarification can help the nurse become more conscious of personal values, which is important in developing insight.

As patient advocates, nurses are expected to protect patients from unsafe procedures or situations and to see that their legal rights to safe and equitable health care are not violated.

Registered nurses, by way of being licensed and belonging to the profession, are legally accountable for their actions. The nursing profession is becoming progressively more accountable as the role of the nurse evolves. Student nurses are not exempt from being accountable. There are several indicators of nursing's accountability and competency.

There is an apparent decline in access to health care. This decline is related to more than just lack of insurance. Nursing is concerned with a patient's access to quality health care. It focuses also on activities that promote the social well-being and health of patients. Nursing does not prescribe or dictate health-promotion strategies but clarifies patient goals and their achievement. Through support of self-identified patient goals, nurses empower patients. Although nursing's goal is the achievement of positive health, from a legal standpoint, a mentally competent patient can refuse all nursing interventions.

KEY CONCEPTS

1. Nursing decisions regarding ethical or legal issues must be rooted in the profession's standards and must comply with legal statutes.

2. Ethical principles and ethical theories, such as teleology and deontology, guide nursing decision making by providing a context in which a situation can be viewed.

3. Basic principles of ethics include autonomy, beneficence, nonmaleficence, veracity, confidentiality, justice, fidelity, standard of best interest, and respect for others.

4. The values clarification process, a process critical in decision making, assists nurses in the understanding of their own value systems and those of their patients.

5. Indicators of nursing's accountability and competency include licensure, credentialing, certification, accreditation, and an adherence to standards of care.

6. To prove negligence, the most frequent basis for nursing liability, the nurse's action causing harm must be within the nurse's professional scope, a breach of duty must have occurred, and this breach of duty must have caused the injury or harm.

7. Ethical and legal questions still arise over who can receive health care, who can afford health care services, and who has the right to access health care.

8. The high cost of health care has given rise to extreme cost-cutting measures that result in fragmentation and inadequacy of the care.

9. Nursing promotes practices that foster positive health through healthy living and personal as well as family development.

10. Through support of patients' self-defined health-promotion goals, nurses empower patients.

CHAPTER REVIEW

Learning Activities

1. Look in your favorite nursing journal and find two clinical situations that can potentially require ethical decision making by the nurse.

2. As a nurse you are expected to communicate pertinent information to your patients concerning their diagnosis, prognosis, procedures, and treatments. Think of a clinical situation in which you have provided patient care. Determine which of the ethical principles listed in Table 22.1 were important to your communication with the patient. Provide a rationale for your choice of principles.

3. In your own words, describe why licensure is important to the nursing profession.

4. Describe a situation that you encountered that required values clarification. What steps did you take in the process?

Multiple Choice

1. Ethical dilemmas are defined as which of the following?
   a. Problems that can be solved through the use of research data
   b. Clearly identified needed information
   c. Decisions requiring choices between undesirable alternatives
   d. Decisions requiring legal consultation

2. Which of the following is a legal guide for nursing?
   a. American Nurses Code of Ethics
   b. Hippocratic oath
   c. Nightingale pledge
   d. State Nursing Practice Act

3. Which of the following indicates that the patient has given informed consent?
   a. Accepts the plan of care
   b. Gets a second opinion
   c. Is knowledgeable regarding the choices given
   d. Participates in an experimental procedure

4. The nurse assesses, explores, and determines personal values through the process of:
   a. enrolling in an ethics class.
   b. personal meditation.
   c. reviewing the ANA Code of Ethics.
   d. values clarification.

5. Which ethical principle is reflected when a nurse acts in the best interest of a patient?
   a. Autonomy
   b. Beneficence
   c. Justice
   d. Nonmaleficence

6. The guarantee of equal protection is part of which of the following?
   a. American Nurses Association Standards of Care
   b. Fourteen amendment to the U. S. Constitution
   c. Code of Ethics for Nurses
   d. Patient's Bill of Rights

7. A purpose of the Affordable Care Act is to:
   a. assist the elderly in paying for insurance, medical, and hospital costs.
   b. force insurance companies to offer low-cost insurance to employed and unemployed individuals and families.
   c. help children and eventually all Americans with pre-existing conditions to gain insurance coverage and keep it.
   d. subsidize hospitals agreeing to care for the poor and indigent who otherwise could not have access to care.

8. An ethical theory that justifies actions based on the results attained by those actions is known as:
   a. beneficence.
   b. deontology.
   c. teology.
   d. veracity.

9. You are having a debate with classmates on the decision to limit organ transplant on the basis of age and take the stance that health professionals have a professional and moral obligation not to discriminate on the basis of age. Your stance is reflective of which of the following?
   a. Autonomy
   b. Deontology
   c. Fidelity
   d. Teology

10. Which one of the following is an indicator of accountability that establishes the minimum degree of competency to practice safely?
    a. Accreditation
    b. Certification
    c. Credentialing
    d. Licensure

ORGANIZATIONS AND WEBSITES

American Counseling Association (ACA): Represents professional counselors in various practice settings; provides information on general ethics issues, including ethical issues revolving around health-related problems: **http://www.counseling.org/**

Ethics Resource Center (ERC): The oldest nonprofit in the United States devoted to organizational ethics; advances understanding of the practices that promote ethical conduct through research, measurement of ethics and compliance program effectiveness in individual organizations, and the development of white papers and educational resources based on overall findings includes information on organizational ethics as well as a question-and-answer section dealing with issues related to ethics: **http://www.ethics.org**

REFERENCES

Allender, J. A., & Spradley, B. W. (2009). *Community health nursing: Concepts and practice* (7th ed.). Philadelphia, PA: Lippincott Williams & Wilkins.

American Cancer Society. (2009). *The patient's bill of rights.* Retrieved from http://www.cancer.org

American Hospital Association (AHA). (1992). *A patient's bill of rights.* Chicago, IL: American Hospital Association.

American Nurses Association (ANA). (1998). *Standards of clinical nursing practice.* Washington, DC: American Nurses Publishing.

American Nurses Association (ANA). (2000). *American nurses credentialing center.* Retrieved from http://www.ana.org/ancc

American Nurses Association (ANA). (2001). *Code of ethics for nurses with interpretive statements.* Washington, DC: American Nurses Publishing.

American Nurses Association (ANA). (2004). *Scope and standards of practice.* Washington, DC: Publishing Program of ANA.

Board of Nurse Examiners for the State of Texas. (2011). *Frequently asked questions about taking the NCLEX-RN examination.* Retrieved from http://www.bne.state.tx.us

Catalano, J. T. (2008). *Nursing now! Today's issues, tomorrow's trends* (5th ed.). Philadelphia, PA: F. A. Davis.

Creasia, J., & Parker, B. (2006) (4th ed.). *Conceptual foundations: The bridge to professional nursing practice.* St. Louis, MO: Mosby.

Ellis, J. R., & Hartley, C. L. (2008). *Nursing in today's world: Trends, issues and challenges.* (9th ed.). Philadelphia, PA: Lippincott Williams & Wilkins.

Fowler, M. (ed.). (2008). *Guide to the code of ethics for nurses: Interpretation and application.* Washington, DC: American Nurses Publishing.

Gaudine. A., LeFort, S. M., Lamb, M., & Thorne, L. (2011). Clinical ethical conflicts of nurses and physicians. *Nursing Ethics, 18* (1), 9–19.

Guido, G. W. (2010). *Legal and ethical issues in nursing* (5th ed.). Upper Saddle River, NJ: Prentice Hall.

Joint Commission. (2011). Retrieved from http://www.jointcommission.org

Lunsford v. *Board of Nurse Examiners*, 648 S. W.2d 391 (Tex. Ct. App.1983).

Pender, N. J., Murdaugh, C. L., & Parsons, M. A. (2010). *Health promotion in nursing practice* (6th ed.). Upper Saddle River, NJ: Pearson Prentice Hall.

Philipsen, N. C., & Haynes, D. (2007). Multi-state nurse lisencure compact: Making nurses mobile. (2007). *Journal of Nurse Practitioners, 3*(1), 36–40.

U.S. Department of Health and Human Services (DHHS). (2010). *Patient's Bill of Rights.* Retrieved from http://www.hhs.gov/ociio/regulations/patient/index.html

Willmann, J. H. (2009). *Annotated guide for RNs to the Texas Nursing Practice Act* (9th ed.). Austin, TX: Texas Nurses Association.

Zerwekh, J., & Claborn, J. C. (2009). *Nursing today: Transition and trends* (6th ed.). St. Louis, MO: Saunders Elsevier.

BIBLIOGRAPHY

Berntsen, K. (2005). Looking beyond tort reform toward safer health care systems. *Journal of Nursing Care Quality, 20* (1), 9–12.

Butts, J. B., & Rich, K. L. (2007). *Nursing ethics: Across the curriculum and into practice.* Sudbury, MA: Jones & Bartlett.

Leininger, M. (ed.). (1990). *Ethical and moral dimensions of care.* Detroit, MI: Wayne State University Press.

Mason, D. J., Leavitt, J. K., & Chaffee, M. W. (2012). *Policy & politics in nursing and health care.* St. Louis, MO: Saunders Elsevier.

Milston, C. (2005). Ethical issues: The ethics of respect in nursing. *Nursing Science Quarterly, 18* (1), 20–23.

Wright, D., & Brajtman, S. (2011). Relational and embodied knowing: Nursing ethics within the interprofessional team. *Nursing Ethics, 18* (1), 20–30.

GLOSSARY

A

abuse   Physical, emotional, or sexual maltreatment.

acanthosis nigricans (AN)   A skin condition associated with insulin resistance and type 2 diabetes.

accreditation   A form of certification or licensure that recognizes demonstrated compliance with established criteria.

acculturation   The process of adapting to, adopting, or taking on aspects of another culture; although something may be gained in the process, something is also usually lost; sometimes used interchangeably with *assimilation*.

acne   An inflammatory process of the sebaceous follicles of the skin, characterized by papules, comedones, and pustules.

active listening   The act of perceiving what is communicated verbally as well as nonverbally.

adaptation   The process of changing behavior in response to external or internal stimuli or surroundings.

addiction   A gradual process that occurs when a person has developed both a biological and a psychosocial dependence on the substance of use.

advance directives   Written instructions regarding specific procedures to be followed if the client becomes incapacitated.

advocate   One who takes the patient's side and provides complete information to allow him or her to make decisions concerning individual health care.

ageism   Prejudice against the elderly

agraphia   In a literate person, the inability to coordinate hand muscles sufficiently to produce handwriting.

alogia   An inability to speak in a person who has the ability to think.

alpha brain waves   Rhythmical brain waves recorded on the electroencephalograph, associated with a quiet, resting state in the brain and body

ambiguous loss   Involves physical or psychological losses in families that are not as concrete or identifiable as traditional losses such as death; ambiguous loss can include a miscarriage or loss of a still living spouse to Alzheimer's disease.

amenorrhea   The cessation of menses.

amniocentesis   Sampling of the amniotic fluid through a transabdominal puncture with ultrasound guidance.

andragogy   The education of adults.

andropause   The male climacteric caused by diminished levels of the androgen hormone, testosterone.

anorexia nervosa   An eating disorder in which the individual voluntarily refuses to eat because of excessive concern over body shape or weight.

anosmia   The absence of the sense of smell.

anticipatory guidance   The preparation of patients or clients for an anticipated developmental and/or situational crisis.

assault   Infringement on the mental security or the tranquility or both of another.

assisted living facility (ALF)   A facility designed to provide a special combination of personalized care, supportive services, and health-related services for care of the elderly.

ataxic aphasia   See *Motor aphasia*.

atrophy   Muscle wastage.

attachment   Unique, specific, and enduring relationship involving mutual trust, responsiveness, and caring between the infant and the mother.

attention-deficit/hyperactivity disorder (ADHD)   Neurobehavioral disorder characterized by increased impulsinty, inability to concentrate hyperactivity, and difficulties in school and family relationships.

auditory amnesia   See *Auditory aphasia.*

auditory aphasia (auditory amnesia, word deafness)   Ability to think and hear without the ability to understand the spoken word when heard.

authenticity   Being real and genuine, as opposed to hiding behind a mask of professionalism.

autonomy   Principle based on the right to self-determination; gives an individual the right to choose what will happen to his or her own person.

ayurveda   A form of healing originating in India that focuses on physical health and spiritual growth, using meditation, sound, massage, herbs, the breath, and types of food specific to the individual to help balance the body and its energy field.

B

baby boomers   U.S. adults born between 1946 and 1964.

balance   A term impling that the total energy intake into the body in the form of nutrient calories does not exceed the body's expenditure of energy.

ballistic stretching   Stretching by means of repeated bouncing.

basal metabolic rate   The amount of energy required to carry out involuntary bodily activities at rest.

battery   Physically touching a person; a physical violation.

beneficence   A principle that requires nurses to act in ways that benefit the client.

bereavement   The state of being deprived of something or someone

biomonitoring   Monitoring used in assessing human exposure to chemicals through the measurement of the chemicals or their metabolites in the body from such human specimens as blood or urine.

body composition   The relative amount of fat in the body compared to fat-free weight, such as that of muscle, bone, and other elements in the body.

body image disturbances   A distorted image that a person has of self.

body language   The use of nonverbal communication behaviors that include personal presentation, proxemics, kinesics, and touch.

body mass index (BMI)   A number that shows body weight adjusted for height and that can be calculated using inches and pounds or meters and kilograms; a convenient tool that relates height and weight to determine whether the individual is considered overweight or obese.

breach of duty   A deviation in some manner from the standard of care.

bruising   The discoloration of the skin (blue or purple) resulting from leakage of blood into skin tissue that has been damaged by an injury.

building-related illness   A diagnosable illness that can be directly linked to airborne building contaminants.

bulimia nervosa   An eating disorder characterized by binge eating followed by purging through self-induced vomiting, laxatives, diuretics, or excessive exercise.

burnout   The state of physical and emotional exhaustion that occurs when health care givers deplete their adaptive energy sources.

C

CAM   Complementary and alternative medicine viewed as a group of diverse medical and health care systems, practices, and products that are not currently considered conventional medicine or that is practiced by medical doctors or other health professionals, such as physical therapists, psychologists, and registered nurses. Complementary modalities are used as an adjunct to conventional medicine, whereas alternative modalities are used instead of conventional medicine.

capacity building   A developmental process that results in independence and self-confidence.

capitation   A type of health care in which the insurer or employer pays a provider a set fee for all the medical expenses necessary for each member covered under the plan.

carcinogens   A substance that can cause or promote the growth of cancer.

cardiovascular fitness   Synonymous with cardiorespiratory fitness, aerobic fitness, or cardiorespiratory endurance, terms that refer to the circulatory system and respiratory system and how effectively and efficiently they transport oxygenated blood to working muscles for an extended period of time.

career ladder   A degree completion program focusing on transitioning from one educational level to the next.

caring   Having a personal interest in the client; *feeling* for the client; involves an investment of the self.

centenarians   A person who lives past her or his 100th birthday.

central obesity   A pattern of obesity in which a high proportion of fat is localized around the abdomen and upper body.

certifications   The process by which an individual registered nurse who has met certain established criteria or qualifications is granted recognition for competency.

chakras   Spinning wheels of energy that help move healing energy from the universal field through the layers of the individual field (spiritual, mental, emotional, etheric) to the human body, and back to the universal field.

chemical sensitivity   The physiological response to a toxic substance following long-term exposure to low-level chemicals that were not recognized as harmful in the past.

chi   An Asian concept referring to invisible energy and vitality by which all living things, earth, and sky are interrelated cosmically.

chromotherapy   The use of color in therapeutic ways.

chronic illnesses   A type of disease or disorder that causes limitation of activity for a prolonged period.

climacteric   The change of life.

Code of Hammurabi   The earliest written reference to health that established standards and practices of living for the ancient civilization of Babylonia.

cognitive restructuring   Also known as cognitive reframing; a process of recognizing, challenging, and changing cognitive distortions and negative thought patterns.

cohabitation   Two unrelated adults of the opposite sex living together without a binding social or institutional contract.

communication   Conveying ideas, thoughts, opinions, or facts from one person to another.

community   Refers to a collection of like-minded people who work with each other and who have common traits and interests.

community-level interventions   An activity that occurs at the community level, rather than at the individual or family level, to promote health or to reduce illness or injury. For example, the fluoridation of the water supply is a preventive community-level intervention. Mandating seat belt use is a community-level intervention to reduce the incidence of injury.

comorbidity   Another disability is present in addition to the substance use/abuse/addiction.

complementary and alternative medicine   See *CAM*

concept   A generalized notion or idea useful in describing facts or occurrences.

conceptual framework   Describes the concepts that are interrelated and central to the understanding of a phenomenon.

congenital   Present at birth.

constipation   Difficult or infrequent passage of hard, dry fecal material.

Consumer Information Processing Model (CIP)   A model that incorporates concepts related to the use of information and the motivational effect of using this information in making choices.

context   The conditions under which communication occurs.

cooldown   A warm-down that is gradual and should be the last 5–10 minutes of the completed workout.

coordinator of care   Assures the appropriate sequence of events in the patient's plan of care.

coping strategies   Techniques used by an individual to deal with situations that are perceived as stressful.

couvade   Medical term for sympathetic pregnancy experienced by the father.

credentialing   A process that recognizes professional achievements such as specialty practice knowledge, educational accomplishments, certification, licensure, and accreditation.

crime   A legal wrong committed against a person or property, punishable by the state and involving jail time.

crisis   A situation of severe disorganization resulting when an individual's coping mechanisms are not effective, or when the usual resources are lacking, or a combination of both.

cross-tolerance   Drugs that are similar to each other and produce similar effects on the body and brain.

cultural competence   Incorporating *emic* and *etic* cultural knowledge into holistic and cultural congruent client care. Cultural competence involves nurses' self-awareness of their *own* culture and its myriad influences on their daily life in order to fully appreciate their clients' culture.

cultural congruent care   The care that is provided to fit with the values, beliefs, and lifeways of an individual, a group, or an institution.

cultural tapestry   A beautiful textured pattern representing an individual's unique cultural heritage.

culture   Dynamic adaptation; a learned way of life that includes interrelated attitudes, morals, beliefs, values, ideals, knowledge, symbols, artifacts, customs, traditions, and norms of a particular group that are transmitted intergenerationally, guide behavior, and make life meaningful. Culture represents a particular group's overarching life ways *as well as* each individual's worldview and way of life.

culture broker   A go-between who advocates on behalf of individuals, families, or communities, providing an avenue for informing health care providers about the effects of culture on health and behavior.

D

decoder   The person who receives and is able to interpret an encoded message in order to understand the sender's original idea, thought, opinion, or fact.

dementia   A progressive, organic mental disorder resulting in changes in personality, confusion, and impaired function, memory, and judgment.

dental caries   Progressive decalcification of the enamel of a tooth.

deontology   A theory of moral or professional obligation.

desirable body weight   The weight by achieving a balance between adequate nutrition, proper body fat, and physical activity.

determinants of health   Factors such as biological, social, personal, environmental, and economic factors that influence a person's health status.

detoxification   Taking an individual who is using drugs off the drug.

diagnosing dying   Recognizing some of the major symptoms that someone who is dying may exhibit.

diagnosis-related groups (DRGs)   The diagnosis classification system created in 1983 that contained 468 diagnoses to be used with the prospective payment system for Medicare to pay hospital costs.

diarrhea   Frequent passage of watery, unformed fecal material.

Dietary Guidelines   Recommendations for healthy Americans 2 years and over regarding food choices.

dietary reference intakes (DRIs)   A new system that replaces the recommended dietary allowances and that focuses on the role of certain nutrients in reducing the risk for chronic diseases.

Diffusion of Innovations Model   A model that addresses how new ideas, products, and social practices spread within a society or from one society to another.

disease cluster   A group of individuals experiencing the same disease in greater numbers than would happen by chance.

disease prevention   Measures taken to reduce the occurrence and severity of disease.

domains   Areas of concern affecting optimal health.

dose response   The pattern of physiological response to varied dosage.

drug abuse   The use of a drug or drugs inconsistent with social norms for purposes other than the intended ones, usually to alter feelings or mood and without relation to medical or health reasons.

drug misuse   The use of a drug or drugs inconsistent with social norms for purposes other than the intended ones, usually to alter feelings or mood and without relation to medical or health reasons.

dual diagnosis   The identification of those with both substance abuse and mental or physical health concerns.

dysomnia   Inadequate or dysfunctional sleep patterns.

E

egocentric   Concentrating upon self with little or no regard to others or the external world.

elder abuse   Any knowing, intended, or careless act that causes harm or serious risk of harm to an older person, whether physically, mentally, emotionally, or financially.

electronic health record (EHR)   An electronic version of a patient's medical history that may include key clinical data relevant to the person's care, demographics, progress notes, problems, medications, vital signs, past medical history, immunizations, and laboratory and radiology reports.

embryo   The product of pregnancy from conception to eight weeks.

emic **knowledge**   A subjective view; an insider's perspective; understanding the *emic* perspective is considered a prerequisite for cultural competence.

empathy   The state of being experienced by identifying closely with your client because you are able to imagine yourself in the client's situation and are able to feel the client's feelings as if they were yours.

empowerment   The process of helping others to help themselves; enabling or giving power to your patient.

encoder   The person who initiates communication by placing a message in a form that is understandable to the person meant to receive it.

encopresis   Fecal incontinence in a child 4 years of age or older who has no physical abnormality causing the incontinence

energy   A dynamic quality or power with the capacity for doing work.

energy field   A field of energy that is composed of constantly changing vibrational frequencies and that surrounds and connects all matter. All living things are energy fields that affect and are affected by all other forms of energy, creating health and disease.

enuresis   Involuntary urinary incontinence in a child 5 years of age or older who has no physical abnormality causing the incontinence.

environmental health hazard   A substance or agent that has the ability to cause any type of adverse health effect. The effect can range from a minor illness to a serious illness to death.

environmental health risk   The probability that there will be actual consequences from the potential danger of an environmental hazard.

environmental loss   A change in the familiar, even if the change is perceived as positive, such as a change in job.

environmental tobacco smoke (ETS)   Tobacco smoke in the air; also known as involuntary, sidestream, or secondhand smoke.

epidemiology   A field of study that examines the relationships among the disease, environment, individual, and community. Epidemiology is concerned with the time, place, and person components of disease, defect, disability, or death.

equal protection   A guarantee under U.S. law that all similarly situated individuals are entitled to be treated similarly.

ergonomics   The study and analysis of human work as it relates to an individual's anatomy and other human characteristics; the science of relationships of furniture and tools to the human body.

essential nutrients   A nutrient is considered essential when the body requires it for growth and maintenance but does not manufacture it in sufficient amounts to meet the body's needs.

estimated safe and adequate daily dietary intake (ESADDI)   The estimated safe and adequate daily dietary intake for some nutrients because not enough information is available to set a specific recommended dietary allowance (RDA).

ethical principles   Basic concepts and rules to guide and give direction to nursing practice.

ethics   The branch of philosophy that is related to moral values and actions.

ethnicity   A social term referring to a large group of people classified according to common national, tribal, linguistic, or cultural origin or background *and* who feel a sense of shared identity.

ethnocentrism   Literally, a belief that one's ethnic group is better than or superior to someone else's (inherent is the belief that someone else's ethnicity is inferior); the term's usage has been broadened to refer to a belief that one's particular cultural beliefs, worldview, and way of life are better than someone else's.

etic **knowledge**   An objective view; an outsider's perspective.

eustress   A positive form of stress that mobilizes as to action.

exchange system   A system for classifying foods into numerous lists based on their macronutrient composition and for establishing serving sizes so that one serving of each food on a list contains the same amount of carbohydrate, protein, fat, and energy (calories).

exclusive provider organization (EPO)   A type of managed care service that requires its members to get their services within the network only.

expected outcomes   Measurable goals set by the nurse and the patient and derived from the nursing diagnosis.

expressive aphasia   The ability to think without the ability to speak.

F

feedback   The process by which the effectiveness of communication is determined. This is the encoding and sending of a message from the receiver back to the original sender in order to let the original sender know how the message was received.

feng shui   An ancient Chinese practice of configuring one's environment to promote a healthy flow of chi, or vital energy, for health, happiness, and prosperity.

fetus   The product of pregnancy from the eighth week until delivery.

fidelity   The concept of faithfulness and the practice of keeping promises.

flexibility   The ability of a joint or group of joints to move freely through a range of motion.

folk health sector   The health arena composed of unlicensed, nonprofessional specialists who are usually members of the local community; *folk* is sometimes used to incorporate lay/popular, although it is best to differentiate the terms; *indigenous, generic,* and *traditional* sometimes are used interchangeably with both *lay/popular* and *folk* and usually refer to people's nonprofessional, tried-and-true health practices.

Food Guide Pyramid   A guide to the amounts and kinds of foods that we should eat daily to maintain health and to reduce risks of developing diet-related diseases.

G

general adaptation syndrome (GAS)   An adaptational response to stress consisting of three phases: an alarm reaction, a resistance or adaptation phase, and an exhaustion phase.

general systems theory   Focuses on the exchange of energy between the individual and the environment and has as a central concept that a person is whole and more than a sum of parts.

genetics   Refers to one gene disorder.

genomics   The situation in which multiple genes are interacting with each other and with the environment.

genogram   A tool that diagrams and depicts family relationships over a period of several generations.

geriatrics   Aspecialized branch of medicine that facases on the diagnosis and treatment of diseased affecting the elderly.

gerontology   The study of all aspects of aging, including all domains and their impacts on the elderly and society.

gestational diabetes   Diabetes that occurs during pregnancy as a result of hormonal changes.

global aphasia   The inability to express or receive verbal messages in any form in a person who can think.

gonads   Generic terms for the female sex glands, the ovaries, and the male sex glands, the testes.

grief   A natural response to a loss, the emotional suffering someone feels when a valued something or a loved someone is taken way, dies, or is no longer accessible.

gynecomastia   Enlargement of breast tissue in the young male.

H

half life   Half the time it takes for a drug to be metabolized out of the system.

hardiness   A resilience to stress.

health   A state that encompasses the total functioning of an individual and includes effective physical, psychological, social, cultural, and environmental functioning.

health behavior patterns Health habits that may relate to physical functioning or to the person's psychological, spiritual, and/or professional lives.

Health Belief Model A model developed by four social psychologists—Hochbaum, Kegeles, Leventhal, and Rosenstock—suggesting that a person's susceptibility to a health threat and its seriousness influences his or her decision to engage in a preventive health behavior.

health education A tool or mechanism for health related learning resulting in increased knowledge, skill development, and change in behavior.

health maintenance organization (HMO) A type of managed care service that provides health care to members for a fixed, usually monthly, payment.

health promotion Any process directed at enhancing the quality of health and well-being of individuals, families, groups, communities, and nations through strategies involving supportive environments, the coordination of resources, and respect for personal choice and values.

health-promotion plan A plan that focuses on achieving wellness and that, with the client's participation, determines the activities necessary to achieve optimal health. The plan examines the client's vulnerability to health imbalance, assesses client weaknesses and strengths, and determines the potential for illness.

health protection A phrase frequently used interchangeably with *disease prevention* and reflects a disease-related focus that is consistent with the medical model supported by the discipline of medicine.

Healthy People 2000 A document developed by the U.S. Surgeon General, in conjunction with health care constituents across the nation, that delineates 22 priority areas with 300 specific measurable objectives for health promotion, health protection, and surveillance and data systems for the United States to be achieved by the year 2000.

Healthy People 2010 A national health-promotion and disease prevention initiative that brings together national, state, and local government agencies; nonprofit, voluntary, and professional organizations; businesses; communities; and individuals to improve the health of all Americans, to eliminate disparities in health, and to improve years and quality of healthy life. It is designed to serve as a road map for improving the health of all Americans through two major goals and 467 objectives in 28 focus areas.

Healthy People 2020 A document that continues previous initiatives and that contains revised categories from *Healthy People 2010*, along with 10 new focus areas, 600 objectives, and 1,300 measurements.

heart rate reserve The difference between the resting heart rate and the maximum heart rate.

heliotherapy The use of sunlight for healing.

heterogeneity The quality or state of not being the same throughout; diversity.

high-level wellness A state that is a step above health and that is the dynamic state of wellness occurring at the individual, environmental, cultural, and social levels. Key to achieving this step are the capability and potential of the individual.

holistic A view of people in their complex entirety or totality.

holistic healing Assisting the establishment and maintenance of balance and wholeness in mind, body, and spirit of client and nurse.

holistic medicine An approach to health care that uses social, psychological, and spiritual aspects to bring about wellness.

holistic nursing A view of nursing in which the whole is defined as equal to the sum of the parts.

homeostasis A state of equilibrium within the body.

homosexuality The sexual orientation of a person who is sexually attracted to a person of the same sex.

hospice Considered the model for quality compassionate care for people facing a life-threatening illness, hospice focuses on providing all expects of patient care.

hypnosis An induced, trancelike state of altered perception and memory resulting in heightened suggestiveness whereby the person often follows the instructions given.

hypothalamus The gland in the brain responsible for control of metabolic activities, regulation of body temperature, integration of sympathetic and parasympathetic activities, and secretion of releasing (stimulating) and inhibiting hormones.

I

ideal body weight What a person should reasonably weigh compared to height.

illness trajectory The phases of an illness.

imagery Creating and holding a mental picture of what we want to happen in life using all five senses. It is the communication mechanism between perception, emotion, and bodily change. Using imagery regularly can bring about changes in the body, mind, energy field, and spirit.

immune modulation A factor, either physical, emotional, or treatment variable, that alters the degree of immune functioning.

immunoenhancement A factor that can bring about increased immune function, prevention of disease, and recovery from illness in an individual.

incest Sexual contact with the adolescent by any member of the family or household.

incontinence Inability to retain urine or feces.

infant Live-born individual from the moment of birth until one year of life.

informed consent A clear explanation of procedures to be had along with associated risks and benefits.

intensity   How hard a person must work to improve physical fitness.

interventions   Nursing actions that enable the person to achieve the desired goal.

intimate partner violence   A pattern of assault or coercion to force a partner to comply with the other partner's wishes.

introspection   The ability to look inside oneself and examine thoughts and personal meaning for identified values.

isoimmunization   Rh-negative mothers sensitized by exposure to Rh-positive blood.

J

justice   Fair, equitable, and appropriate treatment according to what is due or owed to persons.

K

kinesics   How we move our bodies or body parts, including conscious and unconscious changes in body posture, facial expressions, and gestures.

L

LaLonde Report   A classic document, created by the Canadian Minister of National Health and Welfare in 1974, that was the first to publicly proclaim health promotion as a major disease prevention strategy.

law   The sum total of rules and regulations by which a society is governed.

lay/popular health sector   The popular health sector; the nonprofessional, nonspecialist health care arena consisting of the individual along with family and friends; *folk* is sometimes used to incorporate lay/popular, although it is best to differentiate the terms; *indigenous*, *generic*, and *traditional* sometimes are used interchangeably with both *lay/popular* and *folk* and usually refer to people's nonprofessional, tried-and-true health practices.

learned helplessness   A phenomenon that has negative physical and psychological consequences and that occurs when an individual believes he or she has no control over an experience, whether a negative or positive experience. The individual becomes helpless or quits trying to affect or change the experience. It can be reversed if control is regained.

loss   Being deprived of or without something that one has had; the undesired change or removal of a valued object, person, or situation.

loss of aspect of self   Loss that involves removal of a body organ, loss of physical functioning, or loss of psychological function, such as losses related to personality, developmental changes, and aging.

M

managed care   A method of delivering health care that integrates and coordinates the delivery of health care with the costs of that service.

managed care organization   A health plan that provides consumers access to quality health care at a reasonable cost.

masturbation   Stimulation to orgasm of the genitals or other erogenous areas.

maximum heart rate   The fastest rate the heart can attain under maximal exercise conditions and still receive benefit.

Medicaid program   A 1965 amendment to the Social Security Act designed to provide a share of payments made by state welfare to health care agencies caring for the poor, medically needy, aged, disabled, and their dependent children and families.

Medicare program   A 1965 amendment to the Social Security Act designed to provide hospital insurance and supplement medical insurance for people over age 65, people with disabilities who receive Social Security benefits, and patients in end-stage renal disease.

medicocentrism   The belief that professional health care practices are better than lay/popular or folk health care practices, reflecting ethnocentrism by members of the professional health care system.

meditation   The intentional focusing of attention on a single object such as one's own breathing, a visual image, a religious symbol, or a phrase repeated silently to oneself; a technique (there are many) to interrupt unconscious, rampant thoughts of the mind. This is often done by noticing and observing what we are thinking or replacing thoughts with more beneficial ones. The body and mind become more relaxed, the stress response ceases, and healing is enhanced.

melanoma   A malignant, darkly pigmented skin lesion which develops from repeated exposure to the sun.

menarche   The initiation of menstruation.

menopause   The cessation of menses; usually considered complete after a year of amenorrhea.

message   The content (idea, thought, opinion, or fact) that one person wishes another person to receive in the process of communication.

metabolic syndrome   An association of obesity, insulin resistance, glucose intolerance, hypertension, and dyslipidemia that predisposes the individual to diabetes and cardiovascular disease.

metaparadigm   Used by an individual discipline to provide a global perspective of the field; for example, nursing's metaparadigm describes the concepts specific to nursing.

mind-body dualism   A philosophy of the separateness of the mind and body, which has existed in medicine at least since 1619 and has allowed the investigation and treatment to focus on the illness of the body, with only a few diseases being thought to have a primary cause related to the mind.

modeling   A nursing theory developed by Helen Erickson, RN, PhD, stating that, for people to heal, their needs must be met.

models   A visual representation of the concepts that work together to become a theory.

morbidity   Illness rate.

mortality   Death rate.

Mosaic Code   Regulations for society developed by ancient Hebrews that included an organized system for disease prevention.

motor aphasia (ataxic aphasia)   An ability to think with an inability to coordinate the muscles responsible for speech (alogia) or writing (agraphia).

multistate licensure   Recognition of a single license allowing registered nurses to practice nursing throughout the country.

mourning   The actual feeling or expression of sorrow; lamentation over someone's death.

muscular endurance   The ability of a muscle or group of muscles to perform or sustain a muscle contraction over an extended period of time.

muscular strength   The ability or capacity to exert force with a muscle against resistance, under maximal conditions in a single effort.

mutagens   A substance that can change genetic material found in chromosomes.

MyPlate   USDA's new icon that represents the new U.S. dietary guidelines and replaces the MY Pyramid food guidance system.

MyPyramid   Replaces the Food Guide Pyramid and is used as a food guidance system.

N

nationality   In general, a term that refers to country of origin or birth.

needs theory   A theory that describes people as whole with many complex needs that motivate behavior.

negative energy balance   A state that occurs when a person's energy needs exceed that produced by the foods consumed.

negligence   The failure to provide the care that a reasonable person would provide in similar circumstances.

nightmares   An anxiety dream to which the child responds by awakening.

night terror   Form of a nightmare in which the child screams out, cries, and does not respond by awakening.

noise   Any loud, discordant, or disagreeable sound or sounds that can decrease body energy or cause auditory damage.

nonessential nutrients   Nutrients that the body can make.

nonmaleficence   A principle that requires nurses to act in such a way as to avoid causing harm to clients.

nonverbal communication   The conveyance of messages without the use of words; consists of body language and paralanguage.

nonverbal vocalizations   Sounds such as grunts, groans, sighs, and sobs that make up one type of paralanguage.

nurse healers   A nurse who helps others to heal or remember their inherent state of wholeness by cherishing, nurturing, and promoting their growth and development. Nurse healers are aware that personal presence with the client is a factor in healing.

Nursing: A Social Policy Statement   The first document, prepared by leaders in the profession, to describe nursing and the profession's responsibility to society.

nursing diagnosis   The actual identification of a patient's need.

nursing process   Method for developing an appropriate plan of care and wellness outcomes for patients that includes assessing and establishing a nursing diagnosis, planning, implementing, and evaluating.

nutrients   Substances found in foods that the body can use for the maintenance of body functions throughout life.

nutrition   The study of food substances or nutrients and their processes that are essential for health.

O

obesity   The condition of being overweight or of being more than 20% over the ideal body weight; weight at or above the 95th percentile for age/sex-specific BMI.

occupational stress   Job-related stress, which leads to extreme tension, anxiety, and possibly even to physical symptoms.

optimal body composition   The proper balance between body fat, muscle mass, and bone.

outcomes   The results of nursing intervention with clients, stated in client-centered, measurable terms.

outgassing   The production of a toxic gas from the breakdown of formaldehyde in synthetic products.

overload principle   Forcing the body to do more than it normally does.

over-the-counter (OTC) drugs   Drugs that can be purchased from pharmacies or supermarkets for use when symptoms are of a minor nature.

overweight   Being between the 85th and 94th percentile for age/sex-specific BMI.

P

palliative care   An approach that improves the quality of life of patients and their families facing the problems associated with life-threatening illness.

Papanicolaou (Pap) test   A laboratory test for cancer in which cells are collected from areas that shed cells to be microscopically examined for early changes that may be related to the development of cancer.

paradigm   An example that serves as a pattern or model for something.

paralanguage   The use of nonverbal components of spoken language.

particulate matter   Small particles or liquid droplets that can be suspended in the air.

paternalism   A system that encourages individuals to make decisions for others.

pedagogy   The education of children.

peers   Individual of the same age.

Pender Health Promotion Model   Developed by nurse researcher Nola Pender, a model that integrates concepts from the expectancy-value model of human motivation and social cognitive theory with self-efficacy as a predominant concept. It is unique to nursing because of its holistic perspective.

perceptions   The process of recognizing and interpreting an illness, a sensation, or an experience in order to gain understanding or give it meaning.

performance-related fitness (PRF)   A type of fitness whose components are agility, reaction time, power, coordination, balance, and speed and, very often, the health-related components.

perimenopause   A time of transition from normal menstrual periods to cessation of menses occurring gradually over 2–15 years.

personal presentation   How we show ourselves to the world, including how we dress, groom ourselves, and use cosmetics, perfumes, and deodorants to create an identity by which we choose to be known.

physical fitness   The ability to be physically active on a regular basis.

phytochemicals   Herbs or plants used to promote and maintain health and cure disease.

pica   Ingestion of substances that have no food value.

plantar fasciitis   Arch pain commonly occurring in walkers and runners.

polypharmacy   The use of multiple medications without the knowledge of a supervising physician or nurse practitioner.

positive energy balance   A state that occurs when the amount of food consumed exceeds the energy used by the body.

postpartum   The time between delivery and the return of a woman's reproductive organs to the nonpregnant state.

posttraumatic stress disorder (PTSD)   The constellation of continuing, long-term detrimental effects resulting from exposure to trauma.

PRECEDE-PROCEED Model   A model to guide the development of health-promotion programs for groups and communities. It is multidimensional, multileveled, and broad-based and is focused on outcomes rather than on inputs.

preferred provider organization (PPO)   A type of managed care service that uses provider networks to deliver health care to its members.

premenstrual syndrome (PMS)   The cyclic recurrence of distressing physical, psychological, and/or behavioral changes related to the menstrual cycle.

prescription drugs   Medications that are prescribed by a physician or nurse practitioner and that contain substances to aid in the prevention of disease, the diagnosis of a condition, or the alleviation of symptoms, or help in the recovery from a disease or disorder.

presence   Being with another in a meaningful way, giving of one's self in the current moment, listening, and providing unconditional acceptance. Presence involves giving of one's self and being open to the experience of another through a reciprocal interpersonal relationship.

primary care providers   Health care providers whom the client sees first for health care services. The primary care provider is a physician, usually a family practice physician.

primary disease prevention   Level of prevention that includes activities and lifestyle factors that can be changed or maximized with high-level wellness as the goal.

primary prevention   Prevention for those who have not used tobacco, alcohol, or other drugs with the goal of preventing exposure to and experimentation with drugs.

principle of progression   Gradually increasing the overload stimulus adaptations to the existing workload occur.

principle of specificity   A principle stating that one must overload the body systems or the specific fitness component to achieve a specific outcome.

professional health sector   The formally organized, modern, scientific health community; much more than only medical care; encompasses professional nursing, medicine, pharmacy, dietetics, and the like.

prospective payment system (PPS)   A fixed predetermined method of payment to hospitals based on the concept that similar medical diagnoses result in the same hospitalization costs.

prospective studies   Research studies that follow subjects without the disease or outcome of interest forward in time. Animal subjects are followed for enough person-years to establish incidence, morbidity, or mortality rates.

Protection Motivation Theory   A fear-driven model proposing that a perceived threat to health activates thought processes regarding the severity of the threatened event, the probability of its occurrence, and coping mechanisms.

protective factors   Situations or conditions or both that build resiliency against substance abuse and increase the likelihood that an individual will resist substance abuse.

proxemics   How we use the personal space around us, including conscious and unconscious changes in the distances we maintain from others and the manner in which we touch and are touched by others.

psychoneuroimmunology (PNI)   The study of the interrelationship of the mind and body.

psychotropic drugs   Drugs that modify mental activity and affect psychic function, behavior, or experience and are normally used to treat mental disorders.

puberty   The period in life during which members of both genders become capable of reproduction.

R

race   A category of humankind that shares certain distinctive physical traits.

rate of perceived exertion   A feeling for the amount of intensity or exertion being attained.

recommended dietary allowance (RDA)   Recommended dietary allowance; daily dietary intake that is sufficient to meet the nutrient requirements of 97–98% of all healthy individuals.

reflexology   A touch therapy using the pad of the thumb to apply pressure to specific points on the feet and hands that correspond to areas of the torso. This technique can enhance relaxation of, stimulate circulation to, and aid healing of the corresponding areas.

registration   The listing of an individual's name and other information on the official roster of a governmental or nongovernmental agency.

relapse prevention   Prevention of the return to substance use.

Relaxation Response   A technique developed by Herbert Benson, MD, that uses focus on a chosen repetition, such as the breath or a word, to interrupt the stress response and promote relaxation.

relaxation techniques   A group of strategies involving breathing or mind control used to decrease stress and tension. Relaxation techniques can be used as an active coping strategy and actually result in changes in heart rate, respiratory rate, and metabolism.

respect for others   The highest ethical principle and incorporates all the other ethical principles; acknowledges that individuals are capable of making decisions for themselves.

retrospective studies   Research studies that identify subjects with the illness or outcome of interest and evaluate their past experiences for postulated causal factors.

RICE   Refers to *r*est, *i*ce, *c*ompression, and *e*levation; a good modality to use with muscle sprains or strains or other minor discomforts.

rickets   A preventable condition resulting in poor bone mineralization increasing the risks for numerous fractures.

risk factors   A characteristic associated with increased likelihood of disease or injury of an individual's vulnerability to substance abuse.

role modeling   To meet their needs, they can look at the stressors in their life and their resources for coping with those stressors.

S

SAD syndrome   Seasonal affective disorder believed to be related to increased melatonin levels. Symptoms associated with SAD syndrome include fatigue, increased craving for carbohydrates in the diet, weight gain, lethargy, and severe clinical depression. Physiological problems such as infertility, alterations in menstrual cycles, and premenstrual syndrome may also occur.

sandwich generation   The middle adult period in which people are sandwiched between their children who need nurturance and support and their aging parents, who also need care.

scoliosis   Abnormal curvature of the spine, usually consisting of an abnormal lateral curvature and a compensatory curve.

screening   The use of a diagnostic procedure such as a laboratory test or an evaluation tool to determine the presence of a particular disease or risk factors known to be associated with a health problem.

secondary prevention   Strategies that involve health screenings to identify abnormalities within a population and that are aimed at preventing substance abuse by individuals at risk for developing problems and those who are already using substances.

self-efficacy   The self-conviction or belief that one can be successful in achieving the desired behavior.

sensitivity of a screening test   The ability of a screening test to correctly give a positive result when the individual has the disease or condition being tested for.

sensory channel   The means by which a message is sent. The three primary routes are the visual (sight), auditory (hearing), and kinesthetic (touch) channels.

set-point of weight control theory   A theory stating that all individuals have a unique, stable, adult body weight that is the result of several biological factors.

severe obesity   The state of being 200% or more over normal body weight.

sexuality   Broad term that includes not only the dimensions of sexual desire and sexual response but also the individual's view of self and presentation of self.

sha   An Asian concept that means bad chi, which is believed to bring bad luck and poor health as well as family and business difficulties.

sick building syndrome   The cluster of vague symptoms that are traced to pollutants in sealed buildings.

simultaneous perception A system used to experience our environment by combining the responses of all our senses.

sleep apnea A sleep disorder characterized by recurrent periods of absence of breathing for 10 seconds or longer, occurring at least five times per hour.

social determinants of health The conditions or environment under which people live, their socioeconomic level, geographic location, and the political and cultural factors that influence their health.

Social Security Act Legislation enacted by the U.S. government in 1935 to provide eligible citizens with public aid, social services, and aid to the elderly.

social support The presence of a group of interconnected, cooperating significant others who provide assistance and help strengthen the individual.

specificity of a screening test The ability of a screening test to correctly give a negative result when the individual being screened does not have the disease.

spiritual health A balance between self and others.

spiritual well-being The affirmation of life in a relationship with God or a higher power, self, community, and environment that nurtures and celebrates wholeness.

spirituality A concept that refers to experiences traditionally considered religious as well as to all states of awarness; the belief in a universal power greater than oneself and a sense of interconnectedness with all living creatures; promotes feelings of hope, comfort, and peace.

sprains An injury to a ligament.

standard of best interest A standard that allows individuals to share in decision making regarding health care.

static stretching Slow and deliberate stretching.

strains An injury to a muscle.

stress An emotional and physiological response to a stressor.

stress response A set of physical changes the human body makes in response to a stressor or threat.

stressors An event, a situation, or a life change perceived as a threat to an individual's physical or psychological well-being; a stress-provoking factor that can impact the health of those who provide health care to others.

substance abuse The habitual use of alcohol and/or illegal substances such as marijuana, cocaine, crack, and numerous others.

T

tao To be connected.

target heart rate The level or zone that one should attain during aerobic activity to obtain training benefit.

taxonomy A common classification structure that links nursing diagnoses, interventions, and outcomes.

teleology An ethical theory that explains phenomena and justifies actions by results, or the doctrine of final causes.

teratogens A substance that can cause abnormal development in embryonic structures.

terrorism The unlawful use of force and violence against persons or property to intimidate or coerce a government, the civilian population, or any segment thereof, in furtherance of political or social objectives.

tertiary prevention Addresses the situation once symptoms have occurred and is directed toward minimizing the disease or disability; the prevention of death and disability of individuals in long-term treatment.

theory A set of relational statements that present a systematic view of a phenomenon. Uses facts, definitions, and propositions to specify relationships among variables.

Theory of Planned Behavior Developed by Icek Ajzen to explain behavior as on a control continuum with total control at one end and absence of control at the other end. Control is viewed as being influenced by resources, support, skills, and self-efficacy needed for a certain behavior.

therapeutic communication The use of verbal and nonverbal techniques focused on client needs and with the avoidance of unhelpful or nontherapeutic techniques.

therapeutic touch A technique developed by Dolores Krieger, RN, PhD, and Dora Kunz that uses the hands to perceive and balance the energy field to enhance relaxation, pain relief, and healing.

tolerance A condition that occurs when more of a drug is required to obtain the desired effects.

tort A legal wrong committed against a person or property and settled in civil court.

touch The manner in which we come into bodily contact with others.

toxins Poisons produced within living cells or organisms that can cause harm or may be fatal to humans in low doses.

transcultural nursing theory A theory that focuses on the individual and describes how culture influences and provides meaning to everything a person does, thinks, feels, or hears.

Transtheoretical Model (TTM) A theory of behavior, developed by Prochaska and DiClemente, asserting that changes in health behaviors progress through five distinct stages containing the elements of thought, action, and time that are influenced by experiential and behavioral processes.

triad diagnosis The presence of a mental health issue, a physical health issue, and a substance abuse issue simultaneously.

U

unconditional positive regard Demonstrating acceptance and respect for the client as a fellow human being, without imposing any conditions for that acceptance.

urinary incontinence   The involuntary leakage of urine.

utter watchfulness   The ability to pay equal attention to everything in the environment at once, emphasizing nothing and omitting nothing.

V

values   A set of personal beliefs and attitudes.

values clarification   The process of becoming more conscious of and naming what one values or considers worthy.

veracity   The practice of telling the truth.

verbal communication   The use of words to convey messages. Often these words are written or spoken, but they may be formed in other ways, such as by the use of sign language.

visual aphasia (word blindness)   The inability of a literate person to decode the written word.

volatile organic chemicals (VOCs)   Gases released from certain solids or liquids.

W

warm-up   Stretching and mild exercise to gradually increase the heart rate, circulation, and body temperature.

weapons of mass destruction (WMDs)   Chemical, biological, and radiological weapons or devices intended to cause death or serious bodily harm to a significant number of people.

weapons of mass effect (WMEs)   Term that denotes the motives of terrorists to cause widespread chaos and despair by whatever method used.

weight control   The change, acquisition, and maintenance of a desirable body weight.

weight cycling   The losing and regaining of weight seen in yo-yo dieting or in the repeated practice of dieting.

word blindness   See *Visual aphasia.*

word deafness   See *Auditory aphasia.*

worldview (also world view)   Reflects values, norms, expressions, taboos, myths, rituals, rites, and so forth; refers to how people perceive the world, including health, wellness, illness, sickness, death, human nature, and the like.

Y

yang   A principal power of Chinese philosophy that works in opposition of yin to regulate the universe and balance the mind, body, and spirit. Yang is the male element associated with positive energy, action, generativity, the sun, light, and the creativity of life.

yin   A principal power of Chinese philosophy that works in opposition to yang to regulate the universe and balance the mind, body, and spirit. Yin is the female element associated with negative energy, passiveness, destruction, the moon, darkness, and death.

INDEX

I

O

P

T